COMPREHENSIVE

Chronic Obstructive Pulmonary Disease

MW01178253

JEAN BOURBEAU, MD, MSc, FRCPC
Assistant Professor
Medicine and Epidemiology
McGill University
Montreal, Quebec

DIANE NAULT, RN, MSc
Head Nurse
Ambulatory Services
McGill University Health Centre
Montreal, Quebec

ELIZABETH BORYCKI, RN, HBScN, MN, GNC (c)
Clinical Informatics Specialist
Informatics
Mount Sinai Hospital
Toronto, Ontario

2002
BC Decker Inc
Hamilton • London

BC Decker Inc
P.O. Box 620, L.C.D. 1
Hamilton, Ontario L8N 3K7
Tel: 800-568-7281
Fax: 888-311-4987
e-mail: info@bcdecker.com
www.bcdecker.com

08 09 10 11/BM/ 9 8 7 6 5 4

ISBN 1-55009-174-3

Printed in the Canada by Ball Media Corporation

Sales and Distribution

United States	UK, Europe, Middle East	Mexico and Central America
BC Decker Inc	McGraw-Hill Education	ETM SA de CV
P.O. Box 785	Shoppenhangers Road	Calle de Tula 59
Lewiston, NY 14092-0785	Maidenhead	Colonia Condesa
Tel: 905-522-7017; 800-568-7281	Berkshire, England SL6 2QL	06140 Mexico DF, Mexico
Fax: 905-522-7839; 888-311-4987	Tel: 44-0-1628-502500	Tel: 52-5-5553-6657
E-mail: info@bcdecker.com	Fax: 44-0-1628-635895	Fax: 52-5-5211-8468
www.bcdecker.com	www.mcgraw-hill.co.uk	E-mail: editoresdetextosmex@prodigy.net.mx
Canada	Singapore, Malaysia,Thailand,	
McGraw-Hill Ryerson Education	Philippines, Indonesia, Vietnam,	Brazil
Customer Care	Pacific Rim, Korea	Tecmedd Importadora E Distribuidora
300 Water St.	McGraw-Hill Education	De Livros Ltda.
Whitby, Ontario L1N 9B6	60 Tuas Basin Link	Avenida Maurílio Biagi, 2850
Tel: 1-800-565-5758	Singapore 638775	City Ribeirão, Ribeirão Preto – SP –
Fax: 1-800-463-5885	Tel: 65-6863-1580	Brasil
	Fax: 65-6862-3354	CEP: 14021-000
		Tel: 0800 992236
Foreign Rights		Fax: (16) 3993-9000
John Scott & Company	Australia, New Zealand	E-mail: tecmedd@tecmedd.com.br
International Publishers' Agency	McGraw-Hill Australia	
P.O. Box 878	Pty LtdLevel 2, 82 Waterloo Road-	
Kimberton, PA 19442	North Ryde, NSW, 2113Australia	India, Bangladesh, Pakistan, Sri Lanka
Tel: 610-827-1640	Customer Service Australia	CBS Publishers & Distributors
Fax: 610-827-1671	Phone: +61 (2) 9900 1800	4596/1A-11, Darya Ganj
E-mail: jsco@voicenet.com	Fax: +61 (2) 9900 1980	New Delhi-2, India
	Email:	Tel: 23271632
	cservice_sydney@mcgraw-hill.com	Fax: 23276712
Japan	Customer Service New Zealand	E-mail: cbspubs@vsnl.com
United Publishers Services Limited	Phone (Free Phone):	
1-32-5 Higashi-Shinagawa	+64 (0) 800 449 312	
Shinagawa-Ku, Tokyo 140-0002	Fax (Free Phone): +64 (0) 800 449 318	
Tel: 03 5479 7251	Email: cservice@mcgraw-hill.co.nz	
Fax: 03 5479 7307		

Notice: The authors and publisher have made every effort to ensure that the patient care recommended herein, including choice of drugs and drug dosages, is in accord with the accepted standard and practice at the time of publication. However, since research and regulation constantly change clinical standards, the reader is urged to check the product information sheet included in the package of each drug, which includes recommended doses, warnings, and contraindications. This is particularly important with new or infrequently used drugs. Any treatment regimen, particularly one involving medication, involves inherent risk that must be weighed on a case-by-case basis against the benefits anticipated. The reader is cautioned that the purpose of this book is to inform and enlighten; the information contained herein is not intended as, and should not be employed as, a substitute for individual diagnosis and treatment.

Contributors

NICHOLAS ANTHONISEN, MD, PhD
Professor of Medicine
University of Manitoba
Winnipeg, Manitoba

BARBARA BARNETT, BA, BMin
Canon, Coordinator of Spiritual Care
Deer Lodge Centre
Winnipeg, Manitoba

DANIELLE BEAUCAGE, RN, BScN
Clinical Instructor
Department of Nursing
McGill University Health Centre
Montreal, Quebec

ALAIN BEAUPRE, MD, FRCPC
Professor of Medicine
University of Montreal
Montreal, Quebec

ELIZABETH BORYCKI, RN, HBScN, MN, GNC (c)
Clinical Informatics Specialist
Department of Informatics
Mount Sinai Hospital
Toronto, Ontario

MARTIN BOULÉ, BPharm, MSc
Clinical Assistant Professor
Faculty of Pharmacy
Laval University
Quebec City, Quebec

JEAN BOURBEAU, MD, MSc, FRCPC
Assistant Professor of Medicine and Epidemiology
McGill University
Montreal, Quebec

SHIRLEY BRYAN, MKin
Research Kinesiologist
Department of Medicine
University of Calgary
Calgary, Alberta

ANNE CATHCART, MSW, RSW
Social Worker
Respiratory Program
Riverview Health Centre
Winnipeg, Manitoba

DAWN CHAITRAM, BSW
Social Worker
Department of Social Work
Deer Lodge Centre
Winnipeg, Manitoba

JOSÉE DAGENAIS, RN, MSc
Clinical Nurse Specialist
Department of Nursing
Maisonneuve-Rosemont Hospital
Montreal, Quebec

TANYA DUTTON, BScPT, MscA
Clinical Manager of Rehabilitation Services
Physiotherapy and Occupational Therapy Department
Queen Elizabeth II Health Science Centre
Halifax, Nova Scotia

GORDON FORD, MD, FRCPC, FACP, FCCP
Professor of Medicine
University of Calgary
Calgary, Alberta

ANDRÉ GERVAIS, MD, FRCPC
Assistant Professor of Medicine
University of Montreal
Montreal, Quebec

ROGER S. GOLDSTEIN, MD, FRCP (C)
Professor of Medicine
University of Toronto
Toronto, Ontario

CATHERINE GRAY-DONALD, PhD
Associate Professor of Dietitics and Human Nutrition
McGill University
Montreal, Quebec

ANN HATZOGLOU, Pht, BSc
Physiotherapist
Physiotherapy and Occupational Therapy
Montreal Chest Institute/McGill University Health Centre
Montreal, Quebec

DOUGLAS HELMERSEN, MD, FRCPC
Respirologist
Department of Medicine
University of Calgary
Calgary, Alberta

PAUL HERNANDEZ, MDCM, FRCPC
Assistant Professor of Medicine
Dalhousie University
Halifax, Nova Scotia

EARL S. HERSHFIELD, BSc, MD, FRCPC
Professor of Medicine
University of Manitoba
Winnipeg, Manitoba

ANGELA JONE, BN, RN, CAE
Clinical Trial Coordinator
Department of Medicine
University of Calgary
Calgary, Alberta

MARCEL JULIEN, MD
Associate Professor of Medicine
University of Montreal
Montreal, Quebec

JOHN KAYSER, RN, BSc
Instructor
Department of Nursing
McGill University
Montreal, Quebec

R. JOHN KIMOFF, MD, FRCP (C)
Associate Professor of Medicine
McGill University
Montreal, Quebec

YVES LACASSE, MD, MSc, FRCP (C)
Assistant Professor of Medicine
Laval University
Quebec City, Quebec

JUDY LAMB, OT, MA, BSc
Guest Lecturer
Department of Occupational Therapy
McGill University
Montreal, Quebec

MARLÈNE LEMIEUX, BSc, RD
Clinical Dietitian
Department of Clinical Nutrition
McGill University Health Centre
Montreal, Quebec

CINDE LITTLE, RRT, CAE
Clinical Trial Coordinator
Department of Medicine
University of Calgary
Calgary, Alberta

BRENDA LOVERIDGE, BPT, PhD
Professor of Medical Rehabilitation
University of Manitoba
Winnipeg, Manitoba

JOSIAH LOWRY, MD, CCFP, FCFP
Assistant Professor of Community and Family Medicine
University of Toronto
Toronto, Ontario

FRANÇOIS MALTAIS, MD
Assistant Professor of Medicine
Laval University
Montreal, Quebec

DARCY MARCINIUK, MD, FRCP (C)
Professor of Medicine
University of Saskatchewan
Saskatoon, Saskatchewan

SUNITA MATHUR, BSc (PT), MSc
Coordinator
Cardiopulmonary program
Atlantic Health and Wellness Institute
Halifax, Nova Scotia

MAUREEN MCGUIRE, BSc, (PT)
Adjunct Staff
Health Sciences Faculty
Queen's University
Kingston, Ontario

ANDREW MCIVOR, MD, MSc, FRCP (C), FRCP (E)
Associate Professor of Medicine
Dalhousie University
Halifax, Nova Scotia

DENISE MELANSON, BSW
Social Worker
Social Services
Montreal Chest Institute/McGill University Health Centre
Montreal, Quebec

DIANE NAULT, RN, MScN
Head Nurse
Ambulatory Services
Montreal Chest Institute/McGill University Health Centre
Montreal, Quebec

SUZANNE NESBITT, RRT
Respiratory Therapist
Respiratory and Anesthesia Technology
McGill University Health Centre
Montreal, Quebec

DENIS E. O'DONNELL, MD, FRCP (I), FRCP (C)
Professor of Medicine
Queen's University
Kingston, Ontario

GISELE PEREIRA, BPT
Senior Instructor
Department of Medical Rehabilitation
University of Manitoba
Winnipeg, Manitoba

VITALIE PERREAULT, RN, MSc
Nurse
Ambulatory Services
Montreal Chest Institute/McGill University Health Centre
Montreal, Quebec

GINETTE POULIN, MSC, RN
Clinical Nurse
Heart Failure Clinic
Institute of Cardiology Montreal
Montreal, Quebec

KATHY RICHES, RN, BScN
Nurse Clinician
Ambulatory Services
Royal Victoria Hospital/McGill University Health Centre
Montreal, Quebec

MICHEL ROULEAU, MD
Clinical Professor of Medicine
Laval University
Quebec City, Quebec

LOUIS ROUSSEAU, MD, RRCP (C)
Liaison Psychiatrist
Department of Psychiatry
Laval University
Quebec City, Quebec

MARY ANN SIOK, RN, BScN, MScA
Nurse Clinician
Ambulatory Services
Montreal Chest Institute/McGill University Health Centre
Montreal, Quebec

JUDITH SOICHER, BSc (PT), MSc
Doctoral Candidate
Epidemiology and Biostatistics
McGill University
Montreal, Quebec

DAVID STUBBING, MD, BS, FRCPC
Associate Professor of Medicine
McMaster University
Hamilton, Ontario

MICHÈLE TREMBLAY, MD
Team Coordinator
Montreal Regional Public Health Department
Montreal, Quebec

RENY VAUGHAN, RRCP, RRT
Clinical Coordinator/COPD Educator/Faciltator
Department of Respiratory Therapy
The Michener Institute for Applied Health Sciences
Toronto, Ontario

PETER WARREN, MB, MA, FRCPC
Professor of Medicine
University of Manitoba
Winnipeg, Manitoba

KATHERINE WEBB, MSc
Research Associate
Department of Medicine
Queen's University
Kingston, Ontario

PETER J. WIJKSTRA, MD, PhD
Chest Physician
Department of Pulmonary Diseases
University Hospital of Groningen
Groningen, Netherlands

PREFACE

T he idea for this book, *Comprehensive Management of Chronic Obstructive Pulmonary Disease* (COPD), started a few years ago when I was leading a multicenter randomized clinical trial assessing the effectiveness of a newly developed education and self-management tool, "Living well with COPD©," for patients with COPD and their families. It became clear from this study that self-care and medical care are enhanced by effective collaboration. However, certain conditions have to be in place if we want to achieve effective collaborative management. For instance, it is essential that patients and care providers have shared goals, a sustained working relationship, mutual understanding of roles, and, furthermore, skills for carrying out their roles.

While taking care of our patients with COPD, we should keep in mind this statement of the World Health Organization: "If you treat your patient, you have helped him for today. If you teach him, you have helped him for a whole lifetime." This is essentially the philosophy of this book.

This book was written to help physicians and the allied health care professionals improve their skills in managing patients with COPD. As physicians or the allied health care professionals, we also have to learn to be facilitators and educators. We must recognize that our patients, who are often elderly, can be complex, with multiple medical and psychosocial problems affecting the way in which they adapt to their COPD. Success in managing these patients depends on the ability of allied health care professionals to create a culture of cooperation among all of the members of the health care team. Furthermore, we have to facilitate the shift from reactive, acute care to planned care, the goal of which is COPD self-management and disease control, for patients to be at their maximum capacity in terms of physical, mental, and social functioning.

This book goes beyond patients' lung function management, beyond pharmacologic intervention, and beyond standard care. One of the unique features of this book is that each chapter has been written by a multidisciplinary team composed of experts and peoples with first-hand experience involved in providing and coordinating patient care. Another feature of the book is the way in which chapters are organized. Each chapter includes the following divisions: objectives and what physicians and the allied health care professionals can expect to learn, introduction, chapter main content, when to refer, summary, case study, key points, references, and suggested readings.

The book is addressed to a large audience: respirologists, physicians, and allied health care professionals who care for patients with COPD. It is not encyclopedic but comprehensive. It integrates knowledge into daily practice, giving health care professionals the information necessary to understand and modify their own activities at a detailed, operational level. The book can be used as a reference or for teaching students, physicians, or allied health care professionals.

I hope you find this book useful. I sincerely believe that implementing the management strategies outlined in this book will improve the care and the quality of life of our patients and optimize health service use. I also hope that this book will provide a framework for future research and innovation to improve COPD care.

Jean Bourbeau
March, 2002

FOREWORD

It is a pleasure to introduce a new text, *Comprehensive Management of Chronic Obstructive Pulmonary Disease* (COPD). The topic is important because COPD is a leading cause of mortality in the Western world; furthermore, it is an even more important cause of morbidity, whether or not the latter is calculated in terms of medical costs, lost productivity, or poor life quality. Chronic obstructive pulmonary disease is a catchall term that describes the clinical manifestations of several abnormalities of the lung, including chronic bronchitis (cough and sputum), small airways obstruction, and pulmonary emphysema. All three of these abnormalities are associated with tobacco use; COPD develops over decades, during which time the disease is often without symptoms severe enough to cause the smoker to seek help. In the vast majority of cases, medical attention is sought only after major, irreversible damage has occurred. Patients with established COPD endure years of gradually progressive shortness of breath with a progressive worsening of exercise capacity and life quality. Their course is often punctuated by exacerbations of their symptoms necessitating medical intervention that can vary all the way from added medication to admission to intensive care units.

Recognition of COPD as a major health problem first occurred about 50 years ago. In the intervening time, a great deal has been learned about its cause and its course, and an armamentarium of management techniques has been developed. It is my belief that these techniques have substantially increased the life expectancy of the average patient. The fact that COPD is caused by smoking has been established beyond question, and one can hope that as smoking decreases, so will the COPD problem. However, even in the most enlightened societies, smoking remains prevalent, and COPD is often a disease of ex-smokers who quit too late to avoid lung damage. These factors ensure that the COPD problem will not disappear soon.

People with COPD have the disease 24 hours a day, 7 days a week for many years. It has only recently been recognized that a team best carries out the medical management of patients with this kind of affliction and that the team's most important member is the patient himself/herself. Although physicians are necessarily part of the team, they are not necessarily the primary contact between the patient and the health care system. Nurses, pharmacists, respiratory therapists, nutritionists, social workers, and physical and occupational therapists all have key roles in COPD care that is truly comprehensive.

This book is aimed at the team caring for COPD patients. It combines features of the "medical" text—symptoms, signs, drugs, and dosages—with practical details concerning smoking cessation, inhalation therapy, and rehabilitation through exercise. Topics such as psychosocial, spiritual, and sexual function are covered, and patient involvement in the care process is emphasized. I believe that these features are the most important aspect of this book, making it unique and justifying the adjective "Comprehensive." The authorship is not only multiple but multidisciplinary, with contributions from representatives of all of the team members enumerated above. All individuals concerned in the care of patients with COPD should find this book useful. It is, in other words, more than the usual medical text.

Another unique feature of this book is its Canadian content. Although many of its authors were born elsewhere, they all currently work in Canada. Obviously, many non-Canadians are as well qualified to write on COPD as the present authors. However, there are several factors that favor the high level of Canadian content. First, it is fair to say that Canadians have contributed disproportionately to the accumulation of knowledge about COPD over the past 50 years. Second, the Canadian health care system is well suited to the team approach to care. Third and most important, Canada is a small country with a relatively small and congenial pulmonary community, facilitating the assembly of a multiauthor text. That is not to say that I believe that putting this book together was easy; it most assuredly was not, and I congratulate the editors and the authors on a job done very well indeed.

Nicholas Anthonisen, Respirologist

FOREWORD

The need to seek medical help has always been faced with anxiety. Inevitably, it starts with a state of vulnerability, whereby the physical environment of the hospital, clinic, and, most of all, the emergency ward, are quite intimidating. Additionally, the nature of the illness itself can be a source of pain or fear. These stresses are all added concern for the patient with chronic obstructive pulmonary disease (COPD) who is already currently faced with the obvious state of turmoil that the medical system has been in for several years now.

Yet somehow, through their medical innovation and against all apparent odds, a number of practitioners have succeeded in breaking through strings of financial cutbacks, armchaired reorganizations, and the institutionalization of mazes of bureaucratic restraints. This new text, *Comprehensive Management of Chronic Obstructive Pulmonary Disease*, is both a convincing example of that success and a tribute to the lasting values of the qualitative practice of medicine for chronic disease.

The starting point of their collaborative effort lies in the commitment to the objective of placing the patient at the center of the practice. This value dominates the entire work and transcends each and all of its parts. Because this objective surpasses the reach of any one individual, it has led its authors to seek contributions from a widened colleague base; in this case, they have gone beyond the traditional borders of their field and have included the patient through an innovative perspective. Here the patient is seen as more than the object of his/her practice; he/she is perceived as a collaborator and as an active member in the application of care itself.

The entire book attests to that perspective of the patient as a colleague; in particular, there are chapters on controlling breathlessness and cough, energy conservation and fatigue, exercise training in patients with COPD, and patient education. The underlying strategy of enabling the patient to become as autonomous as possible in managing his or her own medical situation is a risky step to take at a time when resources are scarce. In addition to the highly pertinent scientific information that is being shared here, all of the sound principles of management seem to have been brought to the forefront in conceiving this project: interdisciplinary perspective, team work, and methodology for imparting medical and pharmaceutical knowledge to patients, as well as new skills to help him/her retain or regain higher states of physical fitness and emotional and psychological health.

Because the patient is a natural ally, the inclusion of the patient as a member of the medical team itself in such an innovative fashion is probably the most promising element of this project. This book fosters a "win-win" strategy for which the practice of medicine is highly qualitative and the increased autonomy of the patient helps in containing the overall cost of the system, and whereby the patient's condition is improved to ultimately attain a higher quality of life.

Henri Tremblay, Patient

ACKNOWLEDGMENTS

In preparing this book, I have been fortunate to have the assistance of two outstanding co-editors, Diane Nault and Elizabeth Borycki. I wish to thank them for their critical reviews and for their many valuable suggestions. I have also been very fortunate to have the collaboration of respirologists, both colleagues and friends, as well as the allied health care professionals highly skilled in the management of chronic obstructive pulmonary disease (COPD) across Canada. Without their significant contributions, it would have been impossible to develop a book with such great content and comprehensive value. I also wish to thank all of my patients with COPD, who really inspired me to undertake this project and gave me the courage and determination to make it come true.

I wish to thank Dr. Nicholas Anthonisen and Mr. Henri Tremblay, a patient with COPD, who each wrote a foreword to the book. I would also like to thank the many external reviewers who contributed to the completion of the different chapters, namely, Dr. M.R. Becklake (Chapter 3), Dr. Frederick Bass (Chapter 4), Vitalie Perreault and William C. Boyle (Chapter 6), Dr. Mayer Balter (Chapter 8), Mme Hélène Boutin and Mme Louise Hagan (Chapter 17), and Dr. Francois Maltais (Chapter 13).

As I look back, I realize that I have been blessed to work with an outstanding team without whom this book could not have been completed. I wish to thank Rame A. Taha, who has reviewed all of the medical references; Vincent Mecca from Mecca Design, who has used his superb skills in computer graphics to refine and finalize many of the illustrations; and, finally, the whole team from the Department of Neurophotography, McGill University Health Centre. My deepest thanks are expressed to Ms. Erica Taylor, who has worked more than a year doing the typing, editing, and seemingly endless revisions of the book, all of which she has done with great skill, dedication, and care. I would also like to thank Ms. Louise Auclair and Ms. Danielle Bastien for their secretarial assistance.

My deep appreciation goes to AstraZeneca, Bayer, Boehringer Ingelheim, and GlaxoSmithKline for their unrestricted educational grant. Their generosity should be duly noted, especially since this book's main focus is not about drugs and they were not involved in any of the steps leading to publication.

I gratefully acknowledge the support of the respiratory network of the Fonds de la recherche en santé du Québec (FRSQ). I am especially thankful to the FRSQ and Boehringer Ingelheim Canada, who support, in partnership, the development and the validation of a self-management program, "Living well with COPD©," from which many pictures have been adapted. This book was written while I was supported by a personal research scholarship from the FRSQ.

Finally, to my wife, parents, and children, I thank you for your constant love, inspiration, encouragement, enthusiasm, and support as I worked on the book. I have learned much from my parents about passion, hard work, and perseverance. They have given me more than can be expressed in words with regard to the completion of this book. The love and support of my wife and children were instrumental in making this book a reality. They have constantly encouraged me even when this involved personal sacrifice on their part. I am truly fortunate and grateful beyond words.

Jean Bourbeau

CONTENTS

CHAPTER 1

OPTIMIZING MEDICAL CARE DELIVERY

*Jean Bourbeau, Mary Ann Siok,
Diane Nault, and Elizabeth Borycki*

OBJECTIVES

The general objective of this chapter is to help physicians and other allied health care professionals become more familiar with the burden of chronic obstructive pulmonary disease (COPD) in our society in order to better respond to the ongoing, continuous needs of the patient and his/her family. This could be done within a new holistic approach of care that favors proactive initiatives instead of the traditional medical model primarily based on reactive responses to acute episodes of disease.

After reading this chapter, the physician and the allied health care professional will be able to

- appreciate the trends in COPD prevalence and mortality over time;
- recognize the impact of COPD over the course of the disease on the patient, family, health care system, and society;
- appreciate the economic burden of COPD;
- differentiate between the traditional acute care and the chronic care trajectory approaches;
- adopt new strategies in clinical practice that include a disease-specific self-management program to optimize the delivery of care to patients with COPD; and
- recognize that there are tools specific to the self-management of COPD; some of these tools, when appropriately used, have been demonstrated to benefit the patient's health and to reduce health service use.

Chronic obstructive pulmonary disease (COPD) is one of the leading causes of morbidity and mortality worldwide.[1,2] The consequences of COPD on individuals, families, health care services, and societies are quite significant. What is most alarming is that the most important risk factor, smoking, is still unacceptably prevalent in developed countries; furthermore, it is definitely increasing parallel to the aging population in both developing and developed countries.[1]

The impact of COPD on our aging population and on the health care system is overwhelming. It is particularly so with respect to emergency departments visits and with hospital re-admission rates, which are often of most concern to politicians,

administrators, and health professionals. There is a clear indication that the current health care system of episodic and acute disease–focused care is not adapted to the global needs of patients with COPD who have a continuum of recurring problems.

Administrators and allied health care professionals must turn toward a long-term or trajectory approach of care and services, which will take the global or biopsychosocial dimensions of the patient more into consideration. This global approach, which is interdisciplinary in nature, has to be based on several factors, including patient self-management, taking an active or maintenance rehabilitation approach, and, finally, adaptation to illness that is reflected in behavior modification or changes.

TABLE 1–1 Estimated Prevalence of Chronic Bronchitis, Emphysema, and Asthma in the United States, 1970, 1986, and 1994*

		Total Population											
		No. (× 1,000)			No. per 1,000			Men No. per 1,000			Women No. per 1,000		
Condition	ICD-9 Code	1970	1986	1994	1970	1986	1994	1970	1986	1994	1970	1986	1994
Chronic bronchitis	490.491	6.529	11.379	14.021	32.7	48.1	54.0	31.2	41.2	44.5	34.0	54.7	63.1
Emphysema	492.0	1.313	1.998	2.208	6.6	8.5	7.8	10.3	10.5	9.7	3.1	6.5	6.0
Asthma	493.0	6.031	9.690	14.562	30.2	41.0	56.1	31.7	40.8	51.7	28.8	41.1	60.2

*Adapted from National Center for Health Statistics, 1973, 1974, 1986a, 1987, 1995, 1997.[4]
ICD-9 = International Classification of Diseases, Ninth Revision.

In this chapter, we review the evidence available on the impact of COPD both on the patient and family, the approach of care that is adapted to chronic disease, and strategies for optimizing care delivery to patients with COPD and examine a program of care designed specifically for COPD.

BURDEN OF COPD

Epidemiology

Epidemiology of COPD is available in developing countries; however, there are wide variations in the data that might be attributable to regional and national differences in sociodemographic and environmental factors. Also, these variations could be the result of the way in which the terms bronchitis, emphysema, and COPD are defined. Furthermore, there is evidence that the prevalence of COPD is greatly underestimated as it is not recognized and diagnosed until it is advanced. The same applies to mortality rates of COPD. Often the precipitating cause of death, usually pneumonia or congestive heart failure, is listed as the principal cause of death rather than the underlying cause of COPD. Thus, this is not captured by the national mortality database. For instance, in a recent study, it was shown that even among patients with at least one hospitalization for COPD, this diagnosis was mentioned on the death certificate for less than 50% of the deaths.[1] The result of this study confirms that COPD is infrequently listed as a contributing cause of death among patients with these diseases.

Prevalence

No data are available about incidence rates that provide a better estimate of time trends. The Global Burden of Disease Study conducted under the auspices of the World Health Organization and the World Bank estimated that the worldwide prevalence of COPD was 9 to 34 in 1,000 men and 7 to 33 in 1,000 women.[1]

In Europe, recent estimates from a survey suggest that the prevalence of COPD may be as high as 80 to 100 in 1,000 in areas in which the prevalence of smoking is high.[3]

In the United States, the National Center for Health estimated the prevalence of the disease based on the responses to standard questions asked of representative samples of a noninstitutionalized, civilian population in the National Health Interview Survey.[4] Table 1–1 shows the estimated prevalence of chronic bronchitis and emphysema in the United States for the years 1970, 1986, and 1994. Reported rates of chronic bronchitis were higher from 1970 to 1994 and for women over men in 1986 and 1994. Reported rates of chronic bronchitis combined with emphysema were also higher from 1970 to 1994 for men and women.

In Canada, the National Center for Health Statistics estimates the prevalence of the disease according to the National Population Health Survey, based on the diagnosis made by physicians, including chronic bronchitis and emphysema. Figure 1–1 shows that the prevalence is higher for men than for women and steadily increases with age, becoming almost twofold over age 75 years.

Mortality

Death rates for COPD in men and women aged 35 to 74 years are shown by country in Figure 1–2.[2] There is substantial variation among countries for both sexes. However, death rates are lower among

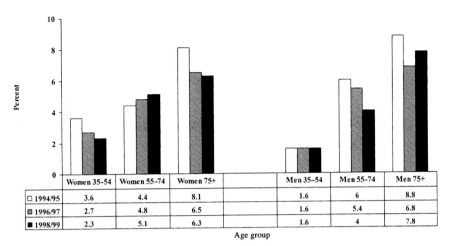

	Women 35-54	Women 55-74	Women 75+	Men 35-54	Men 55-74	Men 75+
□ 1994/95	3.6	4.4	8.1	1.6	6	8.8
▨ 1996/97	2.7	4.8	6.5	1.6	5.4	6.8
■ 1998/99	2.3	5.1	6.3	1.6	4	7.8

Age group

Figure 1–1 Prevalence of physician-diagnosed chronic bronchitis and emphysema by age group, Canada, 1994 to 1995, 1996 to 1997, and 1998 to 1999. (Adapted from the Centre for Chronic Disease Prevention and Control, Health Canada, using data from the National Population Health Survey, Statistics Canada.) (©Editorial board, Respiratory Disease in Canada. Health Canada, Ottawa, Canada, 2001.)

women than men in every nation. Comparison between countries is difficult considering the lack of standardization of death certificates and coding practices, as well as differences in diagnostic practice between countries.

According to projections, COPD will be the third leading cause of death worldwide in 2020, whereas in 1990, it ranked fifth.[1] Chronic obstructive pulmonary disease accounted for 4% of all deaths in the United States in 1996, being fourth highest among causes of death (Table 1–2).[2] From the same sources in 1996, the age-adjusted death rate per 100,000

population was 54.7 for white men, 42.5 for black men, 31.4 for white women, and 15.6 for black women. The rate has remained relatively constant since the 1980s for white men but has increased in black men and doubled in white women.

Chronic obstructive pulmonary disease also accounted for 4% of all deaths in Canada in 1998, making it the fourth leading cause of death for men and the seventh for women. The actual mortality rate may be higher because the primary cause of death may be listed as pneumonia or congestive heart failure, with COPD listed on the death cer-

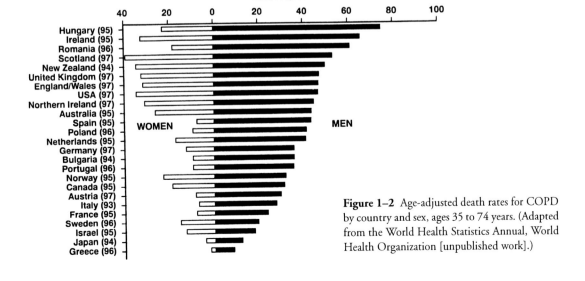

Figure 1–2 Age-adjusted death rates for COPD by country and sex, ages 35 to 74 years. (Adapted from the World Health Statistics Annual, World Health Organization [unpublished work].)

**TABLE 1–2 Leading Causes of Death,
United States, 1996***

Cause of Death	No. of Deaths
Heart disease	733,834
Cancer	544,278
Cerebrovascular disease (stroke)	160,431
COPD and allied conditions	106,146
Accidents	93,874
Pneumonia and influenza	82,579
Diabetes	61,559
Human immunodeficiency virus infections	32,655
Suicide	30,862
Chronic liver disease	25,135
All other causes of death	451,168

*Adapted from Vital Statistics of the US National Center of Health Statistics.[4]

tificate as the underlying cause. Since the National Mortality Database does not capture the underlying cause of death, these COPD cases will not be included in the COPD statistics. Mortality rates increased with age, especially in the over 70 age group (Figure 1–3). Rates were higher for men than women in all of the older age groups; this difference may reflect a higher rate of smoking among men in their younger years.

In the absence of incidence data on COPD, mortality projections can be used as a proxy to assess how COPD will affect people throughout developed countries in the future. The change in the age structure of the population, with an increasing number of people aged over 65, will eventually result in a continued increase in mortality related to COPD. Figure 1–4 illustrates the number of deaths from COPD, actual and projected in Canada, from 1987 to 2016. Increasing mortality rates are expected in both men and women; however, the increasing mortality rates among women compared to men, combined with the higher proportion of women among seniors, will produce a significantly increased rate among women.

In developing countries, it is even more difficult to have an estimate of COPD-related deaths since data are either unavailable or the quantity of medical care curtails its interpretation. However, it is expected that there will be a higher rate of death caused by COPD in view of increasingly aging populations related to improved socioeconomic conditions, combined with an increase in people who smoke.

Impact on the Patient, Family, and Health Care System

Impact on the Patient

Chronic obstructive pulmonary disease is insidious and progresses asymptomatically, with the exception of some cough and sputum production. This is

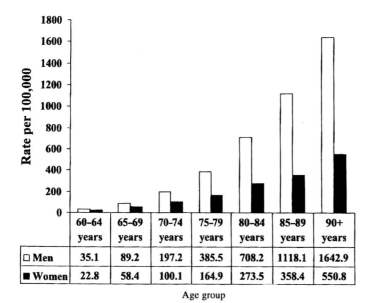

	60–64 years	65–69 years	70–74 years	75–79 years	80–84 years	85–89 years	90+ years
☐ Men	35.1	89.2	197.2	385.5	708.2	1118.1	1642.9
■ Women	22.8	58.4	100.1	164.9	273.5	358.4	550.8

Age group

Figure 1–3 Chronic obstructive pulmonary disease mortality rates per 100,000 by age and sex, Canada, 1998. (Adapted from the Centre for Chronic Disease Prevention and Control, Health Canada, using data from the Hospital Morbidity file. Canadian Institute for Health Information.) (©Editorial board, Respiratory Disease in Canada. Health Canada, Ottawa, Canada, 2001.)

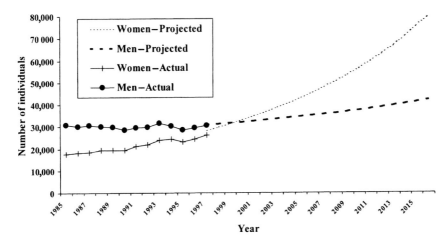

Figure 1–4 Number of chronic obstructive pulmonary disease deaths, actual and projected, Canada, 1987 to 2016. (Adapted from the Centre for Chronic Disease Prevention and Control, Health Canada, using data from the Morbidity Database. Statistics Canada. Population projections from Statistics Canada.) (©Editorial board, Respiratory Disease in Canada. Health Canada, Ottawa, Canada, 2001.)

followed by a period of time when the most common symptom of increased breathlessness on exertion can be ignored or misinterpreted as a natural process of aging. Over the course of the disease, breathlessness on exertion progressively deteriorates to the point where physical activities can become severely limited. The patient then gets into a vicious downward spiral of recurrent breathlessness on exertion, limited physical activity, further deterioration in breathlessness, and reduced exercise capacity as well as quality of life.[5] Although the influence of acute exacerbations on the progression of COPD has not been established, it has recently been reported that exacerbations can further aggravate the symptoms and result in complications, hospitalizations,[6] and a negative impact on health-related quality of life.[7]

Eventually, breathlessness with a constant reduction in exertion capabilities can force the patient to leave work or retire and thus be confined to the home. The patient experiences a whole spectrum of emotions and frustrations, such as anger, anxiety, and fear of dying. Often a mortal fear of breathlessness drives this behavioral response as the patient, losing self-esteem and self-confidence, retreats from almost all activities, becomes progressively isolated, and is thus confined to a sedentary and extremely boring existence. Patients may be embarrassed in public for a variety of reasons. For example, they may

be unwilling to accept the loss of autonomy and the subsequent need for help, they may be frustrated as these handicaps deteriorate, and, finally, they may become angry and increasingly isolated as friends or relatives have difficulty understanding the medical condition itself. Patients with COPD are often elderly, which makes them even more susceptible to isolation and, in turn, further increases the risk of depression. Nutrition is also a factor that may add to the complexity of the problem in that patients may eat less because they are experiencing extreme breathlessness and fatigue or are simply depressed. Certain individuals live with limited financial resources as they may have a poor income either from the inability to work or because of early retirement. In addition, the cost of medications, medical assistance, and various home-care facilities can seriously affect their financial state. Therefore, the whole situation escalates in complexity and spirals into an abstract context of interrelated physical, emotional, and psychosocial problems.

Impact on the Family

As in any advanced chronic disease, family members play an essential role in the life of the patient with COPD.[8] Patients become increasingly dependent on their caregivers for activities of daily living and emotional and social support. Furthermore, in the case of primary caregivers, they may also be put in a situation in which they become progressively isolated and essentially lose their own personal lives, culminating in caretaker fatigue and/or burnout.

However, not all family members are supportive because many do not understand COPD, and often the patient with the disease actually looks well despite advanced disease symptoms. It is a common perception, especially during the early stages of the disease, that the individual can do more than is feasible. As a result, the family may become disinterested and sometimes even hostile.

However, despite these difficulties, and because the demands of the disease are so incredibly overwhelming for the patients to cope with alone, family members must be encouraged to stay involved. Symptoms such as severe breathlessness can be frightening if those surrounding the patient are unaware of how to cope and which precautionary measures to take. Thus, it is clearly beneficial if family members are well educated in the management of the patient's disease. It is also important to listen to family input on the situation, in terms of their opinions, outlook, and desired roles in the patient's life.

Impact on the Health Care System

The patient with COPD requires a wide variety of care and services. Acute exacerbation of COPD and the concomitant development of complications, or comorbid conditions, often require frequent re-evaluation and increased use of health care services, including hospitalization.

Hospitalization rates are rising dramatically in the United States[4]; an estimated 553,000 hospital dis-charges were reported in 1995, a rate of 21.2 per 10,000 of population. Between 1992 and 1995, hospitalization discharge rates for COPD increased by 5.4% (Figure 1–5). Most discharges (67.1% in 1995) are in the population that is 65 years of age or more, which is greater than four times the amount in the 45- to 64-year-old age group. Discrepancies in reported data may exist because of changes in both the design of the National Hospital Discharge Survey in 1988 and in the ninth revision of the International Classification of Diseases code for chronic bronchitis in 1992.

In Canada, COPD is the fourth most common cause of hospitalization for men and the sixth for women. Beginning at about age 55, the hospitalization rates for patients with COPD increase steadily with age. Rates are higher for men than women at all ages (Figure 1–6). This is consistent with the higher smoking rates among men 40 to 50 years ago. Although the rates and duration of hospitalization for COPD have been decreasing, likely attributable to changes in the delivery of health services, the actual numbers themselves have been increasing because of the growing numbers of seniors in the population.

Forty to 50% of patients with COPD discharged from the hospital are re-admitted within the following year,[6,9] and after emergency department management, 17% of patients discharged have relapses that require hospitalization.[10] Using data from the Régie de l'assurance maladie du Québec (RAMQ), it was possible to determine that 39.6% of the patients admitted to the hospital in 1997 to 1998 had been

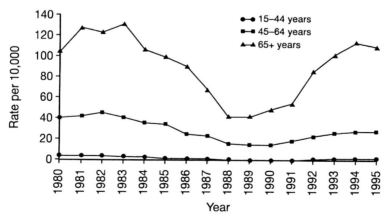

Figure 1–5 Age-specific COPD hospital discharge trends in the United States from 1980 to 1995. (Adapted from Sullivan, et al.[14])

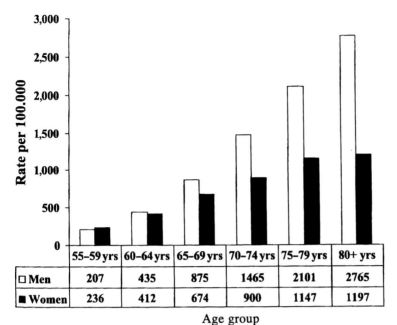

Figure 1–6 Chronic obstructive pulmonary disease hospitalization rate per 100,000 by age group and sex, Canada, 1998 to 1999. (Adapted from the Centre for Chronic Disease Prevention and Control, Health Canada, using data from the Hospital Morbidity File. Canada Institute for Health Information.) (©Editorial board, Respiratory Disease in Canada. Health Canada, Ottawa, Canada, 2001.)

	55–59 yrs	60–64 yrs	65–69 yrs	70–74 yrs	75–79 yrs	80+ yrs
□ Men	207	435	875	1465	2101	2765
■ Women	236	412	674	900	1147	1197

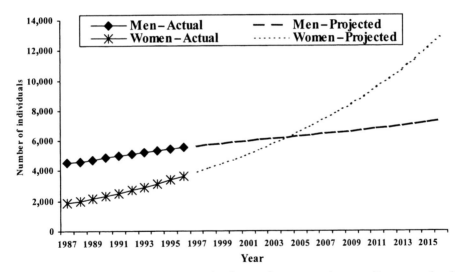

Figure 1–7 Number of individual hospitalizations for chronic obstructive pulmonary disease, actual and projected, Canada, 1985 to 2016. (Adapted from the Centre for Chronic Disease Prevention and Control, Health Canada, using data from the Hospital Morbidity File. Canada Institute for Health Information.) (©Editorial board, Respiratory Disease in Canada. Health Canada, Ottawa, Canada, 2001).

previously hospitalized at least once in the preceding 2 years and had contributed to 58.7% of the total number of days of hospitalization. Hospitalizations for patients with COPD and the phenomenon of multiple hospitalizations create a major burden on the health care system that will continue to bear its weight into the future (Figure 1–7).

The emergency department is the point of entry for most of the patients with COPD who require hospitalization. However, there is very limited data that indicates the importance of the problem or allow for a comparison with other diseases. A recent evaluation of Montreal's emergency departments from the public health department has shown a 20% increase in the daily number of stretchers occupied in emergency departments from April 1995 to March 2000 and an additional 20% increase during peak periods, from December to March (unpublished data). For the most part, pneumonia, COPD, and asthma were responsible for the increases during peak periods and were also the main diseases requiring hospitalization. Respiratory and heart failure also contributed to increased hospitalizaton rates but to a much lesser degree. A breakdown in the number of stretchers occupied in excess during peak periods showed that respiratory health problems were by far the most common cause, accounting for 36%.

Data are also scarce with regard to information on physician visits. Based on the 1995 National Ambulatory Care Survey in the United States, more than 16 million visits were made to doctors' offices for conditions for which the principal diagnoses were listed as COPD and allied conditions; this represents a sharp rise from the 9.3 million reported in 1985.[4] In 1995, chronic bronchitis was the most frequently reported, with chronic airway obstruction coming in second. The same survey indicated that there were 9 million office visits for asthma in 1995. Similarly, in a study carried out in a sociosanitary region of 250,000 people in England,[11] there were more outpatient medical consultations over the course of 1 year for patients with COPD than for asthmatic patients—14,200 compared with 11,900. Although none of these data provide information on the age distribution within the studied populations, with the aging population in the developed countries, it is clear that COPD will place a major burden on the health care system that will even exceed that of asthma.

Economic and Social Burden

Chronic obstructive pulmonary disease progresses through different stages with a major impact on the patient's functional abilities in life, disability,[12] and, finally, premature mortality. The Global Burden of Disease Study estimated the fraction of premature mortality and disability attributable to major disease using a composite score, disability-adjusted life year (DALY).[1] The DALY represents the sum of years lost because of premature mortality and years of life lived with disability adjusted for the severity of that disability. According to some projections, COPD, which ranked twelfth in 1990, will be the fifth leading cause of DALYs worldwide in 2020, behind ischemic heart disease, major depression, traffic acci-

dents, and cerebrovascular disease.

It is evident that COPD exerts a heavy toll on society in that it places a major economic burden on families, the health care system, and the community. There is a distinct difference in costs to be considered when looking at the economic impact of an illness on society; these costs are subdivided into direct and indirect costs. Direct costs are those associated with medical management, including medication. Indirect costs are those associated with individual family costs, which are essentially attributable to the loss of work time and productivity as a consequence of the illness. The lack of comprehensive data makes it difficult to estimate the actual cost of COPD across countries.

In the United States, according to estimates from the National Heart, Lung and Blood Institute,[13] the total annual cost of COPD was 23.9 billion dollars in 1993. This included 14.7 billion dollars in direct costs for medical services, 4.7 billion in indirect costs, and 4.5 billion in costs related to premature mortality. The largest contributor to cost was hospitalization and emergency department care (72.8%).[3] Outpatient clinic and office visits accounted for 15% of expenditures and drug prescriptions for 12.2%. As with other chronic diseases, the more severely affected persons (10% of the Medicare beneficiaries with COPD) incurred nearly 50% of the total Medicare payments.[14] Combining disease prevalence and illness burden, COPD costs an average of $1,522 per person per year, or almost three times the per capita cost of asthma.[14] Treatments that could prevent or limit hospitalizations could have a substantial impact on the overall burden of this disease. The indirect burden of COPD is difficult to assess, and very little information is available in the literature today.

OPTIMIZING MEDICAL CARE DELIVERY

Strategies for Managing Chronic Diseases

As demonstrated by increasing emergency department occupancy and hospital admission rates, the impact of COPD on the health care system is overwhelming, mostly because of the rapidly aging population. The health care system in many developed countries was implemented at a time when the population was younger and thus largely required health care for acute disease. The current system of episodic, acute, and reactionary disease–focused care practiced in many settings does not adequately address the numerous problems brought on by a chronic illness such as COPD. With COPD, one needs to cope with not only the symptoms but also the multiple problems that branch out psychologically, socially, and physically as a result of them. The person is faced with trying to live a normal life with the following goals in mind: to prevent medical crises, to manage the crises that occur, to handle the prescribed regimens, to control symptoms, and to overcome disability, stigma, social isolation, and often economic issues.[15]

We should be reminded that health and illness can coexist. The meaning of health in illness is in part the ability to manage or cope with the illness.[16] This means that the person with the disease and his/her family should (1) work at learning new ways to effectively manage the consequences of a chronic illness, (2) gain some control by actively participating and adjusting their response to the disease, and (3) assume responsibility for these measures. The patient should also set goals and work toward functioning at his or her perceived maximum capacity and satisfaction or quality of life.[17]

Chronic illness such as COPD is long term and should be viewed as having different stages that comprise a trajectory. It should also be understood that the important element of uncertainty is associated with any chronic illness like COPD. As the patient moves through various stages of the disease, it is within the family context. Thus, both the patient and family are in a constant process of learning as they endure, manage, and adapt to these COPD-related changes.

In the acute care approach, the physician focuses on the disease by first diagnosing it, then treating it, and, finally, following up with the patient according to his/her medical needs. The chronic care approach is more adapted to COPD. This approach focuses not only on the disease but also on the patient within the context of his/her family and on health promotion principles being primarily those of adult learning and self-management. The patient learns to engage in self-management activities that promote health and prevent complications, thereby ensuring his/her engagement in daily management decisions. The patient learns how to communicate with the physician and other health professionals as they try to help him/her adapt to changing needs. The differences between acute and chronic care approaches are presented in Table 1–3.

TABLE 1–3 Differences between Acute Care and Chronic Care Approaches

Issue	Standard Acute	Chronic
Underlying philosophy	Diagnosis, medical treatment of the disease, and follow-up with medical complications as the focus	Holistic and interdisciplinary approach based on health prevention and promotion principles
Key values	Best care for episodic and acute exacerbations, medical diagnosis	Taking a long-term or trajectory approach while taking into consideration the environment and a behavior diagnosis
Focus	Pulmonary function control, medical management	Self-management; taking an active or maintenance rehabilitation approach, behavior changes, adaptation to illness
Intervention	Symptoms, drug protocols	Risk factors, integrated care based on consistent and established guidelines, continuity ensured
Drivers	Lung function and acute events	
Patient role	Passive, expected to comply with prescribed medical regimens	Actively collaborates, care goals are established with the patient, self-management is fostered
Health care provider	Reactive—responds	Proactive—initiates
Key outcomes	Physiologic and symptoms	Self-management of symptoms, well-being, quality of life, including the various dimensions; cost effectiveness
Intervention	Pharmacologic and adjunctive therapy	Pharmacologic, exercise, educational, behavioral; community and system change

Common Features of Successful Programs

Mounting evidence indicates that standard medical care often fails to meet the needs of patients with chronic disease.[18–20] In the clinical experience of numerous health professionals involved in the care of patients with COPD, many patients do not receive proven preventive practices such as smoking cessation or vaccination, self-management through education, an exercise training program, and/or psychosocial support.

Most will agree that, we attempt to provide the patient with the best medical care. But it must be stressed that medical care for chronic disease is rarely effective in the absence of adequate self-care or self-management. Patients and their families are the primary caregivers in chronic disease. Medical care and self-care are both enhanced by effective collaboration among chronically ill patients and their families, as well as health care providers. Self-care or self-management refers to (1) setting realistic self-management goals and objectives; (2) engaging in activities that promote health and prevent adverse sequelae; (3) two-way interaction with health care providers; (4) adhering to recommended treatments; (5) making appropriate management decisions based on self-monitoring; (6) controlling the effects of illness on important roles, emotions, on self-esteem, and in relationships with others; and (7) evaluating self-management outcomes to reinforce successful behaviors and facilitate the performance of poorly integrated behaviors.

A landmark study in the successful care of COPD was the Disease Specific Self-Management COPD Trial (Impact/COPD study), which was a self-management program applied in an ambulatory setting and evaluated in a multicenter randomized clinical trial.[21–24] Impact/COPD trial patients in the self-management group saw care-oriented treatment organized very differently from their usual medical care. Patients in both groups of the Impact/COPD study, self-management and usual care groups, were already on maximal drug treatment and were followed up by a respirologist in an outpatient clinic of a secondary or tertiary care hospital. In addition to the usual care, each patient of the intervention group received a disease-specific self-management program, Living Well with COPD©, consisting of the following: (1) approximately 1-hour teaching sessions for 7 to 8 weeks delivered by an experienced and previously trained health professional (nurses in four cen-

ters, inhalation therapists in two, and a physiotherapist in one); (2) 8 weeks of weekly telephone calls, by the same health professional, following the teaching sessions; and (3) additional monthly telephone follow-ups for the remainder of the study. The health professional was also available by telephone for advice and treatment supervision. The program included a flipchart and seven skill-oriented, self-help workbook modules. The net effects of the program were the following: (1) a high level of new skill acquisition and help strategies with respect to activities of daily living[21,22]; (2) a high level of adherence and maintenance of the above-mentioned behavior changes[21,22]; (3) at least a 40% reduction in use of health care services (hospital admission, emergency department, and unscheduled physician visits) in the self-management group as compared with the usual care group[23]; and (4) an overall improvement in health status.[24] The features that distinguished the Impact/COPD trial protocol from the current customary practice are the following:

1. Care was planned with the patient, and clearly delegated roles were assigned to all those involved
2. Philosophy of care was based on principles of patient self-management, adult learning, and empowerment
3. The program provided a consistent educational message
4. Continuity of care was ensured
5. Support case management was provided by a trained health professional who used the same approach, teaching, and follow-up tools so that consistency in care and access to clinical expertise were ensured
6. Interventions were made by clinical experts focused on their patient's needs and patient outcomes or quality-of-care indicators

Indeed, the same aspects of care were associated with improved outcomes in similar intervention studies in other chronic illnesses.[20,25,26] As was the case in the Impact/COPD trial, the plan of care and interventions were based on a comprehensive or "biopsychosocial" assessment. A number of community resources can then be mobilized depending on the patient's needs and his/her personal goals; the care plan can be revised periodically with the patient and the family. A good assessment of the patient's and the family's needs, a realistic patient self-assessment plan of care based on the establishment of mutual goals and objectives, case management for patient follow-up and communication between patients, and finally, families and health care providers are all composites in the foundation on which any organized approach to chronic disease, such as COPD care, should be built.

A common reaction to the Impact/COPD trial care and similar trials with other chronic diseases is that because of the intensity of the intervention, such a system is not realistic in the real world of clinical care. Our argument about the Impact/COPD trial is not based on the intensity of care provided (which we agree is not realistic to every group of patients with COPD) but lies in the proactive system based on consistency and the ongoing monitoring of patients with COPD. We are still awaiting the study results of similar self-management programs for COPD in community settings. However, the intensity of care should be predicated not only on the disease severity but even more importantly on the patient's well-being and on health service use (hospital admission, emergency department visit, etc).

Program of Care Specific to COPD

The key concepts of a care delivery approach for chronic disease are protocol-driven planned care, established in collaboration, and revised periodically. This would include interdisciplinary care with delegated roles, self-management support and empowerment, and care that is accessible and within a continuum. The challenge, of course, is for the existing practitioners and organizations to adapt themselves to this new approach of care. In reorganizing the care for patients with COPD, we should aim to implement those key concepts within a strategy of medical care delivery for chronic disease.

Case management has been proposed as a system of managing complex patients.[27–29] It promotes continuity, communication, and collaboration between the patient, the family, the physicians, and various health care providers. Case management is a systematic process of assessment, planning, service coordination, referrals, and monitoring that meets the multiple care and service needs of patients with COPD. However, it has to be distinguished from the critical pathway established on many acute care units. Critical pathways are helpful tools, but many patients do not follow diagnosis or have multiple chronic diseases that need special care. In addition, the patient with COPD, especially the complex patient, needs someone who is accessible, is able to

provide information, can coordinate the necessary services at different stages of the disease, and can also provide continuity when the patient is back in the community after hospital discharge. In clinical follow-ups, patients tell us that they feel more secure when it is evident that there is good communication between health providers and institutions. Case management has been recommended as particularly useful and successful in optimizing care and in the mobilization of community-based services among a variety of chronically ill and medically fragile patients.[30]

Framework for a Program of Care

These are the possible problems experienced with patients with COPD in institutions prior to the adoption of this new combined care delivery approach of case management and disease-specific self-management comprehensive program:

1. Patients having frequent emergency department visits and hospitalizations
2. Patients exhibiting learned helplessness
3. Patients lacking in follow-up postpulmonary rehabilitation programs
4. Patients with minimal communication, coordination, and limited mobilization of various in-hospital and community resources
5. Often a premature closure of various community and/or home care services

A care delivery approach with case management for chronic disease, like the Impact/COPD study, can be implemented in institutions through outpatient clinic departments using a program delivery specific to COPD, such as Living Well with COPD©. The foundation of such an intervention is through an evaluation by the treating respirologist and a global evaluation by a health professional acting as a case manager. Nurses are in a position to act as case managers as they are trained to assess patients and the family's health needs, plan global patient care, and intervene with the patient, family, and community. Nurse training is based on a global nursing care approach, which considers the person as a whole and as having biopsychosocial health needs. However, the choice of a health professional as a case manager might vary from one institution to the other, depending on the health personnel qualifications and availability. The COPD initial evaluation is critical as the plan of care and services must be established according to the needs of the patient. The evaluation should include (1) a global or "biopsychosocial" assessment of the patient's needs, (2) readiness of the patient to learn, and (3) a collaborative relationship with mutual understanding and agreement on the objectives of care and services.[16]

Following the initial evaluation, a disease-specific program such as Living Well with COPD© is provided to the patient. Depending on the patient's needs and personal goals, the patient can be referred to one of the outpatient programs such as smoking cessation, pulmonary rehabilitation, or a stress management group; alternatively, a consultation may be requested with other health professionals such as a physiotherapist, physical educator, occupational therapist, dietitian, social worker, psychologist, or others. The patient follow-up is done at the outpatient clinic to help him/her integrate and maintain what was learned in the given program and/or the outpatient pulmonary rehabilitation program. The case manager should be part of the rehabilitation program setting because the manager's presence assists in a more prompt recognition of physical and psychosocial problems that often limit the patient's adherence to the program. Furthermore, the case manager facilitates communication between the different health professionals from within the hospital and outward to the community, as well as to the patient's physician. This ensures that the treating physician and other health professionals involved in the care of the patient are at an advantage in being able to support a long-term response. Referrals or liaisons with various community resources are carried out according to patient needs. The ambulatory COPD program must be interdisciplinary, with the work done collaboratively between the patient, family, and various health professionals.

This type of COPD program of care was implemented at the Montreal Chest Institute of the Royal Victoria Hospital McGill University Health Centre. Patients reported that they felt more secure when it was evident that there was good communication between health professionals within and between health institutions. It has been documented that case management can successfully increase the use of community-based services among a variety of chronically ill and medically fragile populations. Furthermore, it can decrease the frequency and length of the hospital stay.[27] We have had success in mobilizing increasingly varied resources for our patients with COPD, such as more community or home care ser-

vices, prompt geriatric assessment, psychiatric services, and others. Although this has been an arduous task, it has also been a genuine learning experience for both ourselves and the various community organizations involved. The process of formalizing some of these relationships has been started with planned meetings to establish proper communication skills with each other, improve the quality of care provided, and, ideally, avoid service duplication.

As previously seen, there is evidence from randomized clinical trials to support comprehensive and coordinated approaches that deal with chronic diseases such as COPD. However, there is also a need to document and assess in the ambulatory and community settings which components of a program are necessary and how intense the intervention should be in different groups of patients with COPD. For example, this might vary with the patient's disease trajectory. Furthermore, we need more comprehensive data to estimate not only the most effective management and care delivery approach but also the most cost-effective approach according to specific disease status.

Target Population

There is an ongoing conflict between trying to achieve the goal of optimizing health care delivery and meeting the goal of minimizing costs. Until more data are available on the cost effectiveness of intervention according to various categories of patients with COPD, there will have to be a reallocation of existing resources, albeit scarce, to the most appropriate treatment approach. Additionally, the resources will also have to target specific patient groups such as those who have significant functional limitation and those who are frequent health care service users.

In the implementation of a new care delivery approach of case management, complemented by a disease-specific self-management comprehensive program, it is necessary to provide physicians and the institution with a guide for patient referral. Thus, ideally, the program should primarily be available to the patients who will be most likely to benefit from additional care and services. It is important to understand that, as a dynamic process, the initially established criteria are in constant revision to be subsequently adjusted, based on documented clinical and health resource indicators. Patients with COPD who are referred to the COPD program at the McGill University Health Centre include: those in whom the disease has a significant impact on their quality of life but who are still relatively autonomous and those who experience a loss of autonomy and decline in their quality of life because of their disease. The COPD program prioritizes those patients who experience hospitalization or emergency department visits. This should be seen as an indicator to prevent such events in the future.

The following patients are usually excluded from the COPD program and have to be seen by a physician or referred to another service:

1. Patients not yet diagnosed with COPD
2. Patients who are in the early phase of their COPD; their requirements are essentially related to smoking cessation management
3. Patients who are in the terminal or preterminal phase of their COPD since their requirements are primarily palliative; because the COPD program and their team members strongly value the principle of continuity of care, they continue to provide services as needed to patients once they become terminal/preterminal
4. Patients who frequently come to the hospital or emergency department but for whom the central issue is placement
5. Patients who have functional impairment and/or loss of autonomy but whose primary issue of concern is not COPD but another illness (eg, Alzheimer's disease, cancer, etc.)

However, patients referred to the pulmonary rehabilitation program are also seen in the COPD program. These are times when a needs assessment is important as it provides an opportunity to marshal increased support and further development. Barriers to maintenance in the community, resulting in frequent emergency department visits and hospitalizations, can be attributable to the following: patients not having learned various COPD self-management skills and health providers not having mobilized appropriate community resources. The cycle of frequent hospitalization can be broken down by referring the patient to a COPD program with integrated care. Recent studies have suggested that for those high-risk patients, an intervention in an outpatient setting with a case manager and a disease-specific self-management program are cost-effective and possibly even cost saving.[31] However, for patients with COPD with mild disease manifestation and a mild degree of risk, the optimal matching with a less intensive intervention has not been well studied in terms of effectiveness and cost.

Clinical Tools for Patient Teaching

The main clinical tool for COPD is a program called Living Well with COPD©. This is an ambulatory care self-management program for patients with COPD that spans the entire continuum of care. All materials are written in simple language with large, easy-to-read type that incorporates friendly, upbeat graphics. All materials have been reviewed and evaluated by patients, caregivers, and educators; furthermore, the program has been evaluated in a randomized clinical trial[23,24,31] and a qualitative study complementary to the clinical trial.[21,22]

The program components include the following:

- Flipchart—teaching tool designed for educators
- Patient workbooks—seven comprehensive modules detailing the management of all facets of the disease
- Inhalation technique sheets for all types of inhalation devices
- A plan of action, including a contact list, regular drugs taken, and a symptom monitoring list linked to appropriate actions and medications
- Relaxation tape—to assist teaching of relaxation and for use at home
  The patient workbooks include the following:
- Module 1—breathing and coughing techniques, energy conservation during day-to-day activities, and relaxation exercises
- Module 2—preventing and controlling symptoms with inhalation technique sheets
- Module 3—understanding and using a plan of action according to situations of stress, environmental change, and respiratory infection
- Module 4—adopting a healthy lifestyle (smoking cessation, nutrition, sexuality, sleep habits, managing emotions)
- Module 5—leisure activities and traveling
- Module 6—home exercise program with warm-up exercises, muscle exercises, and cardiovascular exercises (stationary bicycle, walking, or climbing stairs)
- Module 7—learning to live with long-term home oxygen therapy for those who need home oxygen

SUMMARY

The inefficiency with which our institutions manage chronic diseases is no longer economically supportable. We can no longer afford the luxury of

---

managing diseases such as COPD with a system that is not designed to help patients self-manage but to cure. The health care practice has to be redesigned to facilitate the shift from reactive acute care to plan care, the goal of which is focused on the prevention of exacerbation and on the promotion of healthy behaviors.

Administrators and health professionals have to implement a chronic care approach for patients with COPD that will better respond to the needs of the patient following a chronic disease trajectory. We are convinced that such a change in care will lessen not only the impact of lung disease, which will be reflected by lung function status, but also will lead to a decrease in hospitalization and emergency department visits. More importantly, the patient and family will be more empowered to manage the various aspects of COPD successfully and thus comprehensively improve their quality of life. This approach of care is associated with improved outcomes in chronic illnesses where intervention studies have been carried out, including studies in COPD.

To achieve optimization of care in the continuum of COPD, new strategies have to be implemented in this chronic care approach, namely, education of the patient with COPD with consistent self-management support and service coordination with protocol-driven planned care and delegated roles. In addition, teaching and follow-up must be carried out by trained health professionals who use the same approach in their teaching and follow-up tools to ensure consistency in care and access to clinical expertise.

Ultimately, if we want a long-term solution to the growing problems of chronic illnesses such as COPD, we have to establish a system of care that will eventually reach all individuals with COPD.

CASE STUDY

Mr. Cope, a 74-year-old patient, has been followed for several years primarily for COPD. He had smoked one pack of cigarettes per day for 40 years and quit when he was 55 years old.

His wife was very supportive, and he also had a strong network to rely on. Figure 1–8 demonstrates the patient support network.

As with most patients with COPD, the patient's disease followed a trajectory over time when he experienced various phases requiring revision and adjustment in his plan of care and services. The disease trajectory is illustrated in Figure 1–9 with various disease phases, corresponding biopsychosocial changes, and care delivery in the disease continuum.

A. *Insidious disease onset*
• The patient is 61 years old.
• For the past 2 years, he has had breathlessness that stops him from walking and keeping up with most of his peers.
• He is still autonomous but experiencing a significant impact on his quality of life: walking less, giving up important social activities, and generally less active.

B. *Hospitalization for acute exacerbation*
• He has the feeling that he cannot do activities of daily living.
• He is dependent on his spouse for instrumental activities of daily living, such as banking and shopping.
• He has fear, anxiety, and panic attacks.
• He is essentially coping by "not doing."
• He is housebound and dependent on nebulized bronchodilators.
• There is a change in roles with tension in the family.

C. *Patient participating in a pulmonary rehabilitation program*
• He is learning new coping strategies to deal with periods of breathlessness caused by emotional

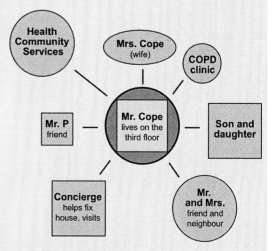

Figure 1–8 Patient support network. ⬭ = essential; ◯ = significant; ▢ = supplemental.

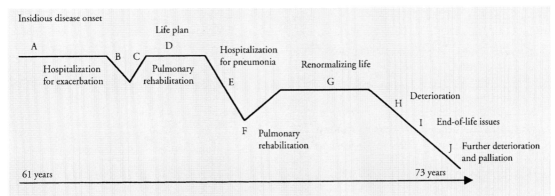

Figure 1–9 Disease trajectory of a patient with COPD.

and environmental stressors and respiratory infections; thus, he is less anxious, is able to analyze why he is experiencing increased breathlessness, and is able to problem solve these various situations effectively.

- Nebulized medication is replaced by a metered-dose inhaler and administered with a spacer device.
- He receives physical strength and endurance training; thus, he feels less breathlessness and has a better exercise tolerance.
- An improved overall sense of well-being.

D. *Life plan*
- He normalizes his life.
- He redefines his life goals: socialization, activities, and leisure (travel and golf).
- He integrates principles of energy conservation and pacing of activities in daily experiences.
- He adopts good nutrition.
- He exercises regularly three to five times per week.
- He has increased autonomy; that is, he is less dependent on a caregiver for activities of daily living and instrumental activities of daily living.
- He communicates with his family and mutual support emerges.

E. *Hospitalization for pneumonia*
- He has an intensive care unit admission.
- He has noninvasive mechanical ventilation for 48 hours.
- He requires a nasal prong oxygen supplement (2 L/min).
- He experiences physical deconditioning, decreased mobility, and loss of autonomy.
- He learns to adapt to breathlessness worsening and disease progression.

F. *Patient participation in a pulmonary rehabilitation program*
- He receives a few sessions of exercise training in hospital with oxygen assessment followed by a home exercise program with telephone monitoring.
- He is mobilizing support in the community: other oxgen-dependent patients, specialized respiratory home care nurse, physiotherapist, and inhalation therapist.

G. *Renormalizing life*
- He modifies his daily activities and gives up some leisure activities such as playing golf.
- He exercises regularly but feels he cannot sustain the same intensity that he used to in previous years.
- He has some weight loss that he cannot get back.

H. *Physical and living status deteriorating*
- He has acute exacerbations averaging twice a year.
- Despite early intervention, the patient deteriorates and an oxygen adjustment is required.
- He is dependent on others for activities of daily living.
- He mobilizes more community support and services, for example, bath help, day center, and community social worker.

I. *End-of-life issues*
- The patient and his family need to address decisions with respect to end-of-life issues.
- He makes decisions on critical interventions and placement.
- He requires home care and social support

J. *Further disease deterioration and palliation*
- He is hospitalized for respiratory infection and an acute exacerbation.
- The patient decides on palliative care.

KEY POINTS

- The prevalence of COPD is highest in countries in which cigarette smoking has been, or still is, very common.
- Data on the prevalence and morbidity of COPD probably greatly underestimate the total burden of the disease because it is not recognized and diagnosed until it is clinically apparent and relatively advanced.
- Patients with COPD use many health services, including ambulatory, hospital, and drugs; the projected increase in cases and resultant deaths will place major demands on health services and a significant cost on society.
- As it progresses, COPD has an impact on numerous aspects of the patient's life and social role and in more advanced disease, it also affects family relations.
- In chronic diseases such as COPD, day-to-day care responsibilities fall most heavily on patients and their families.
- New strategies with a chronic care approach, namely COPD self-management, service coordination, and delegated roles, have been successful in the following respects: they have demonstrated an impact on the patient's quality of life, optimized health service use, and proven to be cost effective.
- A long-term solution to the growing problems of chronic illnesses, such as COPD, entail integrating disease-specific management into the continuum of services that will eventually reach all individuals with COPD.

REFERENCES

1. Murray CJL, Lopez AD. The global burden of disease: a comprehensive assessment of mortality and disability from diseases, injuries and risk factors in 1990 and projected to 2020. Cambridge, MA: Harvard University Press, 1996.
2. Hurd S. The impact of COPD on lung health worldwide. Epidemiology and incidence. Chest 2000;117: 1S–4S.
3. Strassels S, Sullivan D, Smith DH. Characterization of the incidence and cost of COPD in the US. Eur Respir J 1996;9 Suppl 23:421S.
4. NHLBI. Morbidity and mortality chartbook, 1998. Available at http://www.nhlbi.nih.gov/resources/coes/cht.book.htm (last accessed February 2002).
5. Ferrer M, Alonso J, Morra J, et al. Chronic obstructive pulmonary disease stages and health related quality of life. Ann Intern Med 1997;127:1072–9.
6. Osman IM, Godden DJ, Friend JA, et al. Quality of life and hospital re-admission in patients with chronic obstructive pulmonary disease. Thorax 1997;52: 67–71.
7. Seemungal TA, Donaldson GC, Paul EA, et al. Effects of exacerbation on quality of life in patients with chronic obstructive pulmonary disease. Am J Respir Crit Care Med 1998;157:1418–22.
8. Bruhn JG. Effects of chronic illness on the family. J Fam Pract 1977;4:1057–60.
9. Connors AFJ, Dawson NV, Thomas C, et al. Outcomes following acute exacerbation of severe chronic obstructive lung disease. Am J Respir Crit Care Med 1996;154:959–67.
10. Emerman CL, Efrron D, Lukens TW. Spirometric criteria for hospital admission of patients with acute exacerbation of COPD. Chest 1991;99:595–9.
11. Anderson HR, Esmail A, Hollswell J, et al. Epidemiologically based needs assessment: lower respiratory disease. London: Department of Health, 1994.
12. Ashutosh K, Haldipur C, Boucher ML. Clinical and personality profiles and survival in patients with COPD. Chest 1997;111:95–8.
13. Division of Epidemiology, National Heart, Lung and Blood Institute, 1996. Available at http://www/nhlbi.nih.gov (last accessed February 2002).
14. Sullivan SD, Ramsey SD, Lee TA. The economic burden of COPD. Chest 2000;117:5S–9S.
15. Strauss AL. Chronic illness and the quality of life. St. Louis, MO: Mosby, 1975.
16. Gottlieb L, Rowat K. The McGill model of nursing: a practice-derived model. ANS Adv Nurs Sci 1987;9: 51–61.
17. Bruhn JG, Cordova FD. The wellness process. J Community Health 1977;2:209–21.
18. Marrero DG, Moore PS, Langefield CD, Clark CM. Patterns of referral and examination for retinopathy in pregnant women with diabetes by primary care physicians. Ophthalmic Epidemiol 1995;2:57–8.
19. Hiss RG, Anderson RM, Hess GE, et al. Community diabetes care. A 10 year perspective. Diabetes Care 1994;17:1124–34.
20. Rich MW, Beckhman V, Wittenberg C, et al. A multidisciplinary intervention to prevent the re-admission of elderly patients with congestive heart failure. N Engl J Med 1995;333:1190–5.
21. Nault D, Pépin J, Dagenais J, et al. Qualitative evaluation of a self-management program "Living Well with COPD"© offered to patients and their caregivers. Am J Respir Crit Care Med 2000;161:A56.
22. Nault D, Dagenais J, Perrault V, et al. Qualitative evaluation of a disease specific self-management program "Living well with COPD©." Eur Respir J 2000;16:317S.
23. Bourbeau J, Collet JP, Schwartzman K, et al. Integrating rehabilitative elements into a COPD self-management program reduces exacerbations and health

services utilization: a randomized clinical trial. Am J Respir Crit Care Med 2000;161:A254.

24. Bourbeau J, Julien M, Rouleau M, et al. Impact of an integrated rehabilitative management program on health status of COPD patients. A multicentre randomized clinical trial. Eur Respir J 2000;16:159S.

25. Delahanty LM, Halford BN. The role of diet behaviors in achieving improved glycemic control in intensively treated patients in the Diabetes Control and Complications Trial. Diabetes Care 1993;16:1453–8.

26. Von Korff M, Gruman J, Schaefer J, et al. Collaborative management of chronic illness. Ann Intern Med 1997;127:1097–102.

27. Erkel EA. The impact of case management in preventative services. J Nurs Adm 1993;23:27–32.

28. Girard N. The case management model of patient care delivery. AORN J 1994;60:403–15.

29. Robinson J, Robinson K, Lewis D. Balancing quality of care and cost effectiveness through case management. ANNA 1992;13:182–9.

30. Trella R. A multi-disciplinary approach to case management of frail, hospitalized older adults. J Nurs Adm 1993;23:20–6.

31. Bourbeau J, Schwartzman K, Collet J-P, et al. Economic impact of a disease specific self-management program in the management of patients with COPD. Am J Respir Crit Care Med 2001;163:A13.

SUGGESTED READINGS

Hodder R, Lightstone S. Every breath I take. A guide to living with COPD. Toronto: Stoddart, 2001. *This book of real-life scenarios shows how people with COPD can live with a debilitating chronic illness and still enjoy a sense of achievement in life. It is informative, realistic, and practical for health professionals, patients with COPD, and their families.*

Von Korff M, Gruman J, Schaefer J, et al. Collaborative management of chronic illness. Ann Intern Med 1997;127:1097–102. *This article presents the importance of an effective collaborative relationship with health care providers to help patients with chronic illness and families better handle self-care tasks. It discusses the essential elements in light of behavioral principles and empiric evidence about effective care in chronic illness.*

Tiep BL. Disease management of COPD with pulmonary rehabilitation. Chest 1997;112:1630–56. *This is a review of COPD management including pulmonary rehabilitation. It suggests that pulmonary rehabilitative components should be integrated in the multidisciplinary continuum of services as defined by the 1994 National Institutes of Health Pulmonary Rehabilitation Research Workshop.*

CHAPTER 2

ASSESSMENT OF COPD

Andrew McIvor, Josiah Lowry,
Jean Bourbeau, and Elizabeth Borycki

OBJECTIVES

The general objective of this chapter is to assist physicians and other allied health care professionals from the hospital and community settings identify and assess the patient's chronic obstructive pulmonary disease (COPD) and subsequent severity stratification by implementation of a thoughtful approach to spirometry. This approach will be based on an assessment of the magnitude of underdiagnosis, the potential effectiveness of intervention, the predictive value of spirometry, and the clinical profile of patients who may have COPD. After reading this chapter, the physician and the allied health care professional will be able to

- improve the early detection of COPD diagnosis based on specific clinical indicators;
- understand the limits of history, physical examination, and radiology in the diagnosis of COPD;
- consider adopting spirometry as the gold standard for diagnosis of airway obstruction;
- differentiate between spirometry and other pulmonary function tests;
- consider the merits of adopting spirometry screening of "at-risk" patients in primary care;
- refer to specific professionals when needed.

Recently published consensus guidelines for the management of asthma and COPD outline markedly different therapeutic approaches to these overtly similar obstructive airway diseases. Chronic obstructive pulmonary disease may be considered as the "forgotten illness" since so much public awareness and educational initiatives have been instead focused around asthma management.

Chronic obstructive pulmonary disease, which represents a mixture of pathologic processes, should not be defined based on symptoms because it is non-specific, nor should it be based on a pathologic definition because this is impractical in clinical practice. The diagnosis is usually made relatively late in the natural history; it is frequently made after the age of 40 years, when symptoms have been in place for a long time, when the patient is restricted from performing certain activities, or, even worse, when this impairment or disability limits fulfilment of a normal role at work and/or at home.

Confirming the diagnosis requires spirometry. Although spirometry is the "gold standard" for diagnosis and disease severity stratification, this tool still remains underused outside specialist practice; consequently, a significant number of individuals remain unidentified. The debate on spirometry as a screening tool used to assist in diagnosis has been raised and dropped on various occasions over the last 30 years.[1,2]

This chapter will explore failings in history recordings, physical examination, and radiologic assessment of patients with suspected COPD; furthermore, it will extol the value of office spirometry over the inappropriate reliance on radiology and will highlight spirometry as an essential screening tool rather than a laborious ritual.

DEFINITION OF COPD

Chronic obstructive pulmonary disease is synonymous with chronic airflow limitation, chronic obstructive lung disease, and chronic airflow obstruction. Chronic obstructive pulmonary disease is characterized by a single physiologic feature, which is the limitation of expiratory airflow owing to obstruction of the airway. This airflow limitation is generally progressive; it may be accompanied by airway hyperreactivity and may also show partial reversibility in response to pharmacologic agents.

Two major pathologic subtypes, chronic bronchitis and emphysema, are embraced under the rubric "COPD" and may be present independently or together, depending on the case. Although not always possible, it is clinically worthwhile to separate asthma from COPD. However, we have to bear in mind that obstructions in many patients with COPD can include a significant and reversible component; moreover, some patients with asthma may go on to develop irreversible airflow obstruction that is indistinguishable from COPD. Other conditions that may lead to the limitation of expiratory airflow, such as upper airway obstruction, bronchiectasis, sarcoidosis, cystic fibrosis, or bronchiolitis obliterans, are usually excluded from the definition.

Chronic bronchitis is defined as a clinical disorder characterized by excessive mucus secretion. It is manifested by a chronic or recurrent productive cough on most days, for a minimum of 3 months in a year and for more than 2 successive years. It is important to remember that not all patients with chronic bronchitis will have airflow obstruction since chronic bronchitis is defined by history, not by spirometry.

In contrast to the clinical description of chronic bronchitis, emphysema has long been defined in anatomic and pathologic terms alone. If a clinical definition of emphysema did exist, it would include the presence of effort dyspnea, which is a nonspecific symptom.

PATHOPHYSIOLOGIC CHANGES

Pathologic changes in the lung lead to corresponding physiologic changes. Mucus hypersecretion in the airways leads to chronic cough and sputum production, which is characteristic of chronic bronchitis. Although these symptoms can be present for years

before other symptoms or physiologic abnormalities of airway obstruction develop, they do not necessarily mean that the patient has an airway obstruction.

In COPD, a variety of pathophysiologic mechanisms can contribute to varying degrees of airflow obstruction. Although contraction of airway smooth muscle is generally regarded as an important mechanism underlying airflow obstruction in asthma, it can also play a role in patients with COPD. This overlap between asthma and COPD has led to some confusion in the clinical classification of patients. Part of the confusion is attributable to the underuse of confirmatory spirometry in primary care practice or the limited access to hospital spirometry for primary care physicians. There are other more important mechanisms independent of smooth muscle contraction that are responsible for airflow obstruction in COPD. Fixed airway obstruction is believed to be primarily owing to fibrosis and alteration in small airway structures. Emphysema, which results in the destruction of alveolar attachments and inhibits the ability of the small airways to maintain patency, plays a smaller role. In addition, patients with COPD can have altered production and clearance of secretions and varying degrees of airway inflammation. All of these contribute to reduced airway caliber and airflow obstruction, especially during exacerbation.[3]

DIAGNOSTIC STRATEGIES

It is important to make a timely diagnosis of COPD to ensure proper triage and appropriate treatment. The most pressing requirement is to be aware of COPD. A firm diagnosis can be made only by an objective assessment of airway obstruction through the use of spirometry. A diagnosis of COPD should be considered in patients who have (1) a history of progressive and persistent dyspnea on exercise, with or without chronic and productive sputum, and (2) previous or current exposure to noxious particles or gases such as tobacco smoke or occupational dust and chemicals.

Patient Medical History

A focused patient history is always a good beginning. Table 2–1 presents some "tips and tricks" to direct a history taking in patients with suspected COPD. Because of the large reserves in lung function and the slowly progressive nature of COPD, patient symptoms, and thus a clinical diagnosis, are often delayed until extensive damage has occurred. Dyspnea is the main symptom that brings the patient to medical attention. It progressively results in decreased exercise tolerance and thus reduces activities of daily living. Increased or chronic sputum production is often present, although some patients may complain only of dyspnea. Other symptoms, such as wheezing and chest congestion or tightness, might be present but are relatively nonspecific. It is important to realize that because many patients have been living with their symptoms for such a long time, they have accordingly learned to adjust to their limitations and may minimize their complaints of dyspnea, cough, and even disability. These symptoms may remain undetected for some time unless the physician proceeds systematically with a careful medical history. In addition to the medical history being specific to the respiratory condition, the physician should also assess the following:

1. Past medical history, childhood illnesses, occupational exposure, etc

2. Presence of comorbid conditions (heart diseases, respiratory diseases such as asthma at a young age, gastroesophageal reflux, chronic sinusitis, obstructive sleep apnea)
3. Impact of disease on work and activities of daily living
4. Family and social support

Although certain elements in the patient's history might seem directly diagnostic of asthma, this is not always the case. These misleading elements can include intermittent symptoms with what appear to be a normal respiratory condition between attacks, asthma at a young age, allergic rhinitis, and/or atopy. Chronic obstructive pulmonary disease can be associated with all of these symptoms and may coexist with asthma.

Physical Examination

Although a physical examination is an essential part of patient assessment, it is a crude and insensitive means of detecting airflow limitation. Regrettably, undergraduate medical education and postgraduate train-

TABLE 2–1 Assessment of Patient Respiratory History

To Be Assessed	Specific Areas to Be Addressed
Smoking habits	Record smoking of cigarette, cigar, or pipe Age patient started to smoke with number of cigarettes smoked per day and estimation of total "pack-years"* of smoking Current smoking status; if patient is an ex-smoker, include date patient stopped smoking; if not, was there any attempt to discontinue smoking in the past
Environment with specific attention to occupational exposure	Ensure a chronologic review Specific environmental and work exposure
Cough	Frequency and duration: intermittent, every day (seldom, only nocturnal) Nature of cough: productive or nonproductive (especially on awakening)
Dyspnea	Progressive and present every day Presence of labored breathing: exercise related, resulting in progressive activity limitation Precipitants other than exercise, especially respiratory infection Perceived severity of dyspnea (ie, activity level/limitation)
Wheezing	Frequency and duration, diurnal pattern Factors precipitating
Acute respiratory infections	Frequency and timing Presence of cough, dyspnea, sputum and sputum purulence, wheezing, and fever Requiring treatment such as antibiotics or systemic corticosteroids; requiring physician visits, emergency department, and hospitalization

*Number of pack-years = number of packs of cigarettes/day multiplied by number of years of smoking (eg, one pack of 20 cigarettes smoked per day for 1 year = one pack-year).

ing programs continue to emphasize the bedside approach to early detection of disease. This misplaced trust in the physical examination is most evident in recent articles addressing the clinical utility of physical examination. Holleman and Simel reviewed the clinical examination and its ability to predict airflow limitation, examining some 44 articles in the field.[4] Most physical findings considered to represent airflow limitation or hyperinflation showed low levels of agreement among observers. Physicians seldom agree on the absence of the apical pulse, whether a patient has a subxiphoid apical impulse, and, finally, the presence of hyperresonance and the degree of diaphragmatic excursion. Agreement is only slightly increased when clinicians attempt to determine the presence or absence of wheezing or the intensity of breath sounds. Given that these are best-case scenarios, with selected physicians performing under ideal test conditions, it is questionable whether under realistic clinical conditions, the usual physical examination can offer any useful information. Holleman and Simel reported that surrogate measures of airflow by physical examination means are more likely to be agreed on by physicians.[4] Specifically, they recommend the "match test" or the measurement of forced expiratory time. The match test requires patients to extinguish a lighted match held 10 cm from the open mouth. Failure to do so is associated with a "higher likelihood of airflow limitation" being present, but the measurement of forced expiratory time has not been standardized. Apparently, the measurement is most precise and useful when multiple expiratory efforts are made and when a stopwatch is used by the physician.

Holleman and Simel offered the inevitable conclusion that "no single item or combination of items from the clinical examination rules out airflow limitation." However, they failed to move to the next inescapable conclusion: objective measurements of airflow are necessary. Instead, they offered a complex scheme of risk factors and physical findings to estimate the risk that airflow limitation is present. Presumably, a moderate or high likelihood of the presence of airflow limitation would lead to the use of spirometry to quantify the severity of the defect. If the diagnosis is suspected from symptoms and/ or high-risk predisposing factors, spirometry should be ordered regardless of the physical findings. The purpose of prolonged and imprecise physical examination, requiring multiple expiratory maneuvers, stopwatches, and lighted candles, must then be questioned. Can such an approach be cost effective?

It appears, however, that the physical examination remains important to assess alternative diagnoses or associated comorbid conditions that are common in patients with COPD. In acute exacerbation of COPD, there are also important changes on physical examination. One example that should bring the patient to immediate medical attention is the presence of any change in the patient's alertness.

Radiologic Studies

Although it is known to be an insensitive means in detecting airflow obstruction and hyperinflation, the standard posteroanterior and lateral chest radiographs are often performed during the work-up of a patient with suspected COPD. Although the chest radiograph of the patient with mild COPD is likely to be normal, that of a patient with advanced disease may feature a flattened diaphragm, increased retrosternal air space, and apparent hyperlucency, usually considered characteristic of emphysema. Similarly, thickened bronchial walls may be seen in chronic bronchitis. The presence of bullae is strongly suggestive of emphysema. Chest radiographs are primarily useful in identifying or ruling out alternative diagnoses or associated comorbid conditions such as lung cancer. This is especially true in patients with symptoms of acute exacerbation, which could be mimicked by other acute diseases such as pneumonia, pneumothorax, pulmonary edema, or pulmonary emboli.

Computed tomography (CT) of the chest, particularly when using high-resolution techniques, is more useful to make a diagnosis of emphysema but should be reserved for the work-up of patients with only particular interventions in mind. More specifically, the CT scan can be used to detect and quantify the severity of emphysema in patients with decreased carbon monoxide diffusion, increased lung volumes, and/ or impaired gas exchange. Thurlbeck and Muller reviewed the pathologic and CT scan findings of emphysema and noted that significant statistical correlations have been found between the two.[5] In moderate to severe emphysema, the severity may be underestimated by CT scan findings. Nonetheless, the CT scan remains the best way to recognize emphysema in living patients. It is not indicated for routine clinical use but is helpful in the investigation of patients with emphysema if bullectomy or lung volume reduction surgery is being considered. The

CT scan can detect nonhomogeneity in the degree of emphysema and can give some indication of the probable success of resectional surgery, especially when correlated with ventilation/perfusion lung scans. Furthermore, it may be useful in the assessment of patients who have dyspnea and reduced diffusion capacity without evidence of airflow obstruction. There are reports of such patients who have CT scan findings of emphysema. Stern and Frank reported that a CT scan might be as "sensitive as pulmonary functions tests at detecting emphysema, and is more sensitive than the standard chest radiography (96% vs. 68%)."[6] The CT scan can detect regional emphysema, whereas spirometry proves a global indication of lung function.

MEASUREMENT OF AIRFLOW OBSTRUCTION

Peak Expiratory Flow and Spirometry Measurements

Peak Expiratory Flow

The use of peak expiratory flow (PEF) rate measurements has been advocated in the management of asthma but has no utility in managing COPD. Advocates of the physical examination have recently adopted PEF measurements in their quest for indirect measurements that might obviate the need for spirometry or at least help select only high-risk individuals for whom spirometry would be requested.

In COPD, there is a poor relationship between PEF and forced expiratory volume in 1 second (FEV$_1$), and it is impossible to predict FEV$_1$ from the PEF or vice versa.[7] Peak expiratory flow may underestimate the degree of airway obstruction in COPD[7] and is relatively insensitive to obstruction of the small airways (mild or early obstruction). Moreover, PEF is very dependent on patient effort and has about twice the inter- and intrasubject variability with mechanical PEF meters, which are much less accurate than spirometers.[7]

Spirometry

Spirometry is neither invasive nor hazardous and should not be expensive. This simple measurement procedure should be readily available to assess possible airflow limitation in regular smokers and in those with chronic or recurrent respiratory symp-

toms, occupational exposure, or family history. The family physician is in an ideal position to identify the patients at risk because of the long-term relationship and knowledge of the patient's lifestyle and medical history. As an example, consider the patient with comorbid ischemic heart disease who presents to his/her family doctor with increasing dyspnea. That person may have quit smoking years ago before his/her coronary history and worsening of dyspnea was thought to be cardiac in origin, but no one has thought to perform spirometry. That can be very helpful to diagnose airway obstruction instead of focusing on ischemic heart disease as the primary cause of the dyspnea. All too often, patients with chronic dyspnea and comorbid diseases have never had spirometry performed as outpatients or even perioperatively.

Why do primary care physicians underuse spirometry? There are many potential reasons to consider:

1. Lack of understanding/knowledge because of the lack of education in medical schools. Many family physicians have graduated without developing a working knowledge of spirometry.
2. Many offices do not have the equipment, time, or staff requirements to adequately perform or interpret spirometry. This requires an effort to develop easy accessibility to spirometry testing and incorporate it into office protocols.
3. Some family physicians have a negative attitude toward COPD as they are used to diagnosing it only in the late/advanced stages, when therapeutic modalities are of less benefit. Earlier diagnosis and intervention in milder disease must be encouraged.
4. Family physicians are not using spirometry enough for monitoring ongoing treatments and disease follow-up.

Spirometry requires no more effort on the part of the patient than the forced expiratory time measurement recommended by Holleman and Simel.[4] Moreover, reliable volume time and flow volume spirometers have become available at an ever-decreasing cost in the past several years. Given the prevalence of both asthma and COPD, it would seem reasonable for any primary care clinician to have easy access to a spirometer, as they do for an electrocardiogram. Spirometry testing requires some skill and quality control (which is easily learned) to ensure accurate and reproducible testing. Simple guidelines have been set out for performing spirometry by the American Thoracic Society (ATS) Snowbird workshop.[8]

Further Lung Function Assessment

Chronic obstructive pulmonary disease and asthma may be characterized by reduced FEV_1, a reduced ratio of FEV_1 to forced vital capacity (FVC) (FEV_1/FVC $\leq$ 70%), and gas trapping. Spirometry measurement cannot reliably distinguish between broad categories of obstructive airway disease. Measurements of bronchodilator response provide some useful distinguishing information. In the most straightforward example, a return to normal lung function following the inhalation of a β_2 agonist is most compatible with asthma and would rule out COPD. When the postbronchodilator FEV_1 remains subnormal, both asthma and COPD are diagnostic possibilities. Various schemes have been used to qualify the bronchodilator response in an effort to offer diagnostically useful information. The most common rule of thumb is that a response of 15% and 180 cc above baseline indicates significant bronchodilator reversibility and a diagnosis of asthma. Yet, such an approach tends to overestimate the responsiveness of subjects with low baseline FEV_1, so that subjects with severe emphysema will paradoxically appear to have the greatest bronchodilator reversibility. A more reasonable approach would be to express bronchodilator responses as a percentage of the predicted normal value. However, it still seems uncertain as to what degree of reversibility will effectively make one patient asthmatic and another a victim to COPD.

A reduction in diffusion capacity is characteristic of emphysema and may help distinguish it from asthma or chronic bronchitis. Given that COPD is often an admixture of chronic bronchitis and emphysema, any reduction in diffusion capacity is more suggestive of COPD than asthma. This laboratory-based study might be a useful baseline measurement for primary care physicians attempting to make initial diagnostic distinctions. However, it is important to remember that patients with COPD might not have a reduction in diffusion capacity.

OFFICE SPIROMETRY VERSUS LABORATORY PULMONARY FUNCTION

Spirometry should follow the patient history and the physical examination. Other tests of airway function may be performed and should be requested as needed by the physician. It is important, however, to differentiate the need for office spirometry from the more labor-intensive full pulmonary function testing. This testing includes spirometry, assessment of lung volumes and diffusion capacity, and gas exchange (ie, oxygen saturation and sometimes arterial blood gases), all of which are usually performed in the pulmonary function laboratory at a local hospital. Postbronchodilator FEV_1 is the best single measurement to follow a patient's therapy for outpatient/office follow-up assessment and adjustment of medications and treatment (Table 2–2).

STAGING COPD SPIROMETRY AND CLINICAL PRESENTATION

The approach to COPD would be greatly facilitated by the implementation of a staging system that would allow standardization of patients with COPD. Currently, there is no staging system for disease severity that would combine symptoms, impairment in airflow, or functional impairment and health status. Unfortunately, there are also no data defining their interrelationship in a qualitative manner. A decreased FEV_1 correlates best with increased mortality and morbidity. Consequently, COPD severity is still staged on the degree of the airflow obstruction. According to the criteria of the ATS statement on the interpretation of lung function, stage I is $FEV_1 \geq$ 50% of predicted, stage II is FEV_1 35 to 49% of predicted, and stage III is FEV_1 < 35% of predicted.[3] However, as shown in Table 2–3, there is no universal agreement on these FEV_1 cutoff levels between different organizations, that is, the European Respiratory Society (ERS),[9] the British Thoracic Society (BTS),[7] and the new Global Initiative for Chronic Obstructive Lung Disease (GOLD) guidelines.[10] Chronic obstructive pulmonary disease describes a spectrum of disease progressing from the earliest symptomless stages through to respiratory failure. The medical requirement of patients increases with increasing severity. Chronic obstructive pulmonary disease has been divided into three stages that approximate to the health care requirements of the patients at each stage. The precise boundaries chosen differ among the ATS,[3] ERS,[9] BTS,[7] and the ever-evolving GOLD guidelines.[10] It is important to remember that, at best, there is only a modest relationship between FEV_1 and dyspnea, functional impairment,

TABLE 2–2 Spirometry and Laboratory Function Testing

Laboratory Test	Purpose of Test
Spirometry (pre-/postbronchodilator)	Essential for confirming the presence and possible reversibility of airflow obstruction and quantifying airflow obstruction
Pulmonary function test Lung volumes	Measurements other than forced vital capacity may be necessary in moderate to severe cases (eg, presence of giant bullae, mixed ventilatory limitation, etc)
Carbon monoxide Diffusion capacity (DLLO)	In circumstances such as disproportional dyspnea in relation to seriousness of airflow obstruction or in emphysema
Arterial blood gases	Necessary in advanced COPD (FEV_1 < 35% of predicted value or with clinical signs suggestive of respiratory failure or right-sided heart failure) In cases of serious airflow obstruction or during acute deterioration, follow-up measurements are important

COPD = chronic obstructive pulmonary disease; FEV_1 = forced expiratory volume in 1 second.

TABLE 2–3 Staging Chronic Obstructive Pulmonary Disease for Disease Severity*

	FEV_1 Predicted of Normal Value (%)			
Classification of disease severity	ATS[3]	BTS[7]	ERS[9]	GOLD[10]
Stage I (mild)	≥ 50	60–79	≥ 70	≥ 80
Stage II (moderate)	35–49	40–59	50–69	30–80
Stage III (severe)	< 35	< 40	< 50	< 30

*In all patients with a reduced FEV_1/FVC ratio, usually less than 70%, which is the mark of obstructive ventilatory impairment.

FEV_1 = forced expiratory volume in 1 second; FVC = forced vital capacity; ATS = American Thoracic Society; BTS = British Thoracic Society; ERS = European Respiratory Society; GOLD = Global Initiative for Chronic Obstructive Lung Disease.

and health-related quality of life. Disease severity staging based on spirometry value should be regarded only as a general indication of the approach to management. Some patients with stage III lung function (FEV_1 < 35% of predicted) may be relatively asymptomatic with a sedentary lifestyle, whereas other patients will be very symptomatic, with lesser degrees of airway obstruction because of their more active lifestyle. Family physicians tend to adjust therapy according to the portrayed symptoms. It is also well known that all-cause mortality, including coronary heart disease and stroke, increases with decreasing FEV_1.[11]

Mild COPD

In patients with mild COPD, there are often no symptoms and no abnormal physical signs. Morning cough and sputum or breathlessness on vigorous exertion should alert the health professional to the possibility of COPD. Clinical examination and investigation other than pulmonary function tests are likely to be normal in these patients. Often, it is just the history of smoking or other potential lung injury (ie, occupational) that leads to the early diagnosis of COPD. A firm diagnosis will be made only by an objective assessment of airway obstruction through the use of spirometry.

Moderate COPD

In patients with moderate COPD, a wide range of symptoms can be present, although there are usually only a few clinical signs. The patients may have cough and sputum production and sometimes wheezing or breathlessness on moderate exertion such as physical work or climbing hills. Acute worsening of symptoms may be associated with an acute exacerbation. Clinical examination may appear normal, but there may be wheezes, rhonchi, or reduced breath sounds. Investigations such as chest radiography are useful to rule out other diseases such as pneumonia or cancer. Once again, a firm diagnosis will be made only by an objective assessment of airway obstruction through the use of spirometry.

Severe COPD

In patients with severe COPD, a progressive disabling breathlessness on minimal exertion or at rest is present. However, the individual patient's perception of breathlessness can vary considerably for the same degree of airflow obstruction.[12]

Cough, sputum, and wheezing can also be present. Complications may develop, such as cor pulmonale (right-sided heart failure) with cyanosis and peripheral edema. Clinical examination is not always diagnostic, but often there are signs of chronic hyperinflation (loss of cardiac dullness, hyperresonance to percussion, increase of the anteroposterior diameter of the chest). Pursed-lip breathing, use of accessory respiratory muscles, and retraction of the lower intercostal muscles are present in severe COPD. When it is very severe, there may be weight loss, central cyanosis, signs of hypercapnia (flapping tremor, drowsiness), raised jugular venous pressure, and peripheral edema. These signs may not be present in stable severe COPD and may occur only during acute exacerbation. Investigations with chest radiography will show increased bronchial markings and/or hyperinflation. Hypoxemia and hypercapnia may also be seen, but as mentioned previously, it is possible to make a firm diagnosis only through the use of spirometry.

SPIROMETRY SCREENING

Some experts recommend spirometry screening to prevent underdiagnosis and maximize the opportunity to intervene, as is done with hypertension.[1,2] However, mass screening remains controversial because it may result in overdiagnosis and overuse of health resources. Although spirometry results have been shown to correlate with the development of COPD in men who smoke, only a similar correlation has been variably demonstrated in women.[13]

"Normal" readings in smokers may cause undue complacency, whereas "abnormal" spirometry readings, based on predicted ideal values, may cause undue alarm. Finally, even aggressive intervention is unlikely to produce a high smoking cessation rate, and the correlation between screening and smoking cessation remains uncertain.[13] Spirometry is well established as a necessary diagnostic tool.[3,7,14] It also demonstrates and reinforces the doctor's diagnosis and treatment regimen. A thoughtful approach to spirometry screening should include assessment of the magnitude of underdiagnosis, the potential effectiveness of intervention, the predictive accuracy of spirometry, and, finally, an overview of the clinical profile of COPD.

Evidence of Underdiagnosis

It has long been believed that COPD is underdiagnosed and that there appear to be several contributing factors. The first factor is based on the similarity of symptoms between COPD and chronic asthma, which makes them clinically indistinguishable from each other. Many asthmatics smoke or have smoked but are not necessarily smoke susceptible; many patients with COPD have hyperreactive airways but are not necessarily asthmatic. Several studies have also demonstrated that asthma, like COPD, is associated with an accelerated decline in lung function, which is irrespective of smoking status.

The most likely cause of underdiagnosis, however, is that disabling COPD symptoms do not appear until the disease is well advanced and pulmonary function is significantly impaired. Wolkove and coworkers have shown that statistically significant changes in FEV_1 do not necessarily represent important differences in symptoms for patients.[12] These authors also demonstrated that the correlation between acute changes in spirometry values and dyspnea is, in fact, very weak.[12] Thus, COPD patients with an FEV_1 that is significantly lower than the predicted normal value may not perceive symptoms related to airway limitation. Conversely, most asthmatic patients will perceive their symptoms related to the degree of airway obstruction much sooner. It is quite usual for patients to come to the physician's attention in clinic only when their FEV_1 is lower than 50% of predicted normal value.

Effectiveness of Intervention

Smoking is by far the most significant risk factor for COPD, and its effects are potentiated by age. As described by Fletcher and colleagues,[15] FEV_1 in susceptible smokers does not begin to diverge significantly from the normal range of decline until about age 35, typically after 20 years or more of smoking, but then it falls precipitously compared with normal values (the "horse-racing effect"). Fletcher and Peto have developed this horse-racing hypothesis, suggesting that those with the worst function (FEV_1) at a single observation have deteriorated most rapidly prior to measurement and will continue to do so.[16,17]

The Lung Health Study was a triumph in its demonstration of the benefits of smoking cessation in patients with COPD.[13,18,19] However, it did not show that spirometry results themselves are a significant motivating factor in sustained smoking cessation, nor did it conversely evaluate whether the finding of normal spirometric values might encourage smokers in their habit. Moreover, the Lung Health Study's limited objective of screening smokers over the age of 35 years did not afford an opportunity for assessing the social usefulness of mass spirometry screening in the general population at risk. Many studies have shown that the single most effective intervention to help smoking cessation is the influence of the family physician; although unproven in practice, the identification of abnormal spirometry and realization of the consequence should be a powerful motivation for both physician and patient toward smoking cessation and lifestyle modification.

Introducing spirometry into a primary care setting can lead to profound changes in both diagnosis and treatment. One study in primary care found that using spirometry to screen at-risk patients led to a new diagnosis of COPD in 17% of patients, whereas 18% of patients with a previous diagnosis of COPD had normal spirometry and were misdiagnosed. Information from spirometry led to a change in therapeutic regimens in 37% of patients.[20]

Matrix for Spirometry Screening

The Lung Health Study demonstrated that spirometry screening in selected populations is an effective way to identify individuals at risk for COPD and to initiate appropriate interventions. Approximately 15 to 20% of smokers have a rapid decline in FEV_1 and need to be identified for COPD. This is a very large detection rate for a screening test in primary care compared with many screening procedures. Effective interventions, such as smoking cessation, can lead to major improvements in morbidity and mortality.

In 1983, the ATS issued a position statement that discouraged population screening for COPD.[21]

It was felt that a positive "one-to-one" correlation between decreased lung function in smokers and future development of COPD had not been adequately demonstrated. A perfect correlation is rare in preventive medicine, but it can be argued that the association between decreased lung function and smoking established in the Lung Health Study is as sound as that between coronary artery disease and hypertension. The second objection claimed that the screening test must be able to detect disease at a point at which effective intervention can affect the outcome. Again, the resounding success of smoking intervention in mild COPD in the Lung Health Study should adequately address any such concerns.

The topic of spirometry screening for COPD was revised in a consensus statement from the National Lung Health Education Program 2000, which recommends widespread use of office spirometry by primary care providers for smoking patients over 45 years old. Spirometry was also recommend for patients with respiratory symptoms such as chronic cough, episodic wheezing, and exertional dyspnea to detect airway obstruction owing to asthma or COPD. Women represent a potential "tidal wave" of new cases of COPD.[22]

Should routine screening for COPD be considered in primary care with spirometry? Based on the literature, a reasonable approach for surveillance spirometry of the general population at risk is to screen all smokers over the age of 35 or any patients with respiratory symptoms. If this model appears too one-dimensional, COPD screening can also be conceived of in the context of a matrix that shifts through a few straightforward risk factors in connection with the complex pathophysiology of the disease. Smoking is the major risk factor for COPD, but only a small percentage of smokers are at risk.[21,23] Age is a factor, but significant airway limitation may also be present in younger, asymptomatic patients. Methacholine reactivity is a factor, but it is linked to smoking and airflow limitation and does not necessarily indicate an asthmatic constitution. Similarly, occupational and environmental irritants may be risk factors, particularly in individuals who smoke. Target populations for whom spirometry screening is recommended are listed in Table 2–4.[1] In any situation, an underdiagnosis of COPD represents a missed opportunity to permanently intervene. If the results of recently published studies do not address the issue

TABLE 2–4 Target Populations for Spirometry Screening*

- All smokers 35 years of age and over
- Current or past smokers with a 20 pack-year history of smoking, whether or not the patient complains of respiratory symptoms
- Patients with recurrent or chronic respiratory symptoms including cough and breathlessness on exertion
- Patients who have significant occupational exposure to respiratory irritants
- Patients with a family history of obstructive pulmonary disease
- Patients with a history of hyperresponsiveness to provocative agents
- Patients with childhood factors that may be associated with the development of chronic obstructive pulmonary disease: low birth weight, prematurity, bronchopulmonary dysplasia, frequent respiratory infections, exposure to environmental tobacco smoke

*If initial spirometry is normal, repeat spirometry in 2 to 3 years or earlier if patient presents with respiratory symptoms.

of mass screening, they at least provide a compelling rationale for screening that is targeted to populations at risk.

FOLLOW-UP ASSESSMENT

After initial assessment of their COPD, patients are followed up in no systematic manner. The frequency of visits and the need for follow-up investigations vary widely between physicians. It is important to note that the follow-up for monitoring postbronchodilated FEV_1 is the best objective measure of lung function in COPD.

More recently, management of many patients with COPD can be best performed by case management coordinators. These are usually nurses or other health professionals who have additional training and expertise in the management of patients with COPD. They function best as important facilitators and patient advocates, aiding the seamless flow of information to and from the patient, family physician, and specialist, and can become important points of contact for exacerbations rather than the emergency department.

Pulmonary rehabilitation programs with exercise training are becoming more numerous and available to patients with COPD. Widespread availability of these programs in community hospitals, not only at academic centers, is to be encouraged.

Patients' self-directed management plans ("action plans"), which are widely adopted in the asthma population and clinics, are now being adapted for the patient with COPD.

WHEN TO REFER TO A RESPIROLOGIST

No evidence-based guidance can be provided as to which patients in the community should be referred for specific assessment and follow-up by a respirologist apart from unusual features being present. But a generalized description could include the following factors: age under 40 years, smoking history of less than 10 pack-years, when the diagnosis is in doubt, or for disabled patients. Patients with frequent attendance at the emergency department or who have been hospitalized with a COPD exacerbation are also worthy of a respirologist's assessment. Some areas require that patients needing home oxygen therapy be assessed by a respirologist.

SUMMARY

Many patients are troubled by dyspnea, cough, and/or sputum production. Both patients and physicians seem complacent with these symptoms. Although patients may consult physicians with acute episodes of cough and sputum, physicians can be lulled into a sense of security by the absence of textbook physical signs of advanced COPD. Ordering chest radiographs should be superseded by a thorough history and spirometry.

Spirometry is a simple to use, cost-effective instrument that primary care physicians should consider for their practice. Spirometry itself takes little time to perform and provides, as illustrated in this chapter, an objective measurement crucial to the appropriate diagnosis and severity stratification of patients with obstructive lung disease. Physicians should be just as comfortable with performing and interpreting spirometry as with blood pressure and electrocardiograms. Objective tests such as spirometry are significantly underused; therefore, many individuals with COPD remain undiagnosed and untreated.

To become proficient and knowledgeable about spirometry, various workshops have been developed, including full-day Mainpro C workshops endorsed by the College of Family Physicians of Canada. They usually have a significant component of hands-on experience and emphasize quality control issues, along with indications for spirometry and interpretation. These courses are very popular and well attended. A guide to the interpretation of spirometry in primary care, dually endorsed by the College of Family Physicians of Canada and the Canadian Thoracic Society, is available.[24]

Health care workers must emphasize public health policies around smoking cessation; they must consider implementation of screening programs directed toward individuals in high-risk groups with spirometry and provide care in keeping with national guidelines. Spirometry should be easily accessible to patients in the primary care office or in local pulmonary function laboratories. Although we strongly support the widespread use of spirometry, it is important for physicians to order this test and not the full pulmonary function tests for assessment and follow-up.

CASE STUDY

Ms. Cope, a 54-year-old woman, presents at her annual physical examination.

Medical History, Physical Examination, and Test Results

Medical History

- She denies any significant respiratory complaints but does state that during the last three winters, her smoker's cough produced sputum on most days.
- She complains of fatigue, occasional cough, and shortness of breath on exertion essentially when she is trying to keep up with her daughter walking in the mall.
- She is limited in her activities of daily living; however, she states that she is not taking part in any sports.
- She is a current smoker and has smoked approximately half a pack per day for 26 years (13 pack-years).
- She has no asthma, allergies, or gastrointestinal or cardiac symptoms.
- She has a family history as follows: her mother died aged 70 with stroke and her father died aged 67 with lung cancer (both were heavy smokers); one sister aged 42 has breathing difficulties and is taking inhalers.

Physical Examination

- There is no respiratory distress.
- She has a respiratory rate of 18 breaths per minute, temperature 37.2°C, heart rate 70 beats per minute, and blood pressure 140/80 mm Hg.
- She has a clear chest, some wheeze on forced expiration, a normal cardiac examination, and no peripheral edema or cynanosis.

Test Results

- The chest radiograph is normal.
- A blood test for α_1-antitrypsin deficiency is performed because of the family history of a sister in her forties with breathing difficulties: 1.55 g/L (reference range 1.24–1.92 g/L).
- Spirometry is compatible with mild obstruction without significant reversibility (Table 2–5).

Questions and Discussion

Ms Cope has a history compatible with chronic bronchitis and spirometry in keeping with a clinical diagnosis of COPD. There is no history in keeping with asthma. She describes no intermittent episodes of dyspnea, cough, wheeze, or chest tightness with exertion or exposure to allergens. She has no posterior nasal drip or heartburn. There is no family history of asthma or childhood symptoms. This woman's history provides a classic description for diagnosis of chronic bronchitis, that is, daily cough productive of sputum on most days for 3 months for 2 consecutive years.

TABLE 2–5 Spirometry Pre- and Postbronchodilators

	Prebronchodilator		Postbronchodilator	
	Measurement	% Predicted	Measurement	% Change
FVC	4.65 L	109	4.85 L	4
FEV_1	2.60 L	79	2.80 L	8
FEV_1/FVC ratio		56		

FVC = forced vital capacity; FEV_1 = forced expiratory volume in 1 second.

In this case, physical examination would not allow such a certain clinical diagnosis. History and spirometry are the key items to appropriate diagnosis. Office spirometry confirms that she has significant obstruction (FEV_1/FVC ratio $\leq$ 70%) and mild obstructive lung disease (FEV_1 of 79%). The bronchodilator response is not significant, which is in keeping with a diagnosis of COPD.

A chest radiograph is not diagnostic of COPD; however, it does help exclude an alternate diagnosis such as pneumonia, pulmonary fibrosis, and congestive heart failure if suspected clinically. The chest radiograph in this case was normal.

Blood tests are not helpful in making the diagnosis; however, because of the family history and young age of her sibling with respiratory symptoms, a blood test for α_1-antitrypsin deficiency is recommended.

As her spirometry showed mild disease, further detailed pulmonary function tests such as lung volumes and diffusion, along with oxygen saturation or arterial blood gas determination, are not required.

Follow-up

Office follow-up assessment should include a history, assessment of functional status, and postbronchodilator FEV_1.

Inhaler technique should be checked at each visit. Education and information on exercise, diet, and follow-up are important. The patient has only ceased smoking for only 3 months, and it is crucial to emphasize how important it is that she does not restart and to offer assistance if needed. An annual influenza immunization and consideration of a once in a lifetime Pneumovax vaccination, along with institution of bronchodilator therapy for symptom relief on exertion, can be discussed and are reviewed in greater detail elsewhere in this textbook.

KEY POINTS

- Physicians should have a high index of suspicion for the diagnosis of COPD.
- Chronic obstructive pulmonary disease may present insidiously and may be easily confused with disease in other organ systems; patients complaining of chronic respiratory symptoms, especially breathlessness on exertion, should have a spirometry for the purpose of diagnosis.
- Smoking cessation efforts in primary care, along with institution of spirometry screening of individuals in at-risk groups, is paramount.
- Physicians unfamiliar with indications for spirometry or performance and interpretation of spirometry may consider an update as a learning need.
- Public awareness and education campaigns are critical in their direction toward COPD diagnosis and therapy.
- Specialist referral for confirmation of diagnosis should be easily available to patients with advanced disease, severe symptoms, or presentation at a young age.

REFERENCES

1. McIvor RA, Taskin DP. Underdiagnosis of COPD: a rationale for spirometry as a screening tool. Can Respir J 2001;8(3):153–8.
2. Ferguson GT, Enright PL, Buist AS, Higgins MW. Office spirometry for lung health assessment in adults. A consensus statement from the National Lung Health Education Program. Chest 2000;117: 1146–61.
3. American Thoracic Society. Standards for the diagnosis and care of patients with chronic obstructive pulmonary disease (COPD). Am J Respir Crit Care Med 1995;152:S77–120.
4. Holleman DR, Simel DL. Does the clinical examination predict airflow limitation? JAMA 1995;273:313–9.

5. Thurlbeck WM, Muller NL. Emphysema: definition, imaging and quantification. AJR Am J Roentgenol 1994;163:1017–25.
6. Stern EJ, Frank MS. CT of the lungs in patients with pulmonary emphysema: diagnosis quantification and correlation with pathology findings. AJR Am J Roentgenol 1994;182:791–6.
7. British Thoracic Society. Guidelines for the management of chronic obstructive pulmonary disease: the COPD Guideline Group of the Standards of Care Committee of the BTS. Thorax 1997;52 Suppl:S16–28.
8. American Thoracic Society. ATS statement. Snowbird workshop on standardization of spirometry. Am Rev Respir Dis 1979;119:831–9.
9. Siafakas NM, Vermeire P, Price NB, et al. Optimal assessment and management of chronic obstructive pulmonary disease (COPD): the European Respiratory Society Task Force. Eur Respir J 1995;8:1398–420.
10. Pauwels RA, Buist AS, Calverley PMA, et al. National Heart and Blood Institute/WHO Global Initiative for Chronic Obstructive Lung Disease (GOLD) workshop summary: global strategy for the diagnosis, management, and prevention of chronic obstructive lung disease. Am J Respir Crit Care Med 2001;163:1256–76.
11. The National Lung Health Education program. Chest 1998;113:123S–61S.
12. Wolkove N, Dajczman E, Colacone A, Kreisman H. The relationship between pulmonary function tests and dyspnea in obstructive lung disease. Chest 1989;96:1247–51.
13. Scanlon PD, Connet JE, Waller LA, et al. Smoking cessation and lung function in mild-moderate chronic obstructive pulmonary disease: The Lung Health Study. Am J Respir Crit Care Med 2000;161:381–90.
14. Pauwels RA. National and international guidelines for COPD: the need for evidence. Chest 2000;117:20S–2S.
15. Fletcher CM, Peto R, Tinker C, Speizer FE. The natural history of chronic obstructive pulmonary disease in working men in London. New York: Oxford University Press, 1976.
16. Fletcher C, Peto R. The natural history of chronic airflow obstruction. BMJ 1977;1:1645–8.
17. Burrows B, Knudson RJ, Camilli AE, et al. The "horse-racing effect" and predicting decline in forced expiratory volume in one second from screening spirometry. Am Rev Respir Dis 1987;135:788–93.
18. Scanlon M, Kanner RE, Connett JE, et al. Effects of randomized assignement to a smoking cessation intervention and changes in smoking habits on respiratory symptoms in smokers with early chronic obstructive pulmonary disease; the Lung Health Study. Am J Med 1999;106:410–6.
19. Gross NJ. The Lung Health Study. Disappointment and triumph [editorial; comment]. JAMA 1994;272:1539–41.
20. Bosse C. Using spirometry in the primary care office. Postgrad Med 1993;93:122–48.
21. Anonymous. Official statement of the American Thoracic Society: screening for adult respiratory disease. Am Rev Respir Dis 1983;128:768–74.
22. Lacasse Y, Brooks D, Goldstein RS. Trends in the epidemiology of COPD in Canada, 1980 to 1995. COPD and the Rehabilitation Committee of the Candaian Thoracic Society. Chest 1999;116(2):306–13.
23. Barter CE, Campbell AH. Relationship of constitutional factors and cigarette smoking to decrease in 1-second forced expiratory volume. Am Rev Respir Dis 1976;113:305–14.
24. Lowry JB. A guide to the interpretation of spirometry for primary care physicians. Toronto: Boehringer Ingelheim, 1998.

SUGGESTED READINGS

American Thoracic Society. Snowbird workshop on standardization of spirometry. Am Rev Respir Dis 1979;119:831–8. *A reference standard of technique and quality control required to perform spirometry either in the family practice office or hopital laboratory.*

Enright PL, Crapo RO. Controversies in the use of spirometry for early recognition and diagnosis of chronic obstructive pulmonary disease in cigarette smokers. Clin Chest Med 2000;21:645–52. *A review of controversies around initiation of spirometry screening programs for the diagnosis of COPD.*

Lowry JB. A guide to the interpretation of spirometry for primary care physicians. Toronto: Boehringer Ingelheim, 1998. *An introduction and "how-to" guide aimed at assisting nonspecialists comfortable with the performance and interpretation of office spirometry. Includes a step-by-step approach, many examples, and real-life spirometry tracings and interpretation.*

McIvor RA, Chapman KR. Diagnosis of chronic obstructive pulmonary disease and differentiation from asthma. Medicine 1996;2:148–54. *An evidence-based approach to the diagnosis of COPD and differentiation from asthma. This review encompasses clinical history taking, physical examination, radiology, and pulmonary function.*

McIvor RA, Taskin DP. Underdiagnosis of COPD: a rationale for spirometry as a screening tool. Can Respir J 2001;8(3):153–8. *An up-to-date review of the literature on the utility of screening spirometry. Includes a list of characteristics of patients who would best benefit from screening spirometry.*

CHAPTER 3

RISK FACTORS

Douglas Helmersen, Gordon Ford,
Shirley Bryan, Angela Jone, and Cinde Little

OBJECTIVES

This chapter will review the existing literature on risk factors for COPD. The general objective of this chapter is to provide the allied health care professionals with an understanding of the literature, which, in turn, will assist patients with COPD to modify the natural history of their disease.

After reading this chapter, the physician and allied health care professional will be able to

- recognize that smoking, of any type, is the single greatest independent risk factor for the development of COPD;
- appreciate that the effect of smoking is dose related and cumulative;
- recognize that genetic factors can influence the individual's susceptibility to cigarette smoke;
- recognize that environmental risk factors other than smoking have been identified in COPD and that these factors play a role in only a minority of COPD cases, for a given patient they may be important;
- recognize that host factors other than genetics can predispose an individual to COPD;
- appreciate the limited effect of current interventions, with the exception of smoking cessation, in slowing the rate of decline in lung function; and
- identify triggers of acute exacerbation and distinguish these from risk factors in the development of COPD.

In industrialized countries, smoking dominates all other etiologic factors for the development of COPD. Although chronic bronchitis and airway obstruction are both related to cigarette smoke inhalation, the two conditions are distinct with respect to prognosis.[1] Chronic bronchitis without airway obstruction is not associated with increased mortality and, after smoking cessation, will resolve in most patients. Unlike sputum production without airway obstruction, a decline in forced expiratory volume in 1 second (FEV_1) over time is directly related to reduced survival.[2] Smoking cessation in COPD patients results in only small improvements in the FEV_1, but the subsequent fall in FEV_1 slows to the rate found in nonsmokers.

Only a relatively small proportion of smokers will develop symptomatic COPD. Despite the increased risk of developing COPD with respect to total tobacco exposure, the individual susceptibility to cigarette smoking is very variable. As a consequence, there has been considerable interest in identifying those who are most susceptible and the mechanisms of their susceptibility.

The interaction between the human lung and other nonbiologic agents, such as tobacco smoke, is complex. A number of additional factors are currently thought to play a role in the airways disease and the destruction of lung tissue that characterize COPD. These factors include aspects of the external environment (experienced primarily by subjects who work in dusty conditions), genetics and other host characteristics such as childhood viral infection, existing bronchial hyperresponsiveness, and gender differences in airway behavior. Although there remains much to discover about the interactions between biologic systems and the external environment in COPD, new research abounds in this area of medicine.

This chapter reviews the role of tobacco exposure, nonsmoking environmental risk factors, host factors, and interactions between environmental and genetic predisposition in the genesis of COPD. The chapter also reviews the conditions that are not considered risk factors but potential triggers for exacerbation of COPD.

ENVIRONMENTAL RISK FACTORS

Tobacco Smoke

Active Exposure

Cigarette smoking is overwhelmingly the most important etiologic agent in the development of COPD. In every population for which prevalence data are available, respiratory symptoms and airflow obstruction are more prevalent among smokers than nonsmokers.[3] In most multivariate analyses, cigarette smoking has been shown to be an independent predictor of airflow obstruction after adjustment for age and initial FEV_1.[4] Altogether, cigarette smoking accounts for 80 to 90% of cases of COPD.[4] Smokers have a greater rate of decline in FEV_1 compared to age-matched nonsmokers, and this increases further with a higher smoking intensity (Figure 3–1).[1] Smoking also retards the normal increase in expiratory flow that occurs during adolescent growth.[5]

It is not known which of the many components of tobacco smoke are responsible for the lung damage that occurs with COPD. Emphysema is the result of unchecked enzymatic degradation of the elastic and collagen framework of the lungs.[6] Cigarette smoke has been shown both to increase the destructive (proteolytic) factors[7–9] and to decrease the defensive (antiproteolytic) factors in the lungs.[6]

A common misconception among smokers is that "light" cigarettes are less damaging than regular cigarettes. This may not necessarily be the case[10] as research demonstrates that light cigarettes can yield higher levels of tar, nicotine, and carbon monoxide than those indicated on the side of the cigarette package.[11] Light cigarettes have tiny air holes cut into the filter, which allow air to enter and dilute the smoke. The smoker's fingers or lips often cover these holes, yielding higher amounts of toxins.[12] Furthermore, light cigarettes tend to be smoked more intensely than regular cigarettes.[13]

Cigar smoke is also an independent predictor of COPD.[14] However, because of a lower frequency and intensity of the habit, cigar and pipe smokers tend to have less smoke exposure than cigarette smokers. Despite this, switching from cigarettes to pipes or cigars is not a safe alternative. Studies have shown that cigarette smokers who switch over may inhale more than those who have previously smoked only pipes and cigars.[15] Chronic marijuana smoking is also associated with airway inflammation similar to that seen in COPD.[16]

Passive Exposure

Passive exposure to tobacco smoke can impact humans in many stages of life. In 1994 to 1995 a national longitudinal survey on children and youth in Canada reported that 23% of children under age 2 years were born to mothers who smoked during pregnancy.[17] Smoking during pregnancy poses a risk for the fetus as it is associated with low birth weight and affects the growth and development of the lungs in utero.[18]

Passive exposure during childhood can affect lung growth and may also be associated with an increased risk of COPD later in life. Environmental tobacco smoke (ETS) has been associated with functional impairment and lower than expected increases in lung function during growth.[17,19–21] The extent to which this represents an exacerbation of underlying asthma in these children is still unclear.

The evidence that ETS causes COPD in adults is less well defined but is still of great concern. Environmental exposure to tobacco smoke in the household[22] and workplace[23] has been associated with deterioration in pulmonary function; however, epidemiologic reviews in this area remain inconclusive.[24]

Nonsmoking Risk Factors

In only a minority of patients with COPD (10 to 20%) is the habit of smoking not the main cause of the disease.[4] However, there is growing evidence that exposure to other environmental factors can contribute to the development of COPD.

Occupational Exposure

Although the role of exposure to occupational agents in the development of COPD has been debated for years, there is increasing evidence that COPD, manifested by a reduction in measures of airflow, occurs in association with occupational exported fibrogenic dusts (coal, silica, asbestos), as well as mixed exposures (mixed dust, gas and fume combination). This topic has been carefully reviewed in a recent article

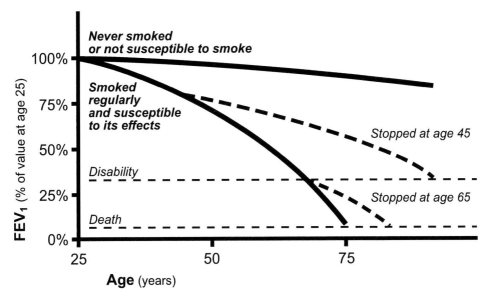

Figure 3–1 Effects of smoking and stopping smoking on the rate of decline of forced expiratory volume in 1 second (FEV₁). (Adapted from Fletcher, et al.[1])

in the textbook *Occupational and Environmental Respiratory Disease.*[25]

In many studies of workers employed in industries with single exposures to potentially fibrogenic dusts, both smokers and nonsmokers have demonstrated that airflow obstruction is a significant outcome.[25] However, the majority of workplace exposures occur in combinations and not through single-element exposure. Epidemiologic study and some pathologic studies have demonstrated that clinically relevant COPD also occurs in many complex and mixed exposure situations, including mineral dust, fumes, and mixtures of organic and inorganic exposure.[25] Recent evidence suggests that although the total dust burden accumulated over time is important in predicting the risk of COPD, other aspects of the exposure are also important such as exposures early in the work career, peak exposures, and a combination of dust plus irritant gas or fume exposure.[25]

Air Pollution

The common urban problem of outdoor air pollution "smog" from automobile emissions is another documented source of environmental sulfur dioxide (SO_2) and nitrogen dioxide (NO_2) gas exposure.[26] It remains controversial as to whether chronic exposure to levels of outdoor pollutants in urban populations can cause COPD in the absence of smoking,

but it is believed by many to be minor compared with that of smoking. Exceptions have included those cities heavily polluted by burning of coal, in which chronic bronchitis may be increased.[27] In developing countries, indoor air pollution from cooking and heating fires in poorly ventilated dwellings can also be an important cause of lung function deterioration.[28,29]

HOST FACTORS

Although cigarette smoking is the most important cause of COPD, many smokers do not develop airflow obstruction. Some sources estimate that approximately 15% of smokers develop clinically significant airflow obstruction.[1] In the Lung Health Study, spirometry, performed on more than 70,000 currently smoking men and women, aged 35 to 59 years (without regard to symptoms), determined that approximately 25% of those tested had borderline to moderate airflow obstruction (FEV₁ < 50% predicted).[30] Because of the aging population and the reduction of mortality from cardiovascular disease, it is anticipated that more smokers may actually develop COPD in the future.[31]

It is becoming evident that host susceptibility factors also explain why some smokers develop COPD,

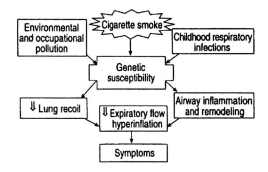

Figure 3–2   Summary of pathogenic mechanisms in chronic obstructive pulmonary disease. (Adapted from Sanford, et al.[46])

whereas others do not (Figure 3–2). The evidence for these proposed host factors is discussed in the following section.

Genetics

Alpha₁-Antitrypsin Deficiency

Some patients who develop COPD have a genetic abnormality known as α_1-antitrypsin (AAT) deficiency. Overall, this accounts for only a very small proportion of cases. Patients with a low AAT level make up no more than 1% of all individuals with emphysema.[32]

Alpha₁-antitrypsin is an enzyme that is normally produced by the body and is important in defending the lung structure against degradation. Alpha₁-antitrypsin deficiency is an autosomal, hereditary disorder in which there are low serum and lung levels of AAT.[32] There are many variations (alleles) for the AAT gene,[33] with more than 100 currently identified.[32] The specific allele denoted "Z," when present in the homozygous state (ZZ), is associated with a very low blood AAT level or activity (approximately 20% of normal). These patients are at high risk (50 to 80%) of developing panacinar emphysema in the third to fifth decades of life,[33] and their disease tends to be most significant in the lower lobes of the lungs.

Cigarette smoking also plays an important role in the development of emphysema in AAT deficiency. Severe airflow obstruction may bring smokers with ZZ AAT deficiency to medical attention very early in life, whereas nonsmokers with the ZZ genotype may not present with symptoms of emphysema until the sixth decade[34] or even later.[35] The risk of emphysema with other alleles of AAT (ie, SZ,

MZ) may also be higher in populations of smokers. However, studies have not revealed an increased risk of emphysema in nonsmokers[36] with AAT genotypes, other than ZZ or an extremely rare genotype labeled "null homozygote."[32]

Other Genetic Factors

Several studies have suggested that genetic factors other than AAT deficiency may be involved in the development of COPD. In the general population, familial studies have shown evidence for a genetic contribution to airflow obstruction[37,38] and studies of pulmonary function in twins have provided additional evidence.[39–41] Family members of patients with COPD have a 1.2 to 3 times increased risk of developing the disease, and several studies report an increased prevalence of airflow obstruction among first-degree relatives of patients with COPD.[42–44] Silverman and colleagues examined a cohort of patients with severe early-onset COPD, not attributable to AAT deficiency, and found increased airflow obstruction in first-degree relatives who were smokers.[45]

Researchers are currently investigating other genes that may be involved in the pathogenesis of COPD. Potential candidates, aside from AAT, include α_1-antichymotrypsin, cystic fibrosis transmembrane regulator, vitamin D–binding protein, α_2-macroglobulin, and cytochrome P-450$_{A1}$.[37,46]

Childhood Viral Infections

Pulmonary viral infections at a young age may result in the alteration of lung function, growth, and defense mechanisms. Cross-sectional studies have suggested increased susceptibility to cigarette smoking and lower FEV_1 levels during adulthood in persons with a history of childhood respiratory infections.[47–49] However, this relationship is not entirely supported by the longitudinal data provided by Fletcher and colleagues.[1]

Research by Hogg suggests that a specific childhood viral infection (adenovirus) may amplify cigarette smoke–induced lung inflammation and contribute to the pathogenesis of some cases of COPD.[50] Studies in a guinea pig model demonstrate that adenoviral deoxyribonucleic acid persists in the lower respiratory tract many weeks after the acute infection has cleared and is associated with persistent bronchiolitis.[51] A study in children with corticosteroid-resistant asthma has shown the presence of adenoviral protein in the lower airways by bronchoscopic biopsy.[52] Research in this area is ongoing.

Bronchial Hyperresponsiveness

The term "Dutch hypothesis" holds that bronchial hyperresponsiveness (BHR) is a risk factor for COPD and a marker of a basic constitution that predisposes the development of fixed airway narrowing.[53] Dutch hypothesis was a term proposed to contrast with the "British hypothesis," which focused on chronic mucus hypersecretion as a marker of recurrent airway infections causing chronic airflow obstruction. This notion of chronic bronchitis as a single disease, progressing from chronic mucus hypersecretion to obstructive bronchitis, proved to be misleading.[1]

Some patients seem predisposed to BHR, and this may relate to atopy or an allergic tendency. Findings that support a potential contribution of atopy to COPD are correlations between deteriorating pulmonary function and an increase in immunoglobulin E levels[54] or eosinophilic bronchial mucosal infiltration[55] in smokers. Clearly, this makes the distinction from asthma difficult. However, this hypothesis is supported by data from the Lung Health Study, which confirms BHR as the third most important independent predictor of declining FEV_1 after smoking and age.[56,57]

Interestingly, female smokers seem to have more demonstrable BHR than male smokers.[56,57] Moreover, in females with BHR due to causes other than asthma (eg, from increased pulmonary venous pressure secondary to mitral valve disease), some clinicians have observed a higher incidence and exaggerated severity of COPD with cigarette smoking. Possible mechanisms have been postulated,[58] yet epidemiologic data are still lacking to support this observation.

Other Potential Risk Factors

Socioeconomic Status

The socioeconomic gradient in COPD is as great, if not greater, than in any other disease.[59] In several studies, a lower socioeconomic status has been shown to predict decreased levels of lung function in both smokers and nonsmokers.[60] It is difficult to separate this effect from smoking habits, ETS, industrial exposure, and other lifestyle factors that are correlated with social class and level of education. In 1996 to 1997, approximately 35% of children aged 6 to 11 years in Canada were regularly exposed to ETS. Children in the lowest income level had the highest exposure to ETS (48%), compared with children in the lower middle (37%), upper middle (29%), and highest income groups (18%).[31] However, several findings indicate that confounding by smoking and occupational exposure does not fully explain the association.[59] Socioeconomic status should not be treated only as a "nuisance parameter" but also as an independent risk factor. It is important because it represents risk factors that are at least partly modifiable.

Alcohol Use

The correlation between alcohol consumption and the development of COPD has been investigated in several studies.[61,62] Both retrospective and prospective studies have shown this effect to be independent of age and smoking habits.[61,62] The potential confounding factors of increased pulmonary infection in this population, along with possible exposure to environmental agents, have not been addressed in scientific literature.

Nutrition

Low body mass index is an independent risk factor for mortality in COPD, and the association is strongest in patients with severe COPD.[63] However, the extent to which nutritional factors actually contribute to the development of COPD versus the correlation with lung disease (as a marker of severity) is still unknown. Interesting evidence is beginning to emerge that suggests a relationship between the intake of certain dietary elements and lung disease. Consumption of fresh fruit in winter was related to improved ventilatory function in smokers and non-smokers without lung disease in Britain.[64] Cross-sectional study have shown that habitual intake of vitamin C may protect against the normal loss of lung function that occurs with age.[65] High dietary intake of n-3 polyunsaturated fatty acids may protect the lungs somewhat from the effects of cigarette smoke.[66] Further research into the importance of specific dietary supplementation is required before any recommendations can be provided.

Gender

The distinction should be made between biologic differences related to genetic factors (sex differences) and differences related to environmental and sociocultural factors (gender differences). Respiratory epidemiology with respect to sex and gender has recently been presented in an extensive and well-documented review by Kauffmann and Becklake.[67]

For the same exposure to smoking, evidence is mounting in favor of a female predisposition to the effects of smoking and various environmental risk factors. Gender differences in environmental factors include personal habits, tobacco and alcohol consumption, and occupational and home environment. In our modern society, the acceptability of smoking among girls and women has significantly modified the pattern of tobacco habits. The clinical pattern of disease may also differ according to sex and/or gender, for example, in the perception and the reporting of symptoms by patients. Although cough and sputum are less reported by women than men, breathlessness has been consistently reported more frequently by women than men. There is also evidence of gender differences in the diagnostic labeling and management of cough and sputum by health care professionals. It is known that a diagnostic bias has existed in women presenting with respiratory complaints and that this has previously contributed to the underreporting of COPD in women.

Recent projections from Statistics Canada anticipate increased COPD-related hospitalizations and deaths in women compared with men in the future (Figure 3–3). However, it is difficult to determine the extent to which this projection can be attributed to biologic predisposition to COPD in women versus an increase in female smoking rates.

Ethnicity

There is limited evidence that ethnic groups vary in their susceptibility to smoking. Almost all of these studies have been hampered by limited statistical power. A recent meta-analysis fails to support the hypothesis of widespread differences in the effects of cigarette smoking on lung function between ethnic subgroups.[68]

CONDITIONS THAT TRIGGER EXACERBATIONS OF COPD

The natural history of COPD varies significantly among individuals and to a large extent is affected by factors that trigger disease exacerbations.[69] Although acute exacerbations of COPD lead to an accelerated decline in FEV_1, it is debated whether there is evidence that exacerbations are associated with a reduction in health-related quality of life[70,71] and thus an increase in health service use.[71,72] The following section deals with triggers of acute exacerbations, which include a variety of environmental agents and medical conditions (pulmonary and nonpulmonary). Although these triggers have not been shown to initiate the pathologic changes seen in COPD, they are

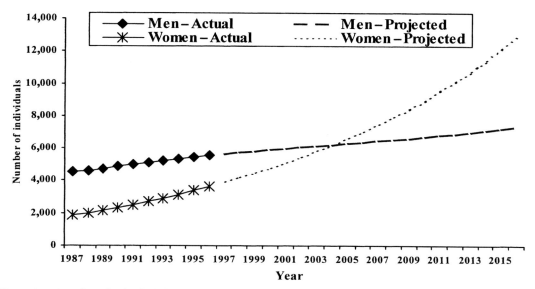

Figure 3–3 Number of individuals hospitalized with chronic obstructive pulmonary disease, actual and projected, in Canada, excluding territories, 1985 to 2016. (Adapted from the Centre for Chronic Disease Prevention and Control, Health Canada, using data from the Hospital Morbidity File, Candian Institute for Health Information.)

nevertheless very important in the clinical course of patients with established COPD.

Environmental Agents

There are indications that elevated levels of dusts and particles, particularly those in the range of 10 to 20 μm, are associated with a wide range of respiratory outcomes.[73] These outcomes may include reduced pulmonary function and an increased incidence of chronic respiratory symptoms, hospitalizations, and mortality[73]; data from Britain in the 1960s showed a sharp increase in the number of deaths in patients with COPD during days with increased air pollution. Current data continue to support this hypothesis.

Decreased humidity and decreased ambient temperature are known to promote BHR. Even patients with normal lungs will develop cough when exposed to cold, dry air. Many patients with COPD notice a deterioration of their disease in conjunction with the changes in season or location that may be related to these mechanisms.

Another common environmental element of change is the ascent to a higher altitude, such as in a commercial airline flight. Increases in altitude result in reductions in barometric pressure and hence the pressure of inspired oxygen. In patients with COPD and borderline blood oxygen saturation, increases in altitude can precipitate a sensation of increased breathlessness.

There are many other environmental agents that have been anecdotally linked to exacerbations of COPD but for which no conclusive epidemiologic or mechanistic link exists at present. For example, many patients describe strong odors as a trigger of their COPD. The true significance of such observations remains unclear at present, but this does not diminish the importance of the association for the individual patient. There is obviously considerable variation in the susceptibility to various triggers among patients with COPD, and there may be existing triggers that are not yet completely understood. For these reasons, advice regarding environmental modification must be individualized for each patient.

Pulmonary Conditions

The most common trigger of an exacerbation of COPD is a superimposed pulmonary diagnosis. Patients with COPD are predisposed to several types of superimposed pulmonary pathology, the most common of which are acute exacerbation of chronic bron-chitis, pneumonia, viral infection, acute or chronic pulmonary hypertension, pneumothorax, lung cancer, and muscular weakness. The investigation and management of many of these conditions are covered here.

Nonpulmonary Conditions

Almost any acute medical condition can tip the precarious balance of stable COPD. Occasionally, an exacerbation of COPD may herald a clue to the diagnosis of an extrapulmonary disorder. Health care professionals should entertain a wide differential diagnosis when faced with any patient who has deteriorating COPD.

Cardiac Disease

The most common and serious extrapulmonary trigger of COPD is cardiovascular disease. Lack of oxygen delivery to the heart, as a result of a blockage in the coronary arteries, can lead to transient dysfunction (ischemia) or permanent damage (infarction) of the heart muscle. Often coronary artery disease goes undiagnosed in patients with COPD. Any patient with recurrent, unexplained exacerbations of lung disease warrants investigation for ischemic heart disease.

A variant of heart disease that commonly causes exacerbations of COPD is called "diastolic dysfunction." This occurs when the heart muscle is stiffened in response to a variety of conditions such as long-standing high blood pressure. Diastolic dysfunction is often undiagnosed in patients with COPD and can be minimized with specific medications to control blood pressure and heart rate.

Any form of cardiovascular disease that results in impaired heart function can lead to exacerbations of COPD. Even when the structure of the heart muscle is intact, abnormal heart rhythms can impair function. A common dysrhythmia in COPD is atrial fibrillation, which typically presents with a rapid, irregular heart rate.

Some medications used to treat various types of heart disease, for example beta-blockers, can cause significant bronchoconstriction in some patients with COPD.[74] A thorough cardiac medication history is essential in the evaluation of all patients with exacerbations of COPD.

Gastrointestinal Disease

Diseases of the alimentary tract can be associated with exacerbations of lung disease. Gastroesophageal reflux occurs when acidic stomach secretions move upward into the esophagus. Gastroesophageal reflux is a common cause of cough and can promote exacerbations of respiratory symptoms.[75] Smoking is a risk factor for the development of the less common malignancies of esophageal and stomach cancer, both of which could potentially tip the balance of stable COPD.

Laryngeal (Upper Airway) Disease

The larynx, a component of the upper airway, is also a site of disease that can mimic or trigger COPD. Dysfunction of the vocal chords can cause sudden breathlessness and loss of voice. This, in turn, can cause anxiety, which promotes rapid shallow breathing and dynamic hyperinflation,[76] similar to the pathophysiology of other types of COPD exacerbation. Causes of vocal chord disease include abnormalities of neck muscle coordination or abnormalities of larynx structure. Smokers are predisposed to the formation of both benign polyps and cancerous lesions, which can distort the laryngeal structure.

Anxiety

Anxiety from sources such as psychological stress may also play an important role in the natural history of COPD. Anxiety may beget the pattern of rapid shallow breathing; thus, exhalation through the (emphysematous) airway is incomplete, causing a progressive increase in lung volumes (dynamic hyperinflation). In addition to becoming short of breath, the patient's work of breathing increases with dynamic hyperinflation, and there is a predisposition to bronchoconstriction.[76] Anxiety management, breathing exercises, and exercise programs can help limit dynamic hyperinflation.

Medications

An often overlooked trigger of COPD exacerbation is respiratory depressant medications. These drugs are available in many different formulations and are common in both the hospital and outpatient settings. They are often marketed as pain relievers or sedatives and as a side effect can suppress the brain's respiratory center. This effect is most pronounced in patients with severe COPD,[77] and, on occasion, these medications can even precipitate a respiratory arrest. All patients with COPD should be cautious with any new pain reliever or sedative medication and should work closely with their physicians and pharmacists to ensure that drugs are used safely. Likewise, the case histories of all patients presenting with COPD exacerbations should be examined for the use of respiratory depressants.

SUMMARY

The most important cause of COPD is active exposure to cigarette smoke. Although only 15 to 25% of smokers actually develop COPD, susceptibility to certain host factors makes some individuals more vulnerable to the effects of cigarette smoke than others. These host factors include a variety of genetic and nongenetic factors such as socioeconomic status and gender; however, the precise role and importance of each factor are not yet fully understood. In only a minority of patients with COPD is smoking not the primary cause of their disease. This group includes patients with AAT deficiency and those exposed to certain occupational agents.

Once COPD has developed, there are many possible disease triggers. These triggers do not cause COPD but play an important role in the disease course and consequently in the patient's life, health care system, and society. Avoidance of environmental agents and the prevention of pulmonary infections and comorbid illnesses (ie, cardiac dysfunction, gastroesophageal reflux, laryngeal disease) can be of significant benefit to the patient with COPD.

An understanding of contributing factors to the development of COPD can enhance the health care professional's ability to care for patients with COPD. It is our hope that this knowledge will assist health care professionals in developing multidisciplinary programs for the management of COPD and thus potentially limit the morbidity and mortality of this condition, which has such a global impact.

CASE STUDIES

Case 1

Ms. Cope, a 40-year-old female park warden, presents at your clinic.

Medical History, Physical Examination, and Test Results

- She describes progressive breathlessness on exertion over several years with no previous acute exacerbation of respiratory disease.
- She is a current smoker with a 25-pack-year smoking history.
- She has no other contributory past medical history.
- Her older sister and mother were heavy smokers and were found to have moderate to severe COPD.
- The physical examination is within normal limits.
- The diagnosis of COPD is confirmed by the presence of fixed airflow obstruction of mild degree on spirometric testing.

Questions and Discussion

How can this patient's disease be modified?

Alpha$_1$-antitrypsin deficiency should be excluded by measurement of serum AAT levels and protease inhibitor (PI) genotyping. If this woman does not have AAT deficiency, based on her positive family history there is a suggestion of another genetic predisposition to emphysema from cigarette smoke. This is the patient for whom aggressive efforts at smoking cessation are most important. Based on the Fletcher and colleagues graphs (see Figure 3–1), the rate of decline of FEV$_1$ in this woman would be expected to return to that of a nonsmoker when smoking cessation occurs—hopefully while the disease is still mild. She is a candidate for pneumococcal 23 and flu vaccinations and will benefit from symptom-relieving medication. She may also benefit from individualized advice regarding trigger avoidance. For example, she may use a scarf to cover her mouth and nose during cold, dry days or change to indoor duties when there are high levels of airborne smoke particles from forest fires.

Case 2

Mr. Cope, a 69-year-old unemployed man, presents at your clinic.

Medical History, Physical Examination, and Test Results

Medical History
- He describes progressive breathlessness on exertion over several years.
- He is a current smoker with a 45-pack-year smoking history.
- He is a heavy alcohol user and has poor nutrition.
- He has a past medical history with recurrent respiratory infections, including pneumonia, some of which required hospitalization.

Physical Examination
- He is a thin man in no respiratory distress.
- He has a regular pulse, 86 beats per minute, and blood pressure, 145/75 mm Hg.
- He has poor hygiene.
- He has decreased air entry but no wheezing.
- His cardiac examination is normal.
- He has no edema and no cyanosis.

Test Results
- On spirometric testing, diagnosis of COPD is confirmed by the presence of fixed airflow obstruction of severe degree.

Questions and Discussion

How can this patient's disease be modified?

Smoking cessation is the most important management to consider for this patient as it is for any patient with COPD. Additionally, socioeconomic supports, which improve nutrition and address alcoholism, may result in reduced pulmonary infections and reduced lung damage. Pneumococcal 23 and influenza vaccinations in this man are paramount. Environmental triggers, such as industrial pollution and exposure to ETS, may be important to address when he is looking for permanent lodging and employment. A combined social, psychological, and medical approach to smoking cessation should be attempted. A multidisciplinary, community-based, rehabilitation program may also help with smoking cessation and improve this patient's quality of life.

KEY POINTS

- Smoking remains the most important risk factor for COPD.
- Host factors play a role in determining susceptibility to cigarette smoke; these factors include genetics, childhood viral infections, bronchial hyperresponsiveness, and gender; these host factors are modulated by environmental factors such as smoking.
- Triggers of COPD exacerbation differ from risk factors in that they do not cause the disease; however, they play an important role in the clinical course of established COPD.

REFERENCES

1. Fletcher C, Peto R, Tinker C. Natural history of chronic bronchitis and emphysema. London: Oxford University Press, 1976.
2. Anthonisen NR. Prognosis in chronic obstructive pulmonary disease: results from multicenter clinical trials. Am Rev Respir Dis 1989;140(3 Pt 2):S95–9.
3. Sethi JM, Rochester CL. Smoking and chronic obstructive pulmonary disease. Clin Chest Med 2000;21(1):67–86.
4. U.S. Surgeon General. The health consequences of smoking: COPD. Washington: U.S. Department of Health and Human Services, 1984.
5. Tager IB, Munoz A, Rosner B, et al. Effect of cigarette smoking on the pulmonary function of children and adolescents. Am Rev Respir Dis 1985;131:752–9.
6. Janoff A. Elastases and emphysema: current assessment of the protese-anti-protese hypothesis. Am Rev Respir Dis 1985;132:417–33.
7. Bridges RB, Wyatt RJ, Rehm SR. Effect of smoking on peripheral blood leukocytes and serum antiproteases. Eur J Respir Dis 1985;139 Suppl: 24–33.
8. Kramps JA, Bakker W, Dijkman JH. A matched-pair study of the leukocyte elastase-like activity in normal persons and in emphysematous patients with and without alpha$_1$-antitrypsin deficiency. Am Rev Respir Dis 1980;121:253.
9. Harris JO, Olsen GN, Castle JR, Maloney AS. Comparison of proteolytic enzyme activity in pulmonary alveolar macrophages and blood leukocytes in smokers and nonsmokers. Am Rev Respir Dis 1975;111:579–86.
10. Health Canada. Health Canada survey on smoking in Canada (cycle 4), "light" cigarettes. Fact sheet 6. Ottawa, ON: Health Canada, 1995.
11. Wald NJ, Boreham J, Bailey A. Relative intakes of tar, nicotine and carbon monoxide from cigarettes of different yields. Thorax 1984;39:361–4.
12. Kessler DA. Statement on nicotine containing cigarettes. Tobacco Control 1994;3:148–58.
13. Djordjevic MV, Fan J, Ferguson S, Hoffmann D. Self-regulation of smoking intensity. Smoke yields of the low-nicotine, low-"tar" cigarettes. Carcinogenesis 1995;16:2015–21.
14. Iribarren C, Tekawa IS, Sidney S, Friedman GD. Effect of cigar smoking on the risk of cardiovascular disease, chronic obstructive pulmonary disease, and cancer in men. N Engl J Med 1999;340:1773–80.
15. Wald NJ, Watt HC. Prospective study of effect of switching from cigarettes to pipes or cigars on mortality from three smoking related diseases. BMJ 1997;314:1860–3.
16. Roth MD, Arora A, Barsky SH, et al. Airway inflammation in young marijuana and tobacco smokers. Am J Respir Crit Care Med 1998;157:928–37.
17. Millar WJ, Chen J. Maternal education and risk factors for small-for-gestational-age births. Health Rep 1998;10:43–51.
18. Todisco T, de Benedictis FM, Iannaci L, et al. Mild prematurity and respiratory functions. Eur J Pediatr 1993;151:55–8.
19. Burchfiel CM, Higgins MW, Keller JB, et al. Passive smoking in childhood: respiratory conditions and pulmonary function in Tecumseh, Michigan. Am Rev Respir Dis 1986;133:966–73.
20. Tsimoyianis GV, Jacobson MS, Feldman JG, et al. Reduction in pulmonary function and increased frequency of cough associated with passive smoking in teenage athletes. Pediatrics 1987;80:32–6.
21. Leuenberger P, Schwartz J, Ackermann-Liebrich U, et al. Passive smoking exposure in adults and chronic respiratory symptoms (SAPALDIA study). Am J Respir Crit Care Med 1994;150:1221–8.
22. Dayal HH, Khuder S, Sharrar R, Trieff N. Passive smoking in obstructive respiratory disease in an industrialized urban population. Environ Res 1994;65:161–71.
23. Masjedi M-R, Kazemi H, Johnson DC. Effects of passive smoking on the pulmonary function of adults. Thorax 1990;45:27–31.
24. Robbins AS, Abbey DE, Lebowitz MD. Passive smoking and chronic respiratory disease symptoms in non-smoking adults. Int J Epidemiol 1993;22:809–17.
25. Kennedy SM. Agents causing chronic airflow obstruction. In: Harber P, Schenker MB, Balmes JR, eds. Occupational and environmental respiratory disease. St. Louis: Mosby, 1996:433–49.
26. Sherk PA, Grossman RF. The chronic obstructive pulmonary disease exacerbation. Clin Chest Med 2000;21:705–21.
27. Buist AS. Smoking and other risk factors. In: Murray JF, Nadel JA, eds. Textbook of respiratory medicine. Vol. 1. Philadelphia: WB Saunders, 1988:1011–2.
28. Pandey MR. Prevalence of chronic bronchitis in a rural community of the hill region of Nepal. Thorax 1984;39:331–6.
29. Xu X, Christiani DC, Dockery DW, Wang L. Exposure-response relationships between occupational exposures and chronic respiratory illness: a community-based study. Am Rev Respir Dis 1992;146:413–8.

30. Enright PL, Johnson LR, Connett JE, et al. Spirometry in the Lung Health Study. 1. Methods and quality control. Am Rev Respir Dis 1991;143:1215–23.
31. Stewart P, Sales P. Strategic plan for the prevention and management of chronic obstructive pulmonary disease in Canada. Canadian Institute for Health Information, Canadian Lung Association Health Canada. Statistics Canada. Respiratory disease in Canada. Ottawa, ON: Health Canada, 2001.
32. Abboud RT, Ford GT, Chapman KR. Alpha$_1$-antitrypsin deficiency: a position statement of the Candian Thoracic Society. Can Respir J 2001;8:81–8.
33. Kueppers F, Black LF. α$_1$-Antitrypsin and its deficiency. Am Rev Respir Dis 1974;110:176–94.
34. Black F, Kueppers F. Alpha $_1$-Antitrypsin deficiency in nonsmokers. Am Rev Respir Dis 1978;117:421–8.
35. Silverman EK, Pierce JA, Province MA, et al. Variability of pulmonary function in alpha-1-anti-trypsin deficiency: clinical correlates. Ann Intern Med 1989;111:982–91.
36. Hutchison DC, Tobin MJ, Cook PJL. Alpha$_1$-antitrypsin deficiency: clinical and physiological features in heterozygotes of Pi type SZ. Br J Dis Chest 1983;77:28–34.
37. Sandford AJ, Pare PD. Genetic risk factors for chronic obstructive pulmonary disease. Clin Chest Med 2000;21:633–43.
38. Lewitter FI, Tager IB, McGue M, et al. Genetic and environmental determinants of level of pulmonary function. Am J Epidemiol 1984;120:518–30.
39. Hankins D, Drage C, Zamel N, Kronenbug R. Pulmonary function in identical twins raised apart. Am Rev Respir Dis 1982;125:119–21.
40. Redline S, Tishler PV, Rosner B, et al. Genotypic and phenotypic similarities in pulmonary function among family members of adult monozygotic and dizygotic twins. Am J Epidemiol 1989;129: 827–36.
41. Webster PM, Lorimer EG, Man SFP. Pulmonary function in identical twins: comparison of nonsmokers and smokers. Am Rev Respir Dis 1979;119:223–8.
42. Larson RK, Barman ML, Kueppers F, Fudenberg HH. Genetic and environmental determinants of chronic obstructive pulmonary disease. Ann Intern Med 1970;72:627–32.
43. Kueppers F, Miller RD, Gordon H, et al. Familial prevalence of COPD in a matched pair study. Am J Med 1977;63:336–42.
44. Cohen BH, Ball NC, Brashears S, et al. Risk factors in chronic obstructive pulmonary disease (COPD). Am J Epidemiol 1977;105:223–32.
45. Silverman EK, Chapman HA, Drazen JM, et al. Genetic epidemiology of severe, early-onset chronic obstructive pulmonary disease. Risk to relatives for airflow obstruction and chronic bronchitis. Am J Respir Crit Care Med 1998;157:1770–8.
46. Sandford AJ, Weir TD, Pare PD. Genetic risk factors for chronic obstructive pulmonary disease. Eur Respir J 1997;10:1380–91.
47. Britten N, Dowies JM, Colley JR. Early respiratory experience and subsequent cough and PEFR in 36-year old men and women. BMJ 1987;294:1317–20.
48. Burrows B, Knudson RJ, Lebowitz MD. The relationship of childhood respiratory illness to adult obstructive airway disease. Am Rev Respir Dis 1977;115: 751–60.
49. Keicho N, Elliot N, Hogg J. Adenovirus E1A upregulates interleukin-8 expression induced by endotoxin in pulmonary epithelial cells. Am J Physiol 1997;272:L1046–52.
50. Hogg JC. Childhood viral infection and the pathogenesis of asthma and chronic obstructive lung disease. Am J Respir Crit Care Med 1999;160(5 Pt 2): S26–8.
51. Vitalis TZ, Kern I, Croome A, et al. The effect of latent adenovirus 5 infection in the guinea pig (Cavia porcellus). Eur Respir J 1998;11:664–9.
52. Macek V, Sorli J, Kopriva S, Marin J. Persistent adenoviral infection and chronic airway obstruction in children. Am J Respir Crit Care Med 1994;150:2–3.
53. Orie NG, Sluiter HJ, De Vries K, et al. The host factor in bronchitis. In: Orie NG, Sluiter HJ, eds. Bronchitis. Assen, Netherlands: Royal Vangorcum, 1961: 43–59.
54. Burrows B, Halonen M, Barbee RA, Lebowitz MD. The relationship of serum immunoglobulin E to cigarette smoking. Am Rev Respir Dis 1981;124:523–5.
55. Saetta M, DiStefano A, Maestrelli P, et al. Airway eosinophilia in chronic bronchitis during exacerbations. Am J Respir Crit Care Med 1994;150: 1646–52.
56. Anthonisen NR, Connett JE, Kiley JP, et al. Effects of smoking intervention and the use of an inhaled anticholinergic bronchodilator on the rate of decline of FEV$_1$. The Lung Health Study. JAMA 1994;272: 1497–505.
57. Buist AS. The US Lung Health Study. Respirology 1997;2:303–7.
58. Snashall PD, Chung KF. Airway obstruction and bronchial hyperresponsiveness in left ventricular failure and mitral stenosis. Am Rev Respir Dis 1991;144:945–56.
59. Prescott E, Vestbo J. Socioeconomic status and chronic obstructive pulmonary disease. Thorax 1999;54: 737–41.
60. Lange P, Groth S, Nyboe J, et al. Chronic obstructive lung disease in Copenhagen: cross-sectional epidemiological aspects. J Intern Med 1989;226: 25–32.
61. Lebowitz MD. Respiratory symptoms and disease related to alcohol consumption. Am Rev Respir Dis 1981;123:16–9.
62. Lange P, Groth S, Mortensen J, et al. Pulmonary function is influenced by heavy alcohol consumption. Am Rev Respir Dis 1988;137:1119–23.
63. Landbo C, Prescott E, Lange P, et al. Prognostic value of nutritional status in chronic obstructive pumonary disease. Am J Respir Crit Care Med 1999;160: 1856–61.
64. Strachan DP, Cox BD, Erzinclioglu SW, et al. Ventilatory function and winter fresh fruit consumption in a random sample of British adults. Thorax 1991;46:624–9.

65. Britton JR, Pavord ID, Richards KA, et al. Dietary antioxidant vitamin intake and lung function in the general population. Am Rev Respir Dis 1995;151: 1383–7.

66. Shahar E, Folsom AR, Melnick SL, et al. Dietary n-3 polyunsaturated fatty acids and smoking related chronic obstructive pulmonary disease. N Engl J Med 1994;331:228–33.

67. Kauffmann F, Becklake MR. Sex and gender. Eur Respir J 2000;5:288–304.

68. Vollmer WM, Enright PL, Pedula KL, et al. Race and gender differences in the effects of smoking on lung function. Chest 2000;117:764–72.

69. Collet JP, Shapiro P, Ernst P, et al. PARI-IS Study Steering Committee and Research Group. Effects of an immunostimulating agent on acute exacerbations and hospitalizations in patients with chronic obstructive pulmonary disease. Prevention of acute respiratory infection by an immunostimulant. Am J Respir Crit Care Med 1997;156:1719–24.

70. Seemungal TA, Donaldson GC, Paul EA, et al. Effects of exacerbation on quality of life in patients with chronic obstructive pulmonary disease. Am J Respir Crit Care Med 1998;157:1418–22.

71. Osman IM, Godden DJ, Friend JA, et al. Quality of life and hospital re-admission in patients with chronic obstructive pulmonary disease. Thorax 1997;52: 67–71.

72. Lacasse Y, Brooks D, Goldstein RS. Trends in the epidemiology of COPD in Canada, 1980 to 1995. COPD and Rehabilitation Committee of the Canadian Thoracic Society. Chest 1999;116: 306–13.

73. American Thoracic Society. Health effects of outdoor air pollution (part 1). Am J Respir Crit Care Med 1996;153:3–50.

74. Ford GT, Borycki EM. Managing chronic obstructive pulmonary disease. Can J CME September 2000; 12:133–51.

75. Irwin RS, Richter JE. Gastroesophageal reflux and chronic cough. Am J Gastroenterol 2000;95(8 Suppl):S9–14.

76. O'Donnell DE. Assessment of bronchodilator efficacy in symptomatic COPD. Chest 2000;117 (2 Suppl):S42–7.

77. Murciano D, Armengaud MH, Cramer PH, et al. Acute effects of zolpidem, triazolam and flunitrazepam on arterial blood gases and control of breathing in severe COPD. Eur Respir J 1993;6:625–9.

SUGGESTED READINGS

Sethi JM, Rochester CL. Smoking and chronic obstructive pulmonary disease. Clin Chest Med 2000;21: 67–86. *This is an extensive review on COPD and smoking as a risk factor.*

Balmes JR. Agents causing chronic airflow obstruction. In: Harber P, Schenker MB, Balmes JR, eds. Occupational and environmental respiratory disease. St. Louis: Mosby, 1996:443–9. *This is an extensive review of mixed exposures causing chronic airflow obstruction from workplace- and population-based studies. It also addresses exposure patterns associated with COPD and controversial questions.*

Sandford AJ, Weir TD, Pare PD. Genetic risk factors for chronic obstructive pulmonary disease. Eur Respir J 1997;10:1380–91. *This is a review of the genetic basis in the development of COPD. Evidence is presented on the propensity to cigarette smoking and the likelihood of quitting influences by genetic factors.*

Abboud RT, Ford GT, Chapman KR. Alpha$_1$-antitrypsin deficiency: a position statement of the CTS. Can Respir J 2001;8:81–8. *This is a position statement of the CTS on patients with AAT deficiency, COPD and replacement therapy.*

Kauffmann F, Becklake MR. Sex and gender. Eur Respir J 2000;5:288–304. *This is a review of gender differences in obstructive airway disease that result from the interactions of sex-dependent genetic factors and those of sociocultural gender-dependent differences in childhood, adolescence, and adulthood.*

MANAGING TOBACCO USE AND ADDICTION

André Gervais,
Michèle Tremblay, and John Kayser

OBJECTIVES

The general objective of this chapter is to help the allied health care professionals and physicians guide their patients with chronic obstructive pulmonary disease (COPD) who smoke through the quitting process. Reduction of personal exposure to tobacco smoke is the most important goal to prevent the onset and progression of COPD.

After reading this chapter, the physician and allied health care professional will be able to

- understand the nature of tobacco addiction,
- highlight the short- and long-term benefits of smoking cessation,
- recognize the efficacy of different cessation methods and strategies,
- use an approach tailored to the level of readiness of the tobacco user,
- make appropriate use of the pharmacotherapy available for smoking cessation, and
- refer to stop smoking resources when needed.

Worldwide, it is estimated that 47% of men and 12% of women smoke. In developing countries, about 48% of men and 7% of women smoke, and in developed countries, the corresponding figures are 42% for men and 24% for women.[1] Some 25% of Americans and Canadians smoke, with men smoking slightly more frequently than women.[2,3]

For those who start smoking in adolescence and continue, there is a 50% risk of dying from a tobacco-related disease, with an average of 15 years lost in life expectancy. Death occurs between the ages of 35 and 69, with an average of 22 years of life lost for the first half, whereas the other half dies after the age of 70, losing 8 years of life.[4] Globally, 3 million people die annually of tobacco-related illness, and it is estimated that by the 2020s, that figure will increase to 10 million deaths per year, with 70% of the burden shifting from developed to developing countries.[5,6] Tobacco use is the leading contributor to mortality, claiming 430,000 lives in the United States and 45,000 in Canada each year.

Chronic obstructive pulmonary disease is one of the 24 tobacco-related causes of death. It is responsible for 15% of all deaths related to smoking in Canada, ranking third after cardiovascular diseases and cancer.[7] Smoking cessation is the single most important therapeutic intervention to reduce the risk of developing COPD and to stop its progression. It is therefore a major goal in the efforts to mitigate the burden of this disease.

In this chapter, we review the basis of nicotine addiction and the benefits of quitting smoking and look at effective ways to guide smoking patients with COPD through the quitting process.

TOBACCO ADDICTION

The smoker inhales more than 4,000 chemicals from a burning cigarette, but it is nicotine addiction that is responsible for maintaining smoking behavior and the use of cigarettes and other tobacco products. Cigarettes are the most efficient nicotine delivery system, with peak levels of this alkaloid reaching brain cell nicotinic receptors within about 10 seconds of inhaling, which is two to three times faster than when nicotine is administered intravenously. Various neurotransmitters are released, including dopamine, resulting in an almost instantaneous effect. A 25-cigarette-per-day smoker repeats the hand-to-mouth gesture, associated with the resulting brain stimulation, some 90,000 times per year, thus creating an ideal situation for fostering addiction. With an approximate half-life of 2 hours, steady-state nicotine levels drop rapidly and produce withdrawal, an unpleasant set of symptoms that compel the smoker to light up again to relieve the discomfort.

Nicotine was thought by many to be a weak reinforcer in comparison with addictive drugs such as cocaine and heroin; thus, for a long time, it has been argued that nicotine is essentially habit forming but not addictive. However, there is compelling evidence that tobacco use is an addictive drug. There are specific neurologic commonalities between nicotine and addictive drugs.[8–11] The addicted brain is qualitatively different from the nonaddicted brain in ways that include glucose use, gene expression, and responsiveness to environmental cues.

Several pieces of evidence suggest that smokers vary in their underlying genetic susceptibility to becoming addicted smokers. Several candidate genes have been associated with smoking behavior. Twin studies estimate that the majority of the liability to become and remain a smoker is explained by additive genetic factors, with a variable remaining portion of the risk related to specific environmental effects.[8] The brain's mesolimbic dopamine system is a common denominator to the addictive properties of nicotine and other substances such as ethanol, cocaine, amphetamine, and morphine. The nucleus accumbens in the mesolimbic system is thought to be involved in the integration and expression of emotions; the stimulation of dopamine transmission in the shell of the nucleus accumbens might induce positive motivational states that could lead to the acquisition of incentive properties by stimuli. This,

associated with the central effects of nicotine stimuli resulting from nicotine use, possibly becomes a powerful determinant in the combined, compulsive tobacco and euphoria effect.

In addition to the euphoric effects of nicotine, smokers might perceive additional benefits through the psychoactive properties of nicotine such as an antidepressant side effect and the ability to enhance task performance. Taken together, this may represent significant benefits for some smokers but obviously creates an additional barrier to quitting smoking.[9,11] Moreover, behavioral science advances have been equally significant in their demonstration of how an addicted brain is abnormally conditioned, so that environmental cues surrounding drug use quickly become part of the addiction. Tobacco addiction is similar to any drug addiction in that it is a brain disease embedded in a social context.

Addiction is now considered a primary, chronic disease characterized by impaired control over the use of a psychoactive substance and/or behavior. Clinically, its manifestations occur along biologic, psychological, social, and spiritual dimensions. Common features include changes in mood, relief from negative emotion, provision of pleasure, preoccupation with the use of substance(s) or ritualistic behavior(s), and continued use of a substance and/or engagement in behavior despite adverse physical, psychological, and/or social consequences. Like other chronic diseases, it can be progressive, relapsing, and fatal. This definition has been adopted by the Canadian Society of Addiction Medicine.[12]

BENEFITS OF QUITTING SMOKING

Respiratory Benefits

The single most important cause of COPD is cigarette smoking.[4,13] The greater the exposure, the greater is the risk of developing airways obstruction.[14] It has been thought that approximately 15% of smokers will develop clinically significant COPD,[15,16] although this may have been underestimated. The loss of the forced expiratory volume in 1 second (FEV_1) is about 45 mL/year in susceptible smokers, compared with 30 mL/year in nonsmokers.[17] Quitting smoking produces only a small improvement in the FEV_1, but the subsequent rate of decline returns to that of a nonsmoker, thus helping to avoid disability or death depending on the time of cessation (Figure 4–1).

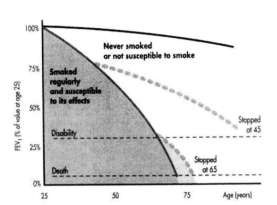

Figure 4–1 Effects of smoking and stopping smoking on forced expiratory volume in 1 second (FEV₁). (Reproduced from Guidelines for the treatment of chronic obstructive pulmonary disease (COPD). 1st ed. Toronto: Canadian Respiratory Review Panel, Medication Use Management, 1998.)

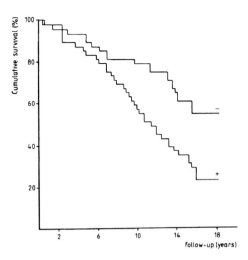

Figure 4–2 Cumulative survival (proportion still alive) curves with respect to smokers (+) and ex-smokers (-) in patients with severe chronic obstructive pulmonary disease. (Reproduced with permission from Postma DS and Sluiter HJ.[19])

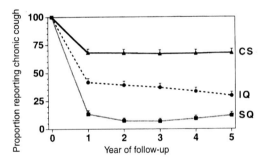

Figure 4–3 Proportion of participants in the Lung Health Study who reported cough at entry into the study reporting chronic cough at each annual follow-up visit by final smoking status. CS = continuous smokers; IQ = intermittent quitters; SQ = sustained quitters. (Reproduced with permission from Kanner RE, et al.[21])

The Lung Health Study, a large multicenter randomized controlled trial, showed that in patients with mild COPD (FEV₁ at 75% of predicted and FEV₁/forced vital capacity [FVC] less than 70%), early detection and smoking cessation intervention altered the course of COPD, as judged by the trend in FEV₁ over a 5-year follow-up. Mortality, however, was not significantly lower in the patients who had successfully quit smoking over that 5-year period.[18] However, in a Dutch study of patients with severe COPD (FEV₁ at 26% of predicted), survival improved progressively in patients who had stopped smoking for more than 15 years of follow-up (Figure 4–2).[19] Furthermore, in male British doctors, a 40-year follow-up study of mortality in relation to smoking showed that the annual death rate from COPD in former smokers was almost half that of those who continued smoking.[4]

The Lung Health Study also showed that those with lower FEV₁ values, lower FEV₁/FVC ratios, and greater methacholine reactivity were more likely to have the symptoms of chronic cough, expectoration, shortness of breath, and wheezing. It also showed that quitting caused symptomatic relief of chronic cough within 1 year of cessation (Figure 4–3). A similar pattern was demonstrated for all symptoms and seemed to be maintained over the 5-year period. This improvement was significant irrespective of the quantity smoked or the length of time the patient smoked. Patients who stopped intermittently had an intermediate improvement of symptoms, better than

those who continued smoking but not as positive as those who stopped completely.[20,21] Cessation also resulted in a decreased rate of acute respiratory infections compared with persons who continued to smoke. In the second American Cancer Society Cancer Prevention Study, mortality from influenza and pneumonia decreased in former smokers when compared with continuous smokers.[22]

Other Health Benefits

There are many other benefits for men and women of all ages with or without smoking-related diseases.

The sense of taste and smell improves, teeth are less stained, and energy levels are restored. Patients who stop smoking feel more in control of their lives, have increased confidence, are good role models for their children, and, in the long run, are protecting people from second-hand smoke to which they would have otherwise been subjected. They also save money by not smoking and enjoy better life insurance premiums.

Nicotine blood levels drop by half 2 hours after quitting and are close to zero after 12 hours. After 5 to 6 hours, carbon monoxide levels drop by half, and by 24 hours, almost all of this poisonous gas is eliminated, thus allowing the body more oxygen. Owing to a decrease in carbon monoxide and catecholamine levels, the risk of sudden cardiac death decreases significantly as soon as smoking stops. Patients will be further reassured by the conclusions made in the U.S. surgeon general's report, "The Health Benefits of Smoking Cessation" (Table 4–1).[22] Smoking cessation increases life expectancy, and people who quit smoking before age 50 have a 50% less risk of dying in the next 15 years compared with continuing smokers.

The benefits of cessation also extend to quitting at older ages. A healthy man aged 60 to 64, smoking a pack of cigarettes or more a day, reduces by 10% the risk of dying during the next 15 years if he quits smoking; smoking cessation reduces not only the risk of lung cancer but the risk of cancers of the larynx, oral cavity, esophagus, pancreas, and urinary bladder.

EFFICACY OF DIFFERENT TREATMENT INTERVENTIONS

Determinants of Cessation Rates

The U.S. Department of Health and Human Services recently examined over 500 trials on tobacco-use treatment interventions.[2] The characteristics of the smokers and the interventions of different clinicians both influenced cessation rates.

The characteristics of smokers associated with high cessation rates are as follows:
• High motivation to stop smoking
• Desire to stop smoking within the next month
• Confidence in their ability to quit and a supportive social network
• A smoke-free workplace and/or having family and friends who do not smoke in the presence of the person quitting

The characteristics of smokers associated with low cessation rates are as follows:
• High nicotine dependence demonstrated by previous, severe withdrawal symptoms
• Smoking more than 20 cigarettes per day and lighting up within 30 minutes of waking in the morning
• History of psychiatric comorbidity, especially schizophrenia or depression and/or high levels of stress

The characteristics of clinical interventions by clinicians that increase cessation rates are as follows:

TABLE 4–1 Health Benefits of Quitting Smoking

	Relative Risk of Disease in Smoker	Number of Years after Quitting	Reduced Risk (%)
Coronary heart disease	1.76–2.27*	1	50
		15	100
Stroke	1.77–2.43*	5–15	100
Lung cancer	12.1–21.3*	10	30–50
		>10	Continues to decline‡
Low birthweight baby	1.7–3.8†	Before pregnancy or during 1st trimester	100

*Risk varies with exposure compared to nonsmoker, an individual who has never smoked, risks from American Cancer Society Cancer Prevention Study-II.

†Risk from a report of the surgeon general, 1990.[22]

‡May never reach the risk of an individual who has never smoked.

(Adapted from The health benefits of smoking cessation. A report of the surgeon general. Washington, DC: U.S. Department of Health and Human Services, 1990.)

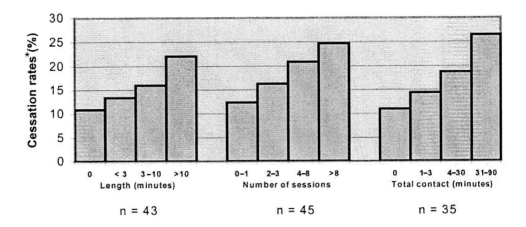

Figure 4–4 Cessation rates according to characteristic of intervention. (Adapted from Fiore MC, et al.[2])
*Minimum 5 months; n = number of studies

- Individual and group counseling are superior to self-help
- Psychologist, nurse, dentist, counselor, or physician intervention is better than self-help
- Amount of person-to-person contact time spent with a smoker increases cessation rates over no intervention (Figure 4–4)
- The number of sessions shows a dose-response relationship, with more than eight sessions proving superior to a total of two or three (see Figure 4–4)
- A total contact time between 31 and 90 minutes increases cessation rates compared with 1 to 3 minutes, without evidence of further effect beyond 90 minutes (see Figure 4–4) (the high quit rate in the control groups is probably due to the patient consenting to participate in such studies, this being an intervention in itself)
- Discussing dangerous situations, developing coping skills, and anticipating relapse all increase cessation rates
- Intratreatment support provided by the clinician also substantially increases cessation rates
- Extratreatment and social support from the social environment help cessation
- Use of stop-smoking medication has consistently been shown to approximately double cessation rates 6 months or later in comparison with placebo[2]

Minimal interventions lasting less than 3 minutes should be offered to every smoker with the understanding that more intensive therapy (individually or in group settings) results in the highest cessation rates. Every smoker should have ready access to smoking cessation counseling.

Smoking Cessation in COPD

Smokers with COPD were compared with healthy smokers in a population-based epidemiologic study in Spain. The smokers with COPD had a higher tobacco consumption, higher dependence on nicotine, and higher concentrations of carbon monoxide in exhaled air, suggesting a different pattern of cigarette smoking. Chronic obstructive pulmonary disease was more likely in smokers if they were males and individuals with lower educational levels. Thirty-four percent of smokers with COPD had never tried to stop smoking and failed to show more motivation to do so than healthy smokers.[23]

Smoking cessation intensive counseling was assessed in the Lung Health Study, in which 5,887 patients with COPD were randomized to special care, with emphasis on smoking cessation, or to usual care by their personal physician during annual visits. The special care intervention comprised a 12-session group intervention program over a 10-week period with behavior modification techniques and the use of nicotine gum. The patients were followed up every 4 months for 5 years, with an extended program for those who were unsuccessful or relapsed. In this special care group, nearly 35% quit at some point during the 5-year period compared with 20%

TABLE 4–2 Cessation Rates According to Different Nicotine Replacement Therapies

Replacement Therapy	Cessation Rates (%)*
	Medication (Placebo)
Nicotine gum	23.7 (17.1)
Nicotine patch	17.7 (10.0)
Nicotine inhaler	22.8 (10.5)
Nicotine nasal spray	30.5 (13.9)

*Minimum 5 months.

(Adapted from Fiore MC, Bailey WC, Cohen SJ, et al. Treating tobacco use and dependence clinical practice guideline. Rockville, MD: U.S. Department of Health and Human Services, Public Health Service, 2000.[2])

in the usual care group; 22% of the special care group and 5% of the usual care group sustained abstinence for 5 years.[20,21]

Bupropion hydrochloride was shown to be an effective means to help patients with COPD quit smoking. In a double-blind, placebo-controlled study of 405 patients with emphysema and chronic bronchitis smoking 15 or more cigarettes per day, 16% of the patients who took bupropion during 12 weeks were continuously tobacco free between weeks 4 to 26 of the study, whereas 9% of those taking placebo quit during that same period. All patients received counseling to help them quit. [24]

Pharmacologic Intervention Efficacy

Pharmacotherapy studies usually involve subjects who are motivated to quit smoking and who receive substantial counseling. Different clinical trials show that nicotine gum, the patch, inhaler, and nasal spray approximately double cessation rates 6 months or later compared with placebo (Table 4–2).[2] However, there is no study that directly compares these modalities with one another. All four nicotine replacement therapies are approved and used in the United States, but in Canada, only the gum and the patch are currently available.[2] The combination of the nicotine patch supplemented with nicotine gum or spray helps more smokers quit than a single modality of nicotine replacement. It is unknown whether this success rate is attributable to combining two delivery systems or simply to higher nicotine blood levels. The combination strategy functions better in suppressing nicotine withdrawal, but it remains unknown as to whether it is more efficacious in patients with high nicotine dependence.[2]

The use of 300 mg/day of bupropion (Zyban™) for 7 and 9 weeks doubled abstinence rates at 1 year compared with placebo, 23.1% versus 12.4% in one study and 30.3% versus 15.6% in the other.[25,26] Bupropion was shown to be effective in treating cigarette smokers independently of all patient characteristics studied: gender, age, number of cigarettes smoked per day, nicotine dependence scale, marital status, education, recovery from alcoholism, history of depression, depression inventory score, prior cessation attempts, prior nicotine replacement therapy, and use of group therapy. A lower number of cigarettes smoked per day, brief (less than 24 hours) or long periods (more than 4 weeks) of abstinence with previous attempts to stop smoking, and male gender were predictive of better outcomes independent of the dose of bupropion used.[27]

The combination of bupropion and a 21-mg nicotine patch for 9 weeks showed a somewhat, but not significantly, higher abstinence rate at 1 year over using bupropion alone; however, the study sample was not large enough to prove or disprove any advantages to the combination. Bupropion showed a higher cessation rate than a 21-mg nicotine patch in one study.[26]

In the U.S. guidelines, published in 2000, clonidine and nortriptyline are also recommended as second-line therapies to be considered for use on a case-by-case basis after first-line treatments have been used or considered. Although these drugs were shown to be efficacious in some studies, there are concerns about more potential side effects than with the medications already discussed. Furthermore, they are not yet approved for smoking cessation by the Food and Drug Administration in the United States,[2] nor are they recommended in Canada or Great Britain.[28–30]

TABLE 4–3 Stages of Readiness to Stop Smoking among Smokers

Stage of Change	Does the Patient Think of Quitting?	Proportion of All Smokers Still Smoking (%)
Precontemplation	Not in the next 6 months	48
Contemplation	Considers stopping in the next 6 months	37
Preparation	Decides to stop in the next month and has spent 24 hours not smoking in the past year	15
Action	Has stopped for less than 6 months and faces withdrawal symptoms	
Maintenance	Has stopped for 6 months or more	

(Adapted from Health Canada. Canadian Tobacco Use Monitoring Survey, Phase II. Ottawa, 1999.[3])

INTERVENTION FOR PATIENTS WHO SMOKE

Data in the United States show that about 70% of smokers visit a physician each year, and more than 70% of smokers have made at least one prior attempt to quit; the results show that 46% try to quit each year, but only about 7% are still abstinent 1 year later.[2] Tobacco dependence is now accepted as a chronic addiction characterized by numerous relapses and requiring treatment with repeated interventions.[2,28,29,30] Smoking cessation counseling is recognized as one of the most cost-effective measures and compares favorably with interventions for treatment of hypertension and hypercholesterolemia; furthermore, it is considered good medical practice.[2,31,32]

Different recommendations have been issued to help physicians and other health professionals integrate quick, effective smoking cessation counseling into their practice.[2,28–30,33,34]

Counseling entails identification of the smoking status of every patient, assessment of the readiness to quit, and the provision of advice and also involves offering assistance to every smoker in the process of cessation.

It is essential to identify smoking as a significant health issue and to ensure consistent follow-up. All patients should be asked whether they smoke. Noting their smoking status prominently on their medical record acknowledges the importance of smoking as a problem to the patient and to the health professional. For example, a sticker placed at the beginning of the examination note, a rubber stamp with a space to indicate the smoking status, adding smoking status to the vital signs, writing it routinely

in the list of medical problems, or using a computerized flagging method can all be used to identify and stress smoking as an issue.

Intervention and Stages of Change

Readiness can be evaluated by asking whether the smoker is considering quitting and when he/she plans to do so. Clear personalized smoking cessation counseling repeated each time a patient is seen, is an effective means of underlining the importance of the issue and providing help to progress to the next stage of change. The clinician is most likely to be successful when demonstrating empathy, promoting patient autonomy, avoiding arguments, and supporting self-efficacy by identifying previous successes in behavior change efforts.

Behavior changes in smokers have been described to proceed through five stages: precontemplation, contemplation, preparation, action, and maintenance (Table 4–3). In the 1999 Canadian Tobacco Use Monitoring Survey, fewer than one in five smokers was ready to quit within the next 30 days and had quit at least once for 24 hours in the previous year. Usually, a smoker goes through three to five serious attempts before completing a year without a cigarette; relapse is part of the process but is not considered a stage as such.[35–38] It has not been demonstrated whether stage-based treatment developed with this model significantly improves outcome. Nevertheless, the model has enjoyed empiric support as an aid to help health professionals tailor their interventions to the smoker's stage in the cessation process.[2,28,30,39–41] The approach outlined below is summarized in Figure 4–5.[42]

In **precontemplation**, the goal is to understand

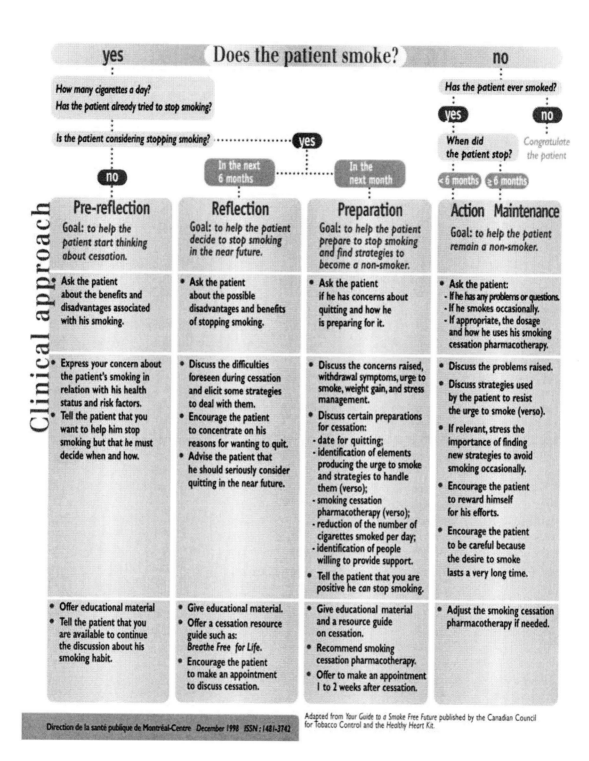

Figure 4–5 Intervention according to the stage of change. (Adapted from Régie Régionale de la Santé et des Services Sociaux de Montréal-Centre. Direction de la santé publique. Prévention en pratique médicale: tobacco use. Montreal: Association des Médecins Omnipraticiens de Montréal, 1998[42])

the reasons why the smoker continues to smoke and to help the smoker consider quitting. This intervention should be built around the risks and rewards that are relevant to the patient. By asking open-ended questions about what the smoker likes and dislikes about smoking, the situation can be assessed and advice personalized. For example, "What do you like and dislike about smoking?" is open ended, whereas "Does smoking relax you?" is close ended. Although smokers are generally nicotine dependent, they may not always realize the full depth and dependency of their addiction to it. While the smoker usually believes that smoking is harmful, the extent of the health risks involved and the benefits of stopping are often underestimated. Smoking is often used to manage stress, control mood, focus attention, and control weight. Although the rapid and significant benefits with respect to mortality and morbidity are positive incentives for many to quit, some younger patients may be more responsive to the negative effects of smoking on their physical appearance; these include wrinkles, bad oral hygiene, tooth decay, decreased fitness, or sexual impotence in the male. Showing concern and repeatedly offering support at different visits are crucial in motivating smokers to quit. A clear message must be given that quitting smoking will have a major impact on physical health and that the health professional is available for help.

In **contemplation**, the reasons for continuing smoking hamper the patient's willingness to take action. Asking about the benefits and disadvantages of stopping smoking will help reinforce the reasons to stop, identify fears, and ideally find ways to deal with them. The smoker can then begin to resolve this "ambiguous characteristic" of cigarette addiction and ultimately make the decision to prepare to quit. Severe withdrawal symptoms, depression, or weight gain experienced in the past may discourage the smoker from attempting to quit again. Smokers often fear failure, and listening to their concerns and offering educational material, or a list of the smoking cessation programs available in the area, might be helpful. For some contemplators, suggesting a follow-up appointment to discuss the matter further can prompt change.

For smokers in **preparation**, setting a target date for quitting and signing a written commitment to quit (a sample of which can be found in various smoking cessation guides) can emphasize the importance of the decision to quit smoking. The smoker

Cigarette	Time	What I'm doing	How I feel ☺ ☹
1			
2			
3			
4			
5			
6			
7			
8			
9			
10			
11			
12			

Figure 4–6 A smoker's journal to document smoking behavior and start planning strategies to quit. (Reproduced with permission from Régie Régionale de la Santé et des Services Sociaux de Montréal-Centre.[43])

prepares by discussing any concerns about quitting, withdrawal, strong desire to smoke, weight gain, social relationships, triggers, and stress. A smoker's journal (Figure 4–6) tied to the cigarette pack with an elastic or inserted inside the pack can be used to note the times of day, circumstances, and emotions associated with smoking.[43] This will block the automatism of smoking and lead to a better understanding of the relationship between smoking and different triggers and feelings; it can be helpful for planning useful strategies to avoid lighting up.

The use of medications (see the following section) should always be considered at this stage. Educational material and or local resource guides might help the smoker obtain more information and support. Discussing what the smoker plans to do when faced with difficult situations is an important step in intervening in the quitting plan; challenging situations include avoiding places where smokers tend to congregate and coping with circumstances that trigger the desire to smoke (Table 4–4). Such times and places are waking up in the morning, after meals, or when drinking alcoholic beverages. Since a weight gain of 2 to 4 kg (5–10 lb) is to be expected, the patient should

TABLE 4–4 Frequent Concerns about Smoking Cessation and Strategies to Suggest

Concerns	Strategies
Withdrawal symptoms	Use appropriate pharmacotherapy
Strong desire to smoke	Drink some water, eat some raw vegetables, chew gum, put a straw or a cinnamon stick in your mouth Do something else Breathe deeply Wait 5 minutes before deciding to light up Be sure enough stop-smoking medication is being taken
Weight gain	Maintain a balanced diet Increase physical activity Use nicotine gum or bupropion
Social relationships	Tell smoker friends about the decision to stop and tell them how they can help (ask smoking friends not to offer you a cigarette) Ask for support from family members, friends, and colleagues at work Plan ahead for difficult social situations (in short term, stay away from social situations where others will be smoking)
Trigger factors	Reduce alcohol and coffee intake (choose water or fruit juices instead) Alter habits related to smoking (telephone, sitting on favorite couch, after meals) Avoid pubs, bars, taverns Get rid of all cigarettes and related items
Stress control	Avoid or modify sources of stress Practice handling stressful situations that cannot be avoided Use relaxation techniques

(Adapted from Your guide to a smoke free future. Ottawa: Canadian Council on Smoking and Health, 1996.[33])

be advised to focus on quitting rather than on the weight issue. Because dieting, in addition to smoking cessation, decreases the chances of successfully quitting, maintaining a balanced diet and increasing physical activity should be recommended.[2]

When the patient is in the **action** stage after stopping, congratulate him or her. Inquire about withdrawal, cravings, and the effects of the medication and adjust the dosage of stop-smoking medication if necessary. Discuss the patient's urges to smoke and review difficult social and emotional situations. By ensuring a follow-up, the health professional will increase the likelihood of success. Slips where one or more cigarettes are smoked without resuming smoking can lead to relapse. Discuss the circumstances when the slips occur and help the patient find new strategies to deal with the situation.

The smoker deserves praise and encouragement for any success in avoiding smoking for a given period of time. It is important to remember that relapses are a natural part of the smoking cessation process. The circumstances that lead to relapse deserve to be reviewed and discussed to prepare for future dealings in similar situations. It is also important to review the reasons that motivated the smoker to quit initially and to always offer encouragement with the intent of stirring up further motivation to try again.

The **maintenance** period begins 6 months after smoking cessation. The desire to smoke persists for a long time, and one cigarette is all it takes to start over; strategies to deal with difficult circumstances need to be planned. Reviewing the reasons to quit smoking, discussing current and future benefits, and encouraging lifestyle changes are helpful. Avoiding difficult situations and places, improving stress management skills, obtaining support from family and friends, and paying attention to diet and exercise are all ways to improve the chances of remaining smoke free.

Pharmacologic Tools

All patients attempting to quit should be encouraged to use effective pharmacotherapies for smoking cessation. Medication alleviates withdrawal symptoms such as insomnia, irritability, frustration and anger, difficulty concentrating, restlessness, strong urges to smoke, increased appetite and weight gain, dysphoria, or depressed mood that occur in most smokers attempting to quit. Those symptoms reach a peak in the first 48 hours and eventually subside within 1 to 3 weeks. This is why most smokers find the first days or even the first weeks after quitting to be the most difficult. Some of the symptoms, such as the inability to concentrate, may last 2 to 3 months. Nicotine replacement therapy (NRT) in the form of gum or the patch and bupropion hydrochloride are approved means of smoking cessation therapy in the United States and Canada.

Smokers are often reluctant to use nicotine replacement or bupropion because they fear harmful effects and do not want to perpetuate their dependency. However, these treatments approximately double their chances of success and usually do not create dependency. The choice of medication is a matter of the patient's personal preference and medication availability, past experience, medical history, and the presence of contraindications for specific drugs. Consideration, before prescribing, is also required with patients who smoke less than 10 cigarettes a day, for pregnant/breastfeeding women, and adolescent smokers.[2]

Nicotine Replacement Therapy

According to the product monographs, NRT is contraindicated under the following conditions: recent myocardial infarction, unstable angina, severe cardiac arrhythmia, recent stroke, pregnancy, lactation, and in patients under 18 years of age.[44] Smokers should also be warned that it is not recommended to smoke while undergoing NRT.

Cases of myocardial infarction in patch users reported by the media in 1992 have created a myth concerning the risks of NRT. Subsequent studies have shown no evidence of toxicity. Nicotine is a stimulant that increases pulse rate and cardiac contractility. This effect is no greater, however, whether the nicotine comes from the two sources simultaneously, such as smoking and using the gum or the patch.[5] Studies carried out in patients suffering from cardiovascular diseases treated with the nicotine patch did not show more myocardial infarcts, cardiac arrests, or admissions to hospital than smokers on placebo.[45] Patches supplying up to 63 mg of nicotine in a 24-hour period have not been shown to cause short-term adverse effects.[46] The Lung Health Study found no

increased risk to the cardiovascular system for patients who smoked while undergoing NRT.[47]

According to recent guidelines, caution has been recommended while using NRT among particular cardiovascular patient groups: those in the immediate (within 2 weeks) post–myocardial infarction period, those with serious arrhythmias, and those with serious or worsening angina pectoris.[2] It should be noted that nicotine gum and the nicotine patch produce lower blood nicotine levels than a-pack-a-day smoking; NRT is much less dangerous than tobacco smoke, which contains more than 4,000 toxic constituents, including carbon monoxide, which interferes with oxygen delivery, carcinogens, and components known to affect coagulation. Considering all of the risks of smoking previously mentioned, NRT can be considered in these medical conditions.[48]

Although nicotine is potentially harmful to the fetus during pregnancy, tobacco smoke is considered even more dangerous, and many experts believe that the use of NRT is preferable to smoking during pregnancy. However, there is no solid proof that NRT is safer than smoking during pregnancy.[48] Thus, if nonpharmacologic treatments fail and NRT is recommended, it is important to warn the patient to avoid exposing the fetus to higher nicotine levels than while smoking; pregnant patients should not simultaneously smoke and use nicotine gums or patches. Nicotine gums should be used during the day only and the patch removed at night to decrease exposure to the fetus.

Explaining how to use NRT is very important (Table 4–5). If chewed too quickly, nicotine gum will provoke adverse side effects such as hiccups, dyspepsia, or jaw cramps. It is often taken in insufficient amounts to decrease withdrawal symptoms. The nicotine patch provides a constant blood nicotine level for 24 hours. It is easy to use and simply needs to be applied to a clean, dry, and hairless surface. Some local skin reaction may occur in up to 50% of all cases, but it can usually be managed by changing the site of application daily. Other side effects include vivid dreams or nightmares, which trouble about 15% of patch users. It may be necessary to remove the patch before bedtime to avoid sleep disturbances. However, the negative aspect of this is that it deprives the patient of nicotine on wakening, which is the most difficult time of the day for the cravings. Although 8 weeks of treatment have proven as effective as 12 weeks, it is recommended

TABLE 4–5 Pharmacologic Tools

Medication	Dosage	Duration, Use, and Advantage	Contraindications	Adverse Reactions
Nicotine gum				
Nicorette^{MD}	2-mg gum if < 25 cigarettes/day maximum 24 gums/day	Up to 12 weeks but longer if required A gum per hour or as needed	Recent myocardial infarction* Unstable angina* Severe cardiac arrhythmia*	Burning in throat Jaw pain Hiccups
Nicorette Plus^{MD}	4-mg gum if ≥ 25 cigarettes/day maximum 24 gums/day	Chew two to three times and park gum between gingiva and cheek for 30 to 60 seconds Repeat this process for 30 minutes Do not eat or drink 15 minutes before or after to allow nicotine absorption Delays weight gain while using it	Recent stroke Pregnancy and breast feeding† Patients under 18 years of age	
Nicotine patch Nicoderm^{MD} or Habitrol^{MD}	21 mg/24 h 14 mg/24 h 7 mg/24 h	Suggested use: 4 weeks 2 weeks 2 weeks Place patch on relatively hairless location typically between neck and waist Tapering and duration should be individualized If < 10 cigarettes/d, start with lower dose	Recent myocardial infarction* Unstable angina* Severe cardiac arrhythmia* Recent stroke Pregnancy and breast feeding† Patients under 18 years of age Allergy to tape Generalized skin disease	Local skin reaction Vivid dreams
Bupropion (Zyban)	150 mg PO once a day, mornings × 3 days 150 mg PO bid At least 8 hours between two successive doses	7–12 wk Smoking cessation advised between days 8 and 14 In case of insomnia, the second dose should not be taken as close to bedtime; if insomnia persists, reduce dosage to 150 mg every morning Consider longer treatment for smokers who are subject to significant mood swings or who continue to experience strong urges to smoke after discontinuing bupropion Monitor blood pressure if used with NRT Decreases weight gain while using it	Current seizure disorder Current or prior diagnosis of bulimia or anorexia nervosa Use of another medication containing bupropion such as Wellbutrin® an antidepressant Undergoing abrupt withdrawal from alcohol or benzodiazepines or other sedatives Known hypersensitivity to bupropion Curent use of antidepressants of the monoamine oxidase inhibitors (MAOIs) or thioridazine within 14 days of discontinuation Not recommended in patients with severe hepatic impairment Caution in situations that may reduce seizure threshold‡ and drug interactions	Insomnia Dry mouth Tremors Skin rashes Serious allergic reactions

Nicotine replacement therapy should be used with caution among particular cardiovascular patient groups: those in the immediate (within 2 weeks) postmyocardial infarction period, those with serious arrhythmias, and those with serious or worsening angina pectoris.[2]

[†]Many experts believe that the use of NRT is preferable to smoking during pregnancy.[2]

[‡]History of head trauma or prior seizures, central nervous system tumor, excessive use of alcohol, addiction to opiates, cocaine or stimulants, use of over-the-counter stimulants or anorectics, hypoglycemics or insulin, medications that lower the seizure threshold (theophylline, systemic steroids, antipsychotics, and antidepressants), St. John's wort.[2,28]

NRT = nicotine replacement therapy; n = number of studies in the meta-analysis; PO = by mouth; bid = twice a day.

Nicorette and Nicoderm are registered trademarks of Aventis Pharma Inc. Habitrol is a registered trademark of Novartis Consumer Health Canda Inc. Zyban is a registered trademark of GlaxoSmithKline Inc.

that the duration of treatment and dosage be adjusted according to the needs of the patient. Start at lower doses of NRT with smokers of less than 10 cigarettes per day. Although the combined use of the patch and gum is not approved in Canada or the United States, the U.S. guidelines recommend this treatment for patients unable to quit using a single type of pharmacotherapy.[2] Obtaining written informed consent before writing a prescription for the nonapproved use of stop-smoking medications will protect the patient and the physician.

Bupropion Hydrochloride

Bupropion hydrochloride is available in sustained-release tablet form as an antidepressant (Wellbutrin) or as a smoking cessation aid (Zyban). The action mechanism seems linked to the drug's effects on neurotransmitters by blocking noradrenaline and dopamine reuptake.[25]

The two most common adverse effects of bupropion are insomnia and dry mouth. Insomnia is reported in 34.6% and 42.4% in two treatment arms compared with 20% in the placebo; dry mouth is reported in 12.8% and 10.7% of treated cases versus 4.5% in placebo.[25,26] An incidence of seizures of 1:1,000 was initially reported in trials of the drug used as an antidepressant with doses of up to 300 mg per day. No seizures have been reported in the studies on smoking cessation. The physician should respect the contraindications, take into account any clinical situation that lowers the threshold for seizures, and always warn the patient of possible side effects before prescribing bupropion (see Table 4–5).

Following agreement with Health Canada, Glaxo-SmithKline, the manufacturer of bupropion, informed Canadian health care professionals in 2001 of important safety information regarding bupropion. It had

been estimated that 1,245,000 patients had been prescribed Zyban® and 699,000 patients had been prescribed Wellbutrin since it became available in Canada in 1998. The Canadian Adverse Reaction Monitoring Programme (CADRMP) had received a total of 1,127 reports of suspected adverse reactions associated with the use of bupropion; 682 were considered serious, 19 had a fatal outcome, 172 involved seizures/convulsions, and 37 were reports of serum sickness/serum sickness-like reactions. Cause and effect relationships had not been established or speculated in the vast majority of reports submitted. To ensure optimal prescription, contraindications were revised and caution was advised when treating patients with risk factors (see Table 4–5). It was recommended not to use bupropion in patients with severe hepatic impairment and to discontinue it immediately if any hypersensitivity reactions were experienced. Table 4–6 is a summary of potential drug interactions with bupropion and their management.[49]

The drug's efficacy and safety have not been established for pregnant women, patients under 18 years of age, and patients with a recent history of heart attacks or unstable heart disease. The product monograph lists precautions rather than contraindications for these patient categories. Since bupropion is secreted in human milk, a mother must choose between breast-feeding and using bupropion when it comes to lactation.

WHEN TO REFER

Since more intense interventions result in higher quitting rates, specialized clinics should be recommended whenever necessary. Certain clinical situations such as psychiatric disorders, alcoholism, addic-

TABLE 4-6 Important Drug Interaction with Bupropion*†

Drugs	Level and Effects of Interaction	Suggested Management
Thioridazine	CONTRAINDICATION Bupropion is a CYP2D6 inhibitor and may increase plasma levels of thioridazine, which may increase the risk of QT prolongation and ventricular arrhythmia	At least 14 days should elapse between discontinuation of thioridazine and bupropion initiation
Monoamine oxidase inhibitors	CONTRAINDICATION Potentiation of monoamine levels	At least 14 days should elapse between discontinuation of MAOIs and intiation of treatment with bupropion
Drugs that reduce seizure threshold Antipsychotics Antidepressants Antimalarials Hypoglycemics/insulin for diabetics Theophylline Tramadol‡ Systemic corticosteroids Lithium Quinolone antibiotics OTC stimulants/anorectic agents	WARNING Increased risk for seizure	Bupropion should be used with extreme caution
Drugs metabolized by CYP2D6 Antidepressants (eg, amitriptyline, desipramine, imipramine, nortriptyline, paroxetine, fluoxetine, fluvoxamine, sertraline, venlafaxine), antipsychotics (eg, risperidone, haloperidol, perphenazine: see also thioridazine under Contraindications), beta-blockers (eg, metoprolol), type 1C antiarrhythmics (eg, propafenone, flecainide)	PRECAUTION Bupropion may increase the plasma level of these drugs	Concomitant therapy with medicinal products predominantly metabolized by this isoenzyme with narrow therapeutic indices should be initiated at the lower end of the dose range of the concomitant medicinal product. If bupropion is added to the treatment regimen of a patient already receiving a medicinal product metabolized by CYP2D6, the need to decrease the dose of the original medicinal product should be considered, particularly for those concomitant medicinal products with a narrow therapeutic index
Drugs that may affect CYP2B6 Orphenadrine, cyclophosphamide, ifosfamide, nelfinavir, ritonavir, efavirenz	PRECAUTION Potential for increased plasma levels of bupropion and associated adverse effects	Monitor for increase in adverse events of bupropion
Drugs that are general inducers of the metabolism of bupropion Carbamazepine Phenobarbital Phenytoin	PRECAUTION Potential for reduced plasma levels of bupropion	Monitor for changes in clinical activity of bupropion

| Levodopa | PRECAUTION
Both bupropion and levodopa increase dopamine availability | Administration of bupropion in patients receiving levodopa should be undertaken with caution, using small initial doses and gradual dose increases. Monitor for increase in adverse events of bupropion |
| Transdermal nicotine | PRECAUTION
Potential to increase blood pressure | Monitoring of blood pressure is recommended in patients who receive the combination of bupropion and nicotine replacement |

*This list is not an exhaustive list of all potential drug interactions with bupropion. It is meant to serve as a guide only. For each patient, all potential drug interactions and predisposing factors must be carefully considered.

†It should be noted that drugs metabolized by CYP1A2 isoenzymes (ie, theophylline, tacrine, and clozapine) should be monitored on smoking cessation. Tobacco may induce CYP1A2 isoenzymes; on its withdrawal, the increased plasma levels of CYP1A2 substrates may result in greater adverse effects associated with smoking cessation following bupropion administration.

‡Not marketed in Canada.

MAOI = monoamine oxidase inhibitor; OTC = over the counter.

(Reproduced with permission from Important Safety Information.[49])

tion to other drugs, or intense stress and repeated relapse further decrease the likelihood of successfully quitting smoking. These situations can be addressed by concomitant referrals to the appropriate resources. Improper use of stop-smoking medication, noncompliance, and adverse effects should be reported and discussed to ensure safety and the best cessation rates.

To obtain more information about local resources to help patients stop smoking (cessation telephone lines, Web sites, specialized clinics or programs), contact a local public health department, professional association, or an organization such as the Lung Association, Cancer Society, and Heart and Stroke Foundation.

SUMMARY

Tobacco addiction is a chronic disease characterized by impaired control over the use of the psychoactive substance nicotine, with manifestations occurring along biologic, psychological, social, and spiritual dimensions. Cigarette smoking is the most important preventable cause of COPD and of many other diseases. Health professionals must play a central role in eradicating this cause of morbidity and mortality. Regardless of the reason for the visit, every patient should repeatedly be asked about smoking and his/her status should be identified. Smokers should be advised to stop and motivated to do so according to their readiness for change; the health professional should be sure that different resources are made available to smokers.

Health professionals should also exploit windows of opportunity in which smoking cessation interventions are more likely to be effective. Medications will help the motivated smoker to quit, and appropriate therapy should be offered and then subsequently tailored to each smoker's need. Relapses are part of the cessation process, and follow-up visits with health professionals, as well as support from the environment, will help smokers remain abstinent.

Currently available therapies produce benefits on health and improved respiratory outcomes in patients with COPD, even for those with advanced disease. Hopefully in the future, a better understanding of the nature of nicotine addiction will help to improve outcome.

CASE STUDY

Mr. Cope is a 58-year-old man who comes to the outpatient clinic because of respiratory symptoms.

Medical History, Physical Examination, and Test Results

Medical History

- He is a current smoker; he smoked a pack of cigarettes per day for the last 40 years.
- He has been experiencing daily cough, sputum production, and increasing shortness of breath on exertion over the past 2 years.
- He has never been hospitalized for respiratory disease.
- He has no other relevant medical or surgical condition.

Physical Examination

- He is in no acute distress: respiratory rate 14/minute, pulse 80/minute, and blood pressure 140/80 mm Hg.
- No accessory muscle used in breathing.
- Chest examination confirms the presence of decrease air entry; with no wheezing or crackles.
- Cardiac examination is normal.
- He has no cyanosis and no edema.

Test Results

- He has spirometry compatible with moderate obstruction without significant reversibility. FEV_1 is 1.8 L (40% of predicted normal). FEV_1/FVC ratio is 60%.

Questions and Discussion

The diagnosis of COPD is confirmed by spirometry.

You ask the patient if he has thought of quitting smoking and he answers, "I have lost 60% of my lungs already: whether I smoke or not won't change anything. It's too late." His answer suggests that he is not ready to quit yet, and you consider that he appears to be in precontemplation.

You reply, "What do you like about your smoking?"

He answers, "It relaxes me, and it gives me something to do. I am hooked; I tried to stop 5 years ago, and I became so anxious and irritable that my wife told me to start smoking again."

You ask him, "Are there things you don't like about smoking?"

He replies, "I know it's dangerous for my health; it is already destroying my lungs, it's expensive as well, and it's hard to smoke anywhere these days with all those laws."

You state, "If you stop smoking, you will cough less and produce less sputum; you might breathe more easily and use fewer medications over time. Within approximately 12 hours, most of the nicotine in your bloodstream will have been eliminated, and within 24 hours, more oxygen will be available for your body as most of the carbon monoxide will also be gone. You will get fewer respiratory infections, and you will slow the deterioration of your lung function. Your risk of having a heart attack or cancer will also decrease. I feel that stopping smoking is the most important step you can take for your health and to control your COPD. It's definitely not too late. I understand that you are not quite ready to quit but whenever you want to talk more about it, I am available to help you." Since he is not limited in his daily activities, you recommend a short acting β_2 agonist to be used as needed.

Follow-Up

Your patient returns to your clinic 6 months later following a 5-day hospital admission for acute exacerbation of COPD. He is now on two inhaled bronchodilators that he takes regularly and has just completed a 10-day treatment with an antibiotic and oral corticosteroids.

He seems concerned and tells you, "I have to stop smoking before I end up in a wheelchair with oxygen like my uncle! Can this smoking cessation pill help me stop?" You wonder if he is really ready.

You reply, "I congratulate you for your decision. When do you consider stopping?"

He says, "I stopped for a few days during my admission, but I became very anxious and started again. I plan to stop next month because I will go to the country for 1 week."

You ask him for the date he has chosen, and he says the first Monday of the month. You express your confidence in his ability to stop and explain that there are different medications, gum or a nicotine patch, and a pill that could decrease his withdrawal symptoms and double his chances of stopping. You review the contraindications, explain how they can be used, and encourage him to choose one.

You also address and discuss his personal concerns: difficulties at work, triggers, dealing with friends who smoke, and so on. You encourage him to ask for support from his wife. You offer a cessation guide and orient him to the preparation stage section. You explain how to use the smoker's journal (monitoring form); he signs a contract to quit by a certain date with you as a witness, and you finally plan a follow-up visit 1 week before the set stop date.

At the follow-up visit, he brings his smoker's journal. He says he has tried delaying some cigarettes on waking up and after meals and that he now goes for a walk after his lunch to avoid being with smokers. He says he has decided to stop and prefers to use the nicotine patch rather than the pill because he is worried that the pill may worsen his insomnia.

He stops as planned but returns 1 week after having not smoked to say he is experiencing frequent, bad cravings to smoke and is having the bad dreams about which you had warned him. His desire to smoke is related to watching television on returning home. He decides to take a walk at that specific time in the evening and to remove the patch before bedtime. He schedules a visit to see you 4 weeks later.

He visits you two more times over the next 3 months. His cough disappears, and he feels slightly less short of breath. He is still experiencing cravings in the morning, after meals, and when stressed and is afraid of stopping the patch. You reinforce the benefits that he has felt since stopping and review his strategies to deal with the difficult moments. He decides to go for walks as much as possible in stressful circumstances. He manages to stop his nicotine patch after 12 weeks of treatment.

He returns to your clinic 6 months later and says, "I lost my job last week. I felt discouraged and very angry, and I deperately wanted a smoke. I remembered what we had discussed. I know that it takes just one cigarette for me to start all over again, so I walked instead and I used nicotine gums and avoided starting all over... Now I have to find a new job!"

You congratulate him for his effort and encourage him to talk about his plans. You both agree to a visit 2 weeks later.

KEY POINTS

- Smoking cessation is the single most important therapeutic intervention to reduce the risk of developing COPD and stop its progression.
- Tobacco use is a chronic condition, a drug addiction that often requires many years to control.
- Screening and chart identification should be part of every smoker's visit to health professionals.
- All tobacco users should be evaluated, treated, and have access to counseling; individual counseling, even less than 3 minutes' duration, is effective, but more time will result in more cessation; intensive individual and group programs are effective.
- Intratreatment support provided by direct contact with a clinician during the quitting period increases cessation; extratreatment and social support from surrounding parties also increase abstinence.
- Pharmacotherapies in the form of nicotine replacement or bupropion hydrochloride are more effective than counseling alone and should be encouraged in the absence of contraindications.
- Long-term follow-up is essential.

REFERENCES

1. World Health Organization. Tobacco alert, World Health Organization, World No-Tobacco Day 1996. Geneva: WHO, 1996.
2. Fiore MC, Bailey WC, Cohen SJ, et al. Treating tobacco use and dependence. Clinical practice guideline. Rockville, MD: U.S. Department of Health and Human Services, Public Health Service, 2000.
3. Canadian Tobacco Use Monitoring Survey, Phase II. Ottawa: Health Canada, 1999.
4. Doll R, Peto R, Wheatley K, et al. Mortality in relation to smoking: 40 years' observation on male British doctors. BMJ 1994;309:901–11.
5. Houston T, Kaufman NJ. Tobacco control in the 21st century: searching for answers in a sea of change. JAMA 2000;284:752–3.

6. Peto R, Lopez AD, Boreham J, et al. Mortality from tobacco in developed countries: indirect estimation from national vital statistics. Lancet 1992;339:1268–78.

7. Makomaski IIling EM, Kaiserman MJ. Mortality attributable to tobacco use in Canada and its regions 1994 and 1996. Malad Chron Can 1999;20:111–7.

8. Bergen AW, Caporaso N. Cigarette smoking. J Natl Cancer Inst 1999;91:1365–75.

9. Koob GF, Sanna PP, Bloom FE. Neuroscience of addiction. Neuron 1998;21:467–76.

10. Pontieri F, Tanda G, Orzi F, DiChiara G. Effects of nicotine on the nucleus accumbens and similarity to those of addictive drugs. Nature 1996;382:255–7.

11. Nisell M, Nomikos G, Svensson T. Nicotine dependence, midbrain dopamine systems and psychiatric disorders. Pharmacol Toxicol 1995;76:157–62.

12. Hajela R. Definitions of addiction medicine. Kingston, ON: Canadian Society of Addiction Medicine, June 2000.

13. Ashley MJ, Choi BCK, Pak AWP. Smoking and non-neoplastic lung disease in Canadian men and women. Can Respir J 1997;4:311–7.

14. Burrows B, Knudson RJ, Cline MG, Lebowitz MD. Quantitative relationships between cigarette smoking and ventilatory function. Am Rev Respir Dis 1977;115:195–205.

15. Burrows B. The course and prognosis of different types of chronic airflow limitation in a general population sample from Arizona: comparison with the Chicago "COPD" series. Am Rev Respir Dis 1989;140:S92–4.

16. Tashkin DP, Clark VA, Coulson AH, et al. The UCLA population studies of chronic obstructive respiratory disease. VIII. Effects of smoking cessation on lung function: a prospective study of a free-living population. Am Rev Respir Dis 1984;130:707–15.

17. Fletcher C, Peto R. The natural history of chronic airflow obstruction. BMJ 1977;1:1645–48.

18. Anthonisen NR, Connett JE, Kiley JP, et al. The Lung Health Study: effects of smoking intervention and the use of an inhaled anticholinergic bronchodilator on the rate of decline of FEV_1. JAMA 1994;272:1497–505.

19. Postma DS, Sluiter HJ. Prognosis of chronic obstructive pulmonary disease: the Dutch experience. Am Rev Respir Dis 1989;140:S100–5.

20. Kanner RE. Early Intervention in chronic obstructive pulmonary disease. A review of the Lung Health Study results. Med Clin North Am 1996;80:523–47.

21. Kanner RE, Connett JE, Williams DE, Buist AS. Effects of randomized assignment to a smoking cessation intervention and changes in smoking habits on respiratory symptoms in smokers with early chronic obstructive pulmonary disease: the Lung Health Study. Am J Med 1999;106:410–6.

22. The health benefits of smoking cessation. A report of the surgeon general. Washington, DC: Department of Health and Human Services, 1990.

23. Jiménez-Ruiz CA, Masa F, Miravitlles M, et al. IBER-POC Study Investigators. Smoking characteristics. Differences in attitudes and dependence between healthy smokers and smokers with COPD. Chest 2001;119:1365–70.

24. Tashkin DP, Kanner RE, Bailey K, et al. Smoking cessation in patients with chronic obstructive pulmonary disease: a double-blind, placebo-controlled, randomised trial. Lancet 2001;357:1571–5.

25. Hurt RD, Sachs DP, Glover ED, et al. A comparison of sustained-release bupropion and placebo for smoking cessation. N Engl J Med 1997;337:1195–202.

26. Jorenby DE, Leischow SJ, Nides MA, et al. A controlled trial of sustained-release bupropion, a nicotine patch, or both for smoking cessation. N Engl J Med 1999;340:685–91.

27. Dale LC, Glover ED, Sachs DPL, et al. Buproprion for smoking cessation. Predictors of successful outcome. Chest 2001;119:1357–64.

28. Smoking cessation guidelines. How to treat your patient's tobacco addiction. Pegasus Healthcare International Publication, Optimum Therapy Initiative Department of Family and Community Medicine. Toronto: University of Toronto, 2000.

29. Raw M, McNeill A, West R. Smoking cessation: evidence based recommendations for the health care system. BMJ 1999;318:182–5.

30. Collège des Médecins du Québec. Smoking preventon and cessation. Régie Régionale de la Santé et des Services Sociaux de Montréal-Centre. Direction de la santé publique. Clinical Practice Guidelines. Montreal: Publication of the Collége des Médecins du Québec and direction de la santé publique de la Régie Régionale de la Santé et des Services Sociaux de Montréal-Centre, 1999.

31. Cromwell J, Bartosch WJ, Fiore MC, et al. Cost effectiveness of the clinical practice recommendations in the AHCPR guideline for smoking cessation. Agency for Health Care and Policy and Research. JAMA 1997;278:1759–66.

32. Hopkins DP, Fielding JE, and the Task Force on Community Preventive Services. The guide to community preventative services: tobacco use prevention and control. Reviews, recommendations, and expert commentary. Am J Prev Med 2001;20 Suppl 2:1–87.

33. Canadian Council for Tobacco Control. Guide your patients to a smoke free future. A program of the Canadian Council on Smoking and Health, endorsed by the college of Family Physicians of Canada and the Canadian Medical Association, Ottawa 1992.

34. Bass F. Mobilizing physicians to conduct clinical intervention in tobacco use through a medical-association program: 5 years experience in British Columbia. Can Med Assoc J 1996;154:159–64.

35. Prochaska JO, DiClemente CC, Norcross JC. In search of how people change. Applications to addictive behaviours. Am Psychol 1992;47:1102–14.

36. Prochaska JO, Goldstein MG. Process of smoking cessation. Implications for clinicians. Clin Chest Med 1991;12:727–35.

37. Canadian Council on Smoking and Health. Patient guide to a smoke free future. A program of the Canadian Council on smoking and Health. Endorsed by the College of Family Physicians of Canada and the Canadian Medical Association. Ottawa: 1996.

38. Health Canada. Survey on smoking in Canada (Cycle 3). Ottawa: 1995.

39. Rohren CL, Croghan IT, Hurt RD, et al. Predicting smoking cessation outcome in a medical center from stage of readiness: contemplation versus action. Prev Med 1994;23:335–44.

40. Goldberg DN, Hoffman AM, Farinha MF, et al. Physician delivery of smoking-cessation advice based on the stages-of-change model. Am J Prev Med 1994;10:267–74.

41. Prochaska JO, Prochaska JM. Why don't continents move? Why don't people change? J Psychother Integr 1999;9:83–102.

42. Régie Régionale de la Santé et des Services Sociaux de Montréal-Centre. Direction de la santé publique. Prévention en pratique médicale: tobacco use. Montreal: Association des Médecins Omnipracticiens de Montréal, 1998.

43. Régie Régionale de la Santé et des Services Sociaux de Montréal-Centre. Direction de la santé publique. Montreal: Freedom, 1999.

44. Canadian Pharmacists Association. Compendium of pharmaceuticals and specialties. Ottawa: Canadian Pharmacists Association, 2000.

45. Benowitz NL, Gourlay SG. Cardiovascular toxicity of nicotine: implication for nicotine replacement therapy. J Am Coll Cardiol 1997;29:1422–31.

46. Zevin S, Jacob P, Benowitz NL. Dose-related cardiovascular and endocrine effects of transdermal nicotine. Clin Pharmacol Ther 1998;64:87–95.

47. Murray RP, Daniels K. Long-term nicotine therapy. In: Benowitz NL, ed. Nicotine safety and toxicity. New York: Oxford University Press, 1998:173–82.

48. Ontario Medical Association. Rethinking stop-smoking medications: myths and facts. http:// www.oma.org/ phealth/stopsmoke.htm (accessed February 2002).

49. Important safety information regarding Bupropin. Letter sent to Canadian Health Professionals. Regulatory Affairs & Pharmaceutical Development. GlaxoSmithKline Inc. July 2001.

SUGGESTED READINGS

Fiore MC, Bailey WC, Cohen SJ, et al. Treating tobacco use and dependence. Clinical practice guideline. Rockville, MD: U.S. Department of Health and Human Services, Public Health Service, June 2000. *The latest consensus statement, evidence-based, updated guideline providing specific recommendations regarding tobacco cessation interventions and system-level changes designed to promote the assessment and treatment of tobacco use. http://www.surgeongeneral.gov/tobacco/ smokesum.htm (accessed February 2002)*

Bergen AW, Caporaso N. Cigarette smoking [review]. J Natl Cancer Inst 1999;91:1365–75. *A review of cigarette smoking in relation to addiction to nicotine, genetic factors, motives, personality factors, psychiatric comorbidity, and subtance use.*

Hopkins DP, Fielding JE, and the Task Force on Community Preventive Services. The guide to community preventive services: tobacco use prevention and control. Reviews, recommendations, and expert commentary. Am J Prev Med 2001;20(2S):1–87. *Guidelines to identify, implement, and apply the most effective and cost-effective interventions to combat tobacco use with tables summarizing the recommendations of four different guidelines and reviews.*

Ontario Medical Association. Rethinking stop-smoking medications: myths and facts. http://www.oma.org/ phealth/stopsmoke.htm (accessed February 2002). *A position paper of the Ontario Medical Association reviewing myths and facts about nicotine's role in the toxicity of cigarettes and the safety of nicotine replacement therapy in relation to the smoker's cardiovascular risk. The use of nicotine replacement therapy in pregnancy for those unable to quit using nonpharmacologic methods and for smokers under 18 and the combination of nicotine gum, patch, and bupropion and prolonged use are discussed.*

PHARMACOLOGIC MANAGEMENT OF STABLE COPD

Nicholas Anthonisen and Martin Boulé

OBJECTIVES

The general objective of this chapter is to help the allied health care professionals and physicians become more familiar with the drug therapy commonly employed in patients with stable, symptomatic chronic obstructive pulmonary disease (COPD). Pharmacologic management is often based on an individualized assessment of the disease and patient response to various medications.

After reading this chapter, the physician and allied health care professional will be able to

- identify the different classes of drugs used in COPD: bronchodilators, corticosteroids, and antibiotics;
- appropriately use these drugs according to their benefits and potential adverse effects;
- recognize that, at this time, there are few other pharmacologic considerations;
- recognize that there are many guidelines with differing recommendations; however, most recommendations for pharmacologic management are empiric because of a lack of scientific information;
- recognize that patients can be noncompliant with drug therapy; and
- refer to specific professionals from the health care team when needed.

Pharmacologic therapy is an important part of managing COPD. However, it must be noted at the outset that no drug therapy has been shown to change the course of the disease or to alter its long-term outlook and/or prognosis. Therefore, the rationale for the use of these drugs is that they relieve symptoms and improve quality of life.[1]

Since most patients with COPD seen in clinical practice have less than optimal quality of life, this is an important objective that is best assessed by carefully interviewing the patient. Such interviews must be structured to some extent to ascertain the severity of symptoms such as dyspnea, cough, sputum, and wheeze and the degree of exercise tolerance. Questions should be aimed at determining the possibility of recent changes because improvement in

the health status of patients with COPD is usually reflected by improvements in these areas. Although the management strategy is based on the patient's symptoms and response to various therapies, it may also depend on adverse drug effects, patient skills in using a specific inhalation device, and availability of medications.

In this chapter, we will review the accepted forms of drug therapy for COPD and discuss their use. Recommendations from national and international guidelines will be reviewed. Finally, issues related to drug compliance will be discussed. Since exacerbations are covered elsewhere in this textbook and hospital management is beyond the textbook's scope, the main focus of the discussion will be on the treatment of stable outpatients with COPD.

BRONCHODILATOR THERAPY

Bronchodilators are the most important agents in the pharmacologic treatment of COPD.[2] Bronchodilator agents dilate the intrapulmonary airways, thereby decreasing airway resistance and improving flow rates in and out of the lungs.[3] Essentially, they act as relaxants of the airway smooth muscle,[4] which is arranged so that its constriction, or even a normal amount of muscle tone, tends to decrease the caliber of the airway and increase the resistance of airflow through it. It should not be assumed that patients with COPD have a poor response to bronchodilators, even in those appearing to have essentially fixed airflow obstruction; several studies have demonstrated improvement in airflow following the use of regularly dosed bronchodilators in most patients with COPD, albeit to a lesser degree than in patients with asthma.[5,6]

There are essentially three types of bronchodilator drugs: β_2 agonists like salbutamol, anticholinergic agents like ipratropium bromide, and methylxanthines like theophylline. There is excellent evidence that ipratropium does not change the underlying course of COPD[7] and little reason to believe that the other types of drugs differ from ipratropium in this respect. However, all of these drugs are widely used because they tend to increase expiratory flow rates such as the forced expiratory volume in 1 second (FEV_1), tend to relieve dyspnea, and, finally, increase exercise tolerance.[1] By optimizing bronchodilator treatment, it may be possible to sufficiently reduce symptoms to permit patients to gradually increase their levels of activity as a form of self-directed pulmonary rehabilitation.

β_2 Agonists

Beta agonists directly stimulate receptors on airway smooth muscle, thus causing it to relax. There are several types of beta receptors in the body, including the heart and blood vessels and the airways. Airway smooth muscle contains type 2 beta receptors, and prescribed agents that are specific to these types of receptors have fewer side effects than others. The prototypical short-acting β_2-receptor agonist, or stimulant, is salbutamol; other similar drugs include fenoterol hydrobromide and terbutaline sulfate. These agents cause bronchodilation when administered systemically, orally, or intravenously and when inhaled. Inhaled agents produce fewer side effects

and greater bronchodilation[8] simply because there are higher fractions of the total dosage in the lungs and airways. For this reason, β_2 agonists are very commonly administered by inhalation and should rarely be prescribed by other methods. The usual short-acting β_2 agonists specified above have a relatively short onset of action with noticeable effects in 15 minutes that can last 2 to 6 hours (Table 5–1).[9] Recently, long-acting β_2 agonists such as salmeterol xinafoate and formoterol fumarate have become available. These agents induce bronchodilation that lasts 8 to 12 hours (Table 5–2).[10]

Beta$_2$ agonists have minor side effects such as fine tremor, which is usually apparent only after large doses. With a conventional dose, the risk of side effects is uncommon in patients with COPD (see Table 5–1). Larger than conventional doses of β_2 agonists may produce additional bronchodilation, but further functional or symptomatic benefit from such increased doses is limited to a small group of patients with COPD with a lack of reproducibility for any given patient.[11] Larger than conventional doses also increase the risk of side effects.

Anticholinergic Agents

Anticholinergic drugs block receptors for acetylcholine, a widely distributed substance that transmits impulses from one nerve to another and from nerve to muscle, including airway smooth muscle.[4] As might be expected, anticholinergic agents that gain access to the circulation, like atropine sulfate, have a wide variety of effects, some of which are unpleasant. One effect is the blocking of impulse transmission from the vagus nerve to the airway smooth muscle; this produces bronchodilation since vagal impulses tend to increase the tone or tension in airway smooth muscle. Ipratropium is an agent that is poorly absorbed from the lungs and gastrointestinal tract but does gain access to smooth muscle when inhaled. Therefore, it produces bronchodilation by blocking vagal transmission to airway smooth muscle. The onset of ipratropium action is slower than that of the short-acting β_2 agonists; furthermore, its duration is longer, lasting more than 4 hours (Table 5–3).[12] Inhaled ipratropium has been shown to have virtually no systemic side effects, with the only well-established risk of the drug occurring when it is mistakenly squirted into the eyes (see Table 5–3).

A longer-acting version of ipratropium, tiotropium, is currently undergoing clinical testing. Tiotropium

TABLE 5–1 Pharmacology of Short-Acting β_2 Agonists

Adrenergic Agents	Administration Route and Dosage*	Pharmacodynamics	Adverse Effects Monitoring, and Interactions
Fenoterol hydrobromide (Berotec®)	MDI 100 µg/inh Sig: (dose)1–2 inh tid–qid prn/regularly Max: 8–12 inh/d Nebulization Nebules: 0.5 mg/2 mL 1.25 mg/2 mL Solution: 1 mg/mL Sig: 0.5–1.25 mg qid prn/regularly	Onset: 5–10 min Peak: 30–60 min Duration: 3–6 h	Most frequent side effects Tremor Headache Nervousness Hypotension Flushing Hypokalemia Tachycardia/palpitations Dizziness
Pirbuterol acetate (Maxair®)	MDI 250 µg/inh Sig: 1–2 inh tid–qid prn/regularly Max: 8–12 inh/d	Onset: 5–10 min Peak: 30–60 min Duration: 3–5 h	Monitoring Blood pressure Heart rate Ion values Physical signs
Salbutamol (Ventolin®)	MDI 100 µg/inh Sig: 1–2 inh tid–qid prn/regularly Max: 8–12 inh/d	Onset: 5–15 min Peak: 30–90 min Duration: 3–6 h	Interactions β-blockers
Diskus	MDI 200 µg/inh Sig: 1 inh tid–qid prn/regularly Max: 6 inh/d Nebulization Nebules 1.25 mg/2.5 mL 2.5 mg/2.5 mL 5 mg/2.5 mL Solution: 5 mg/mL Sig: 2.5–5 mg tid–qid prn/regularly	Rotahaler 200 and 400 µg/capsule Sig: 1–2 capsules tid–qid prn/regularly Max: 1,600 µg/d Oral solution 0.4 mg/mL Sig: 2–4 mg (5–10 mL) tid–qid	Choose cardioselective • Atenolol (Tenormin®) • Acebutolol (Sectral®) • Metoprolol tartrate (Lopressor®) • Bisoprolol (Monocor®) Attention: potential cardiac toxicity Monoamine
Diskhaler	MDI 200 and 400 µg/blister Sig:1–2 blisters tid–qid prn/regularly Max: 1,600 µg/d	prn/ regularly Max: 16 mg/d	oxidase inhibitors Tricyclic antidepressants Diuretics Digoxin Systemic corticosteroids Methylxanthines
Salbutamol (Airomir®)	MDI (Hydrofluroalkane-134a) 100 µg/inh Sig: 1–2 inh tid–qid prn/regularly Max: 8–12 inh/d	Onset: 5–15 min Peak: 60–90 min Duration: 3–6 h	
Terbutaline sulfate (Bricanyl®)	Turbuhaler 500 µg/inh Sig: 1–2 inh tid–qid prn/regularly Max: 8–12 inh/d	Onset: 5–15 min Peak: 30–90 min Duration: 3–6 h	

*Dosage in clinical practice can be higher than those recommended in this table.

MDI = metered dose inhaler.

TABLE 5–2 **Pharmacology of Long-Acting β_2 Agonists**

Adrenergic Agents	Administration Route and Dosage*	Pharmacodynamics	Adverse Effects, Monitoring, and Interactions
Salmeterol xinafoate (Serevent®)	MDI 25 µg/inh Sig: 1–2 inh id–bid regularly Max: 100 µg/d	Onset: 10–20 min Duration: 12 h	See short-acting β_2 agonists
	Diskhaler 50 µg/blister Sig: 1 blister id–bid regularly		
	Diskus 50 µg/inh Sig: 1 inh id–bid regularly		
Formoterol fumarate (Foradil®)	Aerolizer 12 µg/capsule Sig: 1 inh id–bid regularly	Onset: 3 min Duration: 12 h	
	Max: 2 inh bid regularly (48 µg/d)		
Oxeze®	Turbuhaler 612 µg/inh Sig: 1 inh id–bid regularly Max: 48 µg/d		

*Dosage in clinical practice can be higher than those recommended in this table.

MDI = metered-dose inhaler.

will be suitable for once-daily dosing.[13] It is undetermined whether its kinetic selectivity for M_1 and M_3 receptors over M_2 receptors will be clinically useful.

Methylxanthines

Methylxanthines such as theophylline are chemically related to caffeine and cause a variety of effects that are of interest in patients with COPD. Although its mechanism of action is uncertain, theophylline is a well-documented bronchodilator. It is also a central nervous system stimulant that causes hyperventilation and has been reported to strengthen the diaphragm.[14] The clinical significance of these latter effects has not been well demonstrated,[15] and thus far, theophylline is employed in COPD largely as a bronchodilator, although it might also elicit improvements in breathlessness.[16,17] Theophyllines are administered orally and are available in long-acting preparations given twice daily (Table 5–4). As might be expected, theophyllines have significant potential for side effects including

convulsions and other serious central nervous system abnormalities. The most common side effects are gastrointestinal and include nausea, vomiting, poor appetite, and even diarrhea (see Table 5–4). The side effects are dose related, as is the degree of bronchodilation achieved with these agents. A problem with the use of this drug is difficulty in predicting its clearance and therefore in establishing the dose that does not cause adverse effects. Theophylline clearance may be modified by factors such as age, cigarette smoking, cardiac failure, liver disease, respiratory failure with cor pulmonale, and drug interactions. Theophylline levels can be measured in the blood; significant bronchodilation is obtained at levels approximating 10 µg/mL, whereas greater bronchodilation, but frequent side effects, is present at levels approximating 15 µg/mL or more. Generally speaking, levels of about 10 µg/mL are obtained when standard doses of theophyllines are given, that is, 300 mg twice a day of long-acting generic theophylline.[16]

TABLE 5–3 Pharmacology of Anticholinergic Agents

Anticholinergics	Administration Route and Dosage*	Pharmacodynamics	Adverse Effects Monitoring

Ipratropium (Atrovent®)	MDI
	20 µg/inh
	Sig: 2–4 inh tid–qid
	  regularly
	Max: 8–12 inh/d
	
	Nebulization
	Nebules: 0.25 mg/2 mL
	    0.50 mg/2 mL
	Solution: 0.25 mg/mL
	Sig: 250–500 µg qid
	  regularly
		Onset: 5–15 min
		
		Peak: 60–120 min
		
		Duration: 4–8 h
			Most frequent side effects
			Dry mouth
			Bad taste
			Headache
			Irritation of upper
			  respiratory airways
			
			Monitoring
			Hydration
			Oral hygiene

Ipratropium/salbutamol (Combivent®)	MDI
	20 µg/inh ipratropium
	100 µg/inh salbutamol
	Sig: 2 inh qid
	  prn/regularly
	Max: 12 inh/d
	
	Nebulization
	0.5 mg/UDV ipratropium
	2.5 mg/UDV salbutamol
	Sig: 1 nebul. tid–qid
	  prn/regularly
		Onset: 5–15 min
		
		Peak: 60–120 min
		
		Duration: 6–8 h
			Side effects
			Good tolerance
			Side effects of both
			  drugs
			Contraindications
			Hypersensitivity
			  to soya, lecithin or
			  similar food products
			  (soybean, peanut)

Ipratropium/fenoterol (Duovent® UDV)	Nebulization 0.125 mg/mL ipratropium 0.3125 mg/mL fenoterol Sig: 4 mL qid prn/regularly	Onset: 5–15 min Peak: 60–120 min Duration: 6–8 h	

*Dosage in clinical practice can be higher than those recommended in this table.

MDI = metered-dose inhaler; UDV = unique dose vial.

Choosing Bronchodilator Therapy

Given this armamentarium, how should bronchodilator therapy be used in patients with COPD? Inhaled bronchodilators should have preference over oral bronchodilators. They should be given to all patients with COPD who obtain symptomatic benefit from this treatment, which, in our experience, applies to virtually all of them. In general, a metered-dose inhaler or powder is used; nebulized therapy for stable patients is usually not necessary unless it has been shown to be more effective than conventional devices. The response to inhaled bronchodilators can be assessed by measuring lung function, usually FEV_1, before and after drug administration. This may be a useful test but should not be used as an absolute guide to therapy; the response to bronchodilators on a particular occasion may not accurately reflect responses at other times.[5] It is better to offer a trial of inhaled bronchodilators to all patients with COPD and discontinue them in the rare individual who does not derive any symptomatic benefit. It is important to listen to patients because they can describe how they feel better than any given test, that is, if there is any reduction in symptoms allowing for an increase in the daily level of activities.

Inhaled Bronchodilators: β₂ Agonists versus Anticholinergic Agents

Considerable energy has been expended by investigators to determine which inhaled bronchodilator

TABLE 5–4 Pharmacology of Methylxanthines

Methylxanthines	Administration Route and Dosage Monitoring	Pharmacology	Adverse Effects Interactions

Theophylline
Theo-Dur®
Quibron-T/SR®
Uniphyl®
Theolair-SR™
Slo-Bid®
Theochron SR®
	Adult dose
	Caution re: purity of
	  the molecule
	
	Theophylline = 100%
	Aminophylline = 80%
	Oxtriphylline = 65%
		Mechanisim of action
		Nonspecific PDE* inhibitor
		Anti-inflammatory and
		  immunoregulatory
		  properties
			Most frequent side effects
			Nausea/vomiting
			Headache
			Anxiety
			Irritability
			Insomnia
			Tremor
			Diarrhea

Aminophylline
Phyllocontin®
Phyllocontin-350®
	Oral route
	Theophylline 200 mg/d or
	  6–8 mg/kg/d
	up to 900 mg/d or
	13 mg/kg/d or
	equivalent conversion
		Metabolism
		Cytochrome P-450$_{1A2}$
		
		Metabolic clearance
		  influenced by
		  Age
		  Cigarette smoking
			Gastroesophageal
			  reflux
			Diuresis
			Tachycardia
			Arrhythmia

Oxtriphylline
Choledyl®
Choledyl SA®
	Monitoring
	Therapeutic deviation
	  10–20 µg/mL
	  Aim: 10–15 µg/mL
	  Dosing: every 6–12 mo
	    when stable
	  Samples
	    Long-acting preparation
	    measure peak concentration
	  12 h preparation: 4–8 h after
	    the dose
	  24 h preparation: 12 h after
	    the dose
	  Short-acting preparation
	    measure through
	    concentration
	  6 hours preparation: before
	    next dose
	  If toxicity suspected, any time
		Diet
		Drugs
		Cardiac disease
		  (congestive heart
		  failure)
		Liver disease
		  (cirrhosis)
		Viral infection
		Influenza vaccine
		
		Absorption influenced by
		Food
		Time of day
		  (slower at night)
		Drugs (antacids)
			Interactions
			(a few examples)
			
			⇑Serum concentrations
			Allopurinol
			Cimetidine
			Ciprofloxacin
			Clarithromycin
			Erythromycin
			Propranolol
			Ticlopidine
			
			⇓Serum concentrations
			Rifampin
			Phenobarbital
			Phenytoin
			Tobacco
			Activated charcoal

*PDE = phosphodiesterase.

should be "first-line therapy." However, the results have not been entirely clear, and there is a general consensus on several issues:

1. Although they are probably not much larger,[18] the responses to ipratropium in patients with COPD are at least as important, if not more so, than those to short-acting β_2 agonists. This implies that bronchodilator response in COPD is essentially owing to the blocking of vagal impulses, which, although an interesting observation, remains of unknown clinical significance.

2. Patients with asthma respond better to β_2 agonists than to anticholinergic agents, implying that bronchoconstriction in asthma is not entirely attributable to vagal influences.[19]

3. The onset of the effect of short-acting β_2 agonists is more rapid than ipratropium so that the former are considered better "rescue" drugs.

4. Concerning the utility of long-term treatment of COPD with β_2 agonists and anticholinergic agents, Colice demonstrated that the acute bronchodilator response to salbutamol on FEV_1

decreased over time but not to ipratropium after an 85-day treatment.[20] As well, there are studies showing that the acute bronchodilator response to salbutamol does not decrease over time. Anthonisen and Wright demonstrated that the bronchodilator response to salbutamol did not decrease over a 3-year period.[5] Therefore, a patient should take his or her bronchodilator as regularly as needed; since COPD is a chronic progressive disease, it usually means that the patient will need to use the bronchodilator for the rest of his/her life.

5. Finally, in many patients with COPD, conventional doses of either ipratropium or short-acting β_2 agonists do not achieve the maximal bronchodilation obtainable. Many patients with COPD are treated with both ipratropium and short-acting β_2 agonists,[18] with the former being used on a regular, four-times-a-day basis and the latter sometimes regularly or simply as a rescue medication.[12] Of the two agents, combinations are also available that can be used both in regular maintenance and as rescue medication, but there is no evidence that these combinations are more effective than larger doses of either of their individual components. Larger doses of both ipratropium and short-acting β_2 agonists are generally well tolerated, with the latter commonly limited by its adverse effects. It is probably safe to say that either type of drug is effective and to allow patients to increase the dose above conventional levels if they perceive added benefits; moreover, in patients with COPD there is little to choose from between ipratropium, short-acting β_2 agonists, and/or combinations of the two.

Long-Acting Inhaled Bronchodilators

Long-acting β_2 agonists are now available. They are effective in COPD,[21,22] although not consistently more effective than the shorter-acting variety. Studies have shown that long-acting β_2 agonists improve FEV_1, attenuate daytime and nighttime symptoms, decrease the use of rescue salbutamol,[10] and improve health-related quality of life.[22] Since the long-acting agents are expensive, their cost-effective use requires that the patient's symptoms or activities of daily living improve and that they are comfortable using smaller amounts of the short-acting drugs, which may not always be the case. Long-acting

agents might also be indicated in patients who experience nocturnal symptoms that disturb their sleep, but this is less common in COPD than in asthma.

Long-acting anticholinergic agents will soon be available, as well. Tiotropium causes an early improvement in FEV_1, which is well maintained[23] and significantly superior to ipratropium at 6 hours.[24] Less salbutamol was used by patients receiving tiotropium, suggesting that the control of COPD was improved. Adverse effects do not appear to be a problem with doses that are clinically useful. To date, there are no published data on direct comparison with long-acting β_2 agonists, measurements of exercise tolerance, symptoms and health status, and effects on acute exacerbations. Tiotropium is an inhaled long-acting anticholinergic drug with a simple treatment regimen of being taken once daily. It may prove to be a more convenient and consistent bronchodilator than the currently recommended four times daily needed for ipratropium.

Methylxanthines: An Add-On Therapy

Theophyllines are not routinely recommended in patients with COPD. However, they may provide distinct benefit to some individuals whose symptoms are not controlled by inhaled bronchodilators.[16] Theophyllines can cause further bronchodilation in patients with COPD who are on maximum inhaled therapy,[25] because as systemically administered drugs, they likely have access to more peripheral airways than inhaled agents. It has also been shown in clinical trials using validated instruments of quality of life, that theophylline does indeed improve dyspnea and health status.[26–28] A recent randomized trial showed that 21% of 34 patients with COPD had improvements in dyspnea as measured by the Chronic Respiratory Questionnaire during theophylline treatment.[17] Thus, there is a rationale for a trial of theophylline in patients with COPD who remain symptomatic and limited in their activities despite having inhaled bronchodilators. It is seldom necessary or advisable to use theophylline doses larger than the standard of 300 mg twice a day or to try to increase serum theophylline levels beyond about 15 µg/mL. It is advisable to check serum theophylline levels in patients who are taking the drug, especially when patients are still symptomatic or other drugs are given that might influence the rate of theophylline metabolism.

CORTICOSTEROID THERAPY

Oral Corticosteroids

The question of whether anti-inflammatory cortico-steroids have a useful role in COPD has a long and controversial history. They are of undoubted benefit in the airway obstruction of asthma, thus making it tempting to think that they might have a comparable effect in the similar airway obstruction of COPD. Until very recently, most studies of corticosteroids in COPD have involved short-term trials of high-dose oral therapy. Most of these studies have shown that a significant minority of patients with COPD, about 15%, show a distinct decrease in obstruction with improvement of FEV_1 on such therapy.[29] It is not known how reproducible these responses are or whether oral corticosteroids are effective in longer-term therapy. Nevertheless, the results of these short-term trials are such that most COPD guidelines recommend that patients who do poorly on bronchodilator therapy be given a therapeutic trial of high-dose oral cortico-steroids, such as prednisone 40 mg per day for 2 weeks. If the trial produces an improvement in the FEV_1 that is greater than 20%, the patient is considered a "steroid responder." In such individuals, long-term cortico-steroid therapy is considered using either low-dose oral prednisone (10 mg/day) or higher-dose inhaled corti-costeroids (see below). However, there is mounting evidence that this approach poorly predicts long-term benefits. There is also evidence that there are undesir-able side effects with either long-term choice.[30] In spite of this, most experts still regard the identification of "steroid responders" and their subsequent treatment with corticosteroids to be justifiable.

As a general rule, chronic treatment with systemic corticosteroids should be avoided, considering their modest beneficial effects, if any, and their well-established long-term adverse effects. It has recently been shown that daily oral corticosteroids can be suc-cessfully discontinued in many "steroid-dependent" patients without apparent harm, thereby reducing cumulative corticosteroid exposure.[31]

Inhaled Corticosteroids

In asthma, inhaled corticosteroids have become the cornerstones of therapy because they are of unques-tionable benefit and are believed to cause no serious side effects. This experience has led to a number of large inhaled corticosteroid trials in patients with COPD.[32–37] For the most part, these trials have been confined to patients who demonstrated little response to oral corticosteroids and/or an inhaled bronchodilator, which, in other words, refers to peo-ple who were unlikely to be "steroid responders." At the present time, it seems clear that in such patients with COPD, substantial doses of inhaled cortico-steroids do not have a worthwhile effect on the rate of change of lung function, which is often thought to represent the course of the disease.[34]

On the other hand, there are at least two trials that indicate that in severely ill patients with COPD, high-dose inhaled corticosteroids reduce the number and severity of exacerbations such as episodes of increased dyspnea, cough, sputum, and wheeze.[33] Exacerbations can have major negative effects on the quality of life and health care costs in such patients, so that decreasing the number and/or severity of such episodes is a worthy goal of ther-apy. However, it remains uncertain if using high-dose inhaled corticosteroids for long periods of time is associated with favorable benefit-to-risk ratios. At present, one could consider the use of relatively high-dose inhaled corticosteroids (500 μg fluticas-one propionate, 800 μg budesonide, or 1,000 μg beclomethasone dipropionate per day) in patients with severe COPD who have frequent exacerbations (Table 5–5). However, it is difficult to determine in a given patient if inhaled corticosteroids actually have an impact on acute exacerbations since the exacerbations are very hard to predict. In addition, since the original studies were done with high doses of inhaled corticosteroids, beclomethasone equivalent to 2,000 μg per day,[33,36] further confir-mation of this approach is needed using lower doses of inhaled corticosteroids. Such high doses may cause significant adverse effects, such as osteoporo-sis in some patients. Moreover, inhaled cortico-steroids in COPD need to be re-examined while taking into account relevant complications of acute exacerbations such as hospitalizations and mortality.

ANTIBIOTICS

Antibiotic therapy of patients with COPD should be reserved for the therapy of exacerbations; there is no evidence that regular antibiotic therapy is of any benefit. This will be covered in more detail else-where in this textbook (Chapter 8, "Managing Acute Exacerbation").

TABLE 5–5 Pharmacology of Oral and Inhaled Corticosteroids

Corticosteroids	Administration Route and Dosage*	Pharmacodynamics	Adverse Effects Monitoring
Oral route			

Prednisone (Deltasone®)	40–60 mg once a day in morning and weaning until minimum effective dose or discontinuation	Onset: a few hours
		
		Maximal response: after several days of treatment
			Most frequent side effects
			⇑ Appetite and weight
			Mood swing
			Dyspepsia
			Hyperglycemia
			Fluid retention
			Acne
			Inhibition of hypophy-
			  seal-pituitary adrenal
			  (HPA)-axis
			Osteoporosis
			Infection
			Muscle wasting

Inhaled			

Beclomethasone (Beclovent®, Vanceril®, QVAR®)	MDI
	50 μg/inh
	Sig: 100–1,000 μg/d
	  bid–qid regularly
	Max: 2,000 μg/d
	
	Diskhaler
	100 and 200 μg/blister
	Rotahaler
	100 and 200 μg/capsule
	
	MDI (HFA134-a)/QVAR®
	Sig: 100–400 μg/d
	  bid regularly
	Max: 800 μg/d
		Mechanism action
		
		Prophylactic and inhibitory action
		Interferes with the metabolism and synthesis of mediators involved in the inflammatory process
		
		Prevents their migration and activation
		
		Decreases vascular permeability caused by inflammatory mediators
			Most frequent side effects
			Hoarseness
			Throat irritation
			Oropharyngeal candidiasis
			Dysphonia
			Increased bruising
			Long term
			Inhibition of HPA axis
			Osteoporosis

Budesonide (Pulmicort®)	Turbuhaler 100–200–400 μg/inh Sig: 200–1,200 μg/d bid–qid regularly Max: 2,400 μg/d Nebulization Nebules 0.25 mg/2 mL 0.5 mg/2 mL 1.0 mg/2 mL Sig: 1–2 mg bid	Increases reactivity of β_2 receptors located in bronchial smooth muscle	Monitoring Oral hygiene Adrenal function Bone loss
Fluticasone (Flovent®)	MDI HFA 134-a 25–50–125–250 μg/inh Diskus 50–100–250–500 μg/inh Sig: 100–500 μg bid Max: 2,000 μg/d		

(continues over...)

TABLE 5–5 Pharmacology of Oral and Inhaled Corticosteroids (continued)

Corticosteroids	Administration Route and Dosage*	Pharmacodynamics	Adverse Effects Monitoring
Triamcinolone (Azmacort®)	MDI 200 µg/inh Sig: 400–600 µg/d bid–qid regularly Max: 3,200 µg/d		
Fluticasone/salmeterol (Advair®)	Diskus 250 µg/50µg/inh 500 µg/50µg/inh Sig: 1 inh bid regularly MDI HFA 134-a 125/250 µg/50µg Sig: 2 inh bid regularly		

*Dosage in clinical practice can be higher than those recommended in this table.

MDI = metered-dose inhaler.

OTHER PHARMACOLOGIC CONSIDERATIONS

The other essentials of COPD management are covered elsewhere in this textbook; this section will primarily focus on the newer but not yet proven methods of treatment.

Other Anti-inflammatory Therapy

There is a need for the development of new anti-inflammatory drugs as evidence shows that the inflammatory process initiated by smoking is not responsive to corticosteroids and may continue even when smoking has ceased. Several new drugs are under development such as leukotriene B_4 inhibitors, 5-lipoxygenase inhibitors, PDE4 inhibitors (phosphodiesterase inhibitors), new antioxidants, neutrophil elastase, and matrix metalloproteinase inhibitors. However, more studies and large trials will be needed to establish the effect of any of these drugs on the rate of decline in lung function.

Mucolytic Therapy

Mucolytic therapy has a long history in the treatment of COPD. Acetylcysteine (Mucomyst) is apparently used in Europe to help patients eliminate secretions but is used very little in North America because it has not been proven beneficial, and we do not recommend its use.[38] Similarly, there is a genetically engineered enzyme that lyses deoxyribonucleic acid (dornase alfa) and unquestionably makes sputum more liquid, but it does not produce improvements in lung function or quality of life in patients with COPD; furthermore, it is expensive and difficult to administer. Because many patients complain of difficulty in raising pulmonary secretions, there is still considerable interest in the development of any agents that will effectively resolve this problem.

Sedatives and Anxiolytic Drugs

A variety of sedatives, tranquilizers, and even narcotics have been used to treat patients with COPD who have severe dyspnea. There is little evidence to suggest that these approaches are helpful; thus, they should be attempted only in special circumstances and under the supervision of specialists.

Proteinase Inhibitors

A small minority of patients with COPD have a genetic deficiency of α_1-antitrypsin, which is a substance that tends to prevent digestion of lung proteins. It is believed that these patients develop emphysema because their lungs are incapable of coping with protein-cleaving enzymes from inflammatory cells, recruited to the lungs by smoke inhalation. This mechanism may apply to patients without α_1-antitrypsin deficiency, with emphysema developing when the normal defenses against protein digestion are overwhelmed.

In patients with α_1-antitrypsin deficiency, intravenous augmentation therapy with naturally derived α_1-antitrypsin has been demonstrated to have biochemical efficacy in achieving and maintaining elevated serum and lung α_1-antitrypsin levels.[39] Published results from registries have suggested that patients with FEV_1 35 to 49% of the predicted normal value who received replacement therapy had a slower rate of decline of lung function than those who did not receive replacement.[40] However, these patients were not randomly assigned to replacement therapy, and the absence of randomized, placebo-controlled trials precludes definitive conclusions regarding intravenous replacement therapy in patients who have the deficiency. In patients without α_1-antitrypsin deficiency, such therapy is even harder to justify.

Leukotriene Antagonist Drugs

There is data to suggest that leukotriene $(LT)B_4$ is a potent chemoattractant of neutrophils and that its concentrations are increased in the sputum of patients with COPD. However, leukotriene antagonist drugs that are available for the treatment of asthma (zafirlukast, montelukast sodium) are not LTB_4 antagonists but involve direct antagonism of the Cys LT_1 receptor for LTC_4 and LTD_4. They will almost certainly be tried in COPD, but, at present, there are essentially no data indicating whether they are helpful. Several potent leukotriene B_4 antagonists may be more promising, but they are now only in early development, and it is not known if they will have clinical significance in COPD.

Complementary/Alternative Medicine

Complementary/alternative medicine has become an increasingly topical theme in respiratory medicine. Alternative medicine comprises hundreds of different therapies that vary in theory and in practice; the most prevalent treatments are acupuncture, aromatherapy, phytotherapy, homeopathy, reflexology, and chiropractics. These alternative therapies are often perceived as effective by those who use them, but their specific and nonspecific effects remain unclear. Nonspecific effects can undoubtedly be an important part of the total therapeutic effect of any treatment; however, because safety is an essential precondition in any treatment, it should be stressed that although alternative medicine is often promoted as entirely risk free, in fact, there is no therapy that is totally devoid of risk. We are uncertain about the benefits of most alternative therapies and ignorant of their potential risks. Some of the possible risks could be the following: (1) acupuncture can cause trauma such as pneumothorax or infections; (2) some herbal medicines are hepatotoxic; and

(3) in some cases, homeopathic remedies might even cause aggravation of symptoms. In addition to these adverse effects, safety issues are sometimes neglected, such as advice against immunizations or conventional drug therapies. Therefore, in light of the absence of evidence-based alternative medicine, these therapies cannot be recommended at this time.

RECOMMENDATIONS FROM INTERNATIONAL AND NATIONAL GUIDELINES

Over the last several years, international and national guidelines on the management of COPD have been produced.[38,41–44] Even though guideline recommendations are based on scientific information as much as possible, except for the Global Initiative for Chronic Obstructive Lung Disease (GOLD) guidelines,[44] none of the guidelines provide evidence-based documentation; in many instances, the recommendations are essentially empiric because of a lack of scientific data. There are many similitudes and some differences in the recommendations for pharmacologic management of stable COPD.

All guidelines recommend inhaled bronchodilators as central to the symptomatic management of stable COPD, with the GOLD guidelines[44] and the European Respiratory Society (ERS)[42,43] offering no preference between β_2 agonists and anticholinergic agents for intitial therapy. The Canadian Thoracic Society (CTS)[41] and the American Thoracic Society (ATS)[38] suggest initial therapy with an anticholinergic drug if regular therapy is needed and a β_2 agonist if therapy as needed is all that is required. All groups discuss the value of combination therapy with a β_2 agonist and an anticholinergic drug compared with increasing the dose of a single drug. The GOLD guidelines consider long-acting inhaled bronchodilators as more convenient; the ERS and the ATS suggest a possible role in patients with nighttime or early morning symptoms, whereas the BTS recommends limited use until more information is available, and the CTS does not provide any mention of it. It is worth noticing that the CTS guidelines were published in 1992, the ERS and ATS in 1995, and the BTS in 1997, well before published studies had reported information on the efficacy and potential convenience of using long-acting bronchodilators. All guidelines place some value on the use of theophylline, but owing to the high risk of drug interaction and its potential toxicity, inhaled bronchodilators are preferred. Theophylline is recommended when patients are still symptomatic despite combined use of inhaled bronchodilators.

The GOLD guidelines recommend that chronic treatment with systemic corticosteroids should be avoided because of an unfavorable benefit-to-risk ratio. When considering regular treatment with inhaled corticosteroids, it should be prescribed only for symptomatic patients with COPD with a documented spirometric response to corticosteroids. It can also be given to those with FEV_1 less than 50% predicted and with repeated exacerbations requiring antibiotic and/or oral corticosteroid therapy. It is worth mentioning that it has also been stated that the dose-response relationship and long-term safety of inhaled corticosteroids in COPD are not known. Other guidelines emphasize the need to document corticosteroid responsiveness before long-term use. Regarding the recommendations on using inhaled corticosteroids, they are of limited value considering that these national guidelines were produced prior to any real research on long-term treatment with inhaled corticosteroids.[34–37]

Other drugs are generally not recommended, such as mucokinetic drugs or the routine use of antibiotics and respiratory stimulants. The use of psychoactive drugs is suggested for the appropriate patients. Alpha₁-antitrypsin replacement therapy is recommended for appropriate patients by the ATS but not by the ERS and BTS. The GOLD guidelines suggest that young patients with severe hereditary α_1-antitrypsin deficiency and established emphysema might be candidates for replacement therapy.

PATIENT NONCOMPLIANCE WITH THERAPY

Successful pharmacologic management of COPD also involves monitoring and reinforcing effective compliance with drug therapy. Compliance can be very poor and should be seen as a significant barrier to improving clinical outcomes for those with COPD. Even in the context of clinical trials, which presumably involved more monitoring than standard care settings, compliance has been reported as low in the past. In the Lung Health Study,[7] patient compliance with inhaled bronchodilator therapy by self-report at 1-year follow-up was slightly over 60%, declining to less than 50% at 5 years. In the same study, compliance measured by canister weight was about 10% below patient-reported compliance. However, these data may not be generalized since patients with COPD participating in the Lung Health Study were largely non symptomatic. Perhaps we should not worry about underuse of drugs that have only symptomatic benefit.

Compliance issues do not refer only to underuse but also to overuse and improper use of the drug or device. Improper use of the inhaled drug devices is an extremely common and important issue. Most commonly, improper patient techniques with inhaled medication result in a suboptimal level of drug delivery.[45,46] Overcompliance in COPD has also been observed.[47] Overuse of inhaled drugs is often a consequence of improper use of the drug delivery system and related drug inefficiency. Patients with severe COPD who often experience breathlessness on exertion may make excessive use of their inhaled β_2 agonist when it is more appropriate and efficient to implement their breathing techniques and appropriately pace their level of activity. It is also important to note that more than one type of noncompliance is possible in the same patient. In patients with unfavorable outcomes, noncompliance should always be considered before concluding that a specific drug therapy is ineffective.

WHEN TO REFER

When to Refer to a Pharmacist

Advice from a pharmacist may be useful when questions arise regarding adverse effects or compliance with drug treatment. Adverse effects are uncommon with most of the drugs used to treat COPD except for theophylline. Theophylline presents a special case whereby the patient's metabolism and consequent blood levels are subject to many drug interactions, including interactions with antibiotics (erythromycin, ciprofloxacin) that may be used to treat exacerbations. It is essential to carefully review the therapy and nonpulmonary conditions of patients with COPD who are considered for theophylline therapy; moreover, consultation with a pharmacist may be of great value in indicating whether these conditions, or drugs to treat comorbid conditions, need to be considered in theophylline dosing and monitoring.

Compliance with drug regimens should always be a consideration in patients with chronic diseases. A dangerous and difficult scenario occurs when a patient with severe disease overuses his/her drugs. This can occur with bronchodilators, corticosteroids, or antibiotics and can cause problems with drug reimbursement plans. In such cases, the clinic and the pharmacist should cooperate to make sure that the appropriate inhaler technique is employed and that proper education is available to the patient in terms of the expectations and effects of these agents. With this in mind, it must be acknowledged that inhaled bronchodilators are given to relieve symptoms and that if they successfully accomplish this, overuse may be occasionally tolerable. However, overuse of corticosteroids or antibiotics can also have serious consequences, and every effort should be made to prevent mistakes; the pharmacist can help by providing the necessary information and education. On the one hand, patients with relatively mild COPD can also fail to comply with drug regimens by under using prescribed therapy. This case, however, is considered less serious since most treatments are aimed at improving symptoms, and one can infer that if the patient chooses not to take a particular drug, it is likely owing to the fact that the drug is reducing symptoms.

When to Refer to a Physician

Generally speaking, physicians should always supervise the care of patients with COPD. Supervision does not always require direct contact between the patient and the physician but does require that the physician know what is going on. Thus, groups of patients with COPD can receive their front-line health care from nonphysicians; this is routine in most clinical research. However, periodic meetings with the responsible physicians and key members of the team are essential so that progress can be monitored. As is always the case in medicine, decisions regarding health care and personal maintenance have to be individualized. Whereas some patients are stable and require little physician input, others need more guidance and supervision. The most comprehensive rule of thumb states that the physician be consulted whenever other caregivers are uncomfortable with the status of a particular patient, which is something that varies according to the individuals involved. Physicians should always be consulted whenever changes in drug therapy are contemplated and whenever a patient does not respond to treatment as anticipated. Furthermore, they should be consulted if a patient appears to be so ill that hospitalization or an emergency department visit may be required. Indicators of this kind of severity include fever and extreme dyspnea, cyanosis, or altered mentation, but no list is completely comprehensive. Physicians should also be consulted whenever a patient with COPD is suspected of developing a nonpulmonary disease.

When to Refer to a Respirologist

This decision varies with the degree of comfort and experience that the practitioner and health care team have in dealing with COPD. Uncertain diagnosis should be an absolute indication for respirologist referral. Although there is no concrete evidence to support this view, it has been suggested that all patients with COPD should see a respirologist at some point in their disease. It is certainly true that patients with COPD should undergo periodic (roughly annual) spirometric testing that is often available only through specialists. Other indications for referral could include patients with cor pulmonale, bullous disease, rapid decline in FEV_1, or disease in relatively young people, such as those under 40 years, and patients who cannot be withdrawn from their oral corticosteroids. Essentially all symptomatic patients with COPD should be given the opportunity to undergo pulmonary rehabilitation under the supervision of established specialists and their programs. Finally, many patients with COPD have such severe symptoms and such a restricted quality of life that consultation with a specialist may be beneficial in serving to reassure both the patient and the person making the referral that everything possible is being done. The vast majority of daily care plans for patients with COPD are successfully delivered by a team of health care workers that does not always include respirologists.

SUMMARY

All patients with COPD should be offered treatment using inhaled bronchodilators with the understanding that the benefits of these agents are confined to the relief of symptoms. The choice of the particular bronchodilator agent is less important than the initiation of inhaled therapy, which should be guided by issues of symptom relief, adverse effects, and cost in individual patients. Combining bronchodilators may improve efficacy and decrease the risk of adverse effects as compared with increasing the dose of a single agent. Many symptomatic patients will derive further symptomatic benefit from theophylline, but some care must be taken with these agents to avoid overdoses and toxicity.

Chronic treatment with oral corticosteroids should be avoided because of an unfavorable benefit-to-risk ratio. Inhaled corticosteroids do not modify the long-term decline in FEV_1 in patients with COPD, but they may reduce the frequency and severity of exacerbations and should thus be considered only in patients with frequent exacerbations. It is important to remember, however, that COPD exacerbations are very difficult to measure, and further validation of this approach is needed. Other than in treating infectious exacerbations of COPD and other bacterial infections, the use of antibiotics is not established.

When a patient is not responding to pharmacologic treatment, it is also essential to consider noncompliance. This is especially a concern as improper patient techniques with inhaled medication result in a suboptimal level of drug delivery.

CASE STUDY

Mr. Cope, a 45-year-old male civil servant, arrives for a check-up.

Medical History, Physical Examination, and Test Results

Medical History

- Morning cough and phlegm production have been present for many years, but he has no wheezing or breathlessness.
- He smoked approximately 20 cigarettes a day for about 30 years.
- He has "chest colds," but not every winter, and he does not miss work because of them; they are characterized by increased cough and purulent sputum, which have been treated with antibiotics.
- He has never been hospitalized for respiratory disease and did not have childhood asthma.
- He is not known to have any medical or surgical condition.

Physical Examination

- Physical examination and chest radiography are normal.

Test Results

- He has spirometry compatible with mild airflow obstruction without significant reversibility; spirometry pre- and postbronchodilators: FEV_1 is 3.11 L (75% of predicted normal) prebronchodilator and 3.30 L postbronchodilator, (FVC) is 4.95 L (101% of predicted normal) prebronchodilator and 5.00 L postbronchodilator, and the FEV_1/FVC ratio is 63%.

Questions and Discussion

Mr. Copd has mild airway obstruction, which is most likely owing to his smoking habit. Alhough he regards himself as asymptomatic, he does, in fact, have COPD. Bronchodilator medication might improve his function, but he is unlikely to comply with treatment. He must be convinced to stop smoking; ideally, his motivation to quit might be increased with the reception of the news on his abnormal pulmonary function. Although this may take several visits, considerable effort should be made to persuade him that quitting smoking is both necessary and urgent. Influenza vaccines can also be recommended for administration in the autumn of every year.

At each encounter, the practicalities of quitting should be discussed; these include drug therapy, group programs available in the community, modifying behaviors associated with cigarettes, and dealing with smokers in the home and the workplace. It is very important that the patient feel that the physician is genuinely interested and concerned. The physician should offer to work with the patient throughout the quitting process.

But what if this same patient has already developed symptoms such as breathlessness on activities at work? A long period of asymptomatic airway obstruction is followed by a gradual worsening of symptoms, such as breathlessness on daily activities. Mr. Copd's FEV_1 would be less than 70% of predicted normal, and he would be experiencing dyspnea on exertion or perhaps even at rest if it is more advanced. Besides making the commitment to stop smoking and administering influenza vaccines in the autumn of every year, this patient should be treated with inhaled bronchodilators. The usual regimen is a regular dose of ipratropium plus an as-needed short-acting β_2 agonist. If the patient regularly uses ipratropium plus a short-acting β_2 agonist to relieve symptoms, prescribing a single metered-dose inhaler that produces both anticholinergic and β_2-agonist bronchodilating effects could be more convenient. Patients could sometimes benefit from a long-acting β_2 agonist combined with ipratropium, although an as-needed short-acting β_2 agonist should still be provided as a rescue medication. In any case, bronchodilator therapy for every patient should be based on the overall assessment of benefit, with the additional goals of achieving compliance with the medication while maintaining a low or tolerable level of adverse effects and an acceptable cost.

In addition to his chronic symptoms, the patient described acute exacerbation of COPD once or twice over the past 5 years. He has required antibiotics but no oral corticosteroid therapy, and he has never been hospitalized for his respiratory condition. Knowing that treatment with inhaled corticosteroids does not modify the long-term decline in FEV_1 in patients with COPD, the use of regular treatment with inhaled corticosteroids would not be required for this patient and should, in fact, be considered inappropriate.

KEY POINTS

Pharmacologic Therapy

- None of the existing medications for COPD have been shown to prevent further decline in lung function; therefore, drug therapy should be used to improve symptoms and/or decrease complications.
- Successful management of COPD also involves monitoring and reinforcing effective compliance with therapy.

Inhaled Bronchodilators

- Inhaled therapy is preferred.
- The choice depends on the availability and cost of the medication, the patient's response, and the adverse effects involved.

β_2 Agonists

- β agonists are effective for reversal (short-acting β_2 agonists) and prevention of bronchospasm.
- β agonists are the most commonly used rescue medication (short-acting β_2 agonists).

Anticholinergic Agents (Ipratropium Bromide)

- Anticholinergic agents have proven value for patients with COPD with chronic symptoms.
- Anticholinergic agents have at least an equal bronchodilation effect in patients with COPD versus β_2 agonists.
- Anticholinergic agents have an excellent side-effect profile regardless of dose administered.

Advice for Patients and Their Families

- Follow the inhalation technique as recommended.
- Encourage use of a spacing device (spacer) for improved therapeutic effects and reduced incidence of adverse effects.
- Rinse mouth after use if tremors or palpitations occur (β_2 agonists).
- Rinse mouth after use to prevent dry mouth and attenuate bad taste (anticholinergic agents).
- Advise patients of the maximum number of inhalations in 1 day.

Oral Bronchodilators

Methylxanthines

- Methylxanthines may be indicated for severe pulmonary obstruction despite optimal use of inhaled bronchodilators.
- Methylxanthines may produce therapeutic benefits unrelated to bronchodilation.
- Dose adjustments may be necessary because metabolic clearance is affected by several diseases, liver dysfunction, and drug interactions.

Advice for Patients and Their Families

- Take theophylline-based preparations at the same time every day with food.
- Avoid taking the medication at bedtime.
- Advise the local pharmacist of any changes in drug regimen (withdrawal or addition of a drug, over-the-counter purchases, new lifestyle changes such as smoking cessation, etc) because of the

very high potential for drug interactions.
- Make patients aware of the importance of requested blood tests to prevent drug toxicity.

Corticosteroids

- There is no clinical evidence that long-term oral administration is justifiable in COPD.
- There is demonstrated efficacy for suppressing inflammatory response and decreasing bronchial hyperreactivity in asthmatics only.
- Inhaled steroids may reduce the frequency and severity of COPD exacerbations and may be of value in patients with frequent exacerbations requiring antibiotic and/or systemic corticosteroid therapy.

Advice for Patients and Their Families

Oral Corticosteroid Therapy
- Encourage patients to take the drug as a single dose in the morning with food.
- Refer elderly patients to a physician or pharmacist for vitamin D and calcium supplements.
- Refer postmenopausal women to a physician for an evaluation of estrogen therapy.
- Evaluate parameters that require monitoring to prevent or control the possibility of numerous adverse effects.

Inhaled Corticosteroid Therapy
- Follow the inhalation technique as recommended.
- Encourage use of a spacing device for improved therapeutic effects and reduced incidence of adverse effects.
- Rinse mouth after use to prevent irritation of the upper respiratory airways or *Candida* infections; do not swallow.
- Advise patients of the maximum number of inhalations in 1 day.
- Refer elderly patients to a physician or pharmacist for calcium and vitamin D supplements when on high doses of inhaled corticosteroids.

REFERENCES

1. Guyatt GH, Townsend M, Pugsley SO, et al. Bronchodilators in chronic air-flow limitation. Effects on airway function, exercise capacity, and quality of life. Am Rev Respir Dis 1987;135:1069–74.
2. Cazzola M, Spina D, Matera MG. The use of bronchodilators in stable chronic obstructive pulmonary disease. Pulm Pharmacol Ther 1997;10:129–44.
3. Calverly PMA. Symptomatic bronchodilator treatment. In: Calverly PMA, Pride NB, eds. Chronic obstructive lung disease. London: Chapman and Hall, 1995:419–45.
4. Barnes PJ. Bronchodilators: basic pharmacology. In: Calverly PMA, Pride NB, eds. Chronic obstructive lung disease. London: Chapman and Hall, 1995: 391–417.
5. Anthonisen NR, Wright EC. Bronchodilator response in chronic obstructive pulmonary disease. Am Rev Respir Dis 1986;133:814–9.
6. Eliasson O, Degraff AC Jr. The use of criteria for reversibility and obstruction to define patient groups for bronchodilator trials. Influence of clinical diagnosis, spirometric, and anthropometric variables. Am Rev Respir Dis 1985;132:858–64.
7. Anthonisen NR, Connet JE, Kiley JP, et al. Effects of smoking intervention and the use of an inhaled bronchodilator on the rate of decline of FEV_1: the Lung Health Study. JAMA 1994;272:1497–505.
8. Shim CS, Williams MH. Bronchodilator response to oral aminophylline and terbutaline versus aerosol albuterol in patients with chronic obstructive lung disease. Am J Med 1983;75:697–701.
9. van Schayck CP, Folgering H, Harbers H, et al. Effects of allergy and age on responses to salbutamol and ipratropium bromide in moderate asthma and chronic bronchitis. Thorax 1991;46:355–9.
10. Boyd G, Morice AH, Pounsford JC, et al. An evaluation of salmeterol in the treatment of chronic obstructive pulmonary disease (COPD). Eur Respir J 1997;10: 815–21.
11. Jaeschke R, Guyatt G, Cook D, et al. The effect of increasing doses of β-agonists on airflow in patients with chronic airflow limitation. Respir Med 1993; 87:433–8.
12. COMBIVENT Inhalation Aerosol Study Group. In chronic obstructive pulmonary disease, a combination of ipratropium and albuterol is more effective than either agent alone. An 85-day multicenter trial. Chest 1994;105:1411–9.
13. Barnes P. Chronic obstructive pulmonary disease. N Engl J Med 2000:343:219–280.
14. Murciano D, Auclair MH, Pariente R, Aubier M. A randomized, controlled trial of theophylline in patients with severe chronic obstructive pulmonary disease. N Engl J Med 1989;320:1521–5.
15. Moxham J. Aminophylline and the respiratory muscles: an alternative view. Clin Chest Med 1988;9:325–36.
16. McKay SE, Howie CA, Thomson AH, et al. The value of theophylline treatment in patients handicapped by chronic obstructive lung disease. Thorax 1993;48:227–32.
17. Mahon JL, Laupacis A, Hodder RV, et al. Theophylline for irreversible chronic airflow limitation. A randomized study comparing "n of 1" trials to standard practice. Chest 1999;115:38–48.
18. Easton PA, Jadue C, Dhingra S, Anthonisen NR. A comparison of the bronchodilating effects of a beta-

2 adrenergic agent (albuterol) and an anticholinergic agent (ipratropium bromide), given by aerosol alone or in sequence. N Engl J Med 1986;315:735–9.

19. Higgins BG, Powell RM, Cooper S, Tattersfield AE. Effect of salbutamol and ipratropium bromide on airway calibre and bronchial reactivity in asthma and chronic bronchitis. Eur Respir J 1991;4:415–20.

20. Colice GL. Nebulized bronchodilators for outpatient management of stable chronic obstructive pulmonary disease. Am J Med 1996;100 Suppl 2A: 11S–8S.

21. Mahler DA, Donohue JF, Barbee RA, et al. Efficacy of salmeterol xinafoate in the treatment of COPD. Chest 1999;115:957–65.

22. Jones P, Bosh T. Quality of life changes in COPD patients treated with salmeterol. Am J Respir Crit Care Med 1997;155:1283–9.

23. Casaburi R, Serby CW, Menjoge SS, et al. The spirometric efficacy of once daily dosing with tiotropium in stable COPD. Am J Respir Crit Care Med 1999;159:A254.

24. Van Noord JA, Bantje T, Eland M, et al. Superior efficacy of tiotropium (TIO) compared to ipra-tropium (IpBr) as a maintenance treatment bronchodilator in COPD. Am J Respir Crit Care Med 1999;159: A525.

25. Filuk RB, Easton PA, Anthonisen NR. Responses to large doses of salbutamol and theophylline in patients with chronic obstructive pulmonary disease. Am Rev Respir Dis 1985;132:871–4.

26. Mahler DA, Matthay RA, Snyder PE, et al. Sustained-release theophylline reduces dyspnea in non-reversible obstructive airway disease. Am Rev Respir Dis 1985;131:22–5.

27. Guyatt GH, Berman LB, Townsend M. Long-term outcome after respiratory rehabilitation. Can Med Assoc J 1987;137:1089–95.

28. Kirsten D, Wegner R, Jorres R, Magmussen H. Effects of theophylline withdrawal in severe chronic obstructive pulmonary disease. Chest 1993;104: 1101–7.

29. Ziment I. Pharmacologic therapy of obstructive airway disease. Clin Chest Med 1990;11:461–86.

30. Decramer M, Lacquet LM, Fagard R, Rogiers P. Corticosteroids contribute to muscle weakness in chronic airflow obstruction. Am Rev Respir Dis 1994;150: 11–6.

31. Rice KL, Rubins JB, Lebahn F, et al. Withdrawal of chronic systemic corticosteroids in patients with COPD. Am J Respir Crit Care Med 2000;162: 174–8.

32. Bourbeau J, Rouleau MY, Boucher S. Randomized controlled trial of inhaled corticosteroids in patients with chronic obstructive pulmonary disease. Thorax 1998;53:477–82.

33. Paggiaro PL, Dahle R, Bakran I, et al. Multicentre randomized placebo-controlled trial of inhaled fluticasone propionate in patients with chronic obstructive pulmonary disease. Lancet 1998;351: 773–80.

34. Vestbo J, Sorensen T, Lange P, et al. Long-term effect of inhaled budesonide in mild and moderate chronic obstructive pulmonary disease: a randomised controlled trial. Lancet 1999;353: 1819–23.

35. Pauwels RA, Lofdahl C-G, Laitinen LA, et al. Long-term treatment with inhaled budesonide in persons with mild chronic obstructive pulmonary disease who continue smoking. N Engl J Med 1999;340:1948–53.

36. Burge PS, Caverley PM, Jones PW, et al. Randomised, double blind, placebo controlled study of fluticasone propionate in patients with moderate to severe chronic obstructive pulmonary disease. The ISOLDE trial. BMJ 2000;320:1297–303.

37. The Lung Health Study Research Group. Effect of inhaled triamcinolone on the decline in pulmonary function in chronic obstructive pulmonary disease. N Engl J Med 2000;343:1902–9.

38. American Thoracic Society. Standards for the diagnosis and care of patients with chronic obstructive pulmonary disease (COPD). Am J Respir Crit Care Med 1995;152:S77–120.

39. Wewers MD, Casolaro MA, Sellers SE, et al. Replacement therapy for alpha$_1$-antitrypsin deficiency associated with emphysema. N Engl J Med 1987; 316:1055–62.

40. Seersholm N, Wencker M, Banik N, et al. Does alpha$_1$-antitrypsin augmentation therapy slow the annual decline in FEV$_1$, in patients with severe hereditary alpha$_1$-antitrypsin deficiency? Eur Respir J 1997;10: 2260–3.

41. Chapman KR, Bowie DM, Goldstein RS et al. Guidelines for the assessment and management of chronic obstructive pulmonary disease. Can Med Assoc J 1992;147:420–8.

42. Siafakas NM, Vermeire P, Price NB, et al. Optimal assessment and management of chronic obstructive pulmonary disease (COPD): the European Respiratory Society Task Force. Eur Respir J 1995;8: 1398–420.

43. British Thoracic Society. Guidelines for the management of chronic obstructive pulmonary disease: the COPD Guideline Group of the Standards of Care Committee of the BTS. Thorax 1997;52 Suppl: S16–28.

44. Pauwels RA, Buist AS, Calverley PMA, et al., on behalf of the GOLD Scientific Committee. National Heart, Lung, and Blood Institute/WHO Global Initiative for Chronic Obstructive Lung Disease (GOLD) workshop summary: global strategy for the diagnosis, management, and prevention of chronic obstructive lung disease. Am J Respir Crit Care Med 2001;163:1256–76.

45. Goodman DE, Isreal E, Rosenberg M, et al. The influence of age, diagnosis and gender on proper use of metered-dose inhalers. Am J Respir Crit Care Med 1994;150:1256–61.

46. McFadden ERJ. Improper patient techniques with metered dose inhalers: clinical consequences and solutions to misuse. J Allergy Clin Immunol 1995; 96:278–83.

47. Dolce JJ, Crisp C, Manzolla B, et al. Medication adherence patterns in chronic obstructive pulmonary disease. Chest 1991;99:837–41.

SUGGESTED READINGS

Barnes PJ. New therapies for chronic obstructive pulmonary disease. Thorax 1998;53:137–47. *This is a review of new therapies for COPD: new bronchodilators, anti-inflammatory treatments, antiproteases, mediator antagonists, pulmonary vasodilators, mucoregulators, and drugs affecting remodeling. It presents some recent advances in the therapy of COPD and several new drugs now in development that may be useful in preventing disease progression.*

Eraker SA, Kirscht JP, Becker MH. Understanding and improving patient compliance. Ann Intern Med 1984;100:258–68. *This review article presents the problem of patient compliance and the ability of the physician and health professional to understand, detect, and improve compliance. A health decision model that combines decision analysis, behavioral decision theory, and health belief is proposed.*

Pauwels RA, Buist AS, Calverley PMA, et al., on behalf of the GOLD Scientific Committee. National Heart, Lung, and Blood Institute/WHO Global Initiative for Chronic Obstructive Lung Disease (GOLD) workshop summary: global strategy for the diagnosis, management, and prevention of chronic obstructive lung disease. Am J Respir Crit Care Med 2001;163:1256–76. *The GOLD guidelines present a COPD management plan with four components: (1) assess and monitor disease, (2) reduce risk factors, (3) manage stable COPD, and (4) manage exacerbations. It has been developed by individuals with expertise in COPD research and patient care and reviewed by many experts and national societies. Levels of evidence are assigned to statements, where appropriate, using a system developed by the NHLBI.*

CHAPTER 6

USING INHALATION DEVICES

Danielle Beaucage and Suzanne Nesbitt

OBJECTIVES

The general objective of this chapter is to help physicians and the allied health care professionals teach the patient and his/her family how to use their inhalation device(s) effectively. The health care team must collaborate with individuals to choose the system that best suits their needs and preferences.

After reading this chapter, the physician and the allied health care professional will be able to

- acquire an in-depth understanding of how the most commonly prescribed inhalation devices function,
- identify the device most appropriate to the individual's needs,
- know correct and effective techniques for the most commonly available devices,
- teach and assess patient's techniques effectively, and,
- when necessary, refer to appropriate professionals from the health care team.

In the administration of treatment medication for chronic obstructive pulmonary disease (COPD), the inhalation route has been favored for the last 20 years. This technique enables the drugs to act directly on the airways, provided that the inhalation device is used correctly.[1] Medication can be delivered as an inhaled aerosol in smaller doses, thus resulting in significantly fewer side effects than drugs delivered orally or intravenously.[2]

The effectiveness of an aerosol is largely dependent on how much of the medication actually reaches the small peripheral airways of the lungs. Particles that are too large or that are traveling too quickly will tend to impact with the walls of the upper airways, such as the throat, and therefore not reach the targeted airways. The size of the particles in an aerosol must be small, between 1 and 5 μm,

to reach the smaller passages.[3] They must also be moving at the right speed to negotiate the changes in the direction of the airways as they travel into the lungs.[4]

Several different types of inhalation devices are available, but not all medications are available in each device. The choice of inhalation device will depend on the medication prescribed and the needs and capabilities of the individual patient.[5]

In this chapter, we explain the characteristics of the various devices most commonly prescribed, including pressurized metered-dose inhalers (pMDIs) with and without spacer devices; the multidose dry powder inhalers (DPIs), including Turbuhaler®, Diskhaler®, and Diskus®, and finally, the nebulizer. We describe how they function, how to use and care for them, and any adjuncts available to facilitate their use.

DIFFICULTIES WITH INHALERS AND NEED FOR TEACHING

It has long been appreciated that many patients have difficulties with inhalers. More than 75% of patients with COPD experience difficulty using metered-dose inhalers.[6,7] There are also other devices that pose difficulties for many patients. Furthermore, some studies show that patients may not maintain a proper technique over time.[8,9] Inhalation technique should therefore be assessed, reviewed, and verified on a periodic basis to ensure appropriate drug delivery and subsequent efficacy.[7]

Patient education should include the following:
- What the treatment is
- Why the treatment is being given
- How it should be administered
- How the devices work
- How to care for and maintain the devices

It is now widely accepted that a demonstration of the inhalation technique is the most effective way to teach and assess patient skills.[10] However, several studies have shown that many health care professionals have a poor understanding of the devices and are unable to demonstrate the correct technique themselves.[5,11,12] It is obvious that to maximize the benefits of inhaled medication, it is essential that the health care professional has the required knowledge and ability to successfully choose the most appropriate device and be an effective teacher.

In the following sections, we present a teaching guide for health professionals that we have developed outlining each technique in easy steps. These steps have been adapted from the evaluation scales previously established for studies assessing inhalation techniques.[5,11,13] We provide detailed explanations for each step and suggestions on how to teach the correct technique for each inhaler, including what to demonstrate, how to coach the patient, and the teaching tools available. In general, placebos and instruction leaflets for all devices are available from the pharmaceutical companies. These should be used for demonstration and for patients to practice and perfect their technique under the supervision of a qualified health care professional.

PRESSURIZED METERED-DOSE INHALER

Without Auxiliary Devices

Design and Operation

The most common device for inhaled drug delivery is the pMDI. The pMDI consists of a pressurized canister and a chamber outfitted with a mouthpiece and protective cover (Figure 6–1). The canister contains a medication, a surfactant and/or a solvent, and a liquid propellant such as chlorofluorocarbons (CFCs). CFCs must be removed from pMDIs according to *The Montreal Protocol on Substances That Deplete the Ozone Layer*.[14] Environmentally friendly propellants such as hydrofluoroalkanes (HFAs) are rapidly replacing CFCs in pMDIs. In Canada, it is

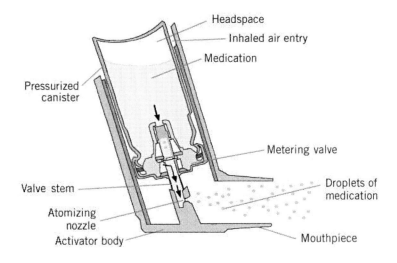

Figure 6–1 Diagram of the pressurized metered-dose inhaler. (Adapted with permission from GlaxoSmithKline, Canada.)

mandated that this transition will be completed by the year 2005.[14]

The inhaler itself is designed to deliver exact doses of medication.[15,16] When the canister is pressed, a one-way metering valve is opened by the trigger mechanism in the activator body. The medication is aerosolized near the opening of the mouthpiece, at which point the patient must inhale it. The aerosol consists of droplets in varying diameters. When the medication is inhaled, large droplets are deposited in the mouth, pharynx, and larynx, whereas smaller droplets make their way toward the lower airways.[15,17]

Manufacturers of HFA-driven devices have improved the design characteristics and drug formulations to address some of the drawbacks of the older pMDIs.[14] They have decreased the velocity and increased fine particle dose in an attempt to improve the therapeutic ratio of the drug. The new designs deliver a more consistent dose throughout the life of the canister, thus eliminating the tailoff effect (reduction of drug output as the device nears empty). Chlorofluorocarbon-driven devices deliver reduced doses when exposed to cold. Hydrofluoroalkane-driven canisters deliver consistent doses even when exposed to temperatures as low as –20°C. The new generation of pMDIs produces a warmer spray, which should alleviate the cold freon effect (interruption of inspiration) experienced by some patients in the past.

It has been proven that pMDIs are a reliable and effective method of delivering inhaled medication, and, when used properly, their efficacy is at least equal to that of other inhalation devices.[18] Their greatest disadvantage, however, is that they are relatively complicated to use effectively. Several studies have revealed that a large number of patients are unable to master the technique.[6,10,19] On the other hand, the use of a pMDI in conjunction with a spacing device, as we will discuss later in this chapter, is a more effective method of delivering medication to the lungs.

The teaching guides for pMDIs are presented in Table 6–1[4,5,16,20–30] and Figure 6–2. The explanations that are provided may be used during patient teaching, but it is important to familiarize yourself with the variations in technique associated with new devices as they enter the marketplace.

Care and Maintenance of the Pressurized Metered-Dose Inhaler

As with any pressurized container, it is best to avoid temperature extremes such as heat and cold; for example, do not place a pMDI on a radiator.[31] Cold temperatures will reduce the efficacy of a CFC-driven pMDI; therefore, the canister should be kept warm (ie, stored close to the body when outside in winter). In case of exposure to cold, one should roll the canister between the palms of the hands to warm it up.

It is important to replace the inhaler's protective cap between uses to avoid aspiration of foreign objects (dust, paperclips, coins, etc). The pMDI's plastic container should be separated from the canister and cleaned once a week. The plastic container and cap should be soaked in warm, soapy water, rinsed, and allowed to air dry.

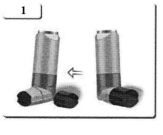

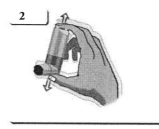

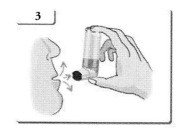

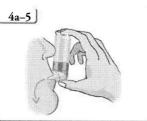

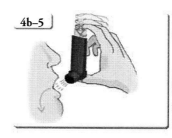

Figure 6–2 Pressurized metered-dose inhaler: illustration of technique. For more explanations, refer to Table 6–1, steps 1 through 5. (Adapted from the self-management program "Living well with COPD©, Inhalation Technique Card, Metered-Dose Inhaler.")

TABLE 6–1 Teaching Guide: Pressurized Metered-Dose Inhaler (pMDI);
Open- and Closed-Mouth Techniques*

Steps to Follow (Suggested Demonstration and Detailed Instructions)	Explanations and References
1. *Remove the cap.* Remove the cap and take your medication while sitting or standing to obtain an adequate dose.	To receive an adequate dose, the device should be held upright. It is recommended that inhaled medications be taken while standing or sitting but never while lying down.[20]
2. *Shake device.** Shake your inhaler 3 to 4 times before each puff to mix the drug particles that have settled in the pump. If you are using your metered-dose inhaler for the first time or if it has not been used for a week or more, spray the pump into the air a few times to "prime" it, then wait 30 seconds to 1 minute before starting again.	Some formulations are in a suspension, and, when not in use, the substances within it separate. It is very important to shake these pumps before each use to ensure a homogeneous and uniform dose.[16] Some new products are in the form of solutions (ie, QVAR™) and do not require shaking.[21] If the pMDI is being used for the first time or has not been used for over 1–2 wk, the dose of medication may have escaped from the metering chamber and a full dose may not be obtained on initial actuation; therefore, the pMDI should be primed.[22]
3. *Exhale to FRC.** Exhale normally. This will help you prepare to take a deep breath in.	Expiration until FRC is reached is sufficient. In fact, research findings indicate that forced expiration is no more effective and is also likely to cause broncho spasm.[23,24]
4.(a) *Closed-mouth technique* (this technique should be used for all anticholinergic metered-dose inhalers). Hold the inhaler upright between your forefinger and thumb. Insert the mouthpiece in your mouth and seal your lips around it.	The "closed-mouth" method is recommended for anticholinergics such as ipratropium bromide because they may precipitate or exacerbate glaucoma if sprayed near or into the eye.[25]
(b) *Open-mouth technique* (CFC-driven pMDIs only). Hold your inhaler upright between your forefinger and thumb about 4 cm away from your lips (about two finger widths). Keep your mouth wide open. Holding the pump away from your mouth gives the mist time to slow down. This way it can be drawn deep into your lungs and less medication will hit the back of your throat.	Some studies indicate that the open-mouth method is superior when using CFC-driven pMDIs because they project the aerosol at a high speed (150 km/h) resulting in greater impact with the upper airways.[26] By placing a greater distance between the mouthpiece and the pharynx, there is time for the aerosol to decelerate and the particles to decrease in size (because of evaporation), allowing for greater penetration into the lungs. HFA-driven pMDIs project medication at a much slower speed, and the particles produced are finer.[27] Manufacturers suggest a closed-mouth technique.
5. *Begin inhaling and actuate canister once.* Begin inhaling slowly through your mouth, pressing down once on the pump at the same time. It is very important to press at the beginning of the inspiration so that you pull the medication into your lungs as it comes out of the puffer.	Lack of coordination between inspiration and the actuation of the pMDI is a common error. Indeed, one study notes that this is a major problem in 51% of patients.[28] A good tip is to practice in front of a mirror. If the patient cannot demonstrate adequate coordination after practice, the use of a spacing device or a different inhaler device should be recommended.

(continues ...)

6. *Inhale slowly until TLC.** Continue to breathe in slowly and deeply until your lungs are full. Try to take 3 are full. Try to take 3 to 5 seconds for the inspiration. If you breathe in too quickly, the drug will hit the back of your throat and mouth instead of reaching your airways. have a tendency to impact in the upper airways.[4]

Optimal therapeutic results demand a slow (inspiratory flow rate < 1 L/s) and deep inspiration, that is, from FRC* to TLC*.[23] Ideally, inspiration should last approximately 3–5 s and have a volume of at least 600 mL.[29] If inspiration is too rapid, the particles

7. *Hold breath for 10 seconds.* Try to hold your breath for 10 seconds. If you cannot, try to hold it for at least 4 seconds. Holding your breath will give the medication time to settle in your airways

Breath holding increases the staying time of the particles in the lungs, thus increasing deposition by means of sedimentation and diffusion.[4] A 10-s pause is more effective than a 4-s pause; however, breath holding longer than 10 s yields no additional benefit.[24]

If the patient cannot breath-hold for at least 4 s, you should recommend the use of a spacing device.

8. *If another dose is required, repeat steps 2 to 8.* If you need more than one dose, wait 30 s to 1 min between puffs and repeat all of the steps again from the beginning. If you do not wait long enough, the next puff will not deliver the correct dose. Shake the puffer (repeat steps 2 to 8). When you are finished, replace the cap on the metered-dose inhaler to help keep it clean.

Failing to wait following each puff of medication may result in little or no medication being delivered during the next actuation because the metering chamber may not have refilled completely and redistribution of the drug and gas propellant will be inadequate.[5,30]

Some new formulations may not require a waiting period (ie, QVAR™). Consult the product monograph for each device.

More than one dose of the same inhaled medication is often prescribed, therefore, it is very important to assess technique for consecutive doses.[5]

*See Figure 6–2 for illustration of technique: steps 1 through 5.

pMDI = pressurized metered-dose inhaler; FRC = functional residual capacity; CFC = chlorofluorocarbon; HFA = hydrofluoroalkane; TLC = total lung capacity.

The inhaler should be replaced when the medication has expired (see date printed on canister) or when the inhaler is nearing empty. One can estimate how much is left by shaking the pump and listening for movement sounds. It should be noted that CFC pMDIs need to be replaced shortly before they are completely empty because the dose delivered becomes inaccurate as it nears empty.[22] This is commonly known as the tailoff effect.

Spacing Devices

Design and Operation

Spacing devices were designed to overcome the difficulties experienced when using a pMDI.[32] Spacing devices are available in varying forms and sizes. The most efficient spacing devices have a holding chamber and a one-way valve that opens during inspiration and closes during expiration, preventing drug loss caused by poor coordination between actuation of the pMDI and inspiration.[33] Spacing devices also improve the deposition of medication in the lower airways. Essentially, they slow down and suspend small droplets of aerosolized medication for approximately 1 to 2 seconds.[34] This allows time for some of the propellant surrounding the particles of medication to evaporate; hence, the inhaled aerosol is made up of a greater proportion of particles small enough to reach the lower airways.[35] The larger particles that would not reach the lungs remain within the spacing device, thus significantly reducing the deposition of medication in the oropharynx and thereby reducing adverse effects.[33,36] The use of a spacing device is recommended for patients who take high doses of inhaled corticosteroids to prevent oropharyngeal candidiasis.[37,38] It does not however, appear to be of benefit against dysphonia, the most common localized adverse effect.[39]

Patients who are unable to hold their breath for 4 seconds should use a spacing device with a one-way valve, allowing the patient to obtain a suitable dose of medication in three to four tidal breaths.[40] Patients who cannot make a tight seal around the mouthpiece—for example, someone suffering from facial paralysis—should use a spacer with a mask attachment.[37] This type of device is also very useful for patients who require assistance in administering their inhaled medication, such as those with a cognitive deficit.

As we have discussed above, the use of a spacing device has many advantages. However, many patients find them embarrassing to use in public or cumbersome to carry.

Spacing devices are therefore indicated as follows:
- To overcome difficulties of patients who are unable to use pMDIs correctly (ie, because of coordination problems, physical or mental handicaps, etc)
- To reduce the risk of adverse effects with inhaled respiratory medications (especially when using high doses of inhaled corticosteroids)
- To decrease or eliminate coughing or arrested inspiration experienced by some patients when using CFC-driven devices[36]
- To administer inhaled medication during severe exacerbations as recommended by the American Thoracic Society

Two commonly used examples of spacing devices that have one-way valves are the Aerochamber Plus™ and the VentaHaler®. *AeroChamber Plus*™ VHC is a 145-mL rigid cylinder made of polyester (Trudell Medical, London, ON) (Figure 6–3). It has a rubber

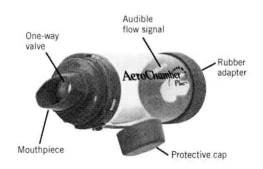

Figure 6–3 Diagram of the *AeroChamber Plus*™ VHC with adult mouthpiece. (Adapted with permission from Trudell Medical International. London ON.)

adapter that makes it compatible with most pMDIs and is available with a mouthpiece or a mask. The *AeroChamber Plus*™ VHC with mouthpiece is also outfitted with an audible flow signal (FlowSignal® whistle) that will sound if the patient inhales too quickly. The VentaHaler® is an elliptical-shaped device made of rigid, transparent plastic with a capacity of 750 mL. The VentaHaler® was designed to fit GlaxoSmithKline products and therefore does not fit all pMDIs.

The teaching guides for the spacing devices are presented in Table 6–2[36,40,38] and Figure 6–4.

Care and Maintenance of Spacing Devices

Spacing devices require regular cleaning. Medication gradually begins to accumulate on the walls of the device in the form of a whitish residue, especially near the valve. This results in an increased variability in the dose available to the patient.[41] Static charge

---

TABLE 6–2 Teaching Guide: Spacing Devices for Pressurized Metered-Dose Inhalers*

Steps to Follow (Suggested Demonstration and Detailed Instructions)	Explanations and References
1. *Remove caps from spacing device and pMDI.* **AeroChamber Plus**™ VHC (valved holding chambers): Remove the caps from your spacing device and inhaler. VentaHaler®: Assemble the two pieces of the spacing device and remove the cap from the inhaler.	
2. *Shake inhaler and connect it to the spacing device, keeping the pMDI upright.* Before taking a puff, you must shake the inhaler 3 to 4 times. Insert the inhaler into the adapter of the spacer with the inhaler in the upright position.	See Table 6–1, step 2, for details.

(continues...)

3. *Exhale to FRC* (functional residual capacity).* Exhale normally. This will help you prepare to take a deep breath in. It is best to take your inhaled medication while standing or sitting.

See Table 6–1, step 3, for explanations.

4.(a) *Spacing device with mouthpiece: insert mouthpiece between lips.* Place the spacing device in your mouth between your teeth and seal your lips around the mouthpiece. Do not block the two slots on either side of the mouthpiece with your lips.

(b) *Spacing device with mask: place mask over face.* Place the mask over the face, making sure that the mouth and nose are covered and that the seal is as airtight as possible without undue discomfort.

5. *Actuate canister once.* Spray one dose of medication into the chamber by squeezing the canister down once between your forefinger and thumb.

6. *Inhale slowly until TLC* (total lung capacity).* Breathe in slowly and deeply through your mouth. Try to take 3 to 5 s to inhale completely. This will open the valve, allowing the drug to leave the spacer. If you breathe in too quickly, the drug will hit the back of your throat and mouth. *AeroChamber Plus*™ VHC: If you hear a whistling sound, you are inhaling too fast. Slow down!

Inspiration should begin no later than 1 to 3 s after actuation of the pump because once the medication is aerosolized, it remains suspended in the holding chamber for less than 10 seconds.[41] As with a pMDI alone, a slow deep breath is recommended (see pMDI, step 6, for an explanation). The *AeroChamber Plus*™ VHC has a special sound feature that indicates when inspiration is too rapid, namely, a flow greater than 45 L/min. We have found in our clinical practice that many patients think the goal is to hear the whistle, so it is important to explain this feature. The *Aero Chamber Plus*™ VHC with mask: Caregivers and teachers can observe the flexible area around the mask compressing as the patient inhales.

7.(a) *Single-breath technique: Hold breath for 5 to 10 seconds.* Try to hold your breath for 10 s. If you cannot, try to hold it for at least 4 s. Holding your breath will give the medication time to settle in your airways.

Breath-holding: see Table 6–1, step 7, for an explanation.

If the patient is unable to maintain an inspiratory pause or continues to have poor coordination despite the spacer, the tidal volume technique should be taught (see below).

(b) *Tidal volume technique:* Breath slowly in and out of the spacing device, 3 or 4 times in a row.

The tidal volume technique is an effective alternative for those who are unable to perform the single-breath technique.[40] Since the one-way valve closes during expiration, there is no risk of drug dispersion.

8. *If another dose is required, repeat steps 2 to 7.* If you need more than one dose, wait 30 s to 1 min between puffs and repeat all of the steps again from the beginning. If you do not wait long enough, the next puff will not deliver the correct dose. Shake puffer (repeat steps 2 to 8). Replace cap on metered-dose inhaler to help keep it clean.

Refer to Table 6–1, step 8, for explanations.

Some patients try to save time by spraying more than one dose into the holding chamber at one time, but this will decrease the total amount of the drug that will reach the lungs.[36]

*See Figure 6–4 for illustration of technique: steps 1 through 6.

pMDI = pressurized metered-dose inhaler; FRC = functional residual capacity; TLC = total lung capacity.

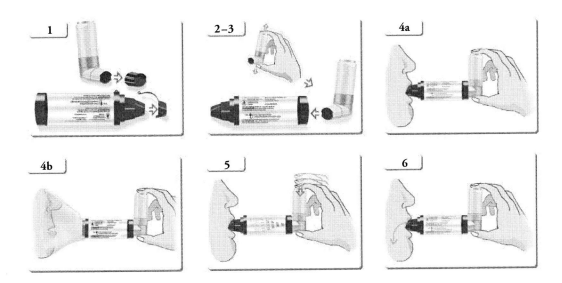

Figure 6–4 Spacing device: illustration of technique. For more explanations, refer to Table 6–2, steps 1 through 6. (Adapted from the self-management program "Living well with COPD©, Inhalation Technique Card, Spacing Device.")

buildup on plastic spacing devices attracts aerosolized particles to the walls of the chamber, thereby decreasing drug output.[42] Leaving a thin film of detergent on the devices (see procedure below) can reduce this effect. Drying with paper towels or cloths will increase static buildup, so it is preferable to allow spacers to drip dry.[38]

The general procedure for cleaning most spacing devices is as follows:

- Take the device apart following the manufacturer's instructions.
- Soak the pieces in a basin of warm, soapy water. Do not rub the interior surfaces with sponges or brushes because this will cause the walls to be roughened and thus increase the amount of medication that will adhere to them.
- Air-dry on a clean surface.

Patients should be advised to check the manufacturer's recommendations on details for each device. Spacing devices should be washed prior to their first use[1] and routinely replaced every year or earlier if damaged.[38]

MULTIDOSE DRY POWDER INHALERS

Alternative methods of aerosol delivery that are effective and easy to use are increasingly in demand.[43] Some patients also have difficulty using pMDIs correctly because of problems synchronizing the activation of the pMDI and inspiration or because of reaction to the propellants used in pMDIs. Breath-activated inhalers were developed in response to these problems.

Dry powder inhalers (DPIs) are portable inspiratory flow-driven devices that deliver dry powder formulations of inhaled drugs to the lungs. Examples include the Turbuhaler®, Diskhaler®, and the Diskus®. As the patient inhales through the device, the medication is released, broken up, and pulled into the bronchial tree. Inspiratory volume and the flows generated by the patient are the main factors that determine drug delivery to the lungs. The minimum inspiratory flow required varies greatly depending on the device.

Dry powder inhalers (DPIs) have both advantages and disadvantages. They do not require coordination because the force of the patient's inspiration activates the aerosol.[36] They do not require propellants and therefore do not cause the "cold freon" effect, are not affected by the cold, and are environmentally friendly. Some devices may not be effective, however, for individuals with severe airflow limitations or in acute situations.[44] Although less dependent on coordination than pMDIs, DPIs nonetheless require a degree of manual dexterity and a basic understanding of how they work. For example, it is important that the patient exhales away from the device to prevent introducing humidity into the medication or blowing away the dose.

In the following sections, we describe in detail the three most frequently prescribed multidose dry powder devices, the Turbuhaler®, the Diskhaler®, and the Diskus®.

Turbuhaler®

Design and Operation

The Turbuhaler® is a multidose breath-actuated metered-dose inhaler that is comprised of 13 components and a metal spring.[45] The medication in the Turbuhaler® is in the form of a fine, additive-free dry powder (eg, budesonide, terbutaline) with the exception of formoterol and Symbicort® (formoterol and budesonide combination), which also contains lactose powder. If the mechanism is activated a second time, either intentionally or inadvertently, the patient cannot inhale a double dose, as only a single dose is aligned at any time with the inhalation channel (Figure 6–5).

The Turbuhaler® uses the force of inspiration to lift particles that are deposited onto a dosing disc within the container into the respiratory system. When a patient inhales through the Turbuhaler®, the fine powder medication moves through the inhalation channel toward a deaggregation zone, which consists of two spiral channels designed to create turbulent air flow in the mouthpiece (hence the name Turbuhaler®). This action further breaks each particle of fine powder into smaller, more therapeutically effective units (particles in diameter < 6 μm).[17]

Studies indicate that the minimum inspiratory flow rate needed to attain a therapeutic dose using the Turbuhaler® is 30 L/min.[46] Because of the low flows required, the Turbuhaler® (Bricanyl®) has been quite successfully used in the treatment of acute severe asthma in the emergency department.[47] It is clear however, that higher inspiratory flows result in greater lung deposition, as illustrated in Table 6–3.[48] Thus, to ensure the highest medication delivery, it is important to encourage patients to inhale forcefully when using a Turbuhaler®.

Because of problems with manual dexterity, patients who experience difficulty loading the device may obtain a larger grip from the pharmaceutical manufacturer.

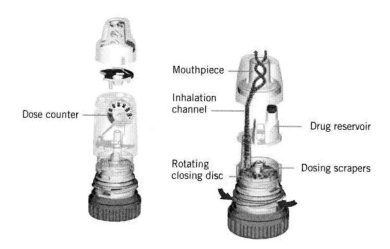

Dose counter

Mouthpiece

Inhalation channel

Drug reservoir

Rotating closing disc

Dosing scrapers

Figure 6–5 Diagram of the Turbuhaler®. (Adapted with permission from AstraZeneca, Canada.)

TABLE 6–3 Relationship between Inspiratory Flow Rate and Drug Deposition Site*

Necessary Inspiratory Flow Rate	Drug Deposition in Lungs (%)	Drug Deposition in Oropharynx
35 L/min	14.8 ± 3.3	66.6 ± 8.0
60 L/min	27.7 ± 9.5	57.9 ± 13.0

*These results were obtained during a trial using Turbuhaler® to deliver budesonide. Similar results were obtained using terbutaline sulfate.[48]

The teaching tools for the Turbuhaler® are presented in Table 6–4 and Figure 6–6.

Care and Maintenance of the Turbuhaler®

The fine powder medication within the Turbuhaler® must be protected from humidity as moisture will cause the medication within the container to clump.[17] A desiccant (drying agent) has been placed in the base of the Turbuhaler® to help protect the medication. The Turbuhaler® should be cleaned by wiping the mouthpiece with a clean dry cloth and should never be immersed in water.[49] The protective cap must be replaced after each use.

The Turbuhaler® has a dose counter that can be seen through a small window below the mouthpiece indicating the amount of doses remaining. When the red mark appears, the device is empty. It is important to mention to patients that the Turbuhaler® will rattle if it is shaken, even when there is no more medication. This is the desiccant rather than the medication.

TABLE 6–4. Teaching Guide: Turbuhaler® *

Steps to Follow (Suggested Demonstration and Detailed Instructions)	Explanations and References
1. *Remove plastic cover.* Unscrew and remove the plastic cover.	
2. *Hold the Turbuhaler® upright (mouthpiece up).* Hold the Turbuhaler® in an upright position when you are loading it, otherwise, the measuring device will not fill properly and you will not have the proper dose.	The Turbuhaler® must be held upright (45°–90°) to load correctly.[45]
3. *Load the device.* Turn the colored handle in one direction as far as possible. Then turn it back until you hear a click. This indicates that the dose is ready. You cannot load more than one dose at a time because the measuring device cannot hold more than one dose.	Note, some patients will shake the Turbuhaler®, a habit associated with the use of pMDIs. This step is useless there is nothing to mix. Furthermore, if the Turbuhaler is loaded, shaking will cause the dose to be lost.
	Patients may actuate the device twice before inhaling thinking they will get two doses at one time. The second dose will be returned to the reservoir and will be wasted because the dosing indicator wheel will still advance each time the handle is turned.[5]
4. *Exhale to FRC: breathe out normally.* Do not blow toward the device for two reasons: (a) you could blow away your dose, and (b) you could introduce humidity into the Turbuhaler® causing the powder to clump.	Expiration until FRC* reached is sufficient (see Table 6–1, step 3, for explanation). Exhaling into the Turbuhaler® will introduce humidity into the system. The small holes of the dosing disk may be partially or totally obstructed because of contact between the powder and humidity, the result being that subsequent doses will be inexact or unobtainable.
5. *Inhale forcefully and deeply through mouth.* Place mouthpiece between your teeth and close your lips around it. Do not put it in too deeply or you will block the air inlets just beneath the mouthpiece. Breathe in deeply and forcefully through your mouth. You will probably not feel or taste the drug since it is such a small amount of very fine powder.	Show the patient the openings on the side of the Turbuhaler®. Air must enter here in order for the patient to inhale the medication and create turbulent flow to break up the particles (see explanation in introduction to Turbuhaler®).

(continues...)

Various teaching tools are available to determine if the inspiratory flow rate is sufficient. Some have auditory indicators, others light indicators. Use of these devices can motivate the patient to adopt a proper technique. These devices are available from AstraZeneca Pharmaceuticals.

It is important to point out to patients that they may be unable to smell, taste, or even feel the sensation of the medication being inhaled because it is such a small amount of very fine powder. Patients must be reassured that proper technique guarantees that the dose will be delivered.

6. *Remove Turbuhaler® from mouth and exhale normally.* Remove the Turbuhaler® from your mouth and breathe normally. When you breathe out, be careful not to blow into your Turbuhaler® or you will introduce humidity into the device.

Recent studies demonstrate that a 10-s inspiratory pause is not be necessary because the powder dissolves as soon as there is contact with the mucous membranes.[20]

7. *If another dose is required, repeat steps 2 to 6.* If you need more than one dose, you must repeat all of the steps again from the beginning. Turn the colored grip (repeat steps 2 to 6).

Often patients require more than one inhalation. It is important that the patient practice the complete sequence of steps in order to simulate what he must do at home and to ensure that he/she does not forget anything.

8. *Put the protective cap back on.* Screw the protective cap back on. This will protect the Turbuhaler® from humidity.

Please note: Caution the patient not to turn the colored grip when replacing the cap as this will reload the device rather than closing it.

*See Figure 6–6 for illustration of technique: steps 1 through 5.

pMDI = pressurized metered-dose inhaler; FRC = functional residual capacity.

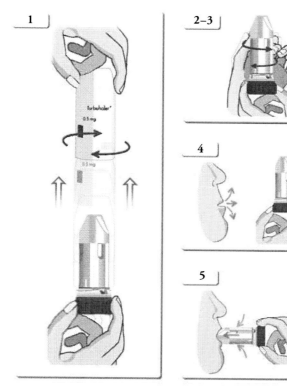

Figure 6–6 Turbuhaler®: illustration of technique. For more explanations, refer to Table 6–4, steps 1 through 5. (Adapted from the self-management program "Living well with COPD©, Inhalation Technique Card, Turbuhaler®.")

Diskhaler®

Design and Operation

The Diskhaler® delivers dry powder formulations of inhaled drugs such as salbutamol, salmeterol, and beclomethasone in a lactose-based drug carrier.[50]

It consists of a case containing a rotating wheel onto which a metallic-filmed medication disk containing four or eight blisters of medication is loaded. A blister is mechanically punctured by lifting the cover. The medication may then be inhaled through the mouth. Subsequent doses are available by rotating the cartridge. Each dose on the blister pack is individually numbered and appears in a small window on the device, allowing the patient to monitor the number of doses taken and how many remain.[51] Every medication disk is hermetically sealed and must remain so to protect the powder medication from humidity that will cause it to clump.

Studies have shown that lung deposition with other dry powder devices, such as the Turbuhaler®, increases with higher flows.[46,52] Unfortunately, there are no data that address the required flow rate for the use of a Diskhaler®.[53,54] Consequently, experts recommend an inspiratory flow rate greater than 60 L/min to achieve an adequate drug deposition in the lungs.[55]

The teaching tools for this device are presented in Table 6–5 and Figure 6–7.

TABLE 6–5 Teaching Guide: Diskhaler®*

Steps to Follow (Suggested Demonstration and Detailed Instructions)	Explanations
1. *Load medication disk.* First you must load a medication disk into the Diskhaler®, as follows: (a) remove the protective cover; (b) slide the white mouthpiece out of the case by pressing gently on the bars on either side of the device; (c) clean the device with a dry cloth and the little brush found inside the case; (d) carefully place a medication disk on the rotating wheel with the numbers side up; (e) push the cartridge back into the case and make sure that the number 8 appears in the window. This will be your first dose.	The Diskhaler® should be cleaned every time the medication disk is changed. A small brush, found inside the case, is provided for cleaning the device. Rotating the disk to the highest number ensures that the patient knows how many doses are left. Each time the disk is rotated, the number that will appear will decrease by one, indicating the number of doses left.
2. *Puncture the blister.* Holding the Diskhaler® in a horizontal position, lift the back of the lid until it is straight up. This will break the blister of medication so that you will be able to inhale the medication. It is very important that you have lifted the lid all the way up to be sure that the blister is pierced completely. It is important that the blisters remain sealed until you are ready to take your medication to protect it from humidity and loss.	The device must not be turned upside down or shaken once the blister has been pierced or the medication may be lost. When the lid is raised to 90 degrees, the blister will be completely pierced all the way to the opposite side, allowing the drug to be inhaled through the mouthpiece via the holding chamber. It is therefore important to advise the patient that it is essential to always lift the lid completely. A blister should never be punctured by any other object; otherwise, it may not be adequately pierced.
3. *Close lid.* Close the lid. The Diskhaler® inhaler is now ready to use. Keep the device horizontal and be careful not to bump or shake the device once it is loaded; otherwise, you may lose your dose.	The lid must be returned to its initial position; otherwise, it will block the opening it has just created.

(continues...)

4. *Exhale to FRC.* Breathe out normally. Keep the Diskhaler® in the horizontal position and do not blow toward the device for two reasons: (a) you could blow away your dose; (b) you could introduce humidity into the Diskhaler, causing the powder to clump.

Exhaling to FRC is sufficient (see Table 6–1, step 3, for an explanation).

It is important not to exhale into the device, especially once the blister has been punctured, because the dose will be lost and humidity may be introduced into the device.

5. *Inhale forcefully and deeply through mouth.* Place the mouthpiece of the Diskhaler® in your mouth between your teeth and seal your lips around it. Be careful not to block the air inlets on either side of the mouthpiece. Inhale as quickly and deeply as you can to ensure that the drug goes directly into your lungs.

Forceful inspiration will break the particles into smaller ones and carry them deep into the lungs.

6. *Remove the device from your mouth and hold breath for 10 seconds.* Remove the Diskhaler® from your mouth. Try to hold your breath for 10 s. If you cannot hold for that long, hold your breath for as long as you can. Breathe out normally. Remember not to exhale into the Diskhaler®

Recent studies demonstrate that a 10-s pause may not be necessary for DPIs because the powder dissolves as soon as there is contact with the mucous membranes.[20] If the patient cannot hold his/her breath for 10 s, ask him/her to try to hold the breath for at least 4 s.

7. *If another dose is required, rotate the dosing wheel to the next full blister and follow steps 2 to 6.* Slide the cartridge out and back in to rotate the drug disk. The disk will advance to the next blister and the number will decrease by one, indicating how many doses you have left. Never use a blister that has been punctured or broken accidentally.

Make sure that the patient punctures the disk only when he/she is ready to inhale the drug. Exposed medication may be exposed to humidity or may be lost.

Patients often require more than one dose. It is important that the patient practice the complete sequence of steps to simulate what he/she must do at home and to ensure that he/she does not forget anything. It is also important for the patient to demonstrate the inhalation technique several times as it can be difficult to master.

8. *Place the protective cover back on the Diskhaler® after use.* Replace the protective cover over the mouthpiece to keep it clean and avoid accidental perforation of the drug disk.

*See Figure 6–7 for illustration of technique: steps 1 through 5.
FRC = functional residual capacity; pMDI = pressurized metered-dose inhaler; DPI = dry powder inhaler.

Care and Maintenance of the Diskhaler®
The Diskhaler® should be replaced every 6 months. Regular checks should be made by the patient to ensure that all pieces are in working order prior to every use. The mouthpiece of the Diskhaler® should be wiped with a clean, dry cloth to prevent moisture from entering the system after each use as it is sensitive to humidity.[17]

After each medication disk is finished, both the internal and external parts of the cartridge should be cleaned using the brush provided by the manufacturer. Patients should be reminded to take note of the expiry dates on each disk and to dispose of those that have expired. Finally, the Diskhaler® should be stored in a dry area.

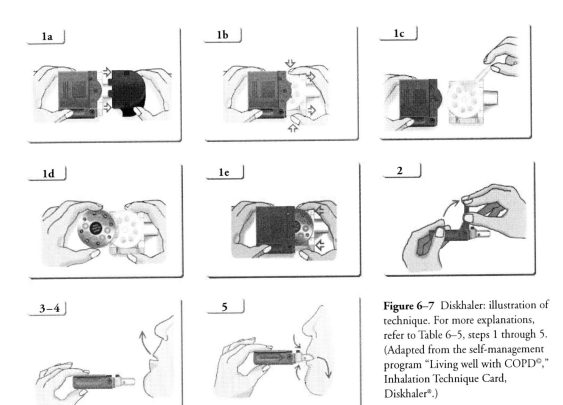

Figure 6–7 Diskhaler: illustration of technique. For more explanations, refer to Table 6–5, steps 1 through 5. (Adapted from the self-management program "Living well with COPD©," Inhalation Technique Card, Diskhaler®.)

Diskus®

Design and Operation

The Diskus® is a new multidose DPI that contains 60 doses of medication in a lactose-based carrier. The Diskus® device currently carries all major classes of inhaled therapy (inhaled corticosteroids, short- and long-acting β_2 agonists, and combination therapy).

The outside of the Diskus® comprises five main parts: an attached cover that slides open, a thumb grip that uncovers the dose-release lever, a mouthpiece, and a dose counter. There are four wheels inside the Diskus® (Figure 6–8). One wheel contains 60 doses of powder medication individually wrapped in blisters on a foil strip. The individual wrapping protects the powder from humidity and other environmental conditions. Sliding the dose-release lever peels the foil off the top of each dose as it is advanced to the mouthpiece. The peeled foil is then wound onto another wheel. The dose is then inhaled, and the empty blister advances to a fourth wheel. Once the Diskus® cover is closed, the lever is automatically returned to the starting position.

The Diskus® provides a relatively consistent dose over a wider range of flow rates than the other DPIs.[56] Inspiratory flow between 30 and 90 L/min ensures delivery of 90% of the dose.[57]

The teaching tools for the Diskus® are presented in Table 6–6 and Figure 6–9.

Care and Maintenance of the Diskus®

The foil blisters protect the medication from humidity and contamination; however, it is important that the device is dry when a dose is being delivered. The mouthpiece of the Diskus® should be wiped with a clean, dry cloth to prevent moisture from entering the system after each use as it is sensitive to humidity.[17] The device should be kept closed when not in use.

The dose-counter window indicates the number of doses left. The numbers from 5 to 0 are indicated in red to remind patients to purchase a new Diskus® before it is empty. The expiry date should be checked and is indicated on the plastic casing.

Conclusion

There are both advantages and disadvantages associated with the use of the various DPIs. All of them share the same important advantage that they do not

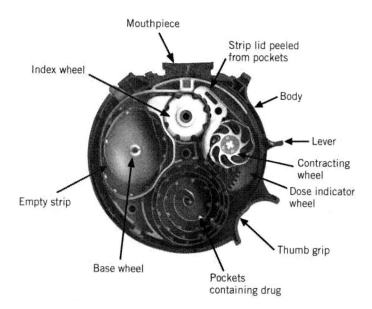

Figure 6–8 Diagram of the Diskus®. (Adapted with permission from GlaxoSmithKline, Canada.)

TABLE 6–6 Teaching Guide: Diskus®*

Steps to Follow (Suggested Demonstration and Detailed Instructions)	Explanations
1. *Open the cover.* Hold the Diskus® flat in one hand and place the thumb of your other hand on the thumb grip. Push the thumb grip away from you toward the back of the Diskus® as far as it will go.	
2. *Slide the lever back.* Hold the Diskus® with the mouthpiece facing you. Slide the lever away from you with your thumb as far back as it will go. You should hear a click.	Sliding the lever back peels the cover off a blister of medication and advances it to the opening in the mouthpiece.
3. *Exhale to FRC, away from the Diskus®.* Exhale normally but not toward or near the Diskus® for two reasons: (a) you could cause the drug dose to blow away; (b) you could introduce humidity into the Diskus®, causing the powder to clump.	Expiration until FRC is sufficient (see Table 6–1, step 3, for an explanation). It is important not to exhale into the device, especially once the blister has been punctured, because the dose will be lost and humidity may be introduced into the device.
4. *Inhale a dose.* Place the mouthpiece between your lips. Inhale steadily and deeply through your mouth to the end breath. The medication will leave a sweet-tasting residue in your mouth.	Ensure that the patient keeps the Diskus flat. This will prevent the patient from losing the dose. The of a full mouthpiece must not be blocked with teeth or lips.
5. *Remove the Diskus® from the mouth and hold breath for 10 seconds.* Remove the Diskus® from your mouth without exhaling. Try to hold your breath for 10 s or for as long as possible, up to 10 s, then exhale normally. Remember not to exhale into the device.	See Table 6–5, step 6, for explanations.

(continues over...)

6. *Close the Diskus® cover.* Close your Diskus®. Put your thumb in the thumb grip and slide the thumb grip back toward you until you hear it click shut. Closing the protective cover over the mouthpiece will keep it clean and dry and automatically return the lever to its starting position ready to deliver another dose.

7. *If another dose is required, follow steps 1 to 6.* If you need more than one dose, you must start by reloading the dose by opening the Diskus® (repeat steps 1 to 6).

Often patients require more than one inhalation. It is important that the patient practice the complete sequence of steps to simulate what he/she must do at home and to ensure that he/she does not forget anything. Be sure to remind the patient to always close the device when finished.

*See Figure 6–9 for illustration of technique: steps 1 through 6.
FRC = functional residual capacity; pMDI = pressurized metered-dose inhaler.

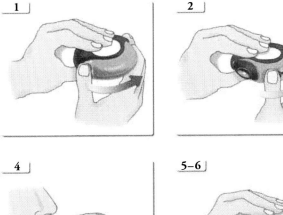
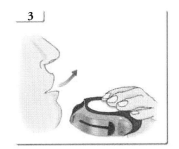
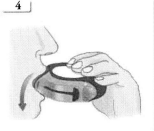
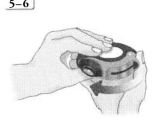

Figure 6–9 Diskus®: illustration of technique. Refer to Table 6–6, steps 1 through 6. (Adapted from "Diskus® Inhaler. Hard to use incorrectly." GlaxoSmithKline, Canada.)

require coordination between actuation and inhalation.[36] Nevertheless, DPIs do require a degree of manual dexterity and a basic understanding of the loading mechanism and the importance of not exhaling into the devices. Studies suggest that the Diskus® is easier to load correctly than either the Turbuhaler® or the Diskhaler®.[58,59] Despite this, there was no significant difference in preference for the Diskus® or the Turbuhaler®. Some subjects preferred the Turbuhaler® because of its smaller size and larger capacity (200 doses). The Diskus®, on the other hand, has a somewhat more precise counting mechanism. The major

disadvantages of the Diskhaler® are that it carries very few doses and requires the highest flows for adequate peripheral deposition. Lactose, the drug carrier used in some DPIs, may be irritating to the upper airways (mouth, throat), thus inducing cough, and also has a taste that some patients find unpleasant.[1] This can, however, be reassuring to many because it signals that they have received their dose.

WET NEBULIZATION

Inhaled medication was delivered most commonly via wet nebulization, until recent years when more efficient portable devices became available. Nebulizers break down measured doses of medication in liquid form into a mist of small droplets, called an aerosol, which can then be inhaled through a mask or a mouthpiece.

Design and Operation

Wet nebulization requires the following:
- An energy source such as a compressor
- Compressed air or oxygen
- A mask or a mouthpiece
- A nebulizer

Compressed air or oxygen is more frequently used in hospitals that have large sources of these gases under pressure. Most patients will use a small portable compressor that is safe and effective for home use. The compressor is powered by electricity and functions by drawing the surrounding air through an external air inlet, forcing it through a small tube to a nebulizer.

In the nebulizer, the driving gas is forced through a very small opening called a Venturi, creating a low-pressure zone (Figure 6–10). As a result of this fall in pressure, the liquid is sucked up from the reservoir through a capillary system, creating droplets.[31] Only the smallest droplets leave the nebulizer, whereas the majority impact on the baffles and walls of the nebulizer and drip back into the reservoir.[36] This process is repeated continuously for several minutes.

During nebulization, the solution used to dilute the medication evaporates resulting in an increasing concentration of the medication. A small amount of solution will remain on the baffles and walls of the

nebulizer (dead volume), even when nebulization continues until no more spray is produced. Because the drug concentration increases during nebulization, up to 50% of the drug may be left in the reservoir.[60]

Several factors will affect drug deposition in the lungs, including the output of the nebulizer and the patient's breathing pattern. Drug output is affected by residual volume and gas flow. The latest nebulizers allow for an initial volume of 2 to 2.5 mL and leave a dead volume of about 0.5 mL.[60] Gas flow affects the size of particles released from the nebulizer and the nebulization time. Studies have shown that optimal flow for most currently used nebulizers is between 6 and 10 L/min. Generally, it takes approximately 5 to 10 minutes to administer 2.5 mL of solution at this flow rate.[61] Breathing should be slow and regular, with an occasional deep breath. Additionally, when inhaling nebulized medication, the patient must learn to breathe through the mouth to reduce drug deposits in the nose and pharynx.

Contrary to popular belief, wet nebulization is not the most effective aerosol delivery system. In fact, only 1 to 5% of the output from most compressed air nebulizers is delivered to the lower branches of the bronchial tree.[62] A large amount of the medication is lost to the air during the exhalation phase because aerosol output is constant during both inspiration and expiration.[60] Medication also lost deposits on the nebulizer walls and baffles, as well as on the mask or mouthpiece and the patient's face. The excessive popularity of nebulizers may be attributable in part to psychological factors. Nebulizers

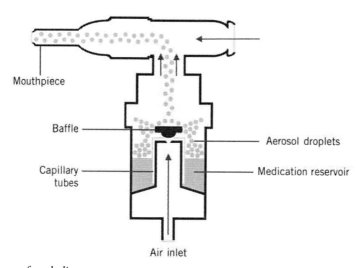

Figure 6–10 Diagram of a nebulizer.

are still widely used in hospitals, and their imposing appearance may suggest to patients that they are receiving the best treatment available.[55]

Many trials have been conducted to compare clinical outcomes (ie, length of stay in the emergency department, spirometric or peak flow measurement, and side effects) of bronchodilator therapy delivered via a pMDI with a spacer and a wet nebulizer. These studies concluded that delivery by either method in the acute treatment of adults with airflow obstruction is equally effective.[63,64] In fact, it has been recommended that pMDIs with spacers replace wet nebulizers for bronchodilator administration in the acute care setting.[55] In hospital settings, some studies have shown that using metered-dose inhalers with holding chambers will probably result in cost savings, mainly related to reduced labor costs.[63]

In the community and for home treatment, wet nebulization is more expensive than treatment with a pMDI and a holding device or other DPIs because of direct costs of medication and equipment. Other disadvantages of wet nebulization include the following: high maintenance requirements, time consuming, noisy, dependent on outside power sources (electricity), and less portable. Furthermore, there is an increased risk of glaucoma when using ipratropium because medication released into the air will come into contact with the eyes.[65]

Close assessment and evaluation of patients who are using a nebulizer at home are essential. Some patients may delay consultation with a physician when they are experiencing an acute crisis because the nebulizer may give them a false sense of security.[66] Furthermore, the typical use of high drug doses in a nebulizer can increase the risk of cardiac complications (angina, rhythm disorders), particularly in elderly patients who are already at risk.[67]

Despite its many drawbacks, the wet nebulization delivery system is still the preferred administration route in some situations. According to the Nebulizer Project Group of the British Thoracic Society Standards of Care Committee[62] and the Quebec Pharmacology Advisory Board,[55] nebulizers are indicated for the following circumstances:

- For those patients who are unable to use other types of inhalation devices, for example, those who suffer from physical or cognitive deficits
- In hospital settings for severe dyspnea and when high doses of medication or oxygen must be administered

Once able to cooperate, individuals should be given another type of inhalation device and their technique should be reassessed.

The teaching tools for the nebulizer are presented in Table 6–7[63,68,69] and Figure 6–11.

Care and Maintenance of Nebulizers

Conscientious care and maintenance of the equipment reduce the risk of infection and increase the life span of the equipment.

Following each use, the nebulizer cup should be disassembled, rinsed, and air-dried to prevent the crystallization of the medication that can clog the nebulizer and thus affect its output. Once a day, the mask or mouthpiece and nebulizer cup should be washed in lukewarm, soapy water, rinsed thoroughly, and air-dried.[62] The nebulizer should be turned on for a few minutes after cleaning to clear the system of water. Various manufacturers recommend that nebulizers should also be periodically disinfected using a solution of water and vinegar.

The mask, nebulizer, tubing, and filter should be replaced regularly according to the manufacturer's recommendation (every 1 to 6 months) or when damaged.

Patients should be sure to have an extra set of the disposable components available at all times in case of equipment failure. They should also have a hand-held inhaler such as a pMDI or DPI with the appropriate medication as a backup. If the compressor begins to make a great deal of noise, runs too slowly, or fails to work, it will need to be repaired. The name and telephone number of the company that supplied the unit should be kept within easy reach to ensure quick repairs or replacement.

WHEN TO REFER

All patients who are prescribed inhaled medications must receive adequate teaching from a knowledgeable physician or allied health professional.

When to Refer to a Respiratory Therapist

If a patient has difficulty mastering a technique or is not responding to treatment, a referral to a respiratory therapist or other knowledgeable health professional may be useful. Improper use of inhaled drug delivery devices is an extremely common problem that frequently results in suboptimal treatment. Even

TABLE 6–7 Teaching Guide: Wet Nebulization*

Steps to Follow (Suggested Demonstration and Detailed Instructions)	Explanations and References
1. *Set up the compressor.* Always make sure that the compressor is resting on a flat, steady surface so that it does not fall. Be careful that none of the air inlets on the sides and back of the compressor are obstructed. Make sure that there is space around it so that it will not overheat. Plug the compressor in.	Placing the unit on a flat, steady surface in compliance with the manufacturer's instructions will prolong the life span of the machine and prevent it from falling and breaking.
2. *Connect the nebulizer to the compressor outlet with the tubing.* Wash your hands. Connect one end of the tubing to the compressor outlet and the other end to the nebulizer inlet port. Make sure that your connections are securely attached and the tubes are in good condition.	It is important that the connections are securely attached and that there are no leaks in the system that may affect nebulizer output.
3. *Prepare medication, place it in the nebulizer cup, and connect the mask or mouthpiece.* Snap off the top of the nebule and squeeze the contents into the nebulizer cup. If you are taking two medications at the same time, pour both into the nebulizer. Block the outlet of the nebulizer and shake to mix the medications. Connect the facemask (or mouthpiece) to the nebulizer cup. Do not open the nebules until ready to use because the medication could evaporate, spill, or become contaminated with bacteria.	Most of the frequently prescribed nebulizer solutions are compatible and therefore can be mixed together in the nebulizer cup as long as the recommended capacity of the nebulizer used is not exceeded. Examples of compatible solutions include salbutamol, ipratropium bromide, and budesonide.[44] It should be noted that some combinations are not recommended, and a pharmacist should be consulted when unsure.
4. *Turn on the compressor and verify output.* While holding the nebulizer upright, turn on the compressor. Check to make sure a fine mist is coming from the mask.	Most compressors are preset at the factory to deliver the optimum flow of 6 to 10 L/min. It is important to verify if the nebulizer output is adequate by observing the mist production. If it is reduced or absent, it could be for several reasons: (1) leaks in the system such as damaged tubing or an improperly closed nebulizer cup; (2) the nebulizer jets may be blocked and the nebulizer needs to be cleaned or replaced; (3) the inlet filter may be blocked and need to be changed; (4) the compressor may need servicing.
5. (a) *Place mask over face or mouthpiece into mouth.* Mask: Place the mask over your nose and mouth. Use the elastic straps to adjust it so that it fits snugly butcomfortably on your face. (b) Mouthpiece: Place the mouthpiece between your teeth and seal your lips around it for the duration of the treatment.	Masks should fit properly to prevent loss of medication. One study demonstrated that if held more than 2 cm away from the face, it will lose 85% of its efficacy in delivering medication.[68] It is worth noting that from the standpoint of efficacy, the mouthpiece is equivalent to a facemask.[69] It can be recommended to use a mouthpiece when taking anticholinergic to prevent these medications from coming into contact with the eyes as it has been found to increase the risk of glaucoma.
6. *Sit upright and breathe normally through mouth, with one deep breath every 10 to 15 breaths, followed by an inspiratory pause of 10 seconds.* Sit upright during treatment because the nebulizer does not work when tilted. Breathe slowly and calmly through your mouth to get the	This breathing method ensures maximum drug distribution within the lungs and reduces the quantity of medication that is deposited within the nose and upper airways.[62]

(continues over...)

most medication deep into your lungs. Every 10 to 15 breaths, take a deep breath and try to hold it for up to 10 seconds if you can or for at least 4 seconds if you cannot. Try not to interrupt your treatment. Avoid pulling the mask away from your face or speaking during the treatment or you will not get your full dose.

7. *Complete the treatment and turn off the compressor. Explain to the patient how to clean and store equipment.* One treatment will take approximately 10 to 15 min. Near the end of the treatment, the nebulizer will begin to splutter. Continue the treatment for 1 more minute, tapping the nebulizer from time to time to knock the droplets clinging to the sides back into the cup. At this point, the mist will have faded. Remove the mask and turn off the compressor. You may notice that a small amount of medication will always remain in the nebulizer cup; this is normal. Do not attempt to run it until dry. Turn off the compressor. Always clean your equipment before putting it away.

Holding the nebulizer upright ensures that the maximum amount of medication will be nebulized because the larger droplets must fall back into the bottom of the nebulizer cup to be nebulized again. See introduction to the nebulizer for details.

The treatment duration for a single dose of medication is approximately 10 min whereas multiple medications may take up to 20 min to administer. The length of treatment duration is often an indicator of the operating condition of the nebulizer and compressor.

Tapping the nebulizer occasionally near the end of the treatment, once the nebulizer begins to splutter, helps to dislodge droplets that are clinging to the walls and baffles and may improve output by up to 50%.[69]

For instructions on cleaning, refer to the previous section. The goal of maintenance is to prevent contamination with microorganisms and to prolong the life of the nebulizer.

*See Figure 6–11 for illustration of technique: steps 1 through 5.

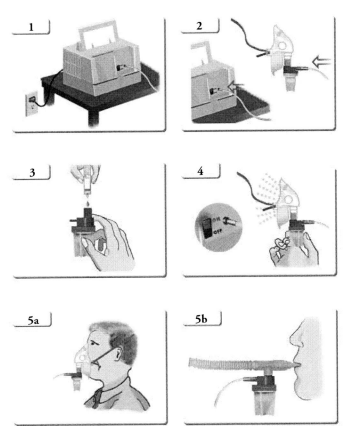

Figure 6–11 Nebulizer: illustration of technique. For more explanations, refer to Table 6–7, steps 1 through 5. (Adapted from the self-management program "Living well with COPD©, Inhalation Technique Card, Nebulizer.")

patients who have been using a device for a long time and have demonstrated adequate technique in the past often contrive to use the device incorrectly because they believe it is as effective.[68,70] Therefore, it is essential to thoroughly assess and review techniques with all patients regularly.

When to Refer to a Physician

Physicians should always supervise the care of patients with COPD; however, front-line health care givers may have more frequent contact with individuals and should alert the physician to potential problems. A physician should be consulted if there is a change in the patient's condition (ie, worsening symptoms despite adequate inhaled drug use, adverse effects, signs of infection, or new symptoms).

SUMMARY

In this chapter we discussed the more commonly found devices presently available on the market. There are approximately 10 to 20 new devices in various stages of development at this time.[14] One of the driving forces behind these changes is the banning of CFC-based propellants from the market. Alternative propellants and propellant-free devices are both options that are being produced and tested. It is expected that Canada will have completed this transition by the year 2005.

There are advantages and disadvantages associated with the various devices. Most are small, portable, and very effective. Pressurized MDIs require good coordination unless accompanied by spacing devices, which some may find inconvenient. Breath-activated devices may require higher inspiratory flow rates and may be difficult for those who have limited capacities. Wet nebulizer systems are cumbersome, expensive, and the least efficient; however, they are often the only choice when patients are unable to use the handheld devices.

The choice of device will depend on the medication prescribed and the abilities of the patient. Furthermore, patients need to be well informed and feel comfortable with the use of the chosen device. Effective delivery of aerosol medication is primarily dependent on correct technique; therefore, it is essential that health professionals keep up to date and proficient with all delivery systems.

CASE STUDY

Mr. Cope is a 65-year-old man who was diagnosed 2 months previously with COPD. He returns to the clinic for his follow-up appointment accompanied by his wife.

Medical History, Physical Examination, Test Results

Medical History

- The patient complains of shortness of breath on mild exertion, such as walking in the apartment, taking his shower, or dressing.
- He is an ex-smoker who smoked approximately 20 cigarettes a day for 50 years.
- The patient was prescribed ipratropium bromide and salbutamol, two puffs four times a day.
- He complains that he has not felt any improvement in his shortness of breath since starting his medication 2 months ago; he claims that the only thing that seems to help him is medication taken by nebulizer, such as the ones he received in hospital.

Physical Examination

- Physical examination is compatible with COPD and shows no evidence of other significant disease or change since his previous visit.

Test Results

- The spirometry results are compatible with moderate airflow obstruction without significant reversibility. Tests repeated today show no change from the initial visit. The spirometry results are as follows:
  Forced expiratory volume in 1 second (FEV_1)— pre- bronchodilator (BD): 1.50 L (55% of predicted normal).
  — postBD: 1.65 L
  Forced vital capacity (FVC)—pre BD: 3.00 L (101% of predicted normal)
  —postBD: 3.10 L
  FEV_1/FVC ratio: 50%

Questions and Discussion

There is no improvement of patient's symptoms from the previous examinaion. You suspect that the lack of improvement in symptoms may be related to inadequate use of the inhaled medication. How should you proceed?

Assess Knowledge of Medication and Adherence to Prescription

- Is he following the prescribed doses and frequency?
- Does he understand when and under what circumstances he should be using his medications?
- Does he understand how his medications work?
- Are his puffers empty or out of date? Does he know how to verify this?

Assessment revealed that his knowledge was adequate and that he was indeed following his medication schedule correctly.

Assess the Patient's Pressurized Metered-Dose Inhaler

Is his technique effective? Have him demonstrate with a placebo.

His technique was found to be ineffective because he was unable to coordinate the actuation of the pump with his inspiration. It was also discovered that he had difficulty depressing the pump because of arthritis in his hands. His wife explained that sometimes she helped him but was worried that he could not take his medication when she was not around. She asked if a nebulizer would be the solution.

How Would You and the Couple Resolve These Issues?

They were informed that because of incorrect pMDI technique, the medication was not getting to his lungs, and this is why he felt that the nebulizer gave him more relief than the pMDI. It was also explained that the nebulizer often seems more effective because higher doses of the same medications are used. Advantages and disadvantages of the nebulizer versus the pMDI were discussed. It was pointed out to the couple that assembling and loading a nebulizer can be quite difficult for somebody with weak hands, and the patient would be more likely to require assistance with this system than with his pMDIs.

Explore Possible Solutions

A DPI may be easier to use in this case because it eliminates coordination problems and may be easier to manipulate. At the present time, however, ipratropium bromide is only available in pMDI. To avoid error and confusion, it is often preferable to give patients only one type of delivery system to learn if possible. In this case, it was decided to add a valved spacer device that fits both inhalers to resolve the coordination problems and to modify his grip to accomodate the weakness in his hands.

It was found that by using both hands together, the patient was able to activate the pMDIs without too much difficulty. The single-breath technique with the valved spacer device was explained. The educator then demonstrated the modified technique, using two hands on the pump while the spacer was held between the teeth. After practicing both by himself and with his wife's assistance, he expressed confidence in this solution and decided to give it a try.

Care and maintenance of the new device were taught. The patient was given education material to review at home. An appointment was scheduled to re-evaluate the effectiveness of the treatment and his technique.

ACKNOWLEDGMENTS

We would like to thank Vitalie Parreault, RN, MSc and William C. Boyle, B.Sc, RRT for their invaluable contributions.

KEY POINTS

- Health professionals must keep abreast of new devices and master the techniques themselves.
- Work with patients to choose the device that best suits their needs and preferences.
- Demonstration, practice, and repetition are the most effective approach to ensure correct technique.
- Written material should be provided to reinforce techniques.
- Understanding how their device works and why each step is important may help patients to be motivated to maintain correct technique.
- Follow-up and periodic re-evaluation by the patient and educator are essential.
- Pressurized MDIs are gas-propelled devices, and inhalation should be slow.
- Dry powder inhalers are breath activated and require an inspiratory effort.
- Patients who encounter coordination difficulties should use a pMDI with a spacer device or a DPI.

REFERENCES

1. Ernst P. Inhaled drug delivery: a practical guide to prescribing inhaler devices. Can Respir J 1998;5: 180–3.
2. American Association for Respiratory Care. Aerosol consensus statement. Respir Care 1991;36:916–21.
3. Burton G, Hodgkin JE, Ward J. Respiratory care: a guide to clinical practice. 3rd Ed. Philadelphia: JB Lippincott, 1992.
4. Dolovich M. Clinical aspects of aerosol physics. Respir Care 1991;36:931–8.
5. Hanania NA, Wittman R, Kesten S, Chapman KR. Medical personnel's knowldge of and ability to use inhaling devices. Metered-dose inhalers, spacing chambers, and breath-actuated dry powder inhalers. Chest 1994;105:111–6.
6. Goodman DE, Isreal E, Rosenberg M, et al. The influence of age, diagnosis and gender on proper use of metered-dose inhalers. Am J Respir Crit Care Med 1994;150:1256–61.
7. Van Beerendonk I, Mesters I, Mudde AN, Tan TD. Assessment of the inhalation technique in outpatients with asthma or chronic obstructive pulmonary disease using a metered-dose inhaler or dry powder device. J Asthma 1998;35:273–9.
8. De Blaquiere P, Christensen DB, Carter WB, Martin TR. Use and misuse of metered-dose inhalers by patients with chronic lung disease. Am Rev Respir Dis 1989;140:910–6.
9. Crompton GK. The adult patient's difficulties with inhalers. Lung 1990;Suppl 168:658–62.
10. Nimmo CJ, Chen DN, Matinusen SM, et al. Assessment of patient acceptance and inhalation technique of a pressurized aerosol inhaler and two breath-actuated devices. Ann Pharmacother 1993;27: 922–7.
11. Kesten S, Zive K, Chapman KR. Pharmacist knowledge and ability to use inhaled medication delivery systems. Chest 1993;104:1737–42.
12. Guidry GG, Brown WD, Stogner SW, Geroge RB. Incorrect use of metered dose inhalers by medical personnel. Chest 1992;101:1256–61.
13. Jackevicius CA, Chapman KR. Inhaler education for hospital based pharmacists: how much is required? Can Respir J 1999;6:23744.
14. Dolovich M. New delivery systems and propellants. Can Respir J 1999;6:290–5.
15. Wilson AF. Aerosol delivery systems. In: Weiss EB, Stein M, eds. Bronchial asthma mechanisms and therapeutics. Toronto, ON: Little Brown and Company, 1993:749–55.
16. Jackson WF. Inhalers in asthma. The new perspective. Oxfordshire, UK: Clinical Visions, 1995.
17. Ganderton D. General factors influencing drug delivery to the lung. Respir Med 1991;Suppl A(91):13–6.
18. Beaupré A, Boucher S, Boulet LP, et al. L'aérosolthérapie. Position officielle de l'Association des pneumologues de la province de Québec. Union Med Can 1986; 115:799–802.
19. Epstein SW, Manning CP, Ashley MJ, Corey PN. Survey of the clinical use of pressurized aerosol inhalers. Can Med Assoc J 1979;120:813–6.
20. Kelcher S, Brownoff R. Teaching residents to use asthma devices. Assessing family residents' skills and a brief intervention. Can Fam Physician 1994;40:2090–5.
21. QVAR™ 50µ and 100µ product monograph. London, ON: 3M Pharmaceuticals, 2000.
22. Schultz R. Drug delivery characteristics of metered-dose inhalers. J Allergy Clin Immunol 1995;96:285–7.
23. Kacmarek RM, Hess D. The interface between patient and aerosol generator. Respir Care 1991;36:952–76.
24. Newman SP, Pavia D, Clarke SW. How should a pressurized beta-adrenergic bronchodilator be inhaled? Eur J Respir Dis 1981;62:3–21.
25. American Thoracic Society. Comprehensive outpatient managment of COPD. Am J Respir Crit Care Med 1995;152:S84–S110.
26. Newhouse MT, Dolovitch M. Control of asthma by aerosols. N Engl J Med 1986;315:870–4.
27. Seale JP, Harrison LI. Effect of changing the fine particle mass of inhaled beclomethasone dipropionate on intrapulmonary deposition and pharmacokinetics. Respir Med 1998;92 Suppl A:9–15.
28. Crompton GK. Problems patients have using pressurized aerosol inhalers. Eur J Respir Dis 1982;63 Suppl 119:101–4.
29. MacIntyre NR, et al. Aerosol consensus statement. Chest 1991;100:1106–9.

30. Barry PW, O'Callaghan C. Multiple actuations of salbutamol MDI into a space device reduces the amount of drugs recovered in the respirable range. Eur Respir J 1994;7:1707–1709.

31. Hess D. Comprehensive respiratoy care. In: Dantzker DR, MacIntyre NR, Bakow ED, eds. Aerosol therapy. Philadelphia: WB Saunders, 1995;539–60.

32. Boulet LP, d'Amours P, Bérubé D, et al. Mise à jour sur l'inhalothérapie dans l'asthme et les bronchopneumopathies obstructives. Union Med Can 1994;123: 23–31.

33. Dolovich M, Ruffin R, Corr D, Newhouse M. Clinical evaluation of a simple demand inhalation MDI aerosol delivery device. Chest 1983;84:36–41.

34. Ahrens R, Lux C, Bahl T, Han SH. Choosing the metered dose inhaler spacer or holding chamber that matches the patient's need: evidence that the specific drug being delivered is an important consideration. J Allergy Clin Immunol 1995;96:288–94.

35. Barry PW, O'Callaghan C. Inhalational drug delivery from seven different spacer devices. Thorax 1996;51: 835–40.

36. Pedersen S. Inhalers and nebulizers: which to choose and why. Respir Med 1996;90:69–77.

37. Conseil consultatif de pharmacologie GdQ. Les bronchopneumopathies obstructive chroniques et l'emploi des bronchodilatateurs chez les personnes agées. Québec: Ministère de la santé et des services sociaux, info-médicament, 1997.

38. British Thoracic Society. The British Guidelines on Asthma Management. 1995 review and position statement. Thorax 1997;52 Suppl 1:S1–S21.

39. Barnes PJ, Pedersen S. Efficacy and safety of inhaled corticosteroids in asthma. Report of a workshop held in Eze, France, October 1992. Am J Respir Crit Care Med 1993;148(Suppl 14, part 2):S1–S26.

40. Gervais AJG, Bégin P. L'aérosolthérapie: pour respirer librement. Clinicien 1990;41–50.

41. Fink JB. Metered-dose inhalers, dry powder inhalers, and transitions. Respir Care 2000;45:623–35.

42. Piérart F, Wildhaber JH, Vrancken I, et al. Washing plastic spacers in household detergent reduces electrostatic charge and greatly imroves delivery. Eur Respir J 1999;13:673–8.

43. The Montreal Protocol. The Montreal protocol on substances that deplete the ozone layer. Final act (Nairobi: UNEP, 1987). Fed Reg 1994;59:56276–98.

44. Kelcher S, Elliott R, Fatum DA, et al. Inhalation devices for obstructive lung disease. A pharmacist's guide to meeting the challenge of patient education. Pegasus Healthcare International Publication: Canadian Pharmaceutical Association, 1996.

45. Crompton GK. Turbuhaler inhalation system. A clinical monograph. Oxford, UK: Oxford Clinical Communications, 1993.

46. Newman SP, Morèn F, Trofast E, et al. Terbutaline sulphate Turbuhaler: effect of inhaled flowrate on drug deposition and efficacy. Int J Pharm 1991;74:209.

47. Tonnesen F, Laursen LC, Evald T, et al. Bronchodilating effect of terbutaline powder in acute severe bronchial obstruction. Chest 1994;105:697–700.

48. Dolovich M, Vanzieleghem M, Hidingerk KG, Newhouse MT. Influence of inspiratory flow rate on the response to terbutaline sulphate inhaled via the Turbuhaler. Am Rev Respir Dis 1988;137:A433.

49. Lindsay DA, Russel NL, Thompson JE, et al. A multicentre comparison of the efficacy of terbutaline turbuhaler and salbutamol pressurized metered dose inhaler in hot, humid regions. Eur Respir J 1994;7: 342–5.

50. Nielsen K, Okamoto L, Shah T. Importance of selected inhaler characteristics and acceptance of a new breath-actuated powder inhalation device. J Asthma 1997;34: 249–53.

51. Meades C, Chucher KM, Palmer JBD. An evaluation of the ease of handling the Diskhaler® dry powder inhaler by asthmatic patients. Eur J Clin Res 1992; 3:43–50.

52. Borgström L, Bondesson E, Morén F, et al. Lung deposition of budesonide inhaled via turbuhaler: a comparison with terbutaline sulphate in normal subjects. Eur Respir J 1994;7:69–73.

53. Biddiscombe M, Marriot RJ, Melchor R, et al. The preparation and evaluation of pressurized metered-dose and dry-powder inhalers containing 99mTc labelled salbutamol. J Aerosol Med 1991;4 Suppl 1:9.

54. Melchor R, Biddiscombe MF, Mak VH, et al. Lung deposition patterns of directly labelled salbutamol in normal subjects and in patients with reversible airflow obstruction. Thorax 1993;48:506–11.

55. Conseil consultatif de pharmacologie GdQ. L'aérosolthérapie dans le traitement de l'asthme et des autres bronchopneumopathies obstructives. Québec: Ministère de la santé et des services sociaux, info-médicament, 1995.

56. Bisgaard H, Klug B, Sumby BS, Burnell PK. Fine particle mass from the Diskus inhaler and Turbuhaler inhaler in children with asthma. Eur Respir J 1998;11:1111–5.

57. Dhand R, Fink J. Dry powder inhalers. Respir Care 1999;44:940–51.

58. Van der Palen J, Klein JJ, Schildkamp AM. Comparison of a new multidose powder inhaler (Diskus - Accuhaler) and the Turbuhaler regarding preference and ease of use. J Asthma 1998;35:147–52.

59. Pieters WR, Stallaert RA, Prins J, et al. A study on the clinical equivalence and patient preference of fluticasone propionate 250 microg twice daily via the Diskus™/ Accuhaler™ inhaler or the Diskhaler™ inhaler in adult asthmatic patients. J Asthma 1998; 35:337–45.

60. O'Callaghan C, Barry PW. The science of nebulised drug delivery. In: Muers MF, Corris PA, eds. Current best practice for nebulizer treatment. The Nebuliser Project Group of the British Thoracic Society Standards of Care Committee. Thorax 1997;52 Suppl 2:S31–S44.

61. Muers MF, Corris PA, eds. Summary of nebulizer guidelines for general practitionners. Current best practice for nebulizer treatment. The nebulizer project group of the British Thoracic Society Standards of Care Committee. Thorax 1997;52 Suppl 2:S20–1.

62. Johnson CE. Principles of nebulizer-delivered drug therapy for asthma. Am J Hosp Pharm 1989;46: 1845–55.

63. Camargo CAJ, Kenney PA. Assessing cost of aerosol therapy. Respir Care 2000;45:756–63.

64. Idris AH, McDermott MF, Raucci JC, et al. Emergency department treatment of severe asthma. Metered-dose inhaler plus holding chamber is equivalent in effectiveness to nebulizer. Chest 1993;103:665–72.

65. Canadian Pharmacists Association. Compendium of pharmaceuticals and speacialties. 36th Ed. Toronto, ON: Webcom Ltd, 2001;157.

66. O'Driscoll BR. Nebulizer for chronic obstructive airwarys disease. In: Muers MF, Corris PA, eds. Current best practice for nebulizer treatment. The Nebulizer Project Group of the British Thoracic Society Standards of Care Committee. Thorax 1997;52 Suppl 2:S49–52.

67. Pounsford JC. Nebulizers for the elderly. In: Muers MF, Corris PA, eds. Current best practice for nebulizer treatment. The Nebulizer Project Group of the British Thoracic Society Standards of Care Committee. Thorax 1997;52 Suppl 2:S53–5.

68. Everard ML, Devadason SG, Summers QA, Le souef PN. Factors affecting total and 'respirable' dose delivered by a salbutamol metered dose inhaler. Thorax 1995;50:746–9.

69. Kendrick AH, Smith EC, Wilson RSE. Selecting and using nebulizer equipment. In: Muers MF, Corris PA, eds. Current best practice for nebulizer treament. The Nebuliser Project Group of the British Thoracic Society Standards of Care Committee. Thorax 1997;52 Suppl 2:S92–S101.

70. Everard ML. Aerosol therapy past, present, and future: a clinician's persepective. Respir Care 2000;45: 769–76.

SUGGESTED READINGS

Respir Care J 2000;45(June). *This volume is dedicated to aerosol therapy and explores a wide range of pertinent topics, including future technologies.*

Abley C. Teaching elderly patients how to use inhalers. A study to evaluate an education programme on inhaler technique, for elderly patients. J Adv Nurs 1997;25: 699–708. *Discusses the difficulties commonly encountered by elderly patients, who make up a large part of the COPD population.*

Ernst P. Inhaled drug delivery: a practical guide to prescribing inhaler devices. Can Respir J 1998;5:180–3. *Concise guide to choosing the appropriate device.*

LONG–TERM OXYGEN TREATMENT

David Stubbing, Alain Beaupre,
and Reny Vaughan

OBJECTIVES

The general objective of this chapter is to help allied health care professionals understand the rationale behind and the safe use of long-term oxygen therapy (LTOT) in patients with chronic obstructive pulmonary disease (COPD). It is important that the health care practitioner teach this knowledge to patients who experience breathlessness so that they can understand why the use of oxygen may or may not be required in their situation.

After reading this chapter, the physician and the allied health care professional will be able to
- understand the use of oxygen and its role in stable patients with COPD;
- know how to assess oxygenation at rest, with exercise, and during sleep;
- prescribe the correct dose of oxygen;
- prescribe the best oxygen delivery system for the patient;
- teach the patient the role of oxygen and how to use it safely; and
- refer to specific professionals from the health care team when needed.

Hypoxemia is a common occurrence in patients with pulmonary impairment caused by COPD. The presence and severity of hypoxemia correlate with the severity of pulmonary impairment[1]; however, the relationships between hypoxemia and the severity of breathlessness,[2] degree of disability,[2] and impact on quality of life[3,4] all appear to be weak. Chronic hypoxemia does have clinical effects, some of which may be improved by treatment with oxygen. As COPD is largely irreversible and medication may have limited effects on respiratory symptoms such as dyspnea, oxygen is often sought by patients, family members, and health professionals when breathlessness occurs, even if hypoxemia is not present. Readily available measurements of oxyhemoglobin saturation (SpO_2) have aggravated the problem by generating a measure of oxygenation that many feel needs correction, when it is abnormal, even if there is no clinical rationale.

Although LTOT has been shown to have a number of physiologic benefits and is one of the few interventions that improves survival in selected patients with COPD,[5,6] it is not always effective in altering breathlessness, improving exercise capacity, or changing quality of life. Because oxygen is a prescription medication with attendant risks as well as possible benefits, the chronic use of it should be reserved for situations for which benefit has been clearly delineated.

In this chapter, we review the mechanisms and effects of hypoxemia, assessment and rationale for therapeutic intervention with LTOT, and oxygen delivery systems available.

MECHANISMS OF HYPOXEMIA

Although not all patients with COPD develop gas exchange abnormalities, the airway narrowing and lung destruction present often result in mismatching of ventilation (V) and perfusion (Q), that is, V/Q mismatch causing hypoxemia. Multiple inert gas studies show that V/Q mismatch is the most frequent and most important cause of hypoxemia in COPD.[7] Other possible causes of hypoxemia in some individuals include diffusion abnormality, true right to left venous to arterial shunt, and areas in the lung where V/Q is 0, which acts like a shunt. Alveolar hypoventilation or the low FIO_2 of altitude may aggravate the hypoxemia in patients. The hypoxemia may also be aggravated by a low mixed venous PO_2, for example, secondary to a low cardiac output, which will magnify the effect of V/Q mismatch on arterial oxygen tension.[8]

In the absence of sleep apnea, a worsening of hypoxemia with sleep is probably attributable to a worsening of the V/Q mismatch,[9] accompanied by alveolar hypoventilation.[10] Hypoxemia seems to be most marked at the onset of sleep and during rapid eye movement (REM) sleep. At the onset of sleep, alveolar ventilation often decreases, causing an increase in $PaCO_2$.[10] In addition, a change in V/Q relationships will also occur if part of the tidal volume falls below closing volume,[8] the lung volume at which airways to the dependent areas of the lung close. This is particularly likely to happen if functional residual capacity falls when individuals assume a supine position.[11] Hypoventilation and change in V/Q relationships in the lung also occur during REM sleep.[10]

Studies using the multiple inert gas method also indicate that V/Q mismatch does not usually change significantly during exercise.[7,12] Similarly, the degree of shunt, defined in these studies as areas of the lung where V/Q was 0, plus true venous to arterial shunt, does not change significantly in most patients with COPD.[7] Worsening hypoxemia during exercise is probably caused by a combination of a rise in arterial PCO_2 and a fall in mixed venous PO_2. Mixed venous PO_2 will fall if the cardiac output does not increase to the same extent as the oxygen consumption, even if V/Q mismatch remains unchanged. A fall in mixed venous PO_2 will aggravate the effects of the V/Q abnormality.[8] Similarly, $PaCO_2$ will rise if ventilation does not increase to the same extent as CO_2 production. This will reduce alveolar oxygen tension (PAO_2) and thereby affect PaO_2 even if the relationship between ventilation and perfusion is stable. The simplified alveolar gas equation

$$PAO_2 = P_IO_2 - PaCO_2/R$$

where P_IO_2 = partial pressure of inspired oxygen and R = respiratory exchange ratio, explains the relationship between $PaCO_2$, P_IO_2, and PAO_2. A higher

$PaCO_2$ will result in a lower alveolar oxygen tension. In addition, as $PaCO_2$ rises, a steady state no longer exists. Therefore, R falls, and this also impacts alveolar oxygen tension, thereby decreasing PaO_2.

In some individuals, hypoxemia during exercise may be worsened by true diffusion impairment or by the opening of a patent foramen ovale when pulmonary artery, right ventricular, and right atrial pressure increase, which occurs with the increase in cardiac output.

EFFECTS OF CHRONIC HYPOXEMIA

There are several well-defined physiologic and clinical effects of chronic hypoxemia (Figure 7–1). Perhaps the most significant ones are the result of vasoconstriction of the pulmonary vessels causing an increase in pulmonary vascular resistance (PVR).[13] If cardiac output is maintained, pulmonary artery pressure (PAP) increases. In the presence of chronic hypoxemia caused by COPD, pulmonary artery hypertension, right ventricular dilatation, and overt cor pulmonale may ensue.[14]

Polycythemia is another result of chronic hypoxemia,[15] and a high hemoglobin should be an indication of the need to assess for oxygenation with sleep and exercise. However, only when the hematocrit increases beyond 55 to 60% does blood viscosity affect perfusion of the major organs.[16]

Other possible effects of chronic hypoxemia are less well defined. Nevertheless, chronic airflow limitation is now recognized as a multisystem disease,[17] and it is possible that the peripheral muscle impairment, nutritional abnormalities, neurologic and cognitive problems, and endocrine changes are to some extent the result of chronic hypoxemia.

The major clinical manifestation of COPD is breathlessness, most prominent with exertion. However, the degree of breathlessness does not usually correlate with the presence or severity of hypoxemia. In the laboratory setting, ventilation increases with induced hypoxemia; however, breathlessness with exertion is more closely related to the work required of the respiratory muscles and the capacity of those muscles to generate force when contraction occurs.[18] The degree of breathlessness does not correlate well with the presence or severity of hypoxemia. Therefore, supplemental oxygen is not the initial treatment for breathlessness even if hypoxemia is present.

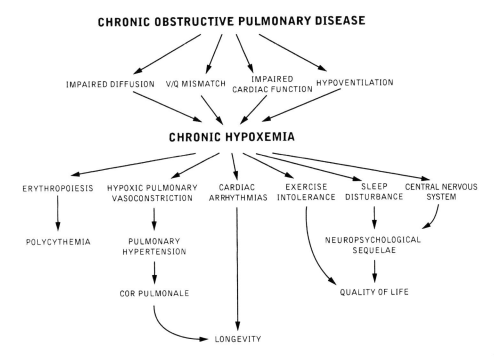

Figure 7–1 Schematic representation of the relationship between chronic obstructive lung disease, hypoxemia, and end organ effects.

ASSESSMENT OF HYPOXEMIA

Measurement of arterial blood gases remains the gold standard for assessing arterial oxygenation. Although this method is the standard for most jurisdictions when determining the need for long-term oxygen therapy,[19–25] the measurement is not practical in many patients, particularly when assessing nocturnal or exercise oxygenation. Noninvasive methods to assess oxygenation using photoplethysmography and spectrophotometry via an oximeter probe are more often used to obtain a continuous measure of oxygenation. Spectrophotometry is used to determine the amounts of oxyhemoglobin and deoxyhemoglobin, whereas photoplethysmography assesses pulse rate.[26] The data obtained are used to calculate a measure of SpO_2. Portable pulse oximeters are accurate ($\pm$ 2 to 4%), particularly when SpO_2 is greater than 80%.[27] Oximeter readings may be less accurate when skin pigmentation is dark.[28] Ambient light,[29] poor peripheral blood flow,[30] certain nail lacquers,[31] and some intravascular dyes[32] may alter light transmission and affect the accuracy of oximeter readings. Elevated carboxyhemoglobin and methemoglobin levels may also affect the accuracy of observed measurements.[30] Some newer models of oximeters use a motion artifact reduction system, which is important when blood flow (pulse volume) is low or when movement occurs frequently, as with exercise.

If the use of long-term oxygen therapy is being considered, oximetry should be used to measure oxygenation continuously during sleep and to determine the appropriate dose of oxygen to prescribe. The patient should sleep overnight with the oximeter probe in place, from which a graphic display of continuous nocturnal oxygenation can be obtained. The testing should be repeated to determine the correct dose of oxygen to prescribe.

If the use of long-term oxygen therapy is being considered, oximetry should be used to assess oxygenation during exercise and the most appropriate dose of oxygen for that individual. Measurements made during steady-state exercise are the most appropriate for determining the dose of oxygen for individuals when they undertake activity or exercise.

Several different methods of exercise have been proposed. Steady-state exercise on either a treadmill or a cycle ergometer, at approximately 60% of the individual's maximum exercise capacity, may be used. However, most patients use oxygen therapy just for ambulation; therefore, we have developed and tested a self-paced walk test where oxygenation is assessed continuously with the individual walking at a pace similar to one they would choose to use outside the home.[33] The traditional maximum 6-minute walk test, which is used as an outcome measure for pulmonary rehabilitation, is less suitable to determine oxygen dose for exercise as it is a maximum exercise test, not steady-state exercise.[34]

MANAGEMENT OF CHRONIC HYPOXEMIA

Principles Of Long-Term Oxygen Therapy

The aim of long-term oxygen therapy should be to prevent or reverse the complications of chronic hypoxemia. Oxygen, however, should be only one part of a comprehensive program of care that also includes other prescription medications, exercise, nutrition, psychosocial adjustment, and education. In patients with COPD, specialist referral should be sought, particularly if the use of LTOT is considered.

When LTOT is prescribed, the dose of oxygen used should aim to increase PaO_2 to approximately 60 mm Hg or SpO_2 to approximately 90%. Different doses or flow rates may be needed for rest, sleep, activity, and exercise. However, because of the risk of inducing or aggravating hypercapnia, care must be taken to ensure that the dose is the lowest required to achieve the goal of correcting hypoxemia. Dose-response curves of the oxygen's effect on hypoxemia should be performed during rest, during sleep, by monitoring nocturnal oximetry, and during exercise comparable to activities usually performed during daily living.

The results of the British Medical Research Council (MRC) Working Party Study[5] and the North American Nocturnal Oxygen Therapy Trial (NOTT)[6] indicate that in the presence of chronic hypoxemia, LTOT should be used for at least 15 continuous hours a day. Using oxygen for sleep alone may not result in any clinical benefit, and oxygen used only when breathlessness occurs is not justified and possible more deleterious than beneficial.

Oxygen may be delivered to the respiratory system at the nose by nasal cannulae, at the oropharynx by a mask, or directly to the trachea by a transtracheal catheter. Controlled oxygen, which provides a constant FIO_2, applied with a mask using the Venturi principle, is the safest method of delivering oxygen to patients, particularly during sleep and in those with an elevated $PaCO_2$. There is less likelihood of an increase in $PaCO_2$ using controlled oxygen than with uncontrolled oxygen applied by nasal cannulae.[35]

An oxygen prescription should include the dose required for resting, sleeping, activity, and exercise. It should also include the duration of use each day, the delivery mechanism both for in-home use and ambulatory oxygen, and the method of application to the respiratory tract whether it is by mask or nasal cannulae. If oxygen-conserving devices or pulsed-dose delivery systems are to be used, dose-finding assessment is required for each patient during rest, sleep, and activity as pulsed-dose units may not provide oxygenation equivalent to continuous flow.[36,37]

Eligibility for funding for long-term oxygen therapy is based on the presence of chronic hypoxemia when patients are optimally treated and free of exacerbation. Nevertheless, in the move toward ambulatory care and a reduction in the length of hospital stays, patients hospitalized for exacerbations of COPD are now being discharged even when their condition is not completely stabilized and they continue to present with significant hypoxemia. It is often felt necessary to prescribe oxygen for these patients at the time of discharge from hospital. If oxygen is to be prescribed for acute use during the recovery phase of an exacerbation, it should be made clear that this is for different reasons than LTOT. The physician, the patient, and the funding source should all be aware that the oxygen is being provided for acute use, hopefully during a short recovery period. Therefore, if oxygen is not discontinued once the patient has recovered from the exacerbation, a reassessment for LTOT is appropriate 2 to 3 months after the initiation of acute home oxygen. If these precautions are not in place, many patients feel dependent on oxygen, and inappropriate long-term use becomes difficult to avoid. Guyatt and colleagues recently assessed patients on LTOT and found that approximately 40% of these patients did not meet eligibility criteria for funding.[38] Many of these patients were probably started on oxygen during an acute exacerbation. Eligibility for LTOT may not have been reassessed when they were clinically stable.

Criteria For Funding Long-Term Oxygen Therapy

General Requirements

Before starting long-term oxygen therapy, the patient should be evaluated by a respirologist to optimize medical treatment and to ensure that hypoxemia is chronic and cannot be corrected otherwise. In collaboration with the patient's attending physician, the patient should be re-evaluated at least once a year by a respirologist to monitor the progress of the disease and the treatment received.

The patient must agree to have home oxygen and comply with the treatment by respecting the medical prescription, particularly the oxygen flow rate, as well as the daily duration of oxygen therapy. The patient must also agree to do minor maintenance on the equipment and to have maintenance visits at home, which are necessary to ensure that the equipment functions correctly. The patient's immediate family should also agree to have the oxygen equipment in the home. The patient's physical environment at home must be such that the equipment can be safely installed, with both the patient and family agreeing to respect the basic safety instructions (Table 7–1).

Specific Criteria

The prescription of LTOT is closely monitored and controlled in most health care jurisdictions. In Canada, provincial ministries of health monitor applications for LTOT and provide funding for those who meet eligibility criteria. The eligibility criteria for funding of LTOT is based on evidence from clinical trials. These criteria are similar in most provinces of Canada and in most other health care jurisdictions (Table 7–2).[19-25]

TABLE 7–1 Oxygen Do's and Don'ts

Description	Do's	Don'ts
Approximately 21% oxygen is naturally found in the air we breathe. It is clear, tasteless, and odorless. It is nonflammable; however, it does support combustion. This means that what may not usually burn in room air will burn in the presence of oxygen or what normally burns will burn much more violently. Oxygen is a safe drug as long as safety guidelines are followed.	Use your oxygen as directed by your doctor. Aim to use your oxygen for a minimum of 15 hours continuous. Clean or change your equipment regularly. Notify your provider if you have any concerns about your equipment. Notify your provider if your prescription is changed. Store your oxygen equipment safely and securely; always ensure the unit cannot fall or tip over. Visibly place a no smoking—oxygen in use sign. Keep your oxygen in a well-ventilated area. Only use water-based lubricants if your nose becomes dry (must not contain oils, ie, Vaseline). Allow only trained individuals to operate the oxygen equipment. Keep a fire extinguisher in your home. Plug concentrators directly to a grounded outlet; when possible use a separate circuit. Ensure cylinders are secure. Carry a spare battery if you use a conserving device that requires one.	Don't adjust the oxygen dose without a prescription from your doctor. Don't permit oil, grease, aerosol sprays, or any other flammable materials to come in contact with oxygen. Don't allow smoking of any kind in the area where oxygen is stored. Don't allow electrical equipment within 5 feet of the oxygen system. Don't allow heat sources or open flames to come within 5 feet of the oxygen. Don't store the oxygen near sources of heat (radiators, fireplaces, ovens, base heaters) Don't attempt to repair the oxygen equipment.

TABLE 7–2 Eligibility Criteria for Long-Term Oxygen Therapy

General Requirements	Specific Criteria	Eligible in Some Jurisdictions
Chronic airflow limitation 　Clinically stable 　Optimal medical treatment 　Nonsmoking	Resting PaO_2 55 mm Hg or less Resting PaO_2 56–60 mm Hg with polycthemia or cor pulmonale as shown by 　P pulmonale 　Edema 　Pulmonary artery hypertension 　Polycythemia	Resting PaO_2 56–60 mm Hg If nocturnal hypoxemia (usually > 30% of the night) or exercise hypoxemia*

*For exercise hypoxemia, oxygen must correct hypoxemia and improve exercise endurance and/or breathlessness with exertion.

Funding is usually provided if resting PaO_2 is 55 mm Hg or less in a stable patient who is receiving optimal therapy. Optimal therapy should include smoking cessation, and stability is usually defined as a patient being free of exacerbation of COPD for at least 3 months.

In the presence of cor pulmonale (as shown by P pulmonale on an electrocardiogram [ECG], edema, or right ventricular dysfunction or dilatation), pulmonary artery hypertension, or polycythemia, funding is also available if resting PaO_2 is greater than 55 mm Hg and not more than 60 mm Hg.

When PaO_2 at rest is greater than 55 mm Hg and not more than 60 mm Hg, a patient may also be eligible for funding when SpO_2 is less than 88% during exercise or sleep. For exercise hypoxemia, most jurisdictions require that oxygen be shown to correct the hypoxemia and to increase exercise endurance.

Special application is required for LTOT if resting PaO_2 is greater than 60 mm Hg. Certain individuals with prolonged nocturnal hypoxemia in the absence of sleep apnea may receive funding. Exercise-induced hypoxemia alone may also be an appropriate indication if oxygen corrects hypoxemia, increases exercise endurance, and decreases symptoms. The effects of oxygen for exercise hypoxemia are variable, and individualized testing will help determine who will benefit. It is important not to further disable or handicap individuals by prescribing long-term oxygen therapy if there is no evidence that a clinical benefit will ensue.

Home Oxygen Therapy and Active Smoking

This is a controversial subject that is generally avoided or ignored. The decision whether to offer home oxygen therapy to a patient who is an active smoker but otherwise meets all of the criteria for oxygen therapy is a dilemma faced by all respirologists.

There are very few studies on the effects of LTOT in individuals who continue to smoke. The MRC study[5] and the NOTT[6] enrolled only nonsmoking patients, and in these studies, polycythemia improved in those who were treated with LTOT. Calverley and colleagues reported that patients with COPD and secondary polycythemia saw no improvement in their polycythemia if they continued to smoke while they were receiving home oxygen therapy.[39] This study suggested that the link between carbon monoxide and hemoglobin decreases the transport of oxygen in smokers and does not enable the oxygen therapy to exercise its long-term beneficial effects. There are no studies showing that LTOT results in long-term beneficial effects for patients with hypoxemia who continue to smoke.

Safety is another important issue with home oxygen therapy. A patient receiving oxygen while simultaneously smoking is exposed to risks of facial and chest burns, especially when lighting a cigarette.[40] A patient who smokes while receiving oxygen also presents a potential fire hazard for the home. The risk is identical if a family member smokes close to the patient who is receiving oxygen. However, the risk of fire and burns can be minimized if the patient smokes only when not using the oxygen.

It could be argued that when the patient simultaneously behaves in a manner that runs completely counter to the treatment, the provision of oxygen is inappropriate. In the absence of a national or international consensus, we recommend giving home oxygen therapy to patients who do not smoke; however, if a patient continues to smoke, we recommend that everything be done to convince him/her to quit smoking by offering a structured, personalized smoking cessation program.

COPD with Isolated Nocturnal Hypoxemia

Nocturnal hypoxemia may occur even in the absence of daytime hypoxemia in patients with COPD. In this population, prior to assessment for LTOT, obstructive sleep apnea should be excluded. In the absence of sleep apnea, the hypoxemia is probably caused by a combination of hypoventilation and an increase in V/Q mismatch during sleep. In some patients, PAP has been found to increase during the episodes of hypoxemia. However, evidence is lacking to indicate that these changes result in chronic pulmonary artery hypertension or cor pulmonale.[41]

Nevertheless, because of these possible effects of hypoxemia during sleep, studies have been undertaken to assess the effects of LTOT in those who exhibit hypoxemia during sleep, despite the absence of significant daytime hypoxemia. In a double-blind, randomized, control trial lasting 3 years, Fletcher and colleagues assessed the effects of oxygen on pulmonary hemodynamics in 16 patients with chronic airflow limitation and nocturnal hypoxemia.[42] Nocturnal hypoxemia was defined as SpO_2 less than 90% for 5 minutes or a nadir SpO_2 less than 85%. Patients were randomized to oxygen at 3 L/min by nasal cannulae or to compressed air at 3 L/min. Primary outcomes were measures of pulmonary hemodynamics.

The pulmonary artery pressure increased from 22.5 to 26.4 mm Hg in the control group and decreased from 26.7 to 23.0 mm Hg in the treatment group. These changes were statistically significant. However, pulmonary vascular resistance, the primary result of hypoxic pulmonary vasoconstriction, increased significantly in both groups, with no difference between treatment and control groups.

In a 2-year randomized control trial, Chaouat and colleagues assessed the effect of long-term oxygen therapy on mortality in patients with nocturnal hypoxemia alone.[43] Seventy-six patients with COPD were studied in whom SpO_2 was less than 90% for 30% of the night. The PaO_2 was greater than 55 mm Hg but less than 70 mm Hg. Mean forced expiratory volume in 1 second (FEV_1) was 0.99 L. Forty-one subjects were randomized to nocturnal oxygen at a flow rate that corrected hypoxemia, whereas 35 were randomized to a control group.

Nocturnal oxygen had no effect on mortality in this study, and the mortality rate was similar in both groups (p = .68). The results of measurements of PAP were available in 46 patients who completed the 2-year follow-up. There were no differences in PAP at entry to the study, and nocturnal oxygen had no effect on the evolution of PAP during the study period.

These trials do not show any effect of LTOT used during sleep in patients who exhibit nocturnal hypoxemia in the absence of daytime hypoxemia. However, a limitation of these studies is the lack of statistical power to enable definitive assessment of the effect of nocturnal oxygen on mortality.

COPD with Isolated Hypoxemia during Exercise

In patients with COPD, breathlessness is heightened by activity or exercise; thus, the question on the role of oxygen to reduce breathlessness during exercise is often raised. Although oxygen may correct hypoxemia and may reduce breathlessness during exercise, the effects are variable, and some patients show no response. Even for those who have chronic hypoxemia and who meet eligibility criteria for funding, oxygen may have no effect during exercise.

Morrison and Stovall assessed the effect of oxygen on exercise in 33 stable patients who were chronically hypoxemic.[44] The exercise protocol was a gradual incremental exercise test, with the workload increasing every 4 minutes. Exercise studies were performed both on room air and with supplemental oxygen. Even though the subjects in the study were not blinded, 11 were considered nonresponders in the sense that exercise endurance did not improve when oxygen was breathed.

In double-blind, randomized trials, the results are similar in that a proportion of subjects show no change in breathlessness or exercise capacity; however, it should be noted that in most of these studies, a significant placebo effect is apparent. In patients who respond to supplemental oxygen as shown by an increased exercise endurance or a decrease in symptoms, the increase in exercise tolerance does not correlate with the degree of decrease in breathlessness. When oxygen is of benefit, the effect is mediated primarily through a decrease in minute ventilation,[45] which may be attributable to improved oxygen delivery or improved use of oxygen in the peripheral muscle.

In the absence of daytime hypoxemia, the effects of oxygen for exercise-induced hypoxemia are also variable. McDonald and colleagues studied 26 patients with COPD and exercise hypoxemia with resting

PaO_2 greater than 60 mm Hg.[46] Mean FEV_1 was 0.9 L, and a randomized, double-blind, crossover design was used. The exercise protocol was a 6-minute walk test. Compared to baseline, both room air and oxygen resulted in small but statistically significant increases in the distance walked. There was a reduction in exercise hypoxemia with oxygen but no change in breathlessness. However, the mean increase in the 6-minute walking distance was approximately 20 meters, much less than the distance considered to have any clinical relevance.[47]

On the other hand, in 12 patients with COPD and resting PaO_2 greater than 55 mm Hg with a mean FEV_1 of 0.9 L, Dean and colleagues reported that oxygen increased exercise endurance by 38%.[48] The exercise testing protocol was a gradual incremental test. However, on close analysis of the results, the use of oxygen resulted in major improvement in exercise endurance in only 4 of the 12 subjects, whereas 3 showed small changes, 4 showed little or no increase, and 1 subject exercised less with oxygen than when breathing room air.

The results of all of these studies indicate that although oxygen may improve exercise hypoxemia and exercise endurance in some individuals with COPD, other patients do not benefit from using oxygen with exercise. Because of this variability, a blanket eligibility statement for the funding of oxygen with exercise is inappropriate; cases must be assessed on an individual basis. There is no role for the use of supplemental oxygen prior to exercise or after activity has induced breathlessness.

In patients with COPD and exercise hypoxemia, the individual assessment should be performed in a laboratory accustomed to the testing procedures. An endurance exercise protocol should be used, ideally one that correlates with the usual activities of daily living. Steady-state exercise at approximately 60% of maximum exercise can be used, either on a cycle ergometer or on a treadmill; alternately, a self-paced walking protocol may be applied.[33] The studies should be blinded, with room air and oxygen applied in random order. A positive response requires correction of exercise hypoxemia and either a significant increase in exercise endurance time or a decrease in symptoms. The magnitude of this change may vary from patient to patient depending on the baseline severity of exercise impairment. When the test is positive, a similar exercise protocol should be used to determine the appropriate dose of oxygen or flow rate to be prescribed.

EFFECTS OF LONG-TERM OXYGEN THERAPY

The role of LTOT in patients with COPD is based on the results of the MRC trial[5] and the NOTT.[6] These landmark studies showed a reduction in mortality with the use of LTOT in patients with COPD, who were chronically hypoxemic. The MRC trial randomized 87 patients either to receive oxygen for 15 hours at 2 L/min by nasal cannulae or to a control group. Entry criteria included a diagnosis of stable irreversible airway obstruction and hypoxemia with PaO_2 between 40 and 60 mm Hg. The mean FEV_1 was 0.68 L. The NOTT used similar entry criteria of PaO_2 less than or equal to 55 mm Hg or PaO_2 less than 60 mm Hg in the presence of edema, P pulmonale on ECG, or hematocrit greater than 55%. The dose of oxygen was titrated to obtain a resting arterial PaO_2 between 60 and 80 mm Hg. Two hundred and three patients were randomized either to nocturnal or continuous oxygen. The mean FEV_1 was 29.7% of predicted.

In the MRC trial, there was a significant reduction in mortality in those treated with oxygen for 15 hours. In the NOTT, continuous oxygen (mean 19.7 hours) conferred a reduction in mortality when compared with nocturnal oxygen alone (mean 12 hours). When the two trials were compared, the mortality rate for nocturnal oxygen in the NOTT was similar to the mortality in the control group (no oxygen) in the MRC trial (Figure 7–2). In addition to a reduction in mortality, both studies showed a reduction in hematocrit in those receiving oxygen for more than 12 hours per day. Pulmonary vascular resistance and PAP increased in the control group (MRC trial) and in those receiving nocturnal oxygen (NOTT), whereas in those using oxygen for more than 15 hours, PVR and PAP did not increase. In those treated with continuous oxygen, pulmonary vascular resistance fell significantly.

There are other potential benefits of supplemental oxygen in those who are chronically hypoxemic. In patients with COPD and chronic hypoxemia, LTOT reverses the nocturnal hypoxemia and may improve sleep quality.[49] Significant cardiac arrhythmia sometimes occurs during sleep hypoxemia and may be reduced in frequency by the use of oxygen during sleep.[50] In both the MRC study[5] and the NOTT,[6] there was a reduction in hematocrit in those treated with oxygen. Oxygen has not been

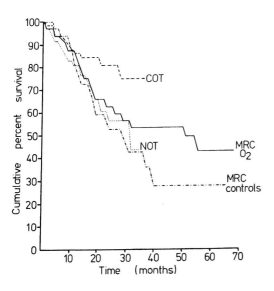

Figure 7–2 Combined results from the Medical Research Council study and Nocturnal Oxygen Therapy Trial showing survival during the study period. The effect of oxygen on survival was greatest in those who used continuous oxygen. Survival using nocturnal oxygen alone was similar to survival in those who used no oxygen. COT = continuous oxygen therapy; MRC O_2 = 15 hours per day of oxygen; NOT = nocturnal oxygen therapy alone (12 hours); MRC controls = no oxygen. (Reproduced with permission from Flenley DC. Chronic obstructive pulmonary disease. In: Cherniack NS. Oxygen therapy in the treatment of COPD. Philadelphia: WB Saunders Company, 1991:468–76.)

shown to have a significant effect on the neuropsychiatric problems that are often present in patients with chronic hypoxemia.[51] Similarly, even though quality of life is often impaired in these patients, the limited studies that have been performed do not show a beneficial effect.[4]

OXYGEN SUPPLY

Oxygen Supply Systems

Oxygen systems have developed over the last decade to better suit both the consumer and the provider (Tables 7–3 and 7–4). Systems are being designed smaller, with the user in mind, while at the same time conserving as much oxygen as possible to allow for the least amount of maintenance, refilling, and cost. Each system will be described with mention of the care and maintenance involved for the various delivery methods. It should be emphasized that the choice of the oxygen delivery system should be based on the patient's needs. However, funding structures may favor less expensive units to maximize profit for the provider. It is therefore incumbent on the prescriber to recommend a unit or to have a respiratory care practitioner assess patient suitability to different oxygen systems to help aid in the decision process. Many factors may be taken into account when deciding not only what is most therapeutic but also what best suits the individual and his/her lifestyle.

Concentrators

Oxygen concentrators are stationary units powered by electricity that produce a high concentration of oxygen from filtered room air (see Table 7–3, Figure 7–3).[26] Either a molecular sieve bed or a permeable plastic membrane is used to obtain nearly pure oxygen. The latter is used infrequently as it is less efficient at extracting the nitrogen from room air. Most manufacturers' specifications state that the oxygen concentrations that concentrators can produce are in the range of 92 to 96 percent, varying somewhat on the set flow rate. The FIO_2 obtained is inversely proportional to the flow rate used. Simply put, the faster the unit has to output oxygen, the less efficient the unit is at extracting all of the nitrogen. The molecular sieve also becomes less efficient with use, resulting in a reduction in FIO_2 generated as the concentrator ages (Figure 7–4).[52]

Concentrators are the most cost-efficient system as they require little maintenance and no refilling. A regular maintenance schedule is needed to monitor the oxygen concentration being produced, the accuracy of the flow rate (to change any necessary filters) and to check the operation of the battery, which operates the audible alarm to notify a power loss. Patients may often have the responsibility of washing an external gross particle filter. This should be performed weekly using a mild dish detergent, rinsing it, and thoroughly drying it before it is replaced. Weekly dusting of the exterior should also be performed with a damp cloth.

TABLE 7–3 Types of Oxygen Supply Systems

Type of Delivery System	Advantages	Disadvantages	Application
Concentrator (see Figure 7–3) A device that uses room air, filters out the nitrogen, and leaves nearly pure O_2 to be delivered to the patient	No fills required Cost efficient Low maintenance Easy to use Low pressure system No O_2 stored when not in use	Requires electricity Low flow range (1–3 Lpm or 1–5 Lpm) Not very portable (37–59 lb) Relatively noisy May generate heat Lower purity of O_2 Back-up system required	Often used in the home when portability is not required or as part of a dual system In rural areas
Cylinders (see Figure 7–5) Oxygen in the gaseous form compressed under a high pressure (2,000–2,200 psi) in an aluminum or steel tank	High flow rates possible Gas does not evaporate Quiet High purity of O_2 Aluminum is lightweight No electricity required	Usage time limited Steel cylinders are heavy Skill required to use and change regulator High-pressure system Special storage required	Smaller cylinders may be used for portability or for back-up for other systems
Liquid (see Figures 7–6 and 7–7) Oxygen stored in its liquid form in an insulated container. Available as a base unit and a portable unit	High storage volume of O_2 Quiet High purity of O_2 Able to transfill into portable units Lightweight portables Low pressure system (~ 25 psi)	Base units require filling Evaporates whether used or not Extremely cold in the liquid state Knowledge and skill required to transfill portables More expensive	Good for portability Can be used for devices requiring higher flow rates

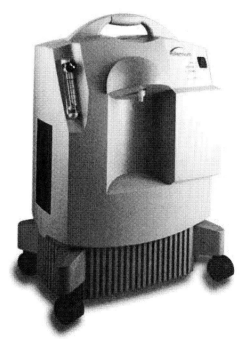

Figure 7–3 Oxygen concentrator (Millineum™). (Reproduced with permission from Respironics®, Pittsburg, PA.)

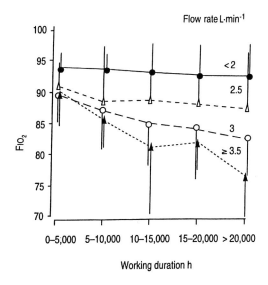

Figure 7–4 FIO$_2$ produced by oxygen concentrators. The FIO$_2$ is seen to vary with flow rate and with the working duration of the concentrator. (Reproduced with permission from Pepin JL, Dautzenberg B, Levy P, Brambilla C. What should we expect from an oxygen concentrator in 1995? Eur Respir Buyers 1995;1:21–6.)

TABLE 7–4 Types of Oxygen-Conserving Devices

Type of Delivery System	Advantages	Disadvantages	Application
Demand/pulse flow systems Oxygen is delivered intermittently during the respiratory cycle. Some deliver O_2 for a portion of inspiration, others throughout inspiration, and some either add a bolus of O_2 or use an algorithm of the set flow rate. Some may do this with each inspiration while others may skip breaths	Increases duration of O_2 supply Less drying/irritation of nasal mucosa Frequency of deliveries reduced Saves oxygen	Devices are expensive Synchronization with breathing pattern may be a concern Many require battery for power Cannot use humidification with unit May not oxygenate as well—patient-dependent variables	Can be used with cylinders or liquid units Greatly extends portability time and allows for smaller lighter O_2 portable units
Conserving cannulae Oxygen delivery devices that incorporate a reservoir that stores O_2 during exhalation and prior to inhalation. This provides a bolus for the next breath	May conserve O_2 by allowing for a lower flow rate to be used May improve oxygenation May increase portable time	Does not work when mouth breathing Obtrusive More expensive than regular nasal cannulae	When a system that may allow for lower flow rates than regular nasal cannulae is desired Refractory hypoxemia on regular nasal cannulae
Transtracheal system Oxygen delivered via a catheter inserted directly into the trachea	O_2 delivered throughout inspiration and expiration May provide effective oxygenation on lower flow rates Increases portable time Obliterates nasal complications Less obtrusive	Invasive Minor surgical procedure More costly to initiate and maintain Potential short- and long-term complications Requires knowledge and skill to care for device	Refractory hypoxemia Cosmetic reasons Noncompliance because of nasal cannulae Complications because of nasal cannulae
High-flow system (eg, Venturi masks, Vickers masks) Oxygen system that provides flow to meet or exceed inspiratory demand and provides a controlled FIO_2	FIO_2 constant irrespective of breathing pattern Able to provide high humidity	Often requires higher flow rates to drive the system Decreases duration of portable O_2 systems	When oxygen requirements exceed capability of low flow systems (ie, nasal cannulae) When hypercarbia/hypoxic drive is a concern Acute exacerbations
Low-flow system (eg, nasal cannulae, simple O_2 mask) The flow from the device does not meet the inspiratory flow rate. Room air is entrained along with the O_2 flow from the system. FIO_2 is variable and depends on the set flow rate and the respiratory pattern	Simple to use Nasal cannulae less obtrusive Can operate with devices that produce only low-flow oxygen Compatible with most home systems	Variable FIO_2 May not be sufficient to oxygenate Nasal cannulae can cause nasal complications	Often used in the home because of the convenience Less obtrusive than mask systems

Many new models of concentrators have the option of having a sensor to monitor the purity of the oxygen being produced. Some refer to it as an oxygen sensing device (Devilbiss™, Somerset, PA) or an oxygen percentage indicator (Respironics®, Pittsburg, PA). These sensing devices do not actually measure the oxygen concentration but use an alternate technology to reference the gas purity, which then translates into an electrical signal that feeds a warning light. The warning and alarm ranges are quite large and may not audibly alarm until oxygen concentration falls below 75%.

Many vendors will provide a concentrator for home use in conjunction with a second system to allow for portability. This will reduce the cost of the consumable oxygen and decrease the number of visits required to replenish stock. It is possible to travel with a concentrator, but assistance may be required to help move the unit. As long as electricity is available at the destination, the patient will have oxygen available. Provisions need to be made for portable oxygen to and from the destination as battery-operated concentrators require special electrical adapters to provide the power needed. It should be noted that patients have had concerns that concentrators produce unwanted noise (average 50 dBA) (Devilbiss™), that they might generate heat, which could be of concern in smaller rooms, and that they will increase the electricity bill. These issues should be discussed with patients prior to initiating treatment to allow for appropriate alternatives if necessary.

Oxygen concentrators commonly used to provide long-term oxygen in the home are an economical and safe method of oxygen delivery. When the unit is not running there is no oxygen stored in the system. The flow rate of oxygen is limited to the range of 1 to 5 liters per minute (Lpm), and it is a low-pressure system. Delivery devices that have a high resistance to flow (eg, mininebulizers or oxygen tubing more than approximately 50 feet in length) should not be used with concentrators as the added resistance makes it impossible for the concentrator to generate adequate flow to drive the device. Oxygen concentrators are best suited for use with nasal cannulae, although the lower FIO_2 range Venturi masks that require less than 5 Lpm of flow can be used with these units even though the resistance is greater than with nasal cannulae. It is important to note that the Venturi is based on the principle that the driving gas is 100% oxygen; the entrainment ratio of air

produces the prescribed amount of oxygen. Since concentrators do not produce 100% oxygen, the entrainment ratio may result in a lower FIO_2 than desired. Hence, it is not only vital to maintain the concentrator efficiency but also to test the patient on the system he/she is using.

Cylinders

One of the first methods used to provide portable oxygen was via a steel cylinder that held many litres of oxygen compressed into it under a high pressure (see Table 7–3, Figure 7–5).[26] Pressures of 2,000 to 2,200 pounds per square inch (psi) are used, which allows for 690 L of gaseous oxygen to be held in an E size cylinder. This would be a typical size used in hospital as a source for transport or emergency. Cylinders under such high pressures pose a safety risk should the cylinder valve break. Hence, safe practice is essential not only with oxygen but also with the handling and storing of the cylinders. Cylinders should always be stored securely in the upright or horizontal position. For ambulation, a cart should be used to secure the cylinder. The cylinders are heavy and, depending on the size, can be quite cumbersome to maneuver. This may impede individuals from venturing far from their main source of oxygen and thus further disable them.

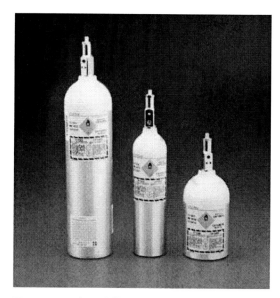

Figure 7–5 Three different size oxygen cylinders. E size (largest), D size, and M6 (smallest). (Reproduced with permission from VitalAire®, Edmonton, AB.)

Originally, large cylinders were used in the home as the primary oxygen source. This method fell out of favor as concentrators became popular. Cylinders may still be needed if high flow rates are required. Smaller cylinders are also often used as a back-up system of oxygen should the primary source fail. Recently, however, an increase in the use of cylinders for portability is occurring as cylinders are being made of aluminum, which is significantly lighter. They are also being made in several smaller sizes: D, M6, C, and so on. These attributes make them attractive for portable use but are limiting because of the smaller gaseous liter capacity (Table 7–5). However, when used in conjunction with a conserving device, the duration increases, making it a very attractive portable option.

Individuals using such a system do require some knowledge and skill to be able to operate the cylinder gauge. A pressure gauge is necessary to control the pressure and flow rate from the cylinder, and skill is required to change the gauge when the cylinder gas has been depleted. To make further use of cylinders applicable for ambulation, some concentrators allow for transfilling of the cylinder directly from the concentrator.

Liquid Oxygen

With the invention of fractional distillation of liquid air by Karl von Linde in 1907, the ability to store oxygen in a liquid form became possible.[26,53] The liquid form allows for the storage of large amounts of oxygen in a relatively small container (see Table 7–3). This is because of the expansion ratio of liquid to gaseous oxygen. One liquid liter of oxygen expands to approximately 862 gaseous liters of oxygen. Because of this expansion ratio, small portable units are able to provide substantial time away from a base unit of liquid oxygen supply. This attribute makes liquid oxygen an ideal method for ambulatory use (Figure 7–6).

Although the favorable characteristics of liquid oxygen make it attractive as a method of providing home oxygen, there are also some drawbacks that require careful attention. Oxygen in its liquid state

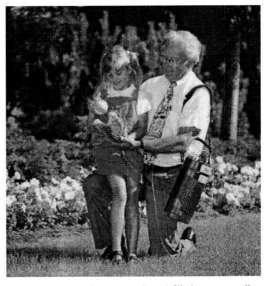

Figure 7–6 Individual using a liquid-filled oxygen stroller. (Reproduced with permission from VitalAire®.)

TABLE 7–5 Portable Oxygen Duration Time for D and E Size Cylinders (h)*

Oxygen Setting (Lpm)	1	2	3	4	5	6
Cylinder Pressure (psi)						
D size						
Full (2,000)	6	3	2	1½	1¼	1
¾ (1,500)	4½	½	1½	1	54 min.	45 min
½ (1,000)	3	1¼	1	45 min	36 min	30 min
¼ (500)	1½	45 min	30 min	22 min	18 min	15 min
E size						
Full (2,000)	10	5	3⅓	2½	2	1¾
¾ (1,500)	7½	3¾	2½	2	1½	1¼
½ (1,000)	5	2½	1¾	1¼	1	50 min
¼ (500)	2½	1¼	50 min	38 min	30 min	25 min

*Hours of duration may vary because of different factors. Always account for a safety margin or have a back-up.
Lpm = liter per minute.

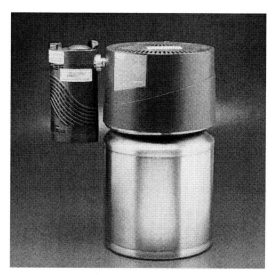

Figure 7–7 Liquid oxygen base unit (Liberator). Stroller unit in position for filling. (Reproduced with permission from VitalAire®.)

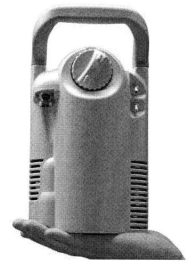

Figure 7–8 Small lightweight liquid oxygen demand flow system (HELiOS™). (Reproduced with permission from Mallinckrodt, Mississauga, ON, Canada, Inc.®.)

has a temperature of –185°C and has to be maintained at this temperature to keep it from turning into gaseous form. Stainless steel, double-walled, vacuum-insulated containers are used to store the liquid oxygen at a pressure of approximately 25 psi (Figure 7–7). The containers act much like a thermos bottle trying to keep the liquid cold. As no thermos is perfect, some warming will occur, and there is a transfer from liquid to gas, resulting in a pressure increase in the container. Therefore, all liquid units are equipped with a pressure relief that continuously bleeds off gas as the liquid oxygen evaporates. The rate of transfer from liquid to gas is referred to as the normal evaporation rate. Because of this evaporation, even if liquid tanks are never turned on, all of the oxygen will eventually bleed out of the system.

Liquid oxygen tends to be more expensive than other delivery systems. The manufacturing of liquid oxygen, equipment required, and need for deliveries all add to the cost. One method of reducing costs is to use liquid oxygen in conjunction with pulse or demand flow devices to conserve the oxygen and increase the portable time. The best method to calculate how long liquid oxygen will last is by its weight; most systems have a gauge or a weight scale to indicate how much oxygen remains in the system (Table 7–6). New technology incorporating oxygen

conservation devices has allowed the development of longer lasting, smaller, lighter weight, portable liquid oxygen canisters, which many patients find more convenient than the usual stroller and less conspicuous for use when walking (Figure 7–8).

Precaution needs to be taken because of the extremely low temperature of liquid oxygen. Contact with the eyes and skin must be avoided as burns are possible even after a brief exposure to liquid oxygen at this temperature. Skill is required to be able to transfill the portable unit from its base unit. Some individuals may not have the ability or the strength to be able to do this on their own. It may also be quite intimidating at first as the process of transfilling can be quite noisy. As for all oxygen systems, proper education with testing of patients and caregivers is essential to ensure that the equipment is used safely and effectively.

Oxygen-Conserving Devices

Conserving Cannula

Reservoir cannula would be a more appropriate name for this type of device, which consists of nasal cannulae, a reservoir, and lariat oxygen tubing (see Table 7–4).[54,55] The reservoirs store approximately 20 to 50 cc of oxygen. The reservoir fills during exhalation, and this oxygen store is accessed at the start of inspi-

TABLE 7–6 Portable Oxygen Duration Time for Liquid Oxygen Stroller (h)*

Oxygen Setting (Lpm)	¼	½	¾	1	1½	2	2½	3	4	5	6
Gauge contents											
Full	62	31	20	15	10	7	6	5	3	3	2½
¾	46	23	15	11	7	5	4	3¾	2¾	2½	1¾
½	31	15	10	7	5	3	3	2½	1¾	1½	1¼
¼	15	7	5	3	2	1¾	1½	1¼	¾	¾	½

*Hours of duration may vary because of different factors. Always account for a safety margin or have a back-up.

Lpm = liter per minute.

ration in addition to the usual oxygen flow through the nasal cannulae. With conserving cannulae, oxygen continues to flow throughout the respiratory cycle. Hence, oxygen is conserved only if the device allows for a lower flow rate. A lower flow rate may oxygenate as effectively as conventional cannulae because of the bolus received from the reservoir.

There are two types of conserving cannulae available. One provides the reservoir under the nose much like a moustache (Figure 7–9), and the other has a pendant further downstream in an attempt to reduce the obtrusive quality of such cannulae (Figure 7–10). The cannulae themselves are larger than usual nasal cannulae, and the weight and comfort of the devices can be a concern. They are more expensive than traditional nasal cannulae, but the savings in oxygen use may outweigh this cost.

The major problem with the reservoir cannulae occurs when the patient breathes through the mouth as the oxygen bolus is accessed only during nasal breathing. Mouth breathing negates the function of the reservoir, thus rendering the conserving cannulae's function similar to that of the standard nasal cannulae. This may become a significant concern only during exercise and sleep. If an increasing FIO_2 is needed, by providing better oxygenation the con-

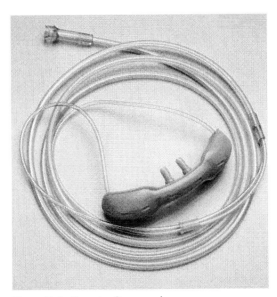

Figure 7–9 Oxymizer® moustache-type oxygen conserving cannulae. (Reproduced with permission from Chad® Therapeutics, Inc., Chatsworth, CA.)

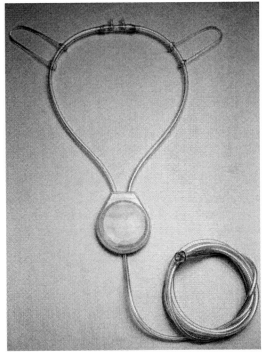

Figure 7–10 Oxymizer® pendant-type oxygen conserving cannulae. (Reproduced with permission from Chad® Therapeutics, Inc., Chatsworth, CA.)

serving cannulae may negate the need to change to a high-flow delivery system.

Pulsers and Demand Flow Systems

The duration for which portable liquid systems and gas cylinders provide oxygen is limited, but pulsers and demand flow systems may provide adequate ambulatory oxygenation for longer duration (see Table 7–4).[54,55] This reduces the amount of oxygen used and the cost of oxygen therapy.

Most pulsers provide a fixed bolus of oxygen at the start of each breath. The size of the bolus can be altered by changing the settings on the device. The size of the bolus differs with different systems, with the oxygen flow rate, and with the respiratory rate. Some pulsers do not provide oxygen with every breath in an attempt to conserve even more oxygen. Even though the volume of oxygen delivered varies with each device, the manufacturers generally claim that the effect on PaO_2 or SpO_2 is equivalent to continuous flow; however, the oxygenation achieved will vary with the different devices, and this variability is attributable at least in part to the size of the bolus. Changes in the pattern of breathing adopted by the patient will also alter the effectiveness of oxygenation with this type of delivery system. In some individuals, the respiratory effort may not be detected by the pulser. If this occurs, no oxygen will be delivered to the patient.

Demand flow systems deliver continuous flow throughout inspiration, often with a bolus of oxygen at the start of the breath. The continuous flow throughout inspiration may provide a greater volume of delivered oxygen than pulser-type devices.

Braun and colleagues assessed the effectiveness of five different oxygen-conserving systems during exercise in patients with COPD; the 12-minute walking distance, average SpO_2, and nadir SpO_2 differed with different conserving devices.[36] Roberts and colleagues compared a demand flow system with continuous flow in 15 patients with COPD.[56] Continuous oxygen provided better oxygenation during exercise. The time with SpO_2 less than 90% and the recovery time were both longer when the demand flow system was used.

The results of bench studies and clinical studies, as well as the differences between the systems provided by each manufacturer, reinforce the need to assess oxygenation with the prescribed delivery system. If the delivery system is changed, a dose-finding study must be performed to ensure effective oxygenation.

Transtracheal Oxygen Delivery

Transtracheal oxygen delivered by a catheter introduced directly into the trachea is a method of delivery that may be applicable for selected patients (see Table 7–4).[57] Continuous oxygen flow during exhalation results in a reservoir of oxygen in the upper airway before the start of the next inspiration, thus resulting in a higher initial FIO_2 and more effective oxygenation. Transtracheal oxygen delivery may be appropriate in those with refractory hypoxemia requiring very high oxygen flow rates.[58] In the United States, transtracheal oxygen is also frequently used for cosmetic reasons as it is less visible than nasal cannulae. In some patients, the fact that the oxygen system is not visible increases compliance with the prescription.

Several complications related to the use of the transtracheal catheter have been reported.[58] These risks include accidental displacement of the catheter, cough, increased sputum production, transitory hoarseness, formation of balls of mucus, and infection at the insertion site. Because of the invasive nature of the delivery system and the attendant risks, it should be used only in specialized respiratory centers where the health professionals are trained in the technique.[59]

WHEN TO REFER

Referral to a physician is essential to evaluate the patient's oxygen requirement. When possible, referral to a respirologist should be considered if long-term oxygen is considered for a patient with COPD. The aim is to ensure that optimal therapy including rehabilitation has been considered and that the patient is clinically stable. Blood gas analysis for determining eligibility should be performed in an accredited hospital-based laboratory. Specific assessments are also necessary to determine the correct dose for rest, sleep, activity, and exercise.

An oxygen vendor or regional/local government health organization will provide oxygen and the delivery equipment. As well, technical support and regular monitoring are provided at home by a team including respiratory/inhalation therapists and nurses. All provinces, states, or countries have programs for funding home oxygen. You may contact these programs or your Lung Association to obtain information regarding the available oxygen services in your area.

SUMMARY

Long-term oxygen therapy improves longevity in patients with COPD who are chronically hypoxemic; it may also decrease morbidity, decrease disability, and improve handicap in some patients. Oxygen should be considered as a pharmaceutical intervention and only one component of a comprehensive plan of management that includes the following: referral to a respiratory specialist, use of other prescribed medications, and pulmonary rehabilitation. The specific criteria for which funding is available for LTOT should be carefully defined based on scientific data from appropriate clinical trials. Only a small proportion of patients who do not meet these criteria seem to benefit from treatment with oxygen. A prescription for LTOT should outline the dose of oxygen for rest, sleep, activity, and exercise; the duration of continuous use; and the delivery devices required.

The delivery systems should be tailored to each patient so that effective correction of hypoxemia is obtained, while at the same time optimizing compliance with the use of oxygen. Ideally, home oxygen therapy should be used within a structured regional program that includes a regular home-based assessment of the patient and technical supervision of the apparatus. Equally important is regular clinical monitoring of oxygen-dependent patients by a multidisciplinary team under the supervision of a respirologist.

CASE STUDY

Ms. Cope, a 60-year-old female, presented for follow-up because of breathlessness.

Medical History, Physical Examination, and Test Results

Medical History

- Her breathlessness had gradually deteriorated over 10 years.
- She is a lifelong nonsmoker.
- She has alpha$_1$-antitrypsin deficiency.
- Self-care activities are not difficult, but household chores occasionally require a rest period; walking quickly results in breathlessness, and recreational activities such as gardening and camping are undertaken less frequently than in the past.
- She has had no previous acute exacerbations or previous need of antibiotics or corticosteroids.
- Medications taken include metered-dose inhalers: ipratropium two puffs four times a day and salbutamol two puffs as needed.

Physical Examination

- Her height is 168 cm and weight is 62 kg.
- She has no acute respiratory distress: pulse regular at 88 bpm and respiratory rate at 22/min.
- JVP (jugular venous pressure) is not elevated.
- Chest wall shows signs of accessory muscle activity, soft tissue indrawing, and hyperinflation.
- Diminished but equal breath sounds throughout

- Cardiac examination with pulmonic second sound is loud.
- She has no peripheral edema but shows the presence of cyanosis.

Test Results

- Hemoglobin is 173 g/L.
- Spirometry is indicative of moderately severe airflow obstruction:
  - FEV$_1$ 1.3 L (48% of predicted)
  - Vital capacity (VC) 2.8 L (82% of predicted)
  - Lung volumes increased with diffusion impaired (diffusion capacity of the lung for carbon monoxide 21% of predicted)
- Chest radiograph shows hyperinflation with areas of diminished vascularity.
- Electrocardiogram shows sinus rhythm and P pulmonale.
- Echocardiogram shows normal right ventricular function and size. Pulmonary artery pressure could not be estimated.
- Oxygenation after optimal pharmacologic treatment is as follows:
  - Resting oximetry on room air showed SpO$_2$ 88%
  - Blood gases showed pH 7.39, PaCO$_2$ 44 mm Hg, HCO$_3$ 25 mmol/L, PaO$_2$ 52 mm Hg, and SaO$_2$ 87%
  - Nocturnal oximetry showed SpO$_2$ less than 88% for 70% of the night. The nadir is 77% (Figure 7–11). Oxygenation during sleep is corrected by oxygen at 2 L/min.

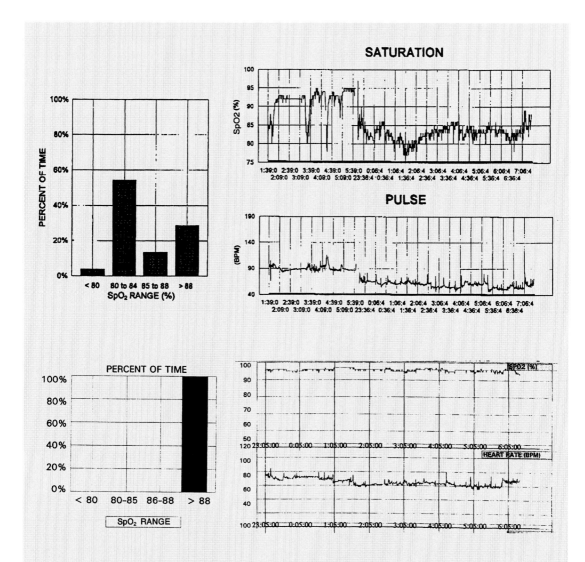

Figure 7–11 Results of nocturnal oximetry on room air and on continuous oxygen at 2 Lpm. The upper panel shows a histogram and continuous oximetry on room air, indicating significant hypoxemia with sleep. The lower panel shows a histogram and continuous oximetry on oxygen at 2 Lpm indicating complete correction of hypoxemia during sleep.

• Walk testing shows significant hypoxemia with walking, even on oxygen. Walking distance during a self-paced walk is 358 m on both 2 L/min and 4 L/min with similar hypoxemia and symptom scores on each occasion.

Questions and Discussion

Ms. Cope has emphysema secondary to α_1-antitrypsin deficiency. There is a family history of

emphysema. The patient is in no acute respiratory distress. She described herself as being in her usual state of health, although her breathlessness has gradually become worse over 10 years.

Is there any urgency to prescribe oxygen?
This patient has a chronic respiratory condition without any evidence of an acute exacerbation. There is no urgency to prescribe oxygen, but it is more than

likely that she will benefit from long-term oxygen treatment; furthermore, considering a primary diagnosis of emphysema in this patient, you will have all of the reasons to expect a nonreversible airflow obstruction. Trials with different combinations of bronchodilators are unsuccessful in improving her breathlessness and her lung function tests.

What is the management that should be recommended in this patient?
Oxygen is indicated for long-term use. It is prescribed as follows: 1 L/min for rest and 2 L/min for sleep and exercise for a minimum of 15 h/day. A concentrator is prescribed with liquid oxygen for portability.

What is the patient's response to the treatment that included long-term oxygen?
After starting home oxygen, there is a noticeable improvement in sleep quality, a general feeling of improved health, and a lower heart rate with exercise. Her lips and fingers are no longer blue. She is more able to undertake activity, can sing with fewer pauses, and notices that her memory has improved. The liquid oxygen stroller caused some difficulty when she performed chores outside of the home.

Is there anything else that could be done for this patient?
You refer the patient for a formal comprehensive pulmonary rehabilitation program. Her 6-minute walking distance improves, as well as breathlessness on exertion. At the time of discharge from the rehabilitation program, the oxygen prescription remained at 1 L/min for rest and 2 L/min for sleep, activity, and exercise. Oxygen 2 L/min is recommended for the regimented exercise program.

Follow-up

One year later, her hemoglobin is 157 g/L, and lung function is unchanged. She is doing well, using oxygen as prescribed for 15 hours continuous, including sleep and for her exercise program.

Three years later, at age 63, further assessment takes place. There has been a slight decline in her ability to undertake activity.

Test Results

- The hemoglobin remains lower at 156 g/L.
- The electrocardiogram shows P pulmonale.

- Right ventricular size is normal but two-dimensional echocardiogram estimation of pulmonary artery pressure is 54 mm Hg.
- Pulmonary function shows FEV_1 1.3 L (50% of predicted) and VC 2.7 L (85% of predicted).
- Maximum 6-minute walking distance is well preserved at 475 meters.
- Oxygenation:
  - Room air SpO_2 is 81 to 82%
  - With walking, on room air SpO_2 falls to 65%; using oxygen at 4 L/min, resting SpO_2 is 96% and falls only to 82% with a 400-meter self-paced 6-minute walk. There is also reduction in symptom scores for both breathlessness and leg effort when walking on oxygen. When tested on continuous oxygen at 6 L/min, there is further correction of the low SpO_2 but no improvement in walking distance, heart rate, or symptoms of breathlessness and leg effort.

What are your recommendations with regard to the above changes?
It is recommended that oxygen be used for as much of the day as possible, but difficulty is still noted with undertaking tasks when having to pull or carry the liquid oxygen system. Liquid oxygen is therefore provided for ambulation using a HELiOS™ (Mallinkrodt, Mississauga, ON) system (see Figure 7–8) following testing to ensure that oxygenation is adequate. The oxygen prescription is 1 L/min for rest, 2 L/min for sleep, 4 L/min on the HELiOS™ demand flow system for exercise, and 2 L/min for simple activities. It is recommended that oxygen be used for as close to 24 hours of the day as possible.

What is the patient's response to the oxygen prescription?
The patient returned to the clinic praising the HELiOS. Her energy is increased, and walking is easier. The HELiOS with a belt pack allows for undertaking activities more easily as both hands are free for carrying garbage or groceries and for performing gardening or other activities (Figure 7–12). The result is that oxygen is used for much more of the day. The system also allows for longer portable use than the usual liquid oxygen stroller.

She continues to use oxygen with the concentrator overnight and with the HELiOS liquid oxygen system for ambulation and exercise. She maintains a regular exercise program and feels better now.

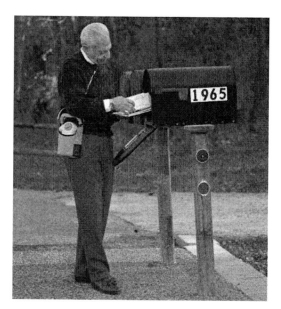

Figure 7–12 Individual using a small portable liquid demand flow oxygen unit (HELiOS™). (Reproduced with permission from Mallinkrodt, Mississauga, ON.)

KEY POINTS TO REMEMBER

- It is essential to ensure that patient treatment is optimized and the lung disease is stable prior to assessing the need for long-term oxygen treatment.
- Respirology assessment should include (1) pulmonary function testing; (2) arterial blood gases; (3) pulse oximetry during rest, sleep, activity, and exercise; (4) electrolytes and complete blood count; (5) ECG; and (6) echocardiogram to measure right ventricular function and PAP.
- There are well-established criteria supported by evidence in the medical literature as to when long-term oxygen treatment should be prescribed and what effect the patient should expect; there are also situations for which it is still unknown if correcting low arterial oxygen level will have an effect on the patient's health.
- Oxygen is a drug; the dose requires proper assessment for each time of day, that is, rest, sleep, activity, and exercise.
- Proper use by the patient is vital for effective therapy; teach the patients to ensure that they understand the proper use, safety, and role of oxygen; and make sure that you address the patient's concerns and fears.

- Long-term oxygen therapy assessment should include the appropriate oxygen system to best suit the patient's needs.

REFERENCES

1. Minh VD, Lee HM, Dolan GF, et al. Hypoxemia during exercise in patients with chronic obstructive pulmonary disease. Am Rev Respir Dis 1979;120: 787–94.
2. Mitlehner W, Kerb W. Exercise hypoxemia and the effects of increased respiratory oxygen concentration in severe chronic obstructive pulmonary disease. Respiration 1994;61:255–62.
3. Prigatano GP, Wright EC, Levin D. Quality of life and its predictors in patients with mild hypoxemia and chronic obstructive pulmonary disease. Arch Intern Med 1984;144:1613–9.
4. Okubadejo AA, Jones PW, Wedzicha JA. Quality of life in patients with chronic obstructive pulmonary disease and severe hypoxemia. Thorax 1996;51:44–7.
5. Report of the Medical Research Council Working Party. Long term domiciliary oxygen therapy in chronic hypoxic cor pulmonale complicating chronic bronchitis and emphysema. Lancet 1981;1:681–6.
6. Nocturnal Oxygen Therapy Trial (NOTT) Group. Continuous or noctural oxygen therapy in hypoxemic chronic obstructive lung disease: a clinical trial. Ann Intern Med 1980;93:391–8.
7. Wagner PD, Dantzker DR, Dueck R. Ventilation-perfusion inequality in chronic obstructive pulmonary disease. J Clin Invest 1977;59:203–16.
8. Morrison SC, Stubbing DG, Zimmerman PV, Campbell EJ. Lung volume, closing volume and gas exchange. J Appl Physiol 1982;52:1453–7.
9. Fletcher EC, Gray BA, Levin DC. Nonapneic mechanisms of arterial oxygen desaturation during rapid-eye-movement sleep. J Appl Physiol 1983;54:632–9.
10. Catterall JR, Claverley PM, MacNee W, et al. Mechanism of transient nocturnal hypoxemia in hypoxic chronic bronchitis and emphysema. J Appl Physiol 1985;59:1698–703.
11. Hudgel DW, Devadatta P. Decrease in functional residual capacity during sleep in normal humans. J Appl Physiol 1984;57:1319–22.
12. Dantzker DR, D'Alonzo GE. The effect of exercise on pulmonary gas exchange in patients with severe chronic obstructive pulmonary disease. Am Rev Respir Dis 1986;134:1135–9.
13. Coccagna G, Lugaresi E. Arterial blood gases and pulmonary and systemic arterial pressure during sleep in chronic obstructive pulmonary disease. Sleep 1978;1:117–24.
14. Wetzenblum E, Apprill M, Oswald M, et al. Pulmonary hemodynamics in patients with chronic obstructive pulmonary disease before and during an episode of peripheral edema. Chest 1994;105:1377–82.

15. Wedzicha JA, Cotes PM, Empey DW, et al. Serum immunoreactive erythropoietin in hypoxic lung disease with and without polycythaemia. Clin Sci (Colch) 1985;69:413–22.

16. York EL, Jones RL, Menon D, Sproule BJ. Effects of secondary polycythmia on cerebral blood flow in chronic obstructive pulmonary disease. Am Rev Respir Dis 1980;121:1813–8.

17. Petty TL. Pulmonary rehabilitation of early COPD. COPD as a systemic disease. Chest 1994;105: 1636–7.

18. El-Manschawi A, Killian KJ, Summers E, Jones NL. Breathlessness during exercise with and without resistive loading. J Appl Physiol 1986;61:896–905.

19. Canadian Thoracic Society Workshop Group. Guidelines for the assessment and management of chronic obstructive pulmonary disease. Can Med Assoc J 1992;147:420–8.

20. Boucher S. Oxygénothérapie à domicile [oxygen therapy at home: criteria for admiministration] : recommandations de l'Association des Pneumologues de la province de Québec. Union Med Can 1984;113: 394–5.

21. Wedzicha JA. Domiciliary oxygen therapy services: clinical guidelines and advice for prescribers. Summary of a report of the Royal College of Physicians. J R Coll Physicians Lond 1999;33:445–7.

22. Petty TL, Casaburi R. Recommendations of the Fifth Oxygen Consensus Conference. Writing and Organizing Committees. Respir Care 2000; 45:957–61.

23. Young IH, Crockett AJ, McDonald CF. Adult domiciliary oxygen therapy. Position statement of the Thoracic Society of Australia and New Zealand. N Z Med J 1999;112:15–8.

24. Celli BR. ATS standards for the optimal management of chronic obstructive pulmonary disease. Respirology 1997;1 Suppl 1:S1–4.

25. Rhodius E, Caneva J, Sivori M. Argentine consensus of home long term oxygen therapy. Medicina (B Aires) 1998;58:85–94.

26. Cairo JM, Pilbeam P. Non-invasive assessment of ABG in respiratory care equipment. In: Mosby's respiratory care equipment. 6th Ed. St. Louis, MO: Mosby, 1999.

27. Pierson DJ. Pulse oximetry versus arterial blood gas specimens in long-term oxygen therapy. Lung 1990; 168:782–8.

28. Emery JR. Skin pigmentation as an influence on the accuracy of pluse oximetry. J Perinatol 1987;7: 329–30.

29. Amar D, Neidzwski J, Wald A, Finck AD. Fluorescent light interferes with pulse oximetry. J Clin Monit 1989;5:135–6.

30. Tremper KK, Barker SJ. Pulse oximetry. Anesthesiology 1989;70:98–108.

31. Cote CJ, Goldstein EA, Fuchsman WH, Hoaglin DC. The effect of nail polish on pulse oximetry. Anesth Analg 1988;67:683–6.

32. Scheller MS, Unger RJ, Kelner MJ. Effects of intravenously administered dyes on pulse oximetry readings. Anesthesiology 1986;65:550–2.

33. Vaughan R, Stubbing DG. The self paced walk test: a better way to determine exercise oxygen prescription. Am J Respir Crit Care Med 2000;161:A503.

34. Zugck C, Kruger C, Durr S, et al. Is the 6 minute walk test a reliable substitute for peak oxygen uptake in patients with dilated cardiomyopathy? Eur Heart J 2000;7:540–9.

35. Campbell EJM. A method of controlled oxygen administration which reduces the risk of carbon-dioxide retention. Lancet 1960;2:12–4.

36. Braun SR, Spratt G, Scott GC, Ellersieck M. Comparison of six oxygen delivery systems for COPD patients at rest and during exercise. Chest 1992;102: 694–8.

37. Cuvelier A, Muir JF, Czernichow P, et al. Nocturnal efficiency and tolerance of a demand oxygen delivery system in COPD patients with nocturnal hypoxemia. Chest 1999;116:22–9.

38. Guyatt GH, McKim DA, Austin P, et al. Appropriateness of domiciliary oxygen delivery. Chest 2000; 118:1303–8.

39. Calverley PM, Brezinova V, Douglas NJ, et al. The effect of oxygenation on sleep quality in chronic bronchitis and emphysema. Am Rev Respir Dis 1982; 126:206–10.

40. Kathawalla S, Mehta A. Risks of home oxygen therapy for cigarette smokers. Chest 1996;110: 1130.

41. Douglas NJ, Weitzenblum E. Sleep and chronic obstructive pulmonary disease. Eur Respir Monit 1988; 7:209–14.

42. Fletcher EC, Luckett RA, Goodnight-White S, et al. A double-blind trial of nocturnal supplemental oxygen for sleep desaturation in patients with chronic obstructive pulmonary disease with a daytime PaO2 above 60 mmHg. Am Rev Respir Dis 1992;145: 1070–6.

43. Chaouat A, Weitzenblum E, Kessler R, et al. A randomized trial of nocturnal oxygen therapy in chronic obstructive pulmonary disease patients. Eur Respir J 1999;14:1002–8.

44. Morrison DA, Stovall JR. Increased exercise capacity in hypoxemic patients after long-term oxygen therapy. Chest 1992;102:542–50.

45. O'Donnell DE, Bain DJ, Webb KA. Factors contributing to relief of exertional breathlessness during hyperoxia in chronic airflow limitation. Am J Respir Crit Care Med 1997;155:530–5.

46. McDonald CF, Blyth CM, Lazarus MD, et al. Exertional oxygen of limited benefit in patients with chronic obstructive pulmonary disease and mild hypoxemia. Am J Respir Crit Care Med 1995; 152:1616–9.

47. Redelmeier DA, Bayoumi AM, Goldstein RS, Guyatt GH. Interpreting small differences in functional status: the six-minute walk test in chronic lung disease patients. Am J Respir Crit Care Med 1997;155: 1278–82.

48. Dean NC, Brown JK, Himelman RB, et al. Oxygen may improve dyspnea and endurance in patients with chronic obstructive pulmonary disease and only

mild hypoxemia. Am Rev Respir Dis 1992;146: 941–5.

49. Calverley PMA, Brezinova V, Douglas NJ, et al. The effect of oxygenation on sleep quality in chronic bronchitis and emphysema. Am Rev Respir Dis 1982;126:206–10.

50. Tirlapur VG, Mir MA. Nocturnal hypoxaemia and associated electrocardiographic changes in patients with chronic obstructive airways disease. N Engl J Med 1982;306:125–30.

51. Krop HD, Block AJ, Cohen E. Neuropsychologic effects of continuous oxygen therapy in chronic obstructive pulmonary disease. Chest 1973;64: 317–22.

52. Pepin JL, Dautzenberg B, Levy P, Brambilla C. What should we expect from an oxygen concentrator in 1995? Eur Respir Buyers 1995;1:21–6.

53. McPherson SP. Respiratory therapy equipment. 3rd ed. St. Louis, MO: CV Mosby, 1985.

54. McCoy R. Oxygen conserving techniques and devices. Respir Care 2000;45:95–103.

55. Tiep BL. Portable oxygen therapy with oxygen conserving devices and methodologies. Monaldi Arch Chest Dis 1995;50:51–7.

56. Roberts CM, Bell J, Wedzicha JA. Comparison of the efficacy of a demand oxygen delivery system with continuous low flow oxygen in subjects with stable COPD and severe oxygen desaturation on walking. Thorax 1996;51:831–4.

57. Christopher KL, Spofford BT, Petrun MD, et al. A program for transtracheal oxygen delivery: assessment of safety and efficacy. Ann Intern Med 1987;107:802–8.

58. Christopher KL, Spofford BT, Brannin PK, Petty TL. Transtracheal oxygen therapy for refractory hypoxemia. JAMA 1986;256:494–7.

59. Orvidas LJ, Kasperbauer JL, Staats BA, Olsen KD. Long-term clinical experience with transtracheal oxygen catheters. Mayo Clin Proc 1998;73:739–44.

SUGGESTED READINGS

Petty TL, Casaburi R. Recommendations of the Fifth Oxygen Consensus Conference. Respir Care 2000; 45:957–61. *This article presents the recommendations of a consensus development conference on the role of LTOT in the management of COPD.*

Respir Care 2000;45:29–245. Issues of January and February. *A series of articles that represent the proceedings of a state-of-the-art conference on LTOT held in 1999. Subjects covered include the effects of hypoxemia, the benefits of LTOT, the adverse effects of low flow oxygen, and the delivery devices that are available.*

Cairo JM, Pilbeam P. Mosby's respiratory care equipment. 6th ed. St. Louis, MO: Mosby, 1999. *This book provides a comprehensive guide of the methods available for the assessment of hypoxemia, and of the equipment available for the provision of home oxygen.*

CHAPTER 8

MANAGING ACUTE EXACERBATION

*Jean Bourbeau, Michel Rouleau, Marcel Julien,
Diane Nault, and Elizabeth Borycki*

OBJECTIVES

The general objective of this chapter is to help physicians and other allied health care professionals from the hospital and community settings teach the patient and family how to prevent and manage acute exacerbation of chronic obstructive pulmonary disease (COPD). Patients with COPD and their family have to be interpreters and managers of their own health. The physician and health professionals must both identify the disease (acute exacerbation) and then remedy it; they also must recognize a chronic illness in addition to an acute problem.

After reading this chapter, the physician and the allied health care professional will be able to

- recognize a patient with an acute exacerbation;
- teach preventive measures to the patient with an acute exacerbation;
- assess the severity of an acute exacerbation according to signs, symptoms, and laboratory tests;
- treat an acute exacerbation and establish the appropriate conditions to its management in terms of locating the patient in hospital or as an outpatient;
- use a written plan of action to avoid, prevent, and/or control an acute exacerbation; and
- refer to specific professionals from the health care team when needed.

The clinical course of COPD is intermittently interrupted by acute exacerbations, especially during the winter months. Patients with symptomatic COPD have been reported to experience one to four exacerbations per year.[1] The frequency of these exacerbations increases with the severity of their pulmonary disease.[2] Exacerbations of COPD reduce quality of life,[3,4] increase resource use, and substantially increase the costs of related diseases. We are awaiting evidence before we can definitively establish that acute exacerbation is a determinant of disease progression in COPD.

During exacerbations, the intensification of treatment is required; there is an increase in the need for physician visits, visits to the emergency department, and hospitalization. In the United States in 1995, there were over 16 million physician visits and 553,000 hospital discharges for COPD.[5] In Canada, between 1981 and 1982 and 1993 and 1994, the total number of hospital separations where COPD was the primary diagnosis increased by 32%, comprising a 14% increase among men and a 67% increase among women.[6] In a survey of all medical admissions in the United Kingdom, 25% of admissions were owing to respiratory diseases, with over half of these being COPD cases.[7] The overall societal and personal burden owing to acute exacerbation of COPD is high despite some variations between countries. It is therefore important to implement the best strategies for preventing and managing exacerbation.

In this chapter, we review the definition, aggravating factors, and preventive practices associated with managing COPD and discuss the importance of self-management. We will examine how to assess the appropriate management of an exacerbation on an outpatient basis or in hospital. Furthermore, we will present a written plan of action to assist patients with decision making. Treatment of stable COPD is covered elsewhere in this volume; hospital treatment is beyond the scope of this textbook.

DEFINITION

There is no universally accepted definition of an acute exacerbation of COPD. Guidelines do not provide a definition of exacerbation, nor do they provide a classification based on clinical parameters. An exacerbation of COPD is usually considered in clinical terms when there is an acute deterioration superimposed on stable COPD; this includes increased dyspnea, cough, and sputum, as well as change in volume, tenacity, and color of sputum. Fever can be present, but it is not considered an exacerbation of COPD and should lead to the consideration of other diagnoses. Exacerbation may also be accompanied by nonspecific complaints such as fatigue, insomnia, sleepiness, and confusion. Acute exacerbation of COPD is also often associated with transient decrements in lung function.

AGGRAVATING FACTORS

Exacerbation has been studied mainly in patients with COPD in whom the exacerbation is severe enough to seek medical attention. Infectious agents are a major cause of acute exacerbations of COPD. It has been estimated that infections play a role in 50% or more, and in 30% of these, the infection is initially of viral (with or without a superimposed bacterial infection), mycoplasmatic, or chlamydial origin.[8] *Haemophilus influenzae*, *Streptococcus pneumoniae*, and *Moraxella catarrhalis* are the most common bacteria found in the lower airway of patients with COPD[9]; the prevalence of positive microbiology samples of bacteria using sputum samples is higher in patients with exacerbated COPD.[10,11] The role of bacterial flora in the lower airways of patients has been examined intensively in recent years. A recent study using the protected specimen brush for microbiology sampling revealed that the prevalence of lower airway bacterial colonization in outpatients

with stable COPD is high (25%) and is mainly attributable to *H. influenzae* and *S. pneumoniae*.[12] In the same study, exacerbated COPD, defined as at least two of the features of increased dyspnea, sputum volume, and sputum purulence, was associated with a significantly higher prevalence (51.7%) of positive results and higher bacterial concentrations in culture grown after sampling of the lower airway. Emerging evidence from molecular epidemiology and measurement of airway inflammation further support the role of bacteria in acute exacerbation.[13]

Air pollution has also been recognized as a trigger for exacerbations of COPD; in addition to this, associations have been made between the level of air pollutants and adverse health effects.[14] Other environmental factors (smoking, cold air, exercise, etc), aspiration, poor adherence to treatment, and emotional stresses are also recognized in patients presenting with exacerbations; however, their frequency and role as independent factors have not been investigated in epidemiologic studies. Many other environmental exposures have been anecdotally linked to exacerbations of COPD; for instance, many patients describe strong odors as an aggravating factor. There is clearly considerable variation in the susceptibility to various triggers that we do not completely understand; this reinforces and justifies advice on the necessity regarding environmental modification and how it has to be individualized.

On other occasions, for example, when the exacerbation is related to an emotional or psychologic factor, the increase in one symptom (especially dyspnea) is not necessarily accompanied by increased coughing or sputum. These factors also have to be recognized as potential triggers, and the patient has to learn how to interpret and manage them.

Unlike asthma, allergies are not usually a trigger for uncontrolled disease. Other health problems such as pneumonia, congestive heart failure, pulmonary embolism, and pneumothorax may mimic the symptoms of an acute exacerbation of COPD.

ASSESSING AND MANAGING EXACERBATIONS

Assessing Exacerbations

The assessment of the severity of an acute exacerbation will usually be based on certain elements: (1) signs and symptoms and (2) laboratory tests.

Signs and Symptoms

The baseline condition of the patient is essential to assess severity. Cough, sputum volume and color, dyspnea, and especially limitation of daily activities have to be evaluated. Dyspnea, when present at rest or when impairing the ability of the patient to complete one sentence, is an indicator of severe exacerbation. The most important signs of severity are the presence of confusion or a change in alertness; when these signals are present, patients require immediate medical attention and evaluation in the hospital. If fever is present, pneumonia should be suspected. Other signs that may indicate a severe, acute exacerbation are paradoxical chest wall movements, worsening of central cyanosis, signs of right congestive heart failure, and hemodynamic instability. Coma and cardiac arrythmia are life threatening and require admission into the intensive care unit.

Laboratory Tests

Spirometric tests might be useful to assess an acute exacerbation of COPD and can be repeated to monitor progress. However, it is not uncommon in patients with severe COPD to detect only minimal spirometric changes despite significant symptom aggravation. Treatment decision should never be based only on the result of a spirometric test in an exacerbation of COPD. Measurement of peak expiratory flow (PEF) has been adopted by some health professionals, but you have to know that it can grossly underestimate the disease severity and is very patient dependent. Serial PEF data are lacking in COPD, which makes interpretation of significant changes difficult. Assessment of arterial oxygen saturation (SaO_2) could also be used, and portable equipment is often supplied by home nurses or inhalation therapists. An SaO_2 level less than 90%, when breathing ambient air, usually indicates respiratory failure in patients when they have had a previously normal SaO_2 level. However, patients with COPD might have chronic respiratory failure with reduced SaO_2, and some of them might already be on long-term home oxygen. When available, prior tests of lung function and arterial blood gases can be very helpful for comparison with those made during acute episodes. Chest radiographs are useful if pneumonia, congestive heart failure, pneumothorax, or pleural effusion is suspected. Sputum culture is not usually recommended as a routine test for acute exacerbation unless there is pneumonia or the patient is unresponsive to the selected antibiotic.

Treating an Acute Exacerbation

Management should include those interventions that both prevent and rapidly treat an exacerbation of COPD. Managing COPD exacerbation depends on the severity of the flare and on the information obtained from the patient when stable. The general principles of managing exacerbation suggest avoiding environmental factors (indoor or outdoor pollutants, temperature variations, etc) that can cause exacerbation, adding or increasing bronchodilator use, and taking an antibiotic if bacterial infection is suspected, and for patients with severe exacerbations or those who have not demonstrated a satisfactory response to bronchodilators and antibiotics in past episodes, taking systemic corticosteroids is advised. One important aspect of the management is to ensure a follow-up of the patient. A follow-up represents an opportunity to help the patient plan for the future, both in terms of preventing exacerbations and in providing advice about prompt treatment of unavoidable flares.

Other aspects of the management include deciding whether to treat an acute exacerbation as an outpatient or in hospital and then monitoring the effects of the treatment. Education, self-management, and use of a suitable plan of action are essential in the follow-up assessment and in any future management planning.

Antibiotic Treatment

With regard to antibiotic treatment of COPD exacerbation, a recent meta-analysis identified only nine randomized, placebo-controlled trials of at least 5 days on antibiotic treatment; the effect score of antibiotics was positive in seven and negative in two.[15] Overall, a small benefit in favor of antibiotic treatment was found. It also appears that antibiotic treatment is linked to accelerated recovery from exacerbation in patients with more severe diseases.[16] From the highest quality clinical study, by Anthonisen and colleagues,[17] Table 8–1 shows the exacerbation resolution and patients requiring additional antibiotics according to symptom features.

The prescription of antibiotics in acute exacerbation has become routine despite unresolved questions about their true benefit for different categories of patients. Based on Anthonisen's study,[17] antibiotics are used if the patient has at least two of three features: increased dyspnea, sputum volume, and purulence. More recent studies are comparing new antibiotics with those used in standard care practice for exacerbation of COPD. The disease is increasingly treated

TABLE 8–1 Exacerbation Resolution and Patients Requiring Additional Antibiotics

	Symptom Types* (%)		
	3	2	1
Exacerbation resolution			
Placebo group	69.7	60.0	43.0
Antibiotic group	74.2	70.1	62.9
Requiring additional therapy			
Placebo group	12.1	10.7	30.5
Antibiotic group	11.4	5.2	14.3

*Type 1: increased dyspnea, sputum volume, and sputum purulence; type 2: two of these three; and type 3: one of these three.
Adapted from Anthonisen, et al.[17]

with newer, large-spectrum, and more expensive antibiotics, even though their superiority over previous antibiotics remains to be proven.[18–20] Increased antibiotic resistance in respiratory tract pathogens in Canada and other countries is becoming a concern. The choice of antibiotic should be based on a variety of factors, such as the likely pathogens, likelihood of antibiotic-resistant bacteria, and cost failure. A recent study has shown that for acute exacerbations of COPD, third-line antimicrobial agents (amoxicillin-clavulanate, azithromycin, and ciprofloxacin hydrochloride) reduce the failure rate, decrease the need for hospitalization, and prolong the time between episodes.[21] There is evidence that as the severity of the exacerbation increases, the bacteriology of the exacerbation changes. One recent study has defined the bacteriology of exacerbation in relation to forced expiratory volume in 1 second (FEV_1) as the percentage of predicted.[22] Enteric gram-negative bacteria were most common in the patients with the most severe lung dysfunction ($FEV_1 < 50\%$), including *Pseudomonas aeruginosa*, particularly in the very severe ones ($FEV_1 < 35\%$), whereas the gram-positives predominated in the exacerbations of the patients with the mildest degree of lung function abnormalities.

Although antibiotic therapy is an important part of treating acute exacerbation, and despite the proof that some preliminary data support the careful selection of specific agents according to specific patients, eventually leading to improved patient outcomes, we still need prospective studies to confirm that different patients may require different antibiotics.

Inhaled Bronchodilators

Inhaled bronchodilators, using a spacer or air-driven nebulizer, are important in the management of acute exacerbations of COPD. During acute exacerbations of the disease, short-acting β_2 agonists are usually the preferred bronchodilators. Although nebulized ipratropium bromide is often added to a nebulized β_2 agonist in hospital emergency settings, the advantage of this combination is less clear than in stable disease treatment.[23]

Corticosteroids

Corticosteroids are widely prescribed, and published data support their efficacy in treating exacerbations of COPD. In the very first randomized, placebo-controlled trial, known as the Albert study,[24] patients treated with 0.5 mg/kg methylprednisolone every 6 hours, for 72 hours, had a greater improvement of pre- and postbronchodilator FEV_1 already detectable after 12 hours of treatment. However, the validity of these results has since been questioned, mainly because of the statistical methods used in the analysis.[25] Recent studies have established that systemic corticosteroids are effective in improving short-term clinical outcomes in acute exacerbations of COPD.[26–28] Compared with placebo, systemic corticosteroids, in addition to bronchodilator and antibiotic therapies, increase FEV_1 more rapidly and also reduce the length of hospital stay by approximately 1 day. However, after 10 to 14 days, the difference in improvement in FEV_1 between placebo and corticosteroids is no longer significant.[27,28] Although these data provide evidence to support the current practice of prescribing high-dose oral corticosteroids to patients with acute exacerbation of COPD, the treatment should be as short as possible. Systemic corticosteroids may reduce the need for additional therapy for up to 90 days after the exacerbation, but they will increase the risk of adverse effects. Furthermore, in the long run, they will not reduce the rate of serious outcomes such as death, intubation, and hospital re-admission.[27,28]

Outpatient or In-Hospital Management

Traditionally, exacerbations of COPD have been treated in hospital. The decision to treat an exacerbation on an outpatient basis or in hospital has essentially been dependent on the severity of the exacerbation, underlying lung disease, and concomitant comorbid conditions. Recently, attempts at managing the patient with alternatives over emergency departments and inpatient wards have been considered.

A respiratory day hospital observation unit staffed by physicians and nurses has been proposed as an alternative to in-hospital and emergency department care.[29] Of 658 patients admitted within 1 year, 431 required acute treatment, including 236 for asthma and 130 for COPD. The COPD patient's mean age was 68 years; the best mean FEV_1 was at 35% of predicted normal value recorded in the previous year and at 28% of predicted on admission. The average length of stay was 5.9 hours per day and 2.2 days per admission. Of the patients admitted for COPD, 94 patients (22%) had to be transferred to an inpatient ward. When necessary, patients were telephoned by the nurse 24 to 48 hours after discharge, and all of the patients had a follow-up visit in the outpatient clinic with their physician within 1 to 2 weeks. Fifteen patients (less than 2%) returned to an emergency department within 24 hours of discharge, and nine patients (1%) had complications; no deaths were reported. From patient satisfaction questionnaires, 100% of the respondents were satisfied to very satisfied overall.

The need to treat patients in hospital could also be reduced by the use of home care services. Proper management of an acute exacerbation of COPD requires information about the patients, their associated diseases, and the severity of the exacerbation. Symptoms and signs that indicate severity include sleeping or eating difficulties, the inability to speak in full sentences, confusion, and an overall poor condition. Additionally, patients may not be able to cope at home. An alternative approach has been reported by Gravil and colleagues,[30] who demonstrated no greater morbidity in patients cared for at home, although there was a significant re-admission rate (12%) in this group. More recently, Davies and colleagues[31] reported the first randomized controlled trial. Patients with acute exacerbation of COPD who met the study criteria for home care (Table 8–2) were randomized (2:1) to home care with a specialist nurse or hospital care. Home care included the patient being escorted by a nurse, nurse visits in the morning and evening for 3 days and thereafter at the discretion of the nurse, immediate social support if required, nebulized bronchodilators, and prednisolone for 10 days and antibiotics for 5 days. Of the 583 patients referred for admission, 192 met the criteria for home care and 150 agreed to participate in the study. No significant difference was demonstrated in postbronchodilator FEV_1 on admission (36.1% predicted normal) at 2 weeks and 3 months. Re-admission rates within a 3-month follow-up were similar between the groups, despite the early re-admission from the home care group, most being attributable to further exacerbations. No patient had called their general practitioner during the exacerbation. No significant difference was demonstrated

TABLE 8–2 Criteria for Home Care in Patients with COPD Exacerbation*

Treatment at Home	Treatment In Hospital
Mini-mental state score > 7	Marked use of accessory muscles
Pulse rate < 100 bpm	Suspected underlying malignancy on chest x-ray film[†]
Systolic blood pressure > 100 mm Hg	Pneumothorax or pneumonia[†]
pH > 7.35	Uncontrolled left ventricular failure
pO_2 > 7.3 kPa	Acute changes on an electrocardiogram
PCO_2 < 8 kPa	Requirement for full-time nursing care[†]
Total white cell count $4-20 \times 10^9$/L	Requirement for intravenous therapy[†]

*Adapted from the Davies, et al. study, a randomized clinical trial.[31]

[†]Treatment in the patient's home will also depend on home service facilities.[46]

in mortality between the groups during these months (9% versus 8%). The limited existing evidence indicates that compared with hospital care, acute home care produces no notable differences in health outcomes. However, to determine whether society would be better served with an increased use of home care services, the effects on patient and caregiver health, as well as the effects on their costs, should be evaluated.

It is worth noticing that often the patient and the family end up in the emergency department because they do not know how to monitor changes in the disease or how to make appropriate management decisions on the basis of self-monitoring results. Patients with COPD need to be taught about their disease and encouraged to be actively involved in its treatment.[32] An effective collaborative relationship with health care providers can help patients and families better handle self-care tasks.[32,33] Bourbeau and colleagues[34] reported the first randomized controlled trial to demonstrate that a disease-specific self–management program that included an action plan reduced health service use owing to COPD exacerbation by 40% or more (unscheduled physician visits, emergency department visits, and hospitalization) as compared with ususal care. Active patient involvement should address issues related to self-assessment of disease, related changes, and self-management of exacerbation symptoms.

PREVENTION OF FUTURE ACUTE EXACERBATIONS

Helping patients to understand their disease and teaching them about factors that contribute to exacerbation is essential; smoking cessation should be promoted as it is central to modifying the natural history of the disease. Other measures have been suggested, such as vaccination and drug treatment. But, more importantly, to effectively reach as many patients as possible, implementation of these measures must be done in primary care.

Vaccination

Influenza Vaccination

Despite long-standing recommendations for annual influenza vaccinations, approximately one-third of elderly persons, including high-risk persons such as those with chronic lung disease, are not vaccinated.[35] Little has been published about the effectiveness of influenza vaccines in persons with underlying respiratory or other serious medical conditions. A recent retrospective, multiseason cohort study has demonstrated that among unvaccinated persons, hospitalization rates for pneumonia and influenza are twice as high during the influenza seasons than they are in the non–influenza seasons.[36] In that study, influenza vaccination was associated with a risk ratio of hospitalization for pneumonia and influenza of 0.48 (95% CI 0.28–0.82) and of death at 0.30 (95% CI 0.21–0.43). These results provide further evidence that the influenza vaccination should be strongly recommended and that every possible effort be made to facilitate its implementation. It is recommended to vaccinate patients with COPD before the start of the influenza season. For people living in long-term care facilities, the recommended time is the month of November since protection conferred by the antibodies sometimes lasts only 4 months. However, the vaccine is indicated as long as the influenza season is in effect; thus, it should still be administered to any latecomers. It is important to remember to vaccinate patients who travel to places where the flu virus can be present (eg, Florida). More information can be obtained by contacting the public health department. Table 8–3 presents information on the dosage, adverse effects, and contraindications for influenza vaccination.

Pneumococcal Vaccination

Streptococcus pneumoniae is the most common cause of community-acquired pneumonia, accounting for approximately 500,000 hospitalizations and 40,000 deaths in the United States each year.[37] The problem, caused by both antimicrobial resistance and the consistently high mortality rate associated with invasive disease, highlights the importance of preventive efforts. Invasive pneumococcal disease affects persons of all ages, with peak incidences in the very young and the very old. The 23 capsular types represented in the pneumococcal polysaccharide vaccine account for nearly 90% of invasive isolates. Because the vaccine is effective against bacteremia among immunocompetent adults,[38,39] persons with underlying chronic diseases should be vaccinated.[37] A recent population-based case-control study has demonstrated that smoking is the strongest independent risk factor for invasive pneumococcal disease among immunocompetent adults.[40] After the authors controlled for potential confounding variables in subjects, such as

TABLE 8–3 Influenza and Pneumococcal Vaccination

Vaccine*	Dosage	Adverse Effects	Contraindications and Precautions
Influenza	One dose of 0.5 mL annually in the fall (intramuscular administration is preferred: deltoid muscle)	Soreness at the injection site; fever, chills, malaise, myalgia; allergic response (rare)	History of previous anaphylactic reaction or hypersensitivity to eggs or egg products; patient with acute febrile illness
Pneumococcal (Pneumovax)	1 dose of 0.5 mL† (subcutaneous or intramuscular)	Local soreness and erythema, low-grade fever occasionally	Hypersensitivity to any component of the vaccine Patient with acute febrile illness Pregnant or nursing women (rarely apply in COPD)

*Vaccines can be given at the same time, at different sites.

†Relative effectiveness of a revaccination is not known specifically for patients with COPD. It is recommended to revaccinate one time only (5 years after the first dose) in patients with COPD with debilitating disease.

the presence or absence of chronic disease and the role of educational levels, current smoking had 4.1 times the odds of invasive infection and second-hand smoke had 2.5 times the odds; furthermore, there was a clear dose-response relation with respect to the amount of smoking, duration of passive exposure, and length of time since the cessation of smoking (increased risk for at least 10 years after quitting). Additional factors associated with invasive disease were chronic disease (including COPD), living with a young child who attended day care, black race, male gender, and low educational and socioeconomic status. Although this study does not address the issue of vaccination specifically in patients with COPD, it provides additional arguments to promote its use in this disease. Advisory bodies responsible for determining its administration are now recommending pneumococcal vaccination for elderly patients with COPD. Therefore, pneumococcal vaccination in COPD for prevention of a condition that causes serious morbidity is justified, especially when the risk of harming an individual patient is extremely small. At present, experience with revaccination is still limited and there are no data on the relative effectiveness of a second dose. It is recommended to revaccinate one time only (5 years after the first dose) in people with the highest risk of serious infection and in those with asplenia, debilitating cardiorespiratory disease, chronic nephrotic syndrome, cirrhosis, and immunoincompetent, whose antibody level could decrease

rapidly. Table 8–3 presents information on dosage, adverse effects, and contraindications for pneumococcal vaccination.

Pharmacologic Treatment

Bronchodilator treatments are essentially for symptom relief as few data are available on the long-term use of pharmacologic treatment and the prevention of acute exacerbations. One recent short-term study of patients with mild COPD (who had a once-a-year exacerbation requiring visits to their physician/hospital for the previous 3 years) showed that fluticasone propionate (1,000 µg per day), in comparison with placebo, did not alter the number of patients who had at least one exacerbation over a 6-month treatment.[41] However, there were significantly fewer patients who had moderate to severe exacerbations of COPD during a 6-month treatment while being treated with fluticasone propionate. More recently, a long-term study showed that fluticasone propionate, again at a relatively high dose (1,000 µg per day), reduced exacerbation rates by 25% from 1.33 exacerbations per year in the placebo group to 0.99 per year in the fluticasone group (p = .023) over a 3-year treatment period.[42] No reductions in exacerbation were demonstrated in patients with a FEV_1 above 1.54 L, and the most important reduction was in patients with FEV_1 below 1.25 L. Exacerbation can have negative effects on the quality of life and health costs, thus making its prevention an important goal of therapy. However, high doses of inhaled corticosteroids might not be without adverse effects. As we await further confirmation of these results, the use of inhaled corticosteroids should be considered only if concomitant asthma is suspected or in patients with severe COPD and frequent exacerbations that require systemic corticosteroid treatment.

Many studies, specifically with new pharmacologic agents under investigation, will be assessing the effects of these drugs on the exacerbation rate in patients with COPD. Physicians should look for those study results, which will be available in the coming years.

SELF-MANAGEMENT AND PLAN OF ACTION

Self-Management

Self-management in COPD is aimed at optimal care and treatment of respiratory symptoms to allow for the best possible quality of life. This involves managing patients through periods of wellness and exacerbations and focusing on the goals of reducing symptoms and improving health.[43] Exacerbations or periods of increased symptom severity occur intermittently. To actively involve patients in the management of their disease, they must be able to recognize signs and symptoms of an exacerbation, and according to changes in symptom and health severity,[32,43] they should be able to respond with immediate adjustments to treatment. The patient also has to be confident enough to manage his/her symptoms because self-efficacy (confidence in ability to cope with disease) is ultimately a large part of the process that determines behavior and outcome.[44]

As an aspect of care, self-management support has been associated with improved outcomes in studies of interventions in chronic disease. Only limited data are available about self-management plans in COPD. In a recent randomized multicentre clinical trial, patients with severe COPD receiving a specific disease self-management program, as compared with usual care, had a number of positive benefits; they had an improvement in health-related quality of life and as previously mentioned, a reduction in unscheduled physician visits, emergency department visits, and hospitalizations over the follow-up year.[34,45] This program included a comprehensive patient education program with components specific to COPD; it also addressed the symptoms and signs of an exacerbation, and a written plan of action. A trained health professional acted as a case-manager and was available by telephone for advice, supervision of treatment, and monitoring of the exacerbation. The health professional was also in close contact with the on-duty physician and the specialist administering the treatment. The relative value of each of these components and the value of single components applied simultaneously are unknown. Many physicians involved in the care of patients with COPD feel that self-management is important; a written plan drawn up with the patient is necessary, as well as having safeguards to call a physician or a trained health professional as part of a group, especially if symptoms become worse.

Plan of Action

A plan of action is a tool that facilitates early recognition of changes in symptoms and accordingly dictates the specific action to be taken by the patient to prevent and manage an exacerbation of COPD. A plan of action needs to be developed to improve patient knowledge, understanding, and management and to aid in decision making with regard to disease symptoms.

Each plan of action is unique; it advocates the use of pharmacologic and nonpharmacologic methods of managing periods of wellness and exacerbations of the disease specific to the patient.[32] The plan of action is written by the patient's physician or respirologist. The health professional, physician, nurse, or inhalation therapist acts as part of the group in his/her responsibility to act as a resource and to teach the patient awareness of the predetermined plan. Additionally, the health professional can help the patient problem solve symptom/medication-related problems and monitor the patient's self-management behaviors. The patient should be able to contact the treating physician or a health professional who acts as a case manager should the symptoms become worse.

In general, the underlying principles of the plan of action for patients with COPD are fivefold in nature. They include

1. appropriate use of pharmacologic and nonpharmacologic treatments during periods of wellness;
2. use of an inhaled bronchodilator (short-acting β_2 agonist) during periods of exacerbation;
3. preventing, avoiding, or controlling environ-

mental factors that cause exacerbation of disease, if possible;

4. treatment with an antibiotic and/or oral corticosteroid depending on the severity and nature of the exacerbation (respiratory infection); and

5. recognizing the importance of comorbid conditions, for example, heart failure, when diagnosing and treating individuals with COPD.

The plan of action helps the patient differentiate between not only managing the disease during periods of wellness and exacerbation but also educating the patient on the varying forms of exacerbation. The patient learns to differentiate between these various periods and is therefore better able to select the most appropriate self-management strategy to diminish symptom presentation and severity.[32]

A written plan of action (adapted from the comprehensive self-management program "Living well with COPD©") is provided as an example (Appendix 1). Each section of the action plan describes the symptoms the patient should be experiencing and the appropriate self-management plan as prescribed by the physician.

For each section, certain considerations have to be taken.

I Feel Well

The first section of the plan of action deals with the patient when he/she is in a state of wellness. Here, the plan of action describes the activities a healthy individual would perform on a daily basis to maintain the current state of wellness—for example, avoiding factors that can exacerbate symptoms, using energy conservation techniques, taking medications as prescribed by your doctor, eating healthily, and performing exercises on a regular basis.

I Feel That My Symptoms Are Getting Worse

This section includes different situations that might trigger an acute exacerbation of COPD: stress factors, environmental factors, and respiratory infection. *Stress Factors.* In the case of emotional stresses, symptoms of disease can be released in the form of anger, fear, and anxiety. This can lead to increased skeletal muscle activity, energy expenditure, and subsequent attacks of dyspnea. Long-term stress relief should also be addressed. Assessing the underlying cause of stress will help both the patient and health professional find successful strategies for managing disease. For example, if a patient's spouse has died and the associated grief

has led to an exacerbation of symptoms, the health professional and patient can discuss the need for counseling. If the underlying cause is more transient or situational in nature, such as an argument with a spouse, relaxation strategies with breathing techniques and exercises may be warranted. Occasionally, an inhaled bronchodilator should be used, especially in an uncontrolled acute situation of emotional stress.

Environmental Factors. In most cases, environmental factors that can cause bronchial irritation should be avoided. For example, patients with COPD who smoke should be encouraged to quit, and friends and family should be asked not to smoke when they are near a person who has COPD. In cases in which exposure to exacerbating environmental factors is unavoidable, an inhaled bronchodilator should be used and attempts made to minimize exposure. There should be an increased administration of a short-acting β_2 agonist: two to four inhalations every 20 to 30 minutes three times and then every 2 to 3 hours may be necessary. The patient should be told that if symptoms are not resolved after a few hours at most, a health professional should be called; if the symptoms still persist, a physician, emergency department, or hospital visit may be warranted. In general, medical treatment should not be used as a substitute for avoiding an environmental factor that can cause an exacerbation of the disease.

In the special situation of exercise, patients will often feel limited and usually complain of severe breathlessness. Many patients will stop exercising because they are breathless and will immediately take a short-acting β_2 agonist when, in fact, just stopping exercise would give the same result. However, it is important to stress that some patients may benefit from taking a short-acting β_2 agonist before doing a specific exercise activity. The health professional should evaluate the patient's level of breathlessness in response to activity on a case-by-case basis.

Respiratory Infection. Patients with upper airway bacterial infection are not easily differentiated from those who do not have infections; thus, antibiotics need to be given more often than is probably necessary. When a respiratory infection does occur, patients will report symptom changes. Changes in sputum color and increases in volume and viscosity of sputum often occur, and dyspnea will usually increase in severity. Symptoms of a cold, pharyngitis, or a fever may or may not accompany respiratory infection. When an infection is suspected, antibiotics should be used as part of the patient's treatment and should be selected according to local procedure guidelines derived from local bacteriologic sensitivity data. Antibiotics are often used if the patient has at least two of three features: increased dyspnea and/or sputum volume and purulence (see Table 8–1). Oral corticosteroids may be needed in the more severe cases and should be used in acute exacerbations in any of the following situations: (1) when the patient is already receiving a maintenance dose, (2) when there has been a previous need for oral corticosteroids and the patient has responded favorably, and (3) when there is a failure to respond with only bronchodilators and antibiotics. Advice on smoking, lifestyle, activity levels, and a review of medication should follow the recommendations for the management of COPD.

I Feel That My Symptoms Are Continuing to Worsen or I Feel I Am in Danger

The last two sections of the plan of action address the role of the patient and his/her decision making when symptoms do not improve, continue to worsen, or rapidly deteriorate. Here, the plan of action acts as a catalyst for seeking immediate medical attention. It advocates either calling the physician, the health professional within a group who has been the patient's advisor, or, in the most severe cases, going to a hospital emergency department. In some cases, an underlying condition can exacerbate the symptoms of COPD and cause a rapid deterioration in health status. As well, some medications may not be effective in treating an exacerbation. In response, the patient should make every effort to address the potential presence of an underlying medical condition or should seek new treatment when this occurs.

WHEN TO REFER

When to Refer to the Physician or Respirologist

An indication for physician and/or respirologist referral should be considered for any patient who is unresponsive to the plan of action, has recurring acute exacerbations requiring antibiotics and/or systemic corticosteroids, or has any change in his/her medical condition. The health professional should not hesitate to contact the physician and/or the respirologist for discussion of any situation involving doubt in the assessment or management of the acute exacerbation. The general practitioner should also consider referring the patient to a respirologist if exacerbations are recurring and if they are associated with progressive deterioration of the respiratory or general condition.

When to Refer to the Hospital

An indication for hospital assessment or admission for acute exacerbation of COPD will depend on the severity of the exacerbation, although local resources will also need to be considered. Alternatives such as day hospital and home care by a specialized nurse to an inpatient ward admission look promising and have been discussed in this chapter. Appropriate resources in the community will facilitate the implementation of home care as an alternative to hospitalization for acute exacerbation or early discharge from the hospital. However, data and cost-benefit analysis with the effect on society as a whole are still awaited.

Patients who should receive immediate medical attention are those who have severe dyspnea with inadequate initial response to emergency treatment, those with severe hypoxemia or worsening hypoxemia, and, lastly, any patients with lethargy or coma. These patients will usually need to be hospitalized and might even need to be admitted to the intensive care unit.

SUMMARY

It is impossible to supply a guide that will apply to all patients suffering from acute exacerbation of COPD. The physician's decision to see patients and either keep them in hospital or send them home will vary according to numerous factors: the severity of the exacerbation, how it compares to the usual health status but also the follow-up, the organization of the health services, and the support that can be given at home by respiratory health professionals and physicians. There is some evidence on which to base the decision process, but more research is needed. Any symptoms or signs suggesting respiratory failure or any doubt should have the patient referred to the hospital or to a specialized clinic. Patient hospitalization can be reduced with particular settings such as a day hospital[29] or if there is a specialized health professional within a health care organization providing home care services.[30,31]

The role of education and self-management has been viewed as increasingly important in the early management and prevention of acute exacerbations.

A recent early control study has shown a reduction in unscheduled physician visits, emergency department visits, and hospitalizations in patients with COPD receiving a disease-specific self-management program when compared with those receiving usual care.[34] Acute exacerbations resulted in an important reduction in emergency department visits and hospital admissions. A plan of action with telephone access to a health professional acting as the case manager offers a distinct possiblity. This health professional can supervise treatment at home and can also offer the perspective of an earlier treatment; furthermore, the health professional provides the potential for preventing deterioration and the chance of reducing the need for subsequent emergency department visits or hospitalizations. Further studies must be done to establish the most cost-effective approach depending on the patient population with acute exacerbation of COPD. However, practice will always have to be adapted according to the stages of the COPD and the health care resources available in a given region.

CASE STUDY

Ms. Cope, a 70-year-old patient with COPD, comes to the outpatient clinic 2 weeks after being discharged from the hospital, where she was admitted for treatment of an acute exacerbation.

Medical History, Physical Examination, and Test Results

Medical History

- Physician has diagnosed COPD for many years.
- No relevant past medical history.
- She lives with her husband in their private residence.
- She is less active in the past 3 years and has a lot of difficulty controlling acute episodes of shortness of breath; she is anxious and worried.
- During the last year, she consulted the emergency department many times and has been hospitalized twice for acute exacerbations.
- When she met her physician in his office, they agreed on a plan of action to prevent and control future exacerbations.

Physical Examination

- She has no respiratory distress.
- Her respiratory rate is 18/minute and has normal vital signs.
- She has a barrel chest, decreased air entry, and no rale; cardiac examination is normal; and no peripheral edema or cyanosis.

Test Results

- She has spirometry compatible with severe airflow obstruction without significant reversibility.

Questions and Discussion

An example of a plan of action template is provided. This plan of action is part of a comprehensive patient education program specific to patients with COPD, "Living Well With COPD©." This can be found at the end of this chapter. (See Appendix 1) We have not included medications in the template for this case study since our objective here is not to do specific commercial drug promotion. Drugs, as part of the plan of action, should be prescribed by the treating physician according to practice guides and specific patient needs.

The physician asked you to teach the patient her plan of action so you did, and she seemed to understand the procedure clearly after practicing the scenarios. A month later, she calls you at the clinic telling you that she is really short of breath and she does not know what to do. How will you evaluate the situation? How will you bring the patient to use her plan of action properly? How will you proceed to do your follow-up?

How Will You Evaluate the Situation? Which Questions Will You Ask?

1. Question the patient on the changes in her daily activities:
   - Are you unusually short of breath?
   - What are you unable to do compared to your normal state?
   - Do you have symptoms other than shortness of breath?
   - How are your sleeping and eating patterns?
   - How effective is your inhaled medication?

2. Question the patient to determine the onset and the duration of the dyspnea episodes:

- How long have you been unusually short of breath?

3. Question the patient on the events preceding the deterioration of symptoms and determine with her which factors exacerbate her disease: a stress situation and/or exposure to an environmental factor and/or a respiratory infection:
   - What do you think provoked this episode of shortness of breath?

4. Question the patient on the symptoms of the respiratory infection such as an increase in secretions or a change in their color:
   - Do you have an increase and/or change in the color of your sputum?

5. Question the patient on any actions taken such as changes in her medication, previous actions and their effectiveness, and the number of physician visits, emergency visits, and hospitalizations. Have the patient analyze her actions, assess the results, decrease her anxiety, and discuss actions that have been successful in the past during similar situations:
   - What measures did you already take at home to control the situation?

6. Question the patient also on the symptoms related to comorbidities (list the comorbid conditions).

How Will You Bring the Patient to Properly Use Her Plan of Action?

Teach the patient the following self-management techniques to alleviate and control the exacerbation:
- identification and duration of the aggravating factors and their symptoms;
- measures to be taken according to the plan of action; and
- medication adjustment according to the physician's prescription: make sure that she can both fill the medication and initiate the treatment.

How Will You Follow-Up with the Patient?

The patient must be advised to call you back within 48 hours following the introduction of an antibiotic or prednisone. If the patient fails to contact you, recontact her as a reminder of the necessity of progress reports in the plan of action. The patient must also be advised to inform you if she sees her family doctor, goes to an emergency department, or is hospitalized. Always give positive reinforcement toward any actions resulting in success.

KEY POINTS

- Managing exacerbation includes (1) avoiding aggravating factors, (2) increasing bronchodilators, (3) taking an antibiotic if infection is suspected, and (4) taking systemic corticosteroids (less than a 2-week course) for those with severe exacerbation or not responsive to previous treatment.
- There are alternatives to hospitalization such as day hospital settings or care with a specialized nurse; appropriate health care organizations have to be in place.
- Managing exacerbation should include those interventions that both prevent (vaccination; inhaled corticosteroids in severe COPD patients with recurrent acute exacerbations, especially those requiring treatment with systemic corticosteroids) and rapidly treat the acute exacerbation when symptoms deteriorate.
- Establish for the patient with COPD an individualized plan of action with the respirologist and/or treating physician.
- Make sure there is a well-established contact between the patient and a resource person acting as a case manager to prevent or control acute exacerbations.
- Review the plan of action, make sure there is a proper follow-up, and, when it is necessary, make a readjustment according to the patient's needs.
- Facilitate patient decision making.

REFERENCES

1. Fletcher C, Peto R. The natural history of chronic airflow obstruction. BMJ 1977;1:1645–8.

2. Collet JP, Shapiro S, Ernst P, et al., and the PARI-IS Study Steering Committee and Research Group. Effects of an immunostimulating agent on acute exacerbations and hospitalizations in patients with chronic obstructive pulmonary disease. Am J Respir Crit Care Med 1997;156:1719–24.

3. Seemungal TA, Donaldson GC, Paul EA, et al. Effects of exacerbation on quality of life in patients with chronic obstructive pulmonary disease. Am J Respir Crit Care Med 1998;157:1418–22.

4. Osman IM, Godden DJ, Friend JA, et al. Quality of life and hospital re-admission in patients with chronic obstructive pulmonary disease. Thorax 1997;32:67–71.

5. NHL BI. Morbidity and mortality chartbook, 1998. Available at http://www.nhlbi.nih.gov/resources/coes/cht.book.htm (last accessed February 2002).

6. Lacasse Y, Brooks D, Goldstein R. Trends in the epidemiology of COPD in Canada, 1980 to 1995. Canadian Thoracic Society Rehabilitation Committee. Chest 1999;116:306–13.

7. Anderson HR, Esmail A, Hollswell J, et al. Epidemiologically based needs assessment: lower respiratory disease. London: Department of Health, 1994.

8. Ball P. Epidemiology and treatment of chronic bronchitis and its exacerbations. Chest 1995;108 Suppl 2:43S–52S.

9. Murphy TF, Sethi S. Bacterial infection in chronic obstructive pulmonary disease. Am Rev Respir Dis 1992;146:1067–83.

10. Philit F, Etienne J, Calvert A, et al. Infectious agents associated with exacerbations of chronic obstructive bronchpneumopathies and attacks of asthma. Rev Mal Respir 1992;9:191–6.

11. Gump DW, Phillips CA, Forsyth BR, et al. Role of infection in chronic bronchitis. Am Rev Respir Dis 1976;113:465–74.

12. Monso E, Ruiz J, Rosell A, et al. Bacterial infection in chronic obstructive pulmonary disease. A study of stable and exacerbated outpatients using the protected specimen brush. Am J Respir Crit Care Med 1995;152:1316–20.

13. Sethi S. Infectious etiology of acute exacerbations of chronic bronchitis. Chest 2000;117:380S–5S.

14. Anderson HR, Spix C, Medina S, et al. Air pollution and daily admissions for chronic obstructive pulmonary disease in 6 European cities: results from the APHEA project. Eur Respir J 1997;10:1064–71.

15. Saint S, Bent S, Vittinghoff E, Grady D. Antibiotics in chronic obstructive pulmonary disease exacer-bations: a meta-analysis. JAMA 1995;273:957–60.

16. Pines A, Raafat H, Plucinski K, et al. Antibiotic regimens in severe and acute purulent exacerbations of chronic bronchitis. BMJ 1968;2:735–8.

17. Anthonisen NR, Manfreda J, Warren CP, et al. Antibiotic therapy in exacerbations of chronic obstructive pulmonary disease. Ann Intern Med 1987;106:196–204.

18. Cazzola M, Vinciguerra A, Beghi G, et al. Comparative evaluation of the clinical and microbiological efficacy of co-amoxiclav vs cefixime or ciprofloxacin in bacterial exacerbation of chronic bronchitis. J Chemother 1995;7:432–41.

19. Chodosh S, Tuck J, Stottmeier KD, Pizzuto D. Comparison of ciprofloxacin with ampicillin in acute infectious exacerbations of chronic bronchitis: a double-blind crossover study. Am J Med 1989;87:107S–12S.

20. Wollschlager C, Raoof S, Khan F, et al. Controlled, comparative study of ciprofloxacin versus amplicillin in treatment of bacterial respiratory tract infections. Am J Med 1987;82:164–8.

21. Destache CJ, Dewan N, O'Donohue WJ, et al. Clinical and economic considerations in the treatment of acute exacerbations of chronic bronchitis. J Antimicrob Chemother 1999;43 Suppl A:107–13.

22. Eller J, Ede A, Schaberg T, et al. Infective exacerbations of chronic bronchitis. Relation between bacteriologic etiology and lung function. Chest 1998;113:1542–8.

23. Karpel JP. Bronchodilator responses to anticholinergic and beta-adrenergic agents in acute and stable COPD. Chest 1991;99:871–6.

24. Albert RK, Martin TR, Lewis SW. Controlled clinical trial of methylprednisolone in patients with chronic bronchitis and acute respiratory insufficiency. Ann Intern Med 1980;92:753–8.

25. Glenny RW. Steroids in COPD. Chest 1987;91:289–90.

26. Thompson WH, Nielson CP, Carvalho P, et al. Controlled trial of oral prednisone in out patients with acute COPD exacerbation. Am J Respir Crit Care Med 1996;154:407–12.

27. Niewoehner DE, Erbland ML, Deupree RH, et al. Effect of systemic glucocorticoids on exacerbations of chronic pulmonary disease. N Engl J Med 1999;340:1941–7.

28. Davies L, Angus RM, Calverley PM. Oral corticosteroids in patients admitted to hospital with exacerbations of chronic obstructive pulmonary disease: a prospective randomized controlled trial. Lancet 1999;354:456–60.

29. Schwartzman K, Duquette G, Dion M-J, et al. Respiratory day hospital: a novel approach to acute respiratory care. Can Med Assoc J 2001;165:1067–71.

30. Gravil JH, Al-Rawas OA, Cotton MM, et al. Home treatment of exacerbations of chronic obstructive pulmonary disease by an acute respiratory assessment service. Lancet 1998;351:1853–5.

31. Davies L, Wilkinson M, Bonner S, et al. "Hospital at home" versus hospital care in patients with exacerbations of chronic obstructive pulmonary disease: prospective randomized controlled trial. BMJ 2000;321:1265–8.

32. Watson PB, Town GI, Holbrook N, et al. Evaluation of a self-management plan for chronic obstructive pulmonary disease. Eur Respir J 1997;10:1267–71.

33. Nault D, Pépin J, Dagenais J, et al. Qualitative evaluation of a self-management program Living Well with COPD© offered to patients and their caregivers. Am J Respir Crit Care Med 2000;161:A56.

34. Bourbeau J, Collet JP, Schwartzman K, et al. Integrating rehabilitative elements into a COPD self-management program reduces exacerbations and health services utilization: a randomized clinical trial. Am J Respir Crit Care Med 2000;161:A254.

35. Influenza and pneumococcal vaccination levels among adults aged ≥ 65 years—United States, 1997. MMWR Morb Mortal Wkly Rep 1998;47:797–802.

36. Nichol KL, Baken L, Nelson A. Relation between influenza vaccination and outpatient visits, hospitalization, and mortality in elderly persons with chronic lung disease. Ann Intern Med 1999;130:397–403.

37. Prevention of pneumococcal disease: recommendations of the Advisory Committee on Immunization Practices. MMWR Morb Mortal Wkly Rep 1997;46(RR-8):1–24.

38. Shapiro ED, Berg AT, Austrian R, et al. The protective efficacy of polyvalent pneumococcal polysaccharide vaccine. N Engl J Med 1991;325:1453–60.

39. Butler JC, Breiman RF, Campbell JF, et al. Pneumococcal polysaccharide vaccine efficacy. An evaluation of current recommendations. JAMA 1993;270:1826–31.

40. Nuorti JP, Butler JC, Farley MM, et al., and the Active Bacterial Core Surveillance Team. Cigarette smoking and invasive pneumococcal disease. N Engl J Med 2000;342:681–9.

41. Paggiaro PL, Dahle R, Bakran I, et al. Multicentre randomized placebo-controlled trial of inhaled fluticasone propionate in patients with chronic obstructive pulmonary disease. Lancet 1998;351:773–80.

42. Burge PS, Caverley PM, Jones PW, et al. Randomised, double blind, placebo controlled study of fluticasone propionate in patients with moderate to severe chronic obstructive pulmonary disease. The ISOLDE trial. BMJ 2000;320:1297–303.

43. Make B. Collaborative self-management strategies for patients with respiratory disease. Respir Care 1994;39:566–79.

44. Bandura A, Adams NE. Analysis of the self-efficacy theory of behavioral changes. Cogn Ther Res 1977;1:287–308.

45. Bourbeau J, Julien M, Rouleau M, et al. Impact of an integrated rehabilitative management program on health status of COPD patients. A multicentre randomized clinical trial. Eur Respir J 2000;16:159S.

46. British Thoracic Society. Guidelines for the management of chronic obstructive pulmonary disease: the COPD Guideline Group of the Standards of Care Committee of the BTS. Thorax 1997;52 Suppl:S16–28.

SUGGESTED READING

Pauwels RA, Buist AS, Calverly PMA, et al., on behalf of the GOLD Scientific Committee. National Heart, Lung, and Blood Institute/WHO Global Initiative for Chronic Obstructive Lung Disease (GOLD) workshop summary: global strategy for the diagnosis, management, and prevention of chronic obstructive lung disease (GOLD) Scientific Committee. Am J Respir Crit Care Med 2001;163:1256–76. *The GOLD guideline is an international guideline on the different aspects of the management of COPD. Recommendations made in the guideline are evidence based; where evidence is lacking, recommendations are based on expert consensus.*

Sherk PA, Grossman RF. The chronic obstructive pulmonary disease exacerbation. Clin Chest Med 2000;21:705–721. *This is an extensive review article with 138 references. The review focuses essentially on the treatment of acute exacerbation: controlled oxygen; pharmacologic treatment, including bronchodilators, corticosteroids, and antibiotics; noninvasive positive pressure ventilation; and outcomes.*

APPENDIX 1

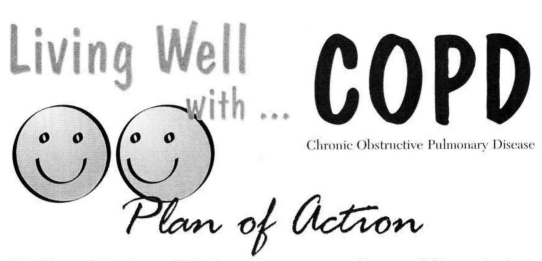

My Plan of Action will help me to treat my disease daily and when my symptoms get worse. It includes:

☞ **Contact names and numbers**

☞ **Daily medications**

☞ **Advice and Medications I will need when my symptoms get worse**

Contact List

Service	Name	Phone Number
Respirologist		
Family Physician		
After 5 p.m. on weekdays/weekends		
Hospital Emergency		
OTHERS:		

I Feel Well

My Symptoms	My Actions
I sleep well and my appetite is good. I am able to do my exercises	• I avoid things that may make my symptoms worse. • I plan each day in advance. • I take my medication as prescribed by my doctor. • I eat healthy food. • I do my exercises on a regular basis

My Regular Treatment

Name of Medication	Dose	Number of Puffs/Pills	Frequency

I Feel Different (environment/stress)

My Symptoms	My Actions
• I am more short of breath than usual. • I may have sputum, a cough or a wheeze.	

I have been exposed to ...

... Stressful Situation.	• I use my breathing techniques and try to relax first. • I position my body so I am less short of breath. • I take _____ puffs of _____.
... Pollutants, Sudden Changes in Temperature, Humidity, Wind or Strong Exercise.	• I take _____ puffs of _____ and repeat each 20 to 45 minutes, for 2 to 3 times. • I avoid or decrease exposure to these factors. • I use my breathing techniques and try to relax.

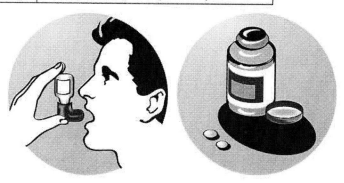

I Feel Different (respiratory infection)

I have at Least 2 of the **Following Symptoms**	My actions
• Increased shortness of breath. • Increased volume of sputum. • Yellow or green sputum.	

I have developed ...	
... a Respiratory Infection	❏ I increase my inhaled bronchodilators as recommended by my doctor. ❏ I notify my contact person or doctor for advice. ❏ I take my antibiotic and my anti-inflammatory as recommended by my doctor.

My Additional Treatment is ...

Bronchodilators	Dose	# of puffs/pills	Frequency	# of days
Antibiotic	Dose	pills	Frequency	# of days
Anti-Inflammatory	Dose	# of puffs/pills	Frequency	# of days

"My Symptoms Continue to Get Worse" or "I am in Danger" ... see reverse

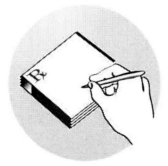

My symptoms continue to get worse

My Symptoms	My Actions
... have not improved or they have become worse	• I call my contact person. • After 5 p.m. or on the weekend, and I am unable to wait, I will go to the hospital or a walk-in clinic.

I Feel I am in Danger

My Symptoms	My Actions
In any situation if: • I am very short of breath, agitated confused and/or drowsy. • I have chest pain.	• **Dial 911 for an ambulance to take you to the nearest hospital emergency**

Other Doctor Recommendations

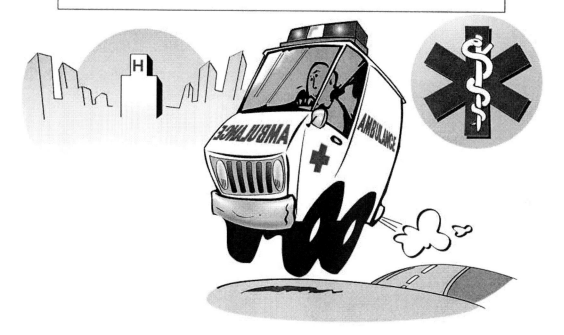

Adapted from: Self-management program "Living well with COPD©".
Supported by: Respiratory network of the fonds de la recherche an santé du Quebec (FRSP) and Boehringer Ingelheim Canada.

CONTROLLING BREATHLESSNESS AND COUGH

Denis E. O'Donnell, Katherine Webb, and Maureen McGuire

OBJECTIVES

The general objective of this chapter is to help physicians and other allied health care professionals understand the pathophysiology of chronic obstructive pulmonary disease (COPD) and develop an approach to assess dyspnea and cough on which to base their interventions in patients with COPD.

After reading this chapter, the physician and the allied health care professional will be able to

- understand the mechanisms of dyspnea in COPD;
- develop a step-by-step approach to the assessment of the dyspneic patient with COPD;
- develop a comprehensive approach to the management of the dyspneic patient with COPD and to understand the beneficial mechanism of therapeutic interventions;
- understand common mechanisms of cough in COPD;
- learn how best to evaluate patients with COPD with cough and to review the role of history, physical examination, and selected investigations;
- develop an effective management strategy for cough control in patients with COPD and, more specifically, the role of pharmacologic therapy and physiotherapy techniques; and
- refer to specific professionals from the health care team.

Breathlessness (dyspnea), the perception of respiratory discomfort, is the most common symptom in patients with COPD. Most patients seek medical attention because of breathlessness as their lung disease progresses; furthermore, it is a major cause of disability and anxiety associated with the disease. The precise neurophysiologic mechanisms of dyspnea are poorly understood, but our knowledge of the pathophysiologic basis of this symptom has advanced considerably.[1–4] This has allowed us to formulate a rational approach to the management of this symptom, which will be the main focus of this chapter.

A second major symptom in many patients with COPD, usually the first symptom to develop, is chronic cough. Cough will often initially be intermittent but with time will present every day, sometime throughout the day, and is seldom entirely nocturnal. Indeed, in some patients, a troublesome cough may be the predominant symptom for which medical attention is sought. A systematic approach to management, which is solidly based on an understanding of the pathophysiology of this symptom, is usually successful.

In this chapter, we review the pathophysiology, clinical assessment, and management strategies of breathlessness and cough, the two most common symptoms of COPD.

CONTROLLING BREATHLESSNESS

Mechanisms of Dyspnea

Dyspnea is provoked or aggravated by activity; therefore, most studies conducted to explore mechanisms of dyspnea have been carried out in exercising patients. These studies have identified several pathophysiologic abnormalities that contribute to dyspnea. These include

1. overloading and weakening of inspiratory muscles,
2. excessive ventilation relative to capacity,
3. gas exchange abnormalities,
4. dynamic collapse of airways in expiration,
5. cardiac factors, and
6. any combination of the above.

The relative importance of these different factors in dyspnea causation varies among individuals with COPD. Generally, as the disease advances, more of these interdependent factors combine to contribute to dyspnea.

The current approach to management of dyspnea involves the search for the most prominent contributory factor(s) so that it can be favorably modified or reversed to achieve symptom relief. There are two recognized factors that will be the primary focus of this discussion: (1) the abnormal mechanical load such as dynamic lung overinflation, which overburdens the inspiratory muscles and (2) the symptom of excessive ventilation. Finally, the neurophysiologic basis of dyspnea will be discussed.

Dyspnea and Dynamic Lung Overinflation

The diagnosis of COPD encompasses wide-ranging pathophysiologic abnormalities. For example, COPD can involve disease of the small and larger airways; it can also involve disease of the lung parenchyma (ie, emphysema) either alone or in highly variable combinations.[5] Although the most obvious and commonly measured abnormality in COPD is expiratory airway obstruction or flow limitation, the most important and often underappreciated mechanical consequence of this is lung overinflation owing to gas trapping (Figure 9–1).[5] Thus, patients with severe expiratory flow limitation are forced to breathe at high lung volumes close to their total lung capacity in order to generate sufficient expiratory flow rates to maintain adequate ventilation. Moreover, under conditions of increased ventilation such as exercise or anxiety, lung emptying is further curtailed by the shortened exhalation time with each breath; this results in even further gas trapping in an already overinflated lung at rest (Figure 9–2). This phenomenon is called dynamic hyperinflation (DH). Average increases in end-expiratory lung volume (EELV) during exercise are 0.3 to 0.6 L, but with considerable variation in the range.[6–8]

It is now recognized that lung overinflation can have disastrous mechanical and sensory consequences:

1. Dynamic hyperinflation restricts thoracic motion and reduces the ability to expand tidal volume

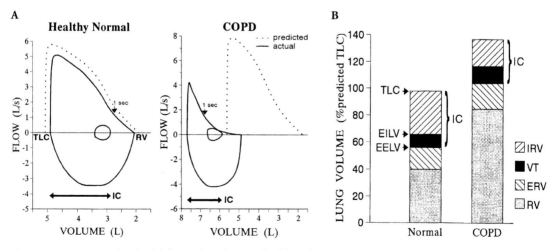

Figure 9–1 *A*, Maximal and tidal flow-volume loops in health and in a patient with COPD. *B*, Volume compartments in health and disease. Note the reduced inspiratory capacity in COPD as a result of resting lung hyperinflation. EELV = end-expiratory lung volume; EILV = end-inspiratory lung volume; TLC = total lung capacity; IC = inspiratory capacity; IRV = inspiratory reserve volume; ERV = expiratory reserve volume; RV = reserve volume.

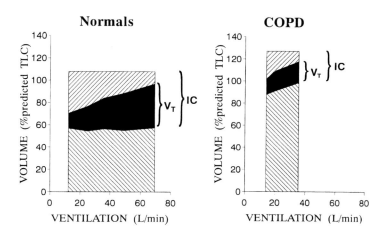

Figure 9–2 Changes in operational lung volume expressed over ventilation during exercise: end-expiratory lung volume (EELV) and end-inspiratory lung volume (EILV) bracket the tidal volume (V_T) in health and in COPD. In contrast with normals, patients with COPD show further dynamic increases in the EELV during exercise. Thus, inspiratory reserve volume (IRV) is relatively diminished in COPD compared with normal, and severe mechanical constraints on V_T expansion are evident. TLC = total lung capacity; IC = inspiratory capacity.

appropriately during exercise,[8–10] thus seriously diminishing the patient's capacity to breathe in (inspiratory capacity) (see Figure 9–2). It burdens the muscles of inspiration (diaphragm, intercostal, and accessory muscles) with additional "elastic" loading. Therefore, because of DH, a much greater pressure must be generated by the inspiratory muscles to achieve a given tidal volume.

2. Dynamic hyperinflation also weakens the inspiratory muscles by seriously compromising their ability to generate pressure.[10] Other important negative effects of lung hyperinflation include inspiratory threshold loading of the inspiratory muscles (auto positive end-expiratory pressure), reduced dynamic compliance of the lung, and impaired cardiac performance.[8–10] The net effect of DH during exercise is that, compared with a normal state, a much greater inspiratory effort must be made in the face of a progressively impaired mechanical response (reduced tidal volume expansion and thoracic motion or displacement). This dissociation between effort (respiratory drive) and thoracic displacement, termed "neuromechanical dissociation," may form the basis for the predominant qualitative dimensions of dyspnea in COPD, that is, the perception of unsatisfied inspiration ("can't get enough air in") and inspiratory difficulty.[9] Neuromechanical dissociation likely contributes to perceived respiratory distress, which is the affective response to respiratory discomfort.

The importance of DH in the causation of dyspnea during activity is confirmed by the findings of a strong correlation between the intensity of dyspnea (measured by a validated category scale) and the reduction in dynamic inspiratory capacity; this reflects the extent of DH and the degree of dissociation between inspiratory effort and the tidal volume response (Figure 9–3).[8] Furthermore, relief of dyspnea following pharmacologic (bronchodilators) and surgical volume reduction has been shown, in several studies, to be explained mainly by the reduced DH and the resultant improvement in inspiratory muscle function (Figure 9–4).[11–13]

Interrelationships at a Standardized Level of Exercise

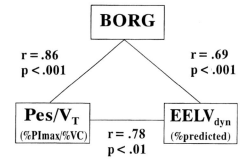

Figure 9–3 Statistical correlations between Borg ratings of inspiratory difficulty, end-expiratory lung volume (EELV) (ie, reduced inspiratory capacity), and the ratio of inspiratory effort (esophageal pressure [Pes] relative to maximum) to tidal volume (V_T standardized for vital capacity) at a standardized level of exercise. (Adapted from O'Donnell, et al.[9])

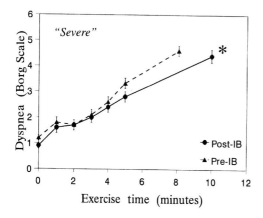
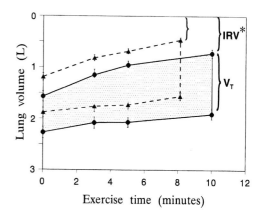

Figure 9–4 Dyspnea and operational lung volumes plotted against time, pre-, and postnebulized ipratropium bromide (IB) in patients with advanced COPD. Note that post-IB, exercise endurance time increased, and dyspnea intensity decreased significantly. These benefits were explained by reduced end-expiratory and end-inspiratory lung volumes (lines bracketing the tidal volume [V_T]) and increased inspiratory reserve volume (IRV). (Adapted from O'Donnell, et al.[12])

Excessive Ventilation and Dyspnea during Exercise

The range of ventilatory response to exercise in patients with COPD is wide. Nevertheless, many studies have shown that submaximal levels of ventilation are often increased compared with normals in patients with COPD.[9,14] Factors that result in accelerated breathing in patients with COPD include a high physiologic deadspace owing to ventilation-perfusion abnormalities, low arterial oxygen concentration (hypoxemia), high cost of breathing, excessive metabolic acidosis that occurs earlier in exercise because of the effects of skeletal muscle deconditioning, and other nonmetabolic sources of ventilatory stimulation such as anxiety and hyperventilation. The intensity of breathlessness during activity in COPD has been shown in several studies to correlate well with the changes in ventilation.[15,16] Increased ventilation relative to normal aggravates the mechanical abnormalities discussed previously; thus, it causes further DH in flow-limited patients and results in earlier attainment of limiting ventilatory constraints on tidal volume and flow generation. Excessive ventilation, therefore, causes a premature termination of exercise because of intolerable dyspnea and ventilatory limitation.

For practical purposes, the most effective way to reduce ventilatory demand in exercising patients with COPD is to alter the metabolic load. This can be done by exercise training[17,18] and, in some

patients, by ambulatory oxygen therapy (Figure 9–5).[19,20] In selected patients, ventilatory demands can be reduced by careful titration of opiates or anxiolytics.[21,22] Dyspnea relief following exercise training and oxygen therapy has been shown to correlate well with reduced submaximal ventilation.[17–19] It has become clear that even modest reductions in ventilation (in the order of 3 to 5 L/min at a standardized work rate) can result in meaningful improvement in dyspnea and exercise performance in severe, mechanically compromised patients with COPD.[17–22]

Neurophysiologic Basis of Dyspnea

In neurophysiologic terms, dyspnea intensity appears to correlate with the amplitude of central respiratory drive from the medulla oblongata; this, in turn, is invariably increased either voluntarily (increased effort) or reflexly in patients with COPD during exercise. Increased central drive is thought to be perceived as the sense of increased inspiratory muscle effort via central corollary discharge from the medulla to the central cortex. In addition to these central mechanisms, peripheral inputs from a multitude of sensory receptors in the lung, chest wall, and respiratory muscles (which are perturbed by mechanical loading) may directly, or indirectly, contribute to perceived respiratory discomfort.[1–4] An attractive hypothesis that is gaining support is that the intensity of dyspnea, or its predominant qualitative dimensions (inspiratory difficulty), results from neuromechanical dis-

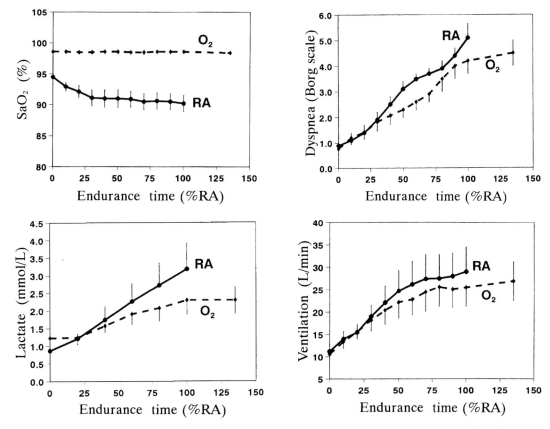

Figure 9–5 Dyspnea intensity (Borg), ventilation, serum lactate concentrations, and oxygen saturations plotted over time fell significantly during constant load cycle exercise tests breathing 60% O_2 compared with room air (%RA = percent of endurance time while breathing room air). (Adapted from O'Donnell, et al.[19])

sociation or uncoupling of the respiratory pump in COPD.[1,19] In this model, sensory inputs from both the central and peripheral nervous systems are processed and integrated; ultimately, they form the basis for the perception of respiratory discomfort and unsatisfied inspiration in COPD.

It must be emphasized that dyspnea is a complex, multidimensional symptom in COPD; the above outlined mechanical factors and/or alterations in ventilatory demand, although common, may not explain dyspnea causation in all patients with COPD. In some patients, other factors may be predominant (eg, inspiratory muscle weakness, arterial oxygen desaturation independent of increased ventilation, or cardiac factors that are currently not very well understood). Therefore, it follows that each patient should be assessed on an individual basis so that identifiable, and potentially reversible, factors can be recognized.

Assessment of the Dyspneic Patient

Patient Interview

The first step in evaluating dyspnea intensity, and the resultant functional disability, in a given patient involves a comprehensive history and physical examination. Generally, dyspnea is first experienced during activity and progresses insidiously over time so that the patient is rarely certain about the precise onset of symptoms. Unfortunately, more often than not, a respiratory tract infection may mark the onset of symptomatic COPD in patients with established advanced disease that was hitherto not clinically recognized. As mentioned in Chapter 2, patients are often unaware that they have made significant lifestyle modifications to avoid dyspnea provocation. Thus, they may learn to accomplish a given physical task at a considerably reduced pace or to avoid certain activities that they know will precipitate dyspnea. Because of this long-term behavioral adaptation, the health professional may have to question the patient extensively to uncover specific circumstances when dyspnea is experienced during common daily activities.

A number of simple questions have traditionally been used to elicit the magnitude of the task required to induce dyspnea in a given individual. These questions include the following:

- How far can you walk on a level surface before experiencing shortness of breath?
- How many flights of stairs can you climb before getting short of breath?
- While walking, can you keep pace with someone who does not have breathing problems?
- Can you talk and walk at the same time?

Patients with COPD describe characteristic qualitative features of their dyspnea such as "can't get enough air in" or "my breathing is too shallow."[9] Questionnaires that list common qualitative descriptors of dyspnea have recently been developed and can help identify particular qualitative aspects of dyspnea in a given individual.[23] However, such descriptor clustering does not permit adequate discrimination between the various cardiopulmonary disorders to justify their routine use for diagnostic purposes.[4]

It is important to establish the factors that are most likely to cause dyspnea in individual patients with COPD, as these can vary considerably between patients. Identification of specific provocation factors permits the health professional to provide helpful advice, or to institute measures in ameliorating dyspnea in each particular individual. The health professional should determine which circumstance commonly causes dyspneic aggravation:

- If unsupported upper limb exercise regularly causes dyspnea, then specific upper limb training may be beneficial.[24,25]
- If climatic extremes (ie, heat, increased humidity, or cold air) precipitate dyspnea, then these can potentially be controlled for the patient's benefit. The finding that diurnal variation in dyspnea is present may influence pharmacologic choices.
- If dyspnea is clearly related to episodes of anxiety or emotional upset, this can be specifically addressed with counseling and pharmacotherapy if necessary.

Factors that relieve dyspnea should also be noted as they may provide insights into the underlying causes. For example, if patients spontaneously resort to pursed-lip breathing (PLB) and/or a forward leaning position (with elbow support) to relieve dyspnea, they are likely to have a more advanced disease, probably with a significant emphysematous component. Patients should be questioned about their symptomatic response to bronchodilators. A consistent immediate response to short-acting β_2 agonists may indicate that bronchoconstriction contributes significantly to dyspnea in that patient. On the other hand, a consistent lack of symptomatic response to bronchodilators may indicate that (1) factors other than bronchoconstriction are contributory, (2) inhaler technique is poor, (3) bronchodilators are not being taken in sufficient dosages, or (4) alternative bronchodilator therapy is required.

Considering that comorbid illness is common, as already mentioned elsewhere in the textbook, the history should include a full review of the systems, particularly in an older population with a history of smoking. The coexistence of other symptoms such as chest discomfort, orthopnea, or ankle swelling may prompt further investigation of cardiac disease. Symptoms of depression should be specifically sought as this is common in patients with advanced COPD and may influence symptom perception.[26] In some patients with advanced disease, episodes of dyspnea may spiral into frank respiratory panic attacks (ie, common features are a feeling of extreme anxiety, a sense of suffocation and impending doom, acute sweating, palpitation, paresthesia, and fear of incontinence or actual incontinence of urine and/or feces). Such patients with respiratory panic may go unrecognized without specific questioning and will require additional therapy such as psychological counseling and/or anxiolytics to control their dyspnea. Concomitant respiratory and nonrespiratory medications should be accurately tabulated since these may need adjustment to optimize symptom control.

Physical Examination

Physical examination is notoriously unreliable in assessing the presence or severity of COPD. The relationship between specific physical findings and dyspnea intensity is poorly defined. Simply observing the patient during the minor activity of undressing or moving to the examination couch may confirm historic information related to the level and intensity of the patient's activity-related dyspnea. Respiratory distress may be evident in an inability to complete sentences. Patients may be seen to spontaneously adopt PLB or to favor the leaning forward position in their efforts to ameliorate dyspnea. Physical findings may give clues to the underlying pathophysiology and source of dyspnea in some patients.

Severe thoracic hyperinflation is readily identified in patients with more advanced disease. However, the physical evaluation of lesser levels of hyperinflation is insensitive. Physical features that are suggestive of lung hyperinflation include an overexpanded chest, accessory muscle use at rest, reduced thoracic motion despite maximal inspiratory efforts, tracheal tug, supraclavicular and intercostal recession during inspiration, indrawing of the lateral aspects of the lower ribs during tidal or deep inspiration (originally described by William Stokes in 1837),[27] and a tympanic percussion note over the thorax with diminished cardiac and liver dullness.

Auscultation of the chest may be insufficiently sensitive to detect airway obstruction in patients with COPD, but markedly reduced breath sounds bilaterally in the face of maximal inspiratory effort are suggestive of emphysema. Prolonged forced expiratory time (measured by stethoscope at the trachea) may be the only auscultatory abnormality in some patients with COPD.[28] Wheeze and crackles are nonspecific but may cause the clinician to suspect additional cardiopulmonary pathology, which, in turn, may contribute to dyspnea in a particular patient.

Investigations

Preliminary investigations in a symptomatic patient with COPD should include hemoglobin concentration; anemia may worsen dyspnea, whereas polycythemia may signal chronic arterial hypoxemia. Urea and electrolyte measurements should be conducted since electrolytic abnormalities may affect inspiratory muscle function and indirectly contribute to dyspnea. An electrocardiogram is necessary if cardiac disease is suspected from the history. Although it is usually more useful to highlight possible comorbid conditions, a chest radiograph may reveal features in advanced COPD of lung overinflation. However, it is important to remember that chest radiographs tend to be insensitive. As previously mentioned in Chapter 2, simple spirometry is useful for diagnostic purposes in the assessment of airway obstruction and severity. The rate of decline of the various pulmonary function parameters over time will help to assess the time course of disease progression in that individual. Bronchodilator responsiveness testing, using bronchodilator combinations while measuring changes in lung volume and expiratory flow rates, may predict sustained clinical benefits of bronchodilators better than the traditional approach (see below).

Management of Dyspnea

In general, dyspnea relief following a therapeutic intervention is achieved by

1. decreasing mechanical impedance;
2. reducing ventilatory demand;
3. strengthening ventilatory muscles;
4. altering central perception of dyspnea-causing stimuli; and
5. any combination of the above.

Putative mechanisms of dyspnea relief for a number of therapeutic interventions are provided in Table 9–1. The relative impact of a number of recently studied therapeutic interventions in patients

TABLE 9–1 Putative Mechanisms of Dyspnea Relief with Various Interventions

	Reduced Ventilation	Reduced Ventilatory Impedance	Ventilatory Muscle Strengthening	Altered Perceptual Response
Bronchodilators	+	+	−	−
Exercise training	+	−	+	+
Oxygen therapy	+	+	−	+
Anxiolytics	+	−	−	+
Opiates	+	−	−	+
CPAP	−	+	−	−
Volume reduction surgery	−	+	+	−
Inspiratory muscle training	−	−	+	−

+ = present; − = absent; CPAP = continuous positive airway pressure.

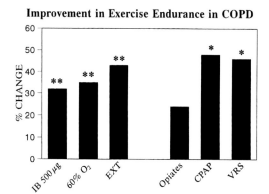

Improvement in Exercise Endurance in COPD

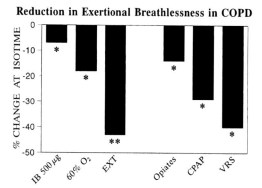

Reduction in Exertional Breathlessness in COPD

* p < 0.05 significant difference from control conditions.
** p < 0.01 significant difference from control conditions.

Figure 9–6 Effects of therapeutic interventions on exercise endurance and exertional dyspnea in patients with advanced COPD. IB = 500 µg of nebulized ipratropium bromide; 60% O_2 = supplemental oxygen; EXT = exercise training; opiates = 15-mg nebulized morphine sulfate; CPAP = continuous positive airway pressure; VRS = volume reduction surgery (either lung reduction or bullectomy). (Adapted from references 12, 17, 19, 52, 75, and 76.)

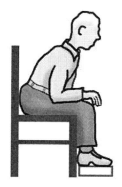

Figure 9–7 Forward lean sitting with elbow resting on thigh: (1) sitting with feet well supported; (2) trunk slightly leaning forward; and (3) elbow resting on thigh and chin resting on hand.

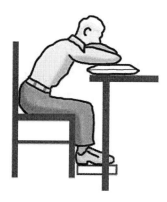

Figure 9–8 Forward lean sitting with forearms resting on table: (1) sitting with feet well supported, (2) trunk leaning slightly forward, (3) arms resting on a table, (4) head resting on pillow, and (5) hands relaxed to avoid increased muscle tension.

with advanced symptomatic COPD is provided in Figure 9–6.

Patients often adopt positions that might serve to facilitate their breathing or promote relaxation. Some of these positions are presented in Figures 9–7 and 9–8. In adopting the forward lean sitting position, the patient should be discouraged from "grabbing the table" as this may promote an increase in muscular tension of the accessory muscles and consequently an increase in breathlessness if the position is prolonged.

Pharmacologic Therapy

Bronchodilator therapy is the first step in the management of patients with symptomatic COPD

(see Chapter 5 for more detail). All classes of bronchodilator therapy (ie, inhaled β_2 agonists, inhaled anticholinergic agents, and oral theophyllines) have been shown to improve exertional dyspnea and increase exercise capacity in patients with COPD when tested in placebo-controlled studies.[29-31] The mechanisms of these beneficial effects are complex and not fully elucidated. From the available literature on the topic, a few generalizations are possible:

1. Meaningful improvements in symptoms, activity levels, and quality of life occur in the presence of only modest changes in forced expiratory volume in 1 second (FEV_1) after bronchodilator therapy.

Dyspnea (Borg scale)

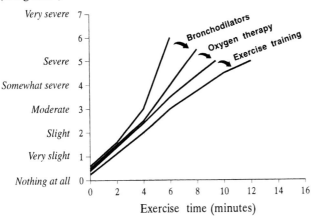

Figure 9–9 Sequential plots of dyspnea intensity over time (Borg scale), during constant load submaximal cycle exercise test in a breathless patient with advanced COPD. Note cumulative effects of various interventions on dyspnea and exercise endurance.[77]

2. The single laboratory bronchodilator reversibility test is not predictive of symptomatic responses to that agent.
3. Different patients respond differently to different classes of bronchodilators or to a single class of bronchodilators over time.
4. Combination bronchodilator therapy may have synergistic effects on respiratory symptoms in COPD.
5. The mode of delivery and doses of bronchodilators must be carefully individualized for maximal benefit.

Several recent control studies have shown that dyspnea relief following all classes of bronchodilators correlates better with the reduction in lung volumes (ie, reduced gas trapping) than with changes in the FEV_1.[11,12] Thus, while assessing bronchodilator responsiveness, it is reasonable to include a consideration of the changes in lung volumes and changes in expiratory flow rates. The inspiratory capacity measurement may prove useful in this regard since it represents a noninvasive measurement of EELV. This measurement is likely to be used more often in the future. In one study, an improvement in inspiratory capacity greater than 10% of predicted resulted in improvement in exercise endurance by 32% in patients with advanced COPD.[12] For patients with more advanced disease, small improvements in airway function with reduced gas trapping can provide meaningful improvements in dyspnea and activity levels.

As mentioned in Chapter 5, bronchodilators are prescribed primarily for symptom relief. The results of a single laboratory reversibility study (change in FEV_1) should not be used as criteria for inhaler prescription by the caregiver, as patients may develop sustained beneficial effects in the presence of a negative laboratory reversibility study. The effectiveness of an inhaler can generally be ascertained on direct questioning:

• Has the new inhaler helped you?
• If so, in what way?

For those patients who describe unequivocal benefits, the decision is simple, if patients are not sure whether the inhaler is helpful, they should simply discontinue its use. If there is symptomatic deterioration, then instruct the patient to reintroduce the inhaler. If there is no noticeable deterioration, then the patient should abandon this medication.

Aerobic Exercise Training

Patients who have persistent activity-related dyspnea and exercise curtailment, despite optimized combination pharmacotherapy, should be encouraged to undergo exercise training (Figure 9–9). The aim of exercise training is to break the vicious cycle of skeletal muscle deconditioning, progressive dyspnea, and immobility to eventually improve symptoms and activity levels and restore patients to the highest level of independent function. All symptomatic patients should be encouraged to engage in regular activity and to avoid the inevitable drift toward an inactive lifestyle. Formal exercise training is generally provided within the context of a comprehensive, multidisciplinary pulmonary rehabilitation program that includes education, psychosocial support, occupational

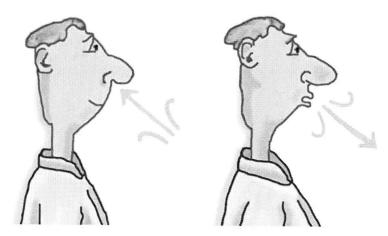

Figure 9–10 Pursed-lip breathing (PLB): (1) take in a normal breath through the nose, and (2) breathe out through pursed lips (expiration should be approximately twice as long as inspiration). If patient has difficulty breathing in through the nose, PLB may consist of both inspiration and expiration through the mouth. Emphasis is placed on expiration through pursed lips. Patient should make sure expiration is prolonged but not forced. (Adapted from the self-management program "Living Well with COPD©").

therapy, and nutritional advice. It is now well established that the exercise training component of the rehabilitation program is pivotal in explaining the benefits of improved exercise capacity and reduced dyspnea.

Upper Limb Training

Many patients with advanced COPD may experience severe breathlessness during upper extremity activity (eg, combing hair, showering, lifting objects, etc).[24,25] In some instances, dyspnea during this type of activity may exceed that experienced during lower limb weight-bearing tasks. Dyspnea during arm exercise may result from the associated high ventilatory demands for a given oxygen consumption (VO_2), which could potentially aggravate DH in flow-limited patients.[24,25] Additionally, the upper limb muscles are anchored to the thorax and can serve as accessory muscles of inspiration. It follows that if these muscles are used for their peripheral locomotor function in patients who depend on their supportive role in ventilation, dyspnea may arise when other inspiratory muscles, such as the diaphragm, are suddenly burdened with a greater share of the work of breathing. In several studies, weight training of upper extremities resulted in greater improvement in endurance and reduced dyspnea during upper limb exercise compared with control in patients with advanced COPD.[24,25] Upper limb training should therefore be incorporated into multimodality exercise

training protocols and may be particularly beneficial in those patients whose dyspnea is regularly provoked by upper extremity exercise.

Breathing Retraining

Various breathing retraining techniques have been advocated for the improvement of dyspnea in symptomatic patients with COPD. Attempts to retrain patients to adopt a slower, deeper breathing pattern are variably successful. The rationale behind retraining is that the adoption of a more efficient breathing pattern, with a reduced relative physiologic deadspace, improves efficiency of CO_2 elimination and consequent V_E (ventilation) reduction; thus, in turn, perceived dyspnea is reduced. Many patients trained in this technique adopt a slower, deeper pattern when supervised but generally resort to their spontaneous faster breathing pattern when they believe they are unobserved. This is not surprising since a rapid, shallow breathing pattern characteristically adopted by patients with more advanced disease, particularly during activity, likely represents the optimal compensatory strategy for intrinsic mechanical loading (ie, elastic loading). A rapid, shallow breathing pattern would act to minimize the intrathoracic pressure perturbations and the associated respiratory discomfort. Moreover, a slower, deeper pattern may actually accentuate mechanical loading and breathing discomfort in some patients, which, in effect, is clearly undesirable.

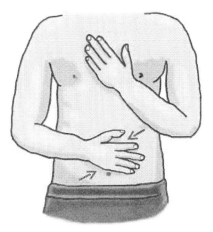

Figure 9–11 Diaphragmatic breathing. This technique follows PLB when the patient is less short of breath and has greater control of his/her breathing pattern. It allows for a deeper, more efficient inspiration, which, in turn, reduces the respiratory rate to facilitate a relaxed breathing pattern. Left hand should stabilize the chest, although movement occurs under the right hand. (Adapted from the self-management program "Living Well with COPD©").

Pursed-Lip Breathing. Pursed-lip breathing is a technique adopted spontaneously by many patients with COPD. It is considered a dyspnea-relieving strategy and is usually used during acute episodes provoked by activity, anxiety, or respiratory distress. Traditionally, patients are taught this technique as a component of pulmonary rehabilitation programs. Pursed-lip breathing involves active expiration through a resistance that is created by constricting or pursing the lips (instruction in the technique is provided in Figure 9–10).[32,33] The nasopharynx has been shown to be occluded during PLB.[34] Expiration is prolonged, and tidal volume generally increases with modest transient improvements in gas exchange. Pursed-lip breathing is thought to be more common in patients with advanced COPD and particularly in patients with emphysema. Although those who spontaneously adopt PLB clearly derive symptomatic relief, symptomatic responses in those who are instructed in the technique are highly variable and unpredictable. Current mechanistic theories are mainly based on clinical observation, and it appears that the mechanisms of dyspnea relief during PLB are conjectural. Attempts have been made to study the possible physiologic mechanisms of dyspnea relief during PLB by applying external resistive loads, but these loads

imperfectly simulate actual PLB. Possible dyspnea-relieving factors during PLB include altered breathing pattern (ie, slower and deeper) with improved ventilation-perfusion relationships, improved arterial oxygen desaturation[35,36] and CO_2 elimination, altered pattern of ventilatory muscle recruitment (ie, more expiratory muscle recruitment, which may optimize diaphragmatic length and assist inspiration), attenuation of dynamic airway compression,[37] and, finally, reduced lung hyperinflation as a result of reduced breathing frequency and prolongation of expiratory time. As with diaphragmatic breathing, PLB may serve as a useful relaxation technique that relieves anxiety and helps patients avoid regression to respiratory panic during acute episodes of dyspnea. Although no consensus exists about the precise neurophysiologic mechanisms of dyspnea relief during PLB, clinical experience has shown that the technique is undoubtedly beneficial in some patients. Thus, instruction in PLB should be provided by skilled instructors as part of the rehabilitation program. Those who derive symptomatic benefit will habitually resort to this technique during episodes of dyspnea.

Diaphragmatic Breathing. Diaphragmatic breathing has been advocated for many years as a dyspnea-relieving strategy in advanced COPD.[38,39] The patient is instructed to allow the abdominal wall to move outward during slow inspiration, which is usually in conjunction with slow expiration through pursed lips (instruction in the technique is provided in Figure 9–11).[38,39] Some studies have provided evidence that this technique offers some alleviation of dyspnea, whereas others have indicated otherwise. The potential mechanisms of dyspnea relief during diaphragmatic breathing are also unclear; putative mechanisms include an altered pattern of ventilatory muscle recruitment, avoidance of excessive increases in breathing frequency during or following activity, and, consequently, a resulting avoidance of DH. Diaphragmatic breathing may serve to distract patients from the distress of dyspnea and may serve as an anxiety-relieving strategy or relaxation technique that hastens recovery from acute dyspneic episodes.

Inspiratory Muscle Training

When inspiratory muscles are functionally weakened, greater motor command output or effort is required to maintain a given ventilation during rest and exercise.[3,40] Intensity of dyspnea has been shown to increase when the inspiratory force required during tidal breathing increases as a fraction of its maximal force-generating capacity.[3] Therefore, theoretically speaking, interventions that increase inspiratory muscle strength should reduce the level of neural activation and inspiratory effort required during tidal breathing, thus consequently reducing dyspnea. In practice, the effectiveness of specific inspiratory muscle training using a variety of techniques (voluntary isocapneic hypercapnea, inspiratory resistive loading, and inspiratory threshold loading) has been inconsistent.[41,42] One meta-analysis of 17 clinical studies concluded that there is insufficient evidence to recommend specific inspiratory muscle training for routine clinical purposes.[42]

Further studies are required to identify the subgroup of patients with COPD who are more likely to benefit from specific inspiratory muscle training. Studies are also needed to define the optimal mode of training involved in training threshold and duration. While we await definitive information on the value of inspiratory muscle training, it seems reasonable to identify patients with severe inspiratory muscle weakness and to institute specific measures to improve function aimed at reversing the underlying problem (ie, nutritional supplementation, correction of electrolytes, withdrawal of high-dose steroid therapy, etc). These measures, in conjunction with an exercise training program in which the training stimulus is targeted to high and sustained ventilation levels, should conjointly improve inspiratory muscle function to a level comparable to that achieved by inspiratory muscle training.[4] Studies are currently under way to assess the effects of anabolic steroid treatment in conjunction with exercise training on ventilatory muscle function, dyspnea, and exercise duration in patients with advanced COPD.

Oxygen Therapy

Although large control studies have provided convincing evidence of the beneficial effects of continuous oxygen therapy on survival in severely hypoxemic patients with COPD, the effects of such therapy on chronic symptoms are unknown.[43,44] As previously mentioned elsewhere in this textbook, the effects of oxygen on dyspnea in a given individual with symptomatic COPD are entirely unpredictable, and the mechanism(s) of dyspnea relief in those who do respond is not fully understood. One potential mechanism is reduced ventilatory drive and ventilation levels as a result of diminished hypoxic drive,

either from peripheral chemoreceptors[16,45] or from reduced activity-generated metabolic acidosis[19] (see Figure 9–5).

Two recent studies have provided evidence that patients with mild exercise hypoxemia, but moderate to severe COPD, can benefit from supplemental oxygen therapy during exercise in terms of reduced exertional dyspnea and improved exercise endurance (see Figures 9–5 and 9–6).[19,20] It follows that ambulatory oxygen may serve as a useful adjunct to exercise reconditioning, promoting increased mobility, and to activity levels in patients with symptomatic COPD. Ambulatory oxygen therapy may be used as an adjunct to formal exercise training, allowing patients to achieve and sustain higher training levels; theoretically, it should help them achieve greater physiologic training effects. There is no consensus on what level of arterial oxygen desaturation warrants consideration for ambulatory oxygen in patients who are not hypoxemic at rest. Reimbursement criteria for ambulatory oxygen from various government agencies and insurance companies varies greatly, and general recommendations cannot be made at this time in the absence of evidence on long-term beneficial effects. Currently, there is no agreement as to what constitutes significant arterial oxygen desaturation during exercise. Since a positive symptomatic response to oxygen therapy is unpredictable in a given patient, a single-blind, case-controlled study should be conducted to identify responders. We employ a treadmill, constant load endurance test at approximately 70% of the patient's predetermined maximum work rate or VO_2; two tests are performed in random order (room air and oxygen) so that endurance times and Borg ratings of dyspnea are recorded. The added oxygen should be sufficient to maintain oxygen saturations greater than 90% during exercise. We recommend ambulatory oxygen for those patients whose endurance times on oxygen are prolonged by greater than 25% of the control value, or whose Borg ratings are diminished by greater than one unit at a standardized exercise time (highest equivalent work rate). Alternative protocols involve stair climbing or walking (including 6-minute walk distance) with a reliable pulse oximeter and a measurement of both endurance time and dyspnea at the end of exercise.

Further studies are required to examine the long-term effects of oxygen (continuous or ambulatory) on chronic activity-related dyspnea, functional status, and quality of life. Studies are under way to assess the value of adjunct ambulatory oxygen therapy during exercise training in COPD. Given the expense of long-term ambulatory oxygen, evidence-based criteria need to be developed for patient selection, oxygen prescription, and optimal mode of delivery.

For patients with COPD who are dyspneic at rest and in the terminal phases of their illness, oxygen therapy may provide some relief regardless of their level of resting hypoxemia.[45,46] Therefore, a trial of oxygen is justified in these patients for palliative purposes, and treatment should be offered to those who are shown to derive benefit.

Adjunct Therapies

Opiates. Opiate therapy has been used for centuries in the treatment of respiratory distress. Over time, the knowledge that these drugs are powerful respiratory depressants has led to their more restricted use as dyspnea-relieving medications. A number of controlled, crossover, randomized studies have shown that oral opiates (morphine, dihydrocodeine, hydrocodone) in small numbers of patients with COPD experience modest, but significant, acute improvements in exertional dyspnea and in exercise capacity compared with placebo.[21,47,48] However, side effects during acute opiate administration are commonly reported and include drowsiness, hypercapnia, hypotension, confusion, and constipation.[21,47–49]

The mechanisms of dyspnea alleviation during opiate therapy in COPD are multifactorial. Opiates have been shown to depress respiratory drive both at rest and during exercise. Reduction in submaximal exercise ventilation and hypercapnia have been reported in a number of acute studies.[21,47] Opiates delivered by nebulizers have not shown superiority over any mode of opiate delivery in patients with symptomatic COPD. Earlier theories that topical opiates may exert their dyspnea-relieving effects via pulmonary opiate receptors are unsubstantiated.[50–52] The efficacy of inhaled opiates appears to be dependent on the degree to which the drug is absorbed into the bloodstream and on the consequent reduction in central ventilatory drive.[52]

Although the role of long-term opiates in advanced symptomatic COPD remains controversial, it is generally accepted that these drugs are very useful as a palliative measure for some patients in the terminal phases of their illness.[53] Dosages must be carefully individualized to obtain maximum symptomatic benefit while minimizing adverse effects to the patient.

From a perusal of the available literature, the routine use of opiates cannot be recommended for patients with symptomatic COPD given their propensity to cause serious side effects. Further studies are required to develop more precise guidelines for their use. Studies are also required to determine if the earlier introduction of lower dosages of opiates in a subpopulation of severely dyspneic COPD patients can diminish the respiratory depressant effects of the drugs that occur when higher dosages are acutely administered to patients with ventilatory compromise. Tolerance to the respiratory depressant effects has been reported in patients in whom long-term, low-dose opiates are prescribed primarily for pain relief.[54] It is not known if similar tolerance could develop in patients with COPD when opiates are prescribed for dyspnea relief.

Anxiolytics. Anxiolytics have the potential to relieve dyspnea by either depressing respiratory drive in response to hypoxemia or hypercapnia or by altering the affective response to perceived respiratory discomfort. Despite the earlier demonstration of a beneficial effect of diazepam in a small, single-blinded study in "pink and puffing" patients with COPD,[55] several subsequent controlled studies have failed to show consistent improvements in dyspnea and exercise tolerance over placebo. Moreover, these drugs caused excessive drowsiness and were often poorly tolerated. Studies using diazepam, alprazolam, and promethazine hydrochloride in patients with symptomatic COPD did not demonstrate improvements in dyspnea or in exercise capacity when examining group responses. However, negative group responses obscured impressive improvements in some individuals.[55–57] The newer anxiolytic agents, such as buspirone hydrochloride, have been tested in dyspneic patients with COPD on the basis of this drug's theoretical advantage in not causing respiratory depression. In a randomized controlled study by Singh and colleagues, a 6-week therapy with buspirone (10 to 20 mg PO) in 11 patients with COPD with mild to moderate anxiety did not result in significant improvements over placebo in dyspnea, exercise tolerance, or anxiety scores.[58] By contrast, Argyropoulou and colleagues showed significant improvements in mood, dyspnea, and exercise endurance using buspirone (20 mg daily) in patients with moderately severe COPD.[22] In this study, the drug was well tolerated, and there was no depression in respiratory drive or deterioration in arterial blood gases.

There is currently insufficient evidence to recommend the routine use of anxiolytics in breathless patients with COPD. However, a trial of anxiolytic therapy is reasonable on an individual basis in dyspneic patients, particularly those with severe anxiety or frequent respiratory panic attacks. Pharmacologic treatment should ideally be provided in conjunction with psychological counseling and instruction in relaxation techniques. Simple measures such as avoidance of excessive β_2-agonist medication, instruction in breathing relaxation techniques, and short-acting anxiolytics such as lorazepam may successfully abort spiraling respiratory panic attacks in those predisposed to them.

CONTROLLING COUGH

Mechanisms of Cough

Chronic cough is a common and often troublesome symptom in patients with COPD.[1] Patients might report prolonged episodes of vigorous and often ineffective coughing, particularly in the morning. This may be associated with dyspnea, fatigue, and considerable frustration or distress at not being able to achieve relief by dislodging impacted bronchial secretions. Other patients with COPD may seek help because of persistent dry coughing, which responds poorly to bronchodilator treatment.

The neural mechanisms of cough are well understood; inhaled irritants, such as cigarette smoke, induce inflammatory changes in the mucosa of the respiratory tract that are associated with slowing mucociliary clearance and excessive mucus secretion.[2-4] Such irritants (ie, smoke, fumes, dust) can activate the afferent limb of the cough reflex by stimulating "irritants" (or rapidly adapting receptors), which are located in abundance in the oropharynx, larynx, and throughout the tracheobronchial tree.[59-61] These irritant receptor endings lie within the epithelium, where, in addition to cigarette smoke, they are sensitive to a wide variety of inflammatory and immunologic mediators.[62,63] Afferent information from these activated irritant receptors is relayed to a collection of neurons in the medulla oblongata of the brain stem known as the "cough centre"; the efferent limb of this reflex consists of motor neurons to the respiratory muscles and to the bronchi.[59-63] Efferent motor output to these sites results in forceful expiratory muscle contraction and variable bronchoconstriction and mucus secretion.[59-63]

The inspiratory phase of the cough consists of deep inspiration through a widely opened glottis. The expiratory phase of the cough consists of two components: (1) the compressive phase, which entails forceful expiration against a closed glottis, and (2) the expulsive phase, when the glottis opens to allow rapid expiratory airflow.[64] Dynamic airway compression during the expulsive phase serves to increase airflow velocity and enhance clearance of secretions. The pattern of coughing among patients with COPD is highly variable and depends on such diverse factors as elastic lung recoil, extent of expiratory airflow obstruction, inspiratory and expiratory muscle strength, degree of airway inflammation, and amount and quality of mucus secretion. Cough may become ineffective in COPD because of a variety of reasons including reduced expiratory muscle strength, excessive dynamic collapse of poorly compliant airways on expiration, localized anatomic airways obstruction, excessive mucus production or increased viscosity of secretions, and damage to the mucociliary escalator as a result of the effects of chronic smoking.

Assessment of the Patient with a Cough

Assessment of the cause of chronic cough in COPD should begin with a comprehensive history and physical examination. The caregiver should ascertain
- duration and frequency,
- characteristics (ie, productive or sustained),
- precipitating or relieving factors, and
- associated clinical features.

The history should also include an inquiry on the adverse consequences of chronic coughing, which include fatigue, dyspnea, disturbed sleep, vasovagal attacks, chest wall and abdominal discomfort, rib fractures, hoarseness, bruising or petechiae, and urinary incontinence.

The health professional should be mindful that other important conditions may coexist with chronic bronchitis as a cause of chronic cough (of greater than 8 weeks' duration); furthermore, systematic questioning and additional targeted investigations may be required (an approach to the investigation of chronic cough is beyond the scope of this review and is detailed elsewhere in a comprehensive review).[65,66] Well-established causes of chronic cough include postnasal drip, asthma, gastroesophageal reflux dis-

TABLE 9–2 Therapeutic Guideline for Managing Cough owing to COPD

Therapeutic Intervention	Potential Effect	Evidence of Their Efficacy
Smoking cessation[64,65]	Disappearance or marked diminution	Within 4 weeks[67]
Antitussive agents (ipratropium bromide, isodopropylidene glycerol)[68]	Decrease volume and alter viscosity of the sputum	Individual therapeutic trial
Protussive agents (acetylcysteine, glyceryl guaiacolate, bromhexine hydrochloride)[69–71]	Alter the volume and consistency of sputum	Evidence lacking that they improve cough clearance or alter clinical outcome
Inhaled bronchodilators	Facilitate sputum clearance and provide symptom benefit	Individual therapeutic trial

ease, bronchiectasis, postinfective cough, angiotensin-converting enzyme inhibitor–induced cough, and, ominously, bronchogenic carcinoma.[65–67] Investigations must be individualized, but appropriate general screening should focus on the most common causes for chronic cough (ie, postnasal drip syndrome, asthma, and gastroesophageal reflux disease), obtaining a chest radiograph, and determining whether the symptoms conform to the clinical profile that it is usually associated with one of the diagnoses just mentioned. In patients who have chronic cough associated with copious sputum production and frequent respiratory tract infections, a localized bronchiectasis should be considered in the differential diagnosis. In such patients, computed tomography is a useful diagnostic tool. Patients with COPD are at high risk for bronchogenic carcinoma, which, according to clinical presentation, is most commonly represented by cough. Therefore, health professionals should have a high index of suspicion for this diagnosis, particularly in patients with COPD who have a recent onset of unexplained cough, persistent change in their cough, or associated hemoptysis.

Management of Cough

The first and most important step in the management of chronic cough in patients with COPD is smoking cessation.[64,65] Studies have shown that in patients seeking medical attention for a troublesome cough, smoking cessation results in the disappearance or marked diminution of cough in the vast majority (ie, 94% and more); furthermore, it shows that these benefits were evident within 4 weeks of quitting smoking.[68] Practical advice should be given about avoidance of dust, fumes, and other triggers of

cough. Coexistent conditions that cause chronic cough will require specific treatment.[65,66]

Pharmacologic Therapy

When a specific cause of cough cannot be identified and smoking cessation is not contemplated by the patient, symptomatic alleviation becomes the main therapeutic goal. Table 9–2 provides a therapeutic guideline for managing cough owing to chronic bronchitis or COPD.

Antitussive agents include drugs such as ipratropium bromide and isodopropylidene glycerol that are theoretically able to alter the afferent limb of the cough reflex in chronic bronchitis by decreasing volume or by altering the viscosity of sputum.[69] If they provide symptomatic relief, individual therapeutic trials of these medications should be initiated and continued with suffering patients.

Prolonged, ineffective morning coughing with sputum inspissation represents some of the most distressing symptoms that patients with COPD may experience. Protussive agents (ie, acetylcysteine, glyceryl guaiacolate, and bromhexine hydrochloride) are rarely prescribed as evidence is lacking that these agents actually improve cough clearance or alter clinical outcomes (ie, pulmonary function improvement, reduced pneumonias, etc).[70–72] Acetylcysteine has been shown to liquify both mucoid and purulent secretions, but the overall clinical benefits of this drug in chronic bronchitis are modest at best.[71] Aerosolized hypertonic saline has been shown to improve the efficacy of cough clearance in patients with chronic bronchitis.[69] Pharmacologic therapy such as combined bronchodilator therapy and inhaled corticosteroids can successfully reduce cough frequency, decrease sputum production, and enhance sputum clearance, but responses are variable, and therapy must be individualized. However, in some patients, bronchodilators may actually aggravate coughing or fail to increase cough effectiveness. Patients with COPD and ineffective cough should be advised to avoid dehydration by drinking adequate fluid, which, in turn, should theoretically reduce sputum viscosity and improve clearance.

Despite the above-outlined pharmacologic and physical therapies, a minority of patients may continue to suffer from intractable cough. This clinical scenario should prompt a search for an alternative diagnosis using a stepwise approach.[66] If no specific diagnosis is uncovered and cough continues unabated, or if it is particularly associated with severe sleep fragmentation, then antitussive agents that reduce "cough center" output may be indicated. Such agents include narcotics (codeine and morphine), and non-narcotics (dextromethorphan hydrobromide, diphenhydramine hydrochloride, and caraminophen). These treatments should be carefully titrated on an individual basis with frequent reevaluation of the patient and vigilance for any adverse effects. Chronic antitussive therapy of this nature is rarely warranted in patients with COPD.

Physiotherapy

The role of chest physiotherapy in improving cough effectiveness has been inconclusive in clinical studies.[73] Nevertheless, there are abundant anecdotal reports that patients may derive immediate symptomatic benefit from techniques such as controlled cough or forced expiration. These techniques enhance sputum clearance and result in avoidance of the sequelae of worsening dyspnea, hypoxemia, and fatigue, which may all accompany ineffective coughing.[74] Instructions on these maneuvers should be provided by a knowledgeable health professional.

Controlled Cough Technique. Ask the patient to
1. Sit comfortably;
2. Lean head forward slightly;
3. Place feet firmly on the ground;
4. Inhale deeply using the diaphragmatic technique, the significant volume of air behind the secretions will help expel them from your lungs;
5. Try to hold his/her breath for 2 seconds; and
6. Cough twice while keeping the mouth slightly open. The first cough will loosen the secretions,

and the second will remove them from the lungs.
7. Take a break and repeat once or twice if not effective.

Tell the patient to stop using the coughing technique if there are few or no secretions.

Forced Expiration Technique. Ask the patient to
1. Sit comfortably;
2. Lean head forward slightly;
3. Place feet firmly on the ground;
4. Inhale deeply using the diaphragmatic technique;
5. Exhale forcefully in short bursts while keeping the mouth open as if about to make mist on a window.
6. Repeat once or twice.

For patients with more advanced disease, single forced expirations may be better tolerated than controlled cough maneuvers.[73] These cough-enhancing procedures should preferably be undertaken each morning at least 10 minutes after short-acting bronchodilators. In some patients for whom sputum inspissation is particularly problematic, these exhalation techniques may be undertaken at regular intervals throughout the day.[73]

WHEN TO REFER

When to Refer to a Respirologist

The decision varies with the degree of comfort and experience that a practitioner and health care team have in dealing with dyspnea and cough in COPD. Patients who seem to have respiratory symptoms that are disproportionate to the degree of COPD severity, unexplained changes in their respiratory symptoms, or disabled respiratory symptoms, either dyspnea or cough, should be referred to a respirologist. Patients should also be referred to a respirologist when a cough persists beyond 8 weeks' duration, if the cough is associated with new chest radiograph abnormalities, and if bronchial malignancy is clinically suspected. An uncertain diagnosis should always be an absolute indication for respirologist referral.

To control dyspnea and cough (especially when symptoms are restricting functional abilities and health-related quality of life), the patient should be given the opportunity to undergo pulmonary rehabilitation under the supervision of established specialists and their program team members.

When to Refer to a Physiotherapist

Ideally, a patient should see a physiotherapist as part of a pulmonary rehabilitation program where the combination of exercise, breathing retraining, and education produces a posititve effect on COPD symptoms, including dyspnea and cough. Referral to a physiotherapist may also be appropriate for patients who may not be able to participate in a formal pulmonary program because of lack of access or a mitigating comorbid illness. A physiotherapist will design an individualized program of activity for each patient based on their specific range of symptoms and goals. Programs of activity can be developed for patients at all stages of COPD. It is often those patients with more severe limitations who make the most dramatic functional gains during pulmonary rehabilitation.

Many patients are frustrated by frequent, unexpected coughing bouts that leave them exhausted, breathless, and embarrassed. Such patients with frequent secretions can benefit from a referral to a physiotherapist where they can be taught to develop a schedule of daily planned coughing sessions in order to cope with their secretions. These sessions may include learning how to use a mechanical vibrator and positioning to help clear secretions. The patient can choose the time and the place when he/she can best clear secretions as comfortably as possible. Repeated practice of these breathing and positioning routines, under supervision, over a period of time will lead to the patient being able to apply these techniques in various situations to successfully control dyspnea and cough and manage his/her daily activities.

Many physiotherapists are skilled educators and patients can benefit enormously from referral for this reason alone. The physiotherapist can instruct the patient on medication use, identification and avoidance of situations where symptoms may be triggered, as well as the use of breathing and positioning techniques as effective methods to gain control over symptoms. The physiotherapist can work with the patient to problem solve difficulties with functional activities and develop strategies that allow the patient to resume a more normal level of daily activity.

SUMMARY

Improvements in our ability to clinically assess the dyspneic patient, together with an increased understanding of the pathophysiologic mechanisms of exertional dyspnea, have resulted in advances in symptom control. The comprehensive management of severely dyspneic patients requires an individualized stepwise approach. In light of the fact that dynamic lung hyperinflation contributes significantly to exertional dyspnea and exercise intolerance, every effort should be made to reduce gas trapping by carefully optimizing combination bronchodilator therapy. Supervised exercise training, which reduces excessive ventilatory demands, remains one of the most effective interventions to reduce dyspnea and increase activity levels in patients in whom pharmacotherapy has been optimized. To sustain these benefits, patients must maintain a home-based exercise program indefinitely. Ambulatory oxygen therapy can reduce dyspnea and improve exercise endurance in some patients with COPD. An individualized, blinded therapeutic trial (oxygen versus room air) is required to identify symptomatic responders. It must be emphasized that small improvements in ventilatory mechanics and ventilatory demand combine in an additive or synergistic manner to achieve important clinical effects in patients with advanced disease (see Figure 9–6). In selected patients, adjunctive pharmacologic (opiates and anxiolytics) and physical therapy (PLB, upper limb and inspiratory muscle training) can provide additional benefits.

Chronic cough and ineffective sputum clearance are also very common symptoms in patients with COPD. A careful history examination and selective investigations can elucidate the nature and the cause of troublesome coughing in the majority of patients. Care must be taken not to overlook coexisting causes of chronic cough in smokers, such as bronchogenic carcinoma. Smoking cessation is an important first step in the management of chronic cough and will yield successful results in the majority of patients. Pharmacologic therapy such as combined bronchodilator therapy and inhaled corticosteroids can successfully reduce cough frequency, decrease sputum production, and enhance sputum clearance, but responses are variable, and therapy must be individualized. Mucolytic agents may provide subjective improvement in some patients, but their overall clinical utility is unproven. Instruction in enhanced coughing techniques by a knowledgeable health professional can benefit many patients with COPD, particularly those with advanced disease who have a demonstrably ineffective cough. Short courses of opiate-based antitussive agents can be prescribed as a last resort for patients whose lives are seriously disrupted by chronic coughing.

CASE STUDIES

Case Study 1

Mr. Cope, a 67-year-old smoker with established COPD, had become disabled over the previous 3 years to a point where he was now housebound. He was referred by his family physician because his symptoms were no longer responding to his inhaler medications.

Medical History, Physical Examination, and Test Results

Medical History.
- Dyspnea was 5/5 on the Medical Research Council (MRC) dyspnea scale (ie, patient has breathlessness dressing or undressing).
- He has no relevant past medical history other than COPD.
- Medications include salmeterol by metered-dose inhaler two puffs per day, ipratropium bromide two puffs four times daily, and fluticasone two puffs four times daily (no spacer device used).

Physical Examination
- He has a barrel-shaped chest with vigorous accessory muscle use.
- Auscultation revealed reduced breath sounds throughout; he appeared in respiratory distress during the minimal activity of walking to the examination couch.

Test Results
- The body mass index was 26.6 kg/m².
- Pulmonary function tests showed an FEV_1 of 37% predicted of normal, residual volume 210% predicted of normal, and diffusion capacity 60% predicted of normal; at rest, PaO_2 was 64 mm Hg, $PaCO_2$ was 41 mm Hg, and pH was 7.4.
- Exercise test results were as follows: the patient stopped after 5 minutes of cycle exercise at a constant work rate of 75% of his achieved maximum primarily because of severe breathlessness (Borg rating = 6); peak exercise ventilation coincided with the estimated maximal breathing capacity, thus indicating ventilatory limitation; during exercise, the lungs became dynamically hyperinflated by an additional 0.5 L above resting values.

Questions and Discussion

How do we control breathlessness in this patient?
Step 1. Optimize Bronchodilators. The optimal dosages are as follows: ipratropium bromide, 4 puffs four times daily; salmeterol, 2 puffs twice daily; salbutamol, as needed. The patient was given an aerochamber and instruction in the proper technique. There was mild oxygen desaturation during the constant workload test.

Step 2. Trial of Ambulatory Oxygen. As previously mentioned, oxygen saturation was normal at rest, but there was a mild arterial oxygen desaturation during the constant workload test. The patient undertook a randomized, controlled, crossover study (n = 1; room air versus oxygen) and was found to improve his exercise endurance by 40%; he was also able to significantly reduce his exertional dyspnea. Ambulatory oxygen was therefore recommended.

Step 3. Refer to Pulmonary Rehabilitation. The patient was enrolled in an 8-week, multimodality, exercise endurance training program. This further improved his exercise capacity and dyspnea, reduced ventilatory demand, improved peripheral and ventilatory muscle strength and endurance, and improved his breathing pattern. The cumulative effects of these three interventions are shown in Figure 9–9.

Case Study 2

Ms. Cope, a 63-year-old woman with a 40-pack-a-year smoking history, was referred for management of her chronic cough.

Medical History, Physical Examination, and Test Results

Medical History
- She reported that she had had a "smoker's cough" for years.
- She had difficulty in expectorating secretions and paroxysms of coughing each morning; in fact, this had become particularly problematic after she suffered respiratory tract infections.
- She reported two respiratory tract infections requiring treatment with antibiotics over the previous year; furthermore, each episode was associated with a persistent, minimally productive cough that lingered for weeks at a time.
- She seldom reported a nocturnal cough.
- No rhinitis, postnasal drip, and no symptoms of

gastroesophageal reflux were reported.
- Apart from her cough, she has few other respiratory symptoms; she did not complain of dyspnea and maintains an active lifestyle.
- Cough syrup was tried to no avail; the patient claimed that her bronchodilators (salbutamol, two puffs four times daily; ipratropium, two puffs four times daily) have little or no impact on her cough.

Physical Examination
- She had a normal ear, nose, and throat examination.
- Cardiac examination was normal.
- She had decreased air entry on both lung bases and a prolonged forced expiratory time (8 seconds); no stigmata of lung malignancy or bronchiectasis were evident.
- She had no edema, cyanosis, or clubbing.

Test Results
- Spirometry compatible with moderate airflow obstruction was not reversible: FEV_1 was 1.4 L (52% predicted of normal pre- and postbronchodilator), and diffusion capacity and residual volume were normal.

- Chest radiography was unremarkable and showed no suspicion of a lung tumor or bronchiectasis.
- Oxygen saturation was 96% at rest.

Questions and Discussion

This patient had a chronic cough for more than 3 months in 2 consecutive years and therefore fit the diagnostic criteria for chronic bronchitis. She had moderate airflow obstruction without features of emphysema and had two acute exacerbations of COPD in the previous year requiring antibiotics but no systemic corticosteroids.

How do we control cough in this patient?

The patient was entered into a smoking cessation program, which has been successful. Because of previous issues related to inhaler compliance, a combination inhaler of salbutamol-ipratropium was prescribed. She was instructed to receive an annual influenza vaccine.

After 4 weeks of the smoking cessation program, she reported a noticeable reduction in her cough and sputum expectoration. She also proudly announced that she had not smoked a cigarette in over 2 weeks. The patient will need to be followed up closely for smoking cessation maintenance.

KEY POINTS

- Dyspnea is the most common symptom in COPD.
- Dyspnea develops insidiously, and its negative impact on the individual's activity levels is often under-recognized by the caregiver.
- Potentially reversible causes of dyspnea in COPD include lung hyperinflation and excessive ventilatory demand during activity.
- Combined bronchodilator therapy reduces operating lung volumes during rest and activity and, as a result, improves inspiratory muscle function, dyspnea, and exercise performance.
- Reduced ventilatory demand can be achieved in patients with COPD with supervised exercise training or ambulatory oxygen in selected individuals.
- A comprehensive management plan that incorporates pharmacologic and nonpharmacologic interventions is required for optimal symptom control in advanced COPD.

- In patients who remain symptomatic despite optimized pharmacotherapy and rehabilitation, surgical options could be considered.
- Smoking cessation is the first step in the management of chronic cough in COPD. Medication can sometimes be useful (see Table 9–2).
- Persistent cough can be the first symptom of lung cancer in patients with COPD.
- Evidence is not conclusive on the role of chest physiotherapy, techniques such as controlled cough or forced expiration may be useful for some patients.

REFERENCES

1. Meek PM, Schwartzstein RMS, Adams L, et al. Dyspnea mechanism, assessment and management: a consensus statement (American Thoracic Society). Am J Respir Crit Care Med 1999;159:321–40.
2. Altose M, Cherniak N, Fishman AP. Respiratory sensations and dyspnea: perspectives. J Appl Physiol 1985;58:1051–4.

3. Killian K, Campbell EJM. Dyspnea. In: Roussos C, Macklem PT, eds. The thorax. Lung biology in health and disease. Vol. 29, part B. New York: Marcel Dekker, 1985:787–828.

4. O' Donnell DE. Exertional breathlessness in chronic respiratory disease. In: Mahler DA, ed. Dyspnea. Lung biology in health and disease. Vol. 2. New York: Marcel Dekker, 1998:97–147.

5. Pride NB, Macklem PT. Lung mechanics in disease. In: Fishman AP, ed. The respiratory system. Handbook of physiology. Vol. 3, part 2. Bethesda, MD: American Physiology Society, 1986:659–92.

6. Potter WA, Olafsson S, Hyatt RE. Ventilation mechanics and expiratory flow limitation during exercise in patients with obstructive lung disease. J Clin Invest 1971;50:910–9.

7. Dodd DS, Brancatisano T, Engel LA. Chest wall mechanics during exercise in patients with severe chronic airflow obstruction. Am Rev Respir Dis 1984;129:33–8.

8. O'Donnell DE, Webb KA. Exertional breathlessness in patients with chronic airflow limitation: the role of lung hyperinflation. Am Rev Respir Dis 1993; 148:1351–7.

9. O'Donnell DE, Bertley JC, Chau LK, Webb KA. Qualitative aspects of exertional breathlessness in chronic airflow limitation: pathophysiologic mechanisms. Am J Respir Crit Care Med 1997;155:109–15.

10. Lougheed MD, Webb KA, O'Donnell DE. Breathlessness during induced lung hyperinflation in asthma: the role of the inspiratory threshold load. Am J Respir Crit Care Med 1995;152:911–20.

11. Belman MJ, Botnick WC, Shin JW. Inhaled bronchodilators reduce dynamic hyperinflation during exercise in patients with chronic obstructive pulmonary disease. Am J Respir Crit Care Med 1996; 153:967–75.

12. O'Donnell DE, Lam M, Webb KA. Spirometric correlates of improvement in exercise performance after anticholinergic therapy in COPD. Am J Respir Crit Care Med 1999;160:542–9.

13. Martinez FJ, Montes de Oca M, Whyte RI, et al. Lung volume reduction improves dyspnea, dynamic hyperinflation and respiratory muscle function. Am J Respir Crit Care Med 1997;155:1984–90.

14. Jones NL, Jones G, Edwards RHT. Exercise tolerance in chronic airway obstruction. Am Respir Crit Care Med 1971;103:477–91.

15. O'Donnell DE, Webb KA. Breathlessness in patients with severe chronic airflow limitation: physiologic correlations. Chest 1992;102:824–31.

16. Swinburn CR, Wakefield JM, Jones PW. Relationship between ventilation and breathlessness during exercise in chronic obstructive airways disease is not altered by prevention of hypoxemia. Clin Sci 1984;67:515–9.

17. O'Donnell DE, McGuire M, Samis L, Webb KA. The impact of exercise reconditioning on breathlessness in severe chronic airflow limitation. Am J Respir Crit Care Med 1995;152:2005–13.

18. Casaburi R. Exercise training in chronic obstructive lung disease. In: Casaburi R, Petty TL, eds. Principles and practice of pulmonary rehabilitation. Philadelphia: WB Saunders, 1993:204–24.

19. O'Donnell DE, Bain DJ, Webb KA. Factors contributing to relief of exertional breathlessness during hyperoxia in chronic airflow limitation. Am J Respir Crit Care Med 1997;155:530–5.

20. Dean NC, Brown JK, Himelman RB, et al. Oxygen may improve dyspnea and endurance in patients with chronic obstructive pulmonary disease and only mild hypoxemia. Am Rev Respir Dis 1992; 146:941–5.

21. Light RW, Muro JR, Sato RI, et al. Effects of oral morphine on breathlessness and exercise tolerance in patients with chronic obstructive pulmonary disease. Am Rev Respir Dis 1989;139:126–33.

22. Argyropoulou P, Patakas D, Koukou A, et al. Buspirone effect on breathlessness and exercise performance in patients with chronic obstructive pulmonary disease. Respiration 1993;60:216–20.

23. Simon PM, Schwartzstein RMS, Weiss JW, et al. Distinguishable types of dyspnea in patients with shortness of breath. Am Rev Respir Dis 1990;142:1009–14.

24. Martinez FJ, Couser JI, Celli BR. Respiratory response to arm elevation in patients with chronic airflow obstruction. Am Rev Respir Dis 1991;143: 476–80.

25. Epstein SK, Celli BR, Martinez FJ, et al. Arm training reduces the VO₂ and VE cost of unsupported arm exercise and elevation in chronic obstructive pulmonary disease. J Cardpulm Rehabil 1997;17: 171–7.

26. Gift AG, Cahill CA. Psychophysiologic aspects of dyspnea in chronic obstructive pulmonary disease: a pilot study. Heart Lung 1990;19:252–7.

27. Stokes WA. A treatise on the diagnosis and treatment of diseases of the chest. In: Stokes WA, ed. Diseases of the lung and windpipe. Vol. 1. London: The New Sydenham Society, 1837:168–9.

28. Stubbing D, Campbell EJM. The physical examination of the chest. Med Clin North Am 1982; 21:2041–4.

29. Hay JG, Stone P, Carter J, et al. Bronchodilator reversibility, exercise performance and breathlessness in stable chronic obstructive pulmonary disease. Eur Respir J 1992;5:659–64.

30. Mahler DA, Matthay RA, Snyder PE, et al. Sustained-release theophylline reduces dyspnea in non-reversible obstructive airway disease. Am Rev Respir Dis 1985;131:22–5.

31. Papiris S, Galavotti V, Sturani C. Effects of beta agonists on breathlessness and exercise tolerance in patients with chronic obstructive pulmonary disease. Respiration 1986;49:101–8.

32. Faling LJ. Pulmonary rehabilitation—physical modalities. Clin Chest Med 1986;7:599–618.

33. Sinclair JD. The effect of breathing exercises in pulmonary emphysema. Thorax 1955;10:246–9.

34. Rodenstein DO, Stanescu DC. Absence of nasal airflow during pursed-lip breathing: the soft palate mechanisms. Am Rev Respir Dis 1983;128:716–8.

35. Thomas R, Stoker G, Ross J. The efficacy of pursed-lips breathing in patients with chronic obstructive pulmonary disease. Am Rev Respir Dis 1966;93:100–6.

36. Tiep BL, Burns M, Kao D, et al. Pursed lip breathing training using ear oximetry. Chest 1986;90:218–21.

37. O'Donnell DE, Sanii R, Anthonisen NR, Younes M. Effect of dynamic airway compression on breathing pattern and respiratory sensation in severe chronic obstructive pulmonary disease. Am Rev Respir Dis 1987;135:912–8.

38. Williams IP, Smith CM, McGavin CR. Diaphragmatic breathing training and walking performance in chronic airways obstruction. Br J Dis Chest 1982; 76:164–6.

39. Gosselink RA, Wagenaar RC, Risjswijk H, et al. Diaphragmatic breathing reduces efficiency of breathing in patients with chronic obstructive pulmonary disease. Am J Respir Crit Care Med 1995; 151:1136–42.

40. Gandevia SC, Macefield G. Projection of low threshold afferents from human intercostal muscles to the cerebral cortex. Respir Physiol 1989;77:203–14.

41. Kim MJ, Larson JL, Covey MK, et al. Inspiratory muscle training in patients with chronic obstructive pulmonary disease. Nurs Res 1993;42:356–62.

42. Smith K, Cook D, Guyatt GH, et al. Respiratory muscle training in chronic airflow limitation: a meta-analysis. Am Rev Respir Dis 1992;145:533–9.

43. Report of the Medical Research Council Working Party. Long term domiciliary oxygen therapy in chronic hypoxic cor pulmonale complicating chronic bronchitis and emphysema. Lancet 1981;1:681–6.

44. Noctural Oxygen Therapy Trial (NOTT) Group. Continuous or nocturnal oxygen therapy in hypoxemic chronic obstructive lung disease. Ann Intern Med 1980;93:391–8.

45. Chronos N, Adams L, Guz A. Effect of hyperoxia and hypoxia on exercise-induced breathlessness in normal subjects. Clin Sci 1988;74:531–7.

46. Bruera E, de Stoutz N, Velasco LA, et al. Effects of oxygen on dyspnoea in hypoxaemic terminal-cancer patients. Lancet 1993;342:13–4.

47. Santiago TV, Johnson J, Riley DJ, Edelman NH. Effects of morphine on ventilatory response to exercise. J Appl Physiol 1979;47:112–8.

48. Woodcock AA, Gross ER, Gellert A, et al. Effects of dihydrocodeine, alcohol, and caffeine on breathlessness and exercise tolerance in patients with chronic obstructive pulmonary disease and normal blood gases. N Engl J Med 1981;305:1611–6.

49. Woodcock AA, Johnson MA, Geddes DM. Breathlessness, alcohol and opiates. N Engl J Med 1982;306: 1363–4.

50. Young IH, Daviskas E, Keena VA. Effect of low dose nebulised morphine on exercise endurance in patients with chronic lung disease. Thorax 1989;44:387–90.

51. Leung R, Hill P, Burdon J. Effect of inhaled morphine on the development of breathlessness during exercise in patients with chronic lung disease. Thorax 1996;51:596–600.

52. Chau LKL, Webb KA, O'Donnell DE. Relief of exertional breathlessness with nebulized morphine sulfate in patients with chronic lung disease. Am J Respir Crit Care Med 1996;153:A656.

53. Saunders C, Baines M. Living with dying: the management of terminal disease. Oxford: Oxford University Press, 1989.

54. Foley KM. Clinical tolerance to opiods. In: Bassbaun AI, Beeson JM, eds. Towards a new pharmacotherapy of pain. UK: John Wiley & Sons, 1991:181–204.

55. Mitchell HP, Murphy K, Minty K, et al. Diazepam in the treatment of dyspnoea in the "pink and puffer" syndrome. QJM 1980;49:9–20.

56. Stark RD, Gambles SA, Lewis JA. Methods to assess breathlessness in healthy subjects: a critical evaluation and application to analyze the acute effects of diazepam and promethazine on breathlessness induced by exercise or by exposure to raised levels of carbon dioxide. Clin Sci 1981;61: 429–39.

57. Rice KL, Kronenburg RS, Hedemark LL, Niewoehner DE. Effects of chronic administration of codeine and promethazine on breathlessness and exercise tolerance in patients with chronic airflow obstruction. Br J Dis Chest 1987;81:287–92.

58. Singh NP, Despars JA, Stansbury DW, et al. Effects of buspirone on anxiety levels and exercise tolerance in patients with chronic airflow obstruction and mild anxiety. Chest 1993;103:800–4.

59. Widdicombe JG. Physiology of cough. In: Braga PC, Allegra L, eds. Cough. New York: Raven Press, 1989:3–25.

60. Coleridge HM, Coleridge JCG. Reflexes evoked from tracheobronchial tree and lungs. In: Cherniak NS, Widdicombe JG, eds. Handbook of physiology: respiration. Vol. (3)2. Bethesda, MD: American Physiology Society, 1986:395–429.

61. Karlsson JA, Sant'Ambrogio G, Widdicombe J. Afferent neural pathways in cough and reflex bronchoconstriction. J Appl Physiol 1988;65:1007–23.

62. Sant'Ambrogio G. Afferent pathways for the cough reflex. Bull Eur Physiopathol Respir 1987; 23 Suppl 10:19S–23S.

63. Coleridge JCG, Coleridge HM. Afferent vagal C-fiber innervation of the lungs and airways and its functional significance. Rev Physiol Biochem Pharmacol 1984;99:1–10.

64. Macklem PT. Physiology of cough. Ann Otol Rhinol Laryngol 1974;83:761–8.

65. Irwin RS, Corrao WM, Pratter MR. Chronic persistent cough in the adult: the spectrum and frequency of causes and successful outcome of specific therapy. Am Rev Respir Dis 1981;123:413–7.

66. Irwin RS, Curley FJ, French CL. Chronic cough. The spectrum and frequency of causes, key components of the diagnostic evaluation, and outcome of specific therapy. Am Rev Respir Dis 1990;141:640–7.

67. Irwin RS, Madison JM. The diagnosis and treatment of cough. N Engl J Med 2001;343:1715–21.

68. Wynder EL, Kaufman PL, Lesser RL. A short-term follow-up study on ex-cigarette smokers. With special

emphasis on persistent cough and weight gain. Am Rev Respir Dis 1967;96:645–55.

69. Irwin RS, Curley FJ. The treatment of cough: a comprehensive review. Chest 1991;99:1477–84.

70. Verstraeten JM. Mucolytic treatment in chronic airways obstruction. Double-blind clinical trial with N-acetylcysteine, bromhexine and placebo. Acta Tuberc Pneumol Belg 1979;61:71–80.

71. Hirsh SR, Viernes PF, Kory RC. The expectorant effect of glyceryl guaiacolate in patients with chronic bronchitis. A controlled in vitro and in vivo study. Chest 1973;63:9–14.

72. Multicenter Study Group. Long-term oral acetylcysteine in chronic bronchitis, a double-blind controlled study. Eur Respir J 1980;61 Suppl 111:93–108.

73. De Boeck C, Zinman R. Cough versus chest physiotherapy: a comparison of the acute effects on pulmonary function in patients with cystic fibrosis. Am Rev Respir Dis 1984;129:182–4.

74. van der Schans CP. Forced expiratory manoeuvres to increase transport of bronchial mucus: a mechanistic approach. Monaldi Arch Chest Dis 1997;52:367–70.

75. O'Donnell DE, Sanii R, Giesbecht G, Younes M. Effect of continuous positive airway pressure on respiratory sensation in patients with chronic obstructive pulmonary disease during submaximal exercise. An Rev Respir Dis 1988;138:1185–91.

76. O'Donnell DE, Webb KA, Bertley JC, et al. Mechanisms of relief of exertional breathlessness following unilateral bullectomy and lung volume reduction surgery for emphysema. Chest 1996;110:18–27.

77. O'Donnell DE. Dyspnea in advanced chronic obstruction pulmonary disease. J Heart Lung Transplant 1998;17:544–54.

SUGGESTED READINGS

American Thoracic Society. Dyspnea. Mechanisms, assessment, and management: a consensus statement. Am J Respir Crit Care Med 1999;159:321–40. *In this state-of-the-art review, current concepts of the origins of breathlessness are discussed. The rationale for the modern management of this symptom is provided, and the evidence for the efficacy of various therapeutic intervention is reviewed in detail.*

Irwin R, Madison JM. The diagnosis and treatment of cough. N Engl J Med 2000;343:1715–21. *This review succinctly summarizes what is known about the pathophysiology of cough and provides a critical analysis of the current scientific literature on the clinical management of chronic cough. It provides evidence-based recommendations on a step-by-step approach to the diagnosis of chronic cough.*

CHAPTER 10

ENERGY CONSERVATION AND FATIGUE

*Judy Lamb, Elizabeth Borycki,
and Darcy Marciniuk*

OBJECTIVES

The general objective of this chapter is to help physicians and allied health care professionals teach patients with chronic obstructive pulmonary disease (COPD) to manage their fatigue and energy limitations. After reading this chapter, the physician and allied health care professional will be able to

- understand the relationship between different dimensions of COPD: impaired pulmonary function, increased effort to breathe, energy limitations, and fatigue;
- develop an approach to appropriately assess and manage this aspect of the patient's care;
- ensure that the patient is able to understand and apply energy conservation principles to reduce fatigue; and
- refer to the appropriate allied health care professional when needed.

Patients with COPD demonstrate impaired pulmonary function, breathlessness, and fatigue that typically interfere with many aspects of daily life, including the ability to work, carry out household tasks, socialize, and engage in leisure activities. In severe cases, the patient's ability to perform basic self-care activities and engage in normal conversation is also affected.[1]

There is a relationship between impaired pulmonary function and the increased work of breathing and fatigue present in these patients. The impact of fatigue and energy limitations on functional capacity and quality of life in patients with COPD is often not recognized or attributed the necessary importance. Energy conservation principles and practical physical and cognitive behavioral strategies that patients can use to minimize their fatigue and adapt to their level of energy, have to be part of the management of COPD. Facilitating the inte-

gration of these new behaviors into the respiratory patient's lifestyle is important to ensure effective self-management of COPD.

In this chapter, we review energy deficiency and fatigue in patients with COPD, along with assessment guidelines and energy conservation principles to reduce fatigue. Other known factors that can impact the fatigue level experienced by a patient are nutrition, sleep, physical exercise, stress management, oxygen therapy, and pharmacologic therapy; they are discussed in detail elsewhere in this book.

ENERGY DEFICIENCY AND FATIGUE

Energy is a biologic phenomenon that manifests itself in human beings as either internal work, such as the energy consumed for maintenance of normal internal body functions, or as external work, which is the energy consumed for movement and physical activity. In the normal population, both the energy requirements and efficiency in energy use vary between individuals; they are dependent on many factors, from age, sex, and body composition to environmental factors and emotional well-being.[2,3]

In patients with COPD, their heart, lungs, and respiratory muscles work harder to overcome the significant airway obstruction and structural changes in the lungs and thorax, to maintain the appropriate gas exchange; in effect, this is the primary responsibility of the respiratory system in humans.[3] When the anaerobic threshold is reached during incremental body exercise, muscle metabolism changes from being principally oxidative to principally glycolytic because the total-body energy supply is inadequate to meet the total-body energy demands. The imbalance between supply and demand leads to fatigue and eventually task failure. Under these circumstances, there is competition between respiratory and locomotor muscles for a supply of energy that is insufficient to meet the needs of both. It appears that neither the respiratory muscles required to breathe nor the skeletal locomotor muscles receive sufficient oxygen to continue metabolizing aerobically. Presumably, some individuals cease exercising because of dyspnea, whereas others stop because of leg effort. In a study of 417 subjects, Killian and colleagues have shown that subjects were limited either by leg fatigue dyspnea (43% and 36%, respectively), or when the two symptoms were of equal intensity then dyspnea was the most prominent symptom limiting exercise performance in only 26% of patients with COPD and 22% of normal subjects.[4] However, we do not yet know why, within the individual, exercise is sometimes limited by dyspnea and other times by leg fatigue.

For patients with COPD, normal activities such as tasks associated with daily living can become restricted and exhausting, thus resulting in a tendency among patients with significant COPD to gradually withdraw from or avoid discomfort-producing activity (Figure 10–1). Typically, the engagement in outside work is the first level of activity to be abandoned, followed thereafter by recreational and social pursuits.[5] This withdrawal can, in turn, lead to other problems including physical deconditioning, social isolation, anxiety, and depression. Such changes in physical and psychosocial well-being can further contribute to the negative impact on breathlessness and quality of life.[6–8] The

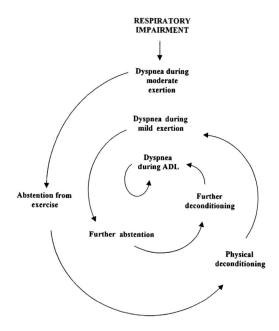

Figure 10–1 Progressive deterioration in COPD resulting from inactivity because of shortness of breath. Exercise-induced dyspnea in chronic pulmonary disease can finally result in severe physical deconditioning; this can occur to a point where activities of daily living (ADL) are compromised out of proportion to the patient's actual cardiorespiratory potential. (Adapted from Haas, et al.[30])

complex interrelationships between these factors is demonstrated in Figure 10–2.

Similar to healthy people, patients with COPD vary widely in their energy metabolism and tendency toward fatigue. However, at some point, patients must learn the difficult lesson that continually pushing themselves beyond their breathing and energy limitations will leave them chronically fatigued and short of breath. Symptoms of fatigue and low energy may be misunderstood by the patient and his/her family, who, with good intention, often believe that if the patient would only try harder, he/she could do more. In this circumstance, it is important for both the patient and the family to realize that balancing activity and rest, rather than further effort, will make the positive difference in mastery of the illness and its unwanted consequences.[7,9,10] The old fable of the tortoise and the hare is a fitting illustration of this point.

When learning to manage their illness, it is important for all respiratory patients to become familiar

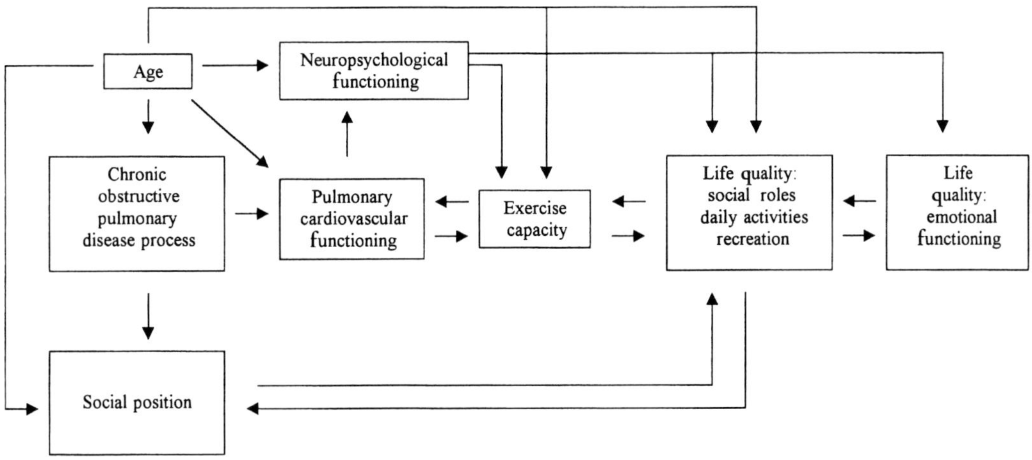

Figure 10–2 The interrelationship of variables affecting quality of life in COPD. Heuristic model relating chronic obstructive pulmonary disease and other variables that affect quality of life. (Reproduced with permission from McSweeney, et al.[31])

with the principles of energy conservation. When learned, practiced, and integrated into one's lifestyle, these principles enable the individual to work toward finding a dynamic balance between internal energetic capacity and the external demands of lifestyle.

ASSESSING THE IMPACT OF ENERGY DEFICIENCY AND FATIGUE

Within the context of their lifestyle and environment, patients with advancing COPD benefit from a thorough evaluation of their functional capacity. The health professional can evaluate with patients what self-care or other daily tasks/interests and responsibilities are causing them more breathlessness or fatigue than is comfortable or tolerable. The following statement by Horne and Corsello is self-explanatory: "Functional capacity it should be noted is not absolute. It is relative to the patient's expectations, priorities, goals and social supports, amongst other factors."[11]

A patient-centered evaluation will typically reflect the primary concerns and motivations of the patient and will include both subjective and objective components. Subjective components of an evaluation may include interview and self-assessment with a formal or informal screening tool. Objective compo-

nents of the evaluation should include a monitored functional assessment.[7,11,12]

Initial Interview

Through directed conversation with the patient, the health professional can begin to formulate an understanding of the disease process impact and make a comparison between this factor and the patient's coping resources. Including the spouse or a close relative in the interview may be valuable in developing a more complete picture of the patient's daily challenges. In an early study,[5] Barstow found the single most important positive resource for adjustment in COPD to be the presence of a helpful support person in the home.

In an initial interview, it is important to first determine what social supports exist for the patient, both inside and outside the home. Family members or friends can also help identify preexisting patterns in the patient's energy level and note changes that they have noticed because of the illness.[13] The patient's emotional status, motivation, and typical coping mechanisms are also useful factors to note.

Other important considerations include the following aspects:
• Where does the person live?
• How accessible is the home in terms of natural environmental barriers such as hills or architectural barriers such as stairs?

- Does the patient have access to a car and a garage to keep it warm in cold weather? If not, does he/she have an available and reliable chauffeur to drive him/her to the store, bank, or medical appointments when needed?
- If the patient does not have access to a car, does he/she have the income to afford taxis? Otherwise, how far does the patient live from the services he/she needs, and how accessible is public transportation?
- How often does the patient go out?

Depending on the circumstance, all of these factors may replenish or drain existing energy resources.[14]

Self-Assessment

How does the patient perceive his/her performance in self-care, domestic, physical, and leisure activities? What is his/her perception of the impact of the illness on functioning? To better assess these factors, and because there are only a few tools that will provide a simple measure of limitation in functional disability, many programs have developed their own unique screening tools to address the specific impact of shortness of breath and fatigue on the patient's self-care and activities of daily living (ADL).

Currently, validated tools are available. The Chronic Respiratory Disease Questionnaire (CRQ), a disease-specific quality of life questionnaire, assesses the specific dimension of fatigue; other subscales of this questionnaire evaluate dimensions of perceived dyspnea as well as emotional function and illness mastery.[15] Although the measure of health-related quality of life has been increasingly conducted in the assessment of COPD, there is little focus on assessment of ADL. There are few tools that will provide a simple measure of limitation in functional disability. In addition to being a time-consuming assessment, the Pulmonary Functional Status and Dyspnea Questionnaire (PFSDQ) contains many items that are no longer feasible for patients with severe COPD.[16] The Nottingham Extended Activities of Daily Living (EADL) scale, originally developed for stroke patients,[17] has been shown in COPD to be a good discriminative tool[18] but was unable to detect changes in ADL performance after a pulmonary rehabilitation program.[19] The London Chest Activity Daily Living (LCADL) scale is a new tool developed specifically for patients with severe COPD. It is a standardized 15-item questionnaire. Studies have shown that the LCADL scale is a valid tool for assessment of

ADL,[20] and data support the use of the LCADL as an outcome measure after 6 weeks of pulmonary rehabilitation.[20] Detailed information regarding these questionnaires and others is provided in Chapter 19.

Monitored Functional Assessment

It is important for the professional to observe activity tolerance and methods employed by the patient to handle the stress associated with various activities. Any activity identified by the patient as problematic could be ideally chosen as the monitored task. Objective parameters measured during a functional assessment should include heart rate, respiration rate, oxygen saturation,[21] number of rests taken, and time for recovery to baseline values at rest. It is useful to have patients contribute both their perceived dyspnea and exertion levels, based on a modified Borg scale.[12,22] Other useful observations by the professional would include the patient's typical breathing pattern and use of pacing, his/her posture and body mechanics in activity, and the emotional states exhibited, such as anxiety or frustration.[7,11] An example of an assessment format used to monitor basic functional capacity is demonstrated in Appendix 10–1.

Basic strength, endurance, and range of motion are also important physical components to evaluate. Assessment with an arm ergometer can provide objective measures of upper extremity endurance.[23] Various walking tests to evaluate the lower extremity are discussed in Chapter 19.

Monitored assessments highlight the patient's functional difficulties and help identify the need for one of the following interventions, to successfully perform the activity:

- Acquisition of a new performance method involving improved pacing and breathing control
- Adapted equipment
- Supplementary oxygen
- Assistance of a caregiver

In surveying the patient's resources and deficits in both subjective and objective ways, it is then possible to develop priorities for treatment.

MANAGING THE ENERGY-DEFICIENT PATIENT

It has been mentioned elsewhere in the textbook that in patients with COPD, regular muscle aerobic training allows improvement in the ability to undertake activities, thereby decreasing disability and ultimately improving quality of life. Thus, an exercise training regimen should be emphasized in every patient with COPD as it aims to improve function for self-care, productive, and recreational activities.

In treating fatigue and energy limitations, an important goal lies in the patient cultivating new lifestyle behaviors that enhance his/her capacity to engage in meaningful activity; the idea is that, in doing so, he/she may achieve maximum functional potential and an improved quality of life. To achieve this goal, patients must (1) develop an awareness and understanding of his/her symptoms and what behaviors they typically use to cope; (2) learn newer, more effective behaviors to help minimize symptoms; and (3) integrate the new behaviors into their lifestyle through practice and problem solving.

Developing Awareness

The most prevalent symptoms reported by patients with COPD are dyspnea and fatigue.[24] The patient's coping behaviors in response to these symptoms are typically ineffective.[25] Patients and their families usually benefit from receiving some basic illness-related information that enables them to make sense of these symptoms. Conducting education sessions in a group setting with other patients with COPD and family members present helps give participants an improved perspective on the illness and provides an opportunity to share experiences and learning. Patients need to understand that there are physiologic reasons for their fatigue and breathlessness and learn self-management strategies that they can apply to garner more control of their symptoms. Identifying what triggers their fatigue and breathlessness and learning to recognize their own energy patterns and personal limitations are essential. Self-knowledge and a healthy acceptance of personal limits can form the basis for an effective lifestyle change.

Learning New Behaviors: Guidelines for Conserving Energy

The focus on treating fatigue usually involves a process of educating respiratory patients to embrace a series of guidelines for conserving energy. These behavioral suggestions draw from the studies of ergonomics and work efficiency, as well as time and stress management.[7,26] Although a useful body of knowledge for many different disabilities, this particular version incorporates suggestions for breathing control during activity for the energy-deficient respiratory patient. The guidelines include the following principles and practices:

1. Practice time management and plan ahead.
2. Slow down the pace: balance work and rest to minimize fatigue.
3. Pay attention to body position and use equipment that reduces the workload.
4. Coordinate breathing with activity to reduce shortness of breath.
5. Control for environmental factors.
6. Recognize personal limitations and ask for help or delegate where indicated.

Although these suggestions are simple in theory, to integrate each one involves complex shifting of a deeply rooted, habitual behavior for most patients. Incorporating these principles into daily activities involves developing new ways of approaching daily plans, with the goal of minimizing fatigue symptoms and shortness of breath and maximizing engagement in meaningful activity.

Practice Time Management and Plan Ahead

Respiratory patients often find that ordinary daily "survival" activities become more difficult and time consuming, and the exertion involved may leave them too tired to devote time to more creative or enjoyable "self-actualizing" activities. Patients become overwhelmed with activities that they have to do, and, as a result, daily pleasures are frequently sacrificed.[2]

The behavioral strategies[10,11,27] to adopt are the following:

- Keep commitments within manageable limits.
- Clarify priorities in terms of "have to do's" and "want to do's" and plan schedules to include both.
- Plan each day to include only what can be realistically accomplished.

Where possible, plan daily schedules so that the most energy-consuming activities are done at the time of day when the patient has the most energy:

- Do one activity at a time and allow ample time to complete each activity.
- Think through challenging tasks in advance. Take into consideration the amount of time needed and where the supplies are located. Assemble all supplies for a task first to avoid extra trips.
- Eliminate unnecessary tasks where possible. For example, wear a terrycloth robe instead of toweling off after bathing. Keep hair short to avoid blow drying time and effort. Let dishes air dry.

Slow Down the Pace: Balance Work and Rest to Minimize Fatigue

A fatigued state can leave the patient with COPD more vulnerable to respiratory infection. Fatigue can also lead to poor body mechanics, decreased attentiveness, and, consequently, an increased risk of injury. It is important for the patient with COPD to incorporate rest periods into the daily work plan.[27]

Behavioral strategies[5,10] to adopt and balance work and rest are the following:

- A slow, steady speed consumes less energy.
- Listen to bodily messages and rest before becoming excessively tired.
- Break difficult activities into manageable parts and take periodic rests, if necessary within activities and between activities.
- Balance heavy and light tasks; do several kinds of activity each day and include time for hobbies, going outside, reading, or other relaxing pursuits.
- Take regular rest breaks throughout the day and learn to let go of physical and mental tension. For example, sit down with eyes closed, head and neck relaxed, and take 10 slow, pursed-lip breaths.
- Pace meals. Eat more frequent small meals or rest between courses to give the body a chance to adjust.
- Allow at least a 30-minute rest period after each meal and after more strenuous activities and outings.
- Get sufficient rest at night. If sleep difficulties are present, develop a routine and try to keep a regular bedtime. Avoid upsetting or exciting activities before bed and practice relaxation techniques.

Pay Attention to Body Position and Use Equipment that Reduces the Workload

For many patients with pulmonary disease, the unsupported upper extremity activities such as washing hair, blow drying it, and shaving cause the most shortness of breath. Often patients must rely heavily on accessory muscles to do the work of breathing, and when these muscles are used for supporting the arms during activity, they are less available to assist with breathing.[9] Other more exertional activities such as reaching, bending, lifting, carrying, pushing, and pulling also tend to stress the respiratory capacities of individuals with COPD. Even maintaining positions such as simple standing for any length of time can be stressful. Proper use of body mechanics can diminish the energy requirements of any task.[25]

Appropriately employing adapted equipment may also assist in conserving energy for the fatigued respiratory patient.

The behavioral strategies[5,10,27] to adopt are the following:

- Sit for as many activities as possible because sitting consumes less energy than standing. For example, use a bath seat and telephone shower while bathing.
- Minimize unsupported arm movements. Adapt activities where possible to provide arm support (ie, sit and brace elbows while shaving).
- When extremely short of breath, assume a forward-leaning position with arms supported and relaxed. Maintain this position until controlled breathing resumes.[28]
- When sitting or standing, choose good work heights (at 2 inches below bent elbows).
- The height of beds or tables can be raised with adjustable blocks if the patient finds the furniture too low, which adds strain to the back or breathing.
- Where possible, avoid reaching, bending, pushing, pulling, and lifting as these functional tasks require more energy.
- Store frequently used items within easy reach (between waist and shoulder level) and keep items in the area where they are used.
- Storing cleaning products on a trolley facilitates their transport.
- When the body is properly aligned, less energy is required to maintain posture. In general (unless you are experiencing shortness of breath and using forward-leaning posture) try to keep the head aligned with the trunk while keeping the shoulders and hips parallel.
- While lifting or carrying, hold the object close to the body and keep the back straight, always bending at the knees.
- Be open to assistive devices; use long-handled utensils (ie, shoe horns, reachers, dressing sticks) and elastic shoelaces if bending over is a problem.
- Investigate innovative products and technologies where possible to save unecessary labor and energy and to achieve maximum independence. A personal computer to do banking, shopping, and pay bills from home; various specialized home and kitchen appliances; frozen foods, and simple and casual clothes can all be energy-saving tools if the individual has the financial means to consider them.

- Mobility aids such as motorized scooters, four-wheel (rollator) walkers with seats, and portable oxygen units can enhance possibilities for independent mobility outside the home.

Coordinate Breathing with Activity to Reduce Shortness of Breath

Respiratory patients frequently carry out activities in a rushed, haphazard way in an attempt to avoid dyspnea. However, in rushing to complete the activity, they actually increase dyspnea and expend more energy. The rapid breathing pattern that accompanies hurrying actually requires more oxygen than a slower, smoother movement. By slowing down and pacing their breathing and movements, patients can work within the oxygen-carrying capacity of their lungs.[25]

The behavioral strategies[7,11,12,25] to adopt are the following:
- Use pursed-lip and diaphragmatic breathing, as discussed in Chapter 9.
- Lengthening the exhalation phase improves lung emptying, which will, in turn, facilitate inhalation.
- When the patient has mastered breathing techniques at rest, begin applying techniques to movement and activity.
- Learn to coordinate the exhalation phase of breathing with the more exertional part of the movement or activity.
- For more exertional activities such as climbing stairs or vacuuming, slow down movements; establish a breathing rhythm with pursed-lip breathing, and exhale on exertion. For example, while climbing stairs, if the patient cannot maintain his/her breathing rhythm, he/she should slow down and go up fewer stairs per breath or stop if necessary until controlled breathing resumes.
- Teach patients to know when to expect disruptions of breathing patterns and to intervene appropriately by adjusting breathing pattern, speed of activity, and/or body position.
- Talking, laughing, eating, and coughing are all exhaling patterns that can interrupt the regular rhythm of breathing and can potentially cause shortness of breath. Accommodate by slowing down, positioning, and breathing at regular intervals. For example, slow down speech by stopping between sentences to breathe and relax.
- Complete heavier tasks right after taking inhaled medications where possible.

- Emphasize the use of oxygen therapy with activity when indicated and prescribed.
- Breathing control must be applied, both at rest and with movement and activity. To provide relief from exertional dyspnea, breathing control must become habitual.

Control for Environmental Factors

Most respiratory patients experience an increase in dyspnea with either hot (and humid) or cold (and dry) ambient weather conditions. Airborne irritants such as paint fumes, dust, chemical odors, industrial pollution, and cigarette smoke can cause increased sensitivity as well.[29]

The behavioral strategies[10] to adopt are the following:
- Consider the weather. Stay indoors when extreme weather conditions or high pollution counts occur.
- In the summer, it is best to do outdoor activity during the coolest part of the day, whereas in the winter, it is preferable to perform outdoor activities during the warmest part of the day.
- Working in a very warm room is less efficient because extra energy must be used by the heart and lungs to cool the body down.
- Avoid extremely hot baths, Jacuzzis, or showers.
- To reduce steam while bathing, turn on the cold water before adding hot water.
- Investigate environmental controls for home use, such as an air conditioner and an air purifier.
- Keep the home a nonsmoking and fragrance-free zone. Patients should help their friends to understand this decision in whatever way possible.
- Use water-based paint when involved in home improvements.
- Shop for odorless cleaning products.
- Use adequate ventilation. Heavy cooking odors, perfumes, or steam (shower) may make breathing more difficult. Keep doors and windows open or get a ceiling fan or air conditioner if necessary to keep air circulating.

Recognize Personal Limitations and Ask for Help or Delegate When Indicated

The patient with COPD is faced with the prospect of an inevitable decline in functional performance. The decline is first evident with respect to work roles and then recreational and social roles. It culminates in difficulty performing the most basic self-care tasks. As the patient's roles contract, the roles of family members must expand, or outside sources will be needed to supplement the patient's ability to function.[5]

Complicating the picture is the value system of work and independence that is prevalent in our culture. This influence may make it difficult for those with a chronic debilitating illness such as COPD to relinquish some of their independence for daily tasks or to give up their own way of performing activities.[2,5] The same value system may make it difficult for the spouse or family members to accept the illness until the symptoms have deteriorated to a point where they must be acknowledged.

Either denial or exaggeration of the illness by the patient or the family will create a dysfunctional situation that interferes with illness management. Healthy redistribution of roles can occur only when the patient and those around him/her are realistic about the extent of the disability and supportive of the patient's needs. A restructuring of attitudes in the family unit and open communication are needed for a successful adjustment to the presence of chronic illness.[5]

The behavioral strategies[5,10,27] to adopt are the following:

- Patients need to discuss their feelings with their health care workers and caregivers; they need to learn to see themselves as active collaborators in the management of their illness as opposed to victims of disease.
- Family members should be encouraged to participate in education sessions to better understand the patient.
- To avoid any emotional buildup, which can quickly oppress the patient's breathing capacity, it is important to deal with interpersonal problems as they arise. Good communication skills cannot be stressed enough and the patient needs to develop a proficiency in emotional management.
- Functional tasks related to homemaking, financial management, and self-care all break down into two components: a managerial component and the actual participation in task performance. The individual who has increasing difficulty in task performance can still be a good manager/collaborator and should be encouraged to maintain an active involvement in whatever way possible.
- Heavy domestic tasks (such as cleaning the oven, washing walls, vacuuming) and outdoor maintenance (mowing the lawn, shoveling snow) should be assigned to other family members, a willing friend, or a hired service.

- If the patient lives alone and is dependent on public transportation, some form of adapted transport may have to be organized for outings.

Integrating New Behaviors

Once the patient understands the symptoms, is aware of how shortness of breath and fatigue impact lifestyle, and has learned newer, more effective coping strategies, these new strategies must be put to the test; integrating new behaviors requires commitment, practice, and problem solving. Because these techniques must be practiced until they become habitual, the patient's initiative and motivation are key to success. Patients require opportunities to think through activities in advance, practice task analysis, and embody physical change strategies while receiving feedback as needed from the therapist. Optimally, the patient should keep a diary documenting difficulties encountered. These experiences could be further explored during teaching and practice sessions. If time permits, the supervised practice setting can progress to the patient's home for a true test of how the patient has integrated the new behaviors. Follow-up sessions at 3 and 6 months are recommended to ensure that these new, effective behaviors are maintained over time.

WHEN TO REFER

It should be understood and emphasized that because of the multilevel involvement and the complexity of the problems associated with COPD and their effects on the patient and family, a complete assessment is necessary with ongoing management by a multidisciplinary team. Effective communication between all members of the team is essential to ensure that the patient attains maximal benefit from the expertise of each individual team member. It would be advisable to consider referring a patient with COPD to pulmonary rehabilitation for an exercise training program when activity and function are reduced secondary to shortness of breath or fatigue.

When to Refer to a Physician

All patients should initially be referred to a physician and when needed a respirologist. Evaluation by a physician complemented by spirometry, or complete pulmonary function tests, will establish the diagnosis of COPD and confirm that no other medical conditions are present to account for the symptoms. During this assessment(s), the physician will also optimize pharmacologic therapy for the management of the patient's disease and his/her symptoms.

When to Refer to an Occupational Therapist

The occupational therapist will evaluate limitations in the patient's ability to perform self-care, domestic, leisure, and work activities and can identify the need for energy conservation training and activity modification. The occupational therapist can also suggest assistive devices that minimize the patient's expenditure of energy and can determine when additional help and support are necessary to maintain independence at home. For example, patients may be able to bathe independently if they are provided with a bath seat, telephone shower, and safety bar. They may be able to manage their own shopping with a rollator walker or a motorized scooter. Home help for heavy housework and bathing may delay long-term care admission.

SUMMARY

In managing COPD, it is essential to consider a team approach. The most appropriate setting to ensure the patient a multidisciplinary assessment and management is a pulmonary rehabilitation program.

Pulmonary rehabilitation offers the advantage of an exercise training program and the expertise of a multidisciplinary team.

The impact of fatigue and energy limitations on the quality of life of the patient with COPD is important to assess. Functional capacity has to be assessed subjectively and objectively within the context of the patient's lifestyle and environment. Then the management strategies should focus on increasing the patient's awareness of his/her strengths and limitations and acceptance of the condition through individual and group interventions. A series of practical guidelines for conserving energy can be employed to help control dyspnea and manage fatigue. These treatment strategies are appropriate for a patient who demonstrates some initiative and motivation. However, if this is not the case, the patient may require prior intervention with a social worker or psychologist.

Although this orientation to evaluation and management may not impact the patient's physiologic pulmonary functions, it can enable patients with COPD to actively collaborate in their treatment with their families and health care providers. They may also learn to live more comfortably and productively within the unfortunate confines of their illness.

CASE STUDY

Mrs. Cope is a 67-year-old woman who was hospitalized for a serious exacerbation of her respiratory condition. Her hospital stay involved an admission to the intensive care unit and a recovery period in the acute care ward.

Medical History, Physical Examination, and Test Results

Mrs. Cope is now medically stable and ready for discharge without oxygen; she is referred to the occupational therapist for follow-up as an outpatient to assist her in managing her illness.

Medical History

- She was diagnosed with COPD and for many years has suffered with dyspnea; she has poor

exercise tolerance that has deteriorated in the last 2 years and, consequently, has a restriction in her ADL.
- She quit smoking 4 years ago after a 40 pack-year history.
- She has no other relevant medical history.
- Medication includes regular use of inhaled bronchodilators (combined β_2 agonist and anticholinergic), a theophylline derivative, prednisone, and an antibiotic for 7 additional days at home.

Physical Examination

- Vital signs are as follows: pulse 92 bpm, respiratory rate 24/min, blood pressure 145/90 mm Hg.
- Accessory muscles used in breathing.
- She has a barrel chest with decreased air entry but no crackle or wheezing.
- Her cardiac examination is normal.

- She has no edema or cyanosis.

Test Results

- Spirometry results are as follows:
  - Forced expiratory volume in 1 second (FEV_1) postbronchodilator 1 L (37% predicted) and FEV_1/forced vital capacity 38%
  - Oxygen saturation at rest on room air is 95%

Mrs. Cope was offered to participate in a pulmonary rehabilitation program. As part of the program, energy deficiency was assessed and managed according to her needs.

Assessment of Impact of Energy Deficiency

Initial Interview

Mrs. Cope was divorced and living alone in a second-floor apartment. There was no elevator in the building and the laundry facilities were in the basement. She had one married daughter with two small children. Her daughter was supportive but busy with her own life and struggled to find the time to help her mother. Mrs. Cope was recently retired from her job as a unit coordinator in a hospital; she was normally efficient and highly independent, thus causing her difficulties in asking for help. Since retirement, she had little contact with her work friends and few other friends to fall back on for support. She had no car and was used to taking public transportation, although in recent years this was getting progressively more difficult. Working and raising her daughter alone had occupied most of Mrs. Cope's energy resources, thus limiting her in her personal pursuit of leisure interests. Mrs. Cope was experiencing increased anxiety and occasional panic attacks in response to her growing restrictions.

Self-Assessment

In assessing herself, Mrs. Cope was able to acknowledge increased difficulties in the area of mobility. In particular, she experienced increased shortness of breath while stair climbing and when walking outdoors for more than a block. Self-care and domestic tasks involving bending (dressing her lower extremity, making the bed) or the unsupported use of her arms (hair washing, vacuuming) also heightened her shortness of breath and triggered anxiety. In particular, bathing was problematic because of the steam factor in the bathroom.

The Chronic Respiratory Disease Questionnaire was conducted and indicated that the patient perceived herself to be compromised on all four dimensions tested: dyspnea, fatigue, emotional factors, and illness mastery. Priority activities for treatment identified by the questionnaire were walking, stair climbing, bathing, dressing, and housework (especially bed making and vacuuming).

Monitored Functional Evaluation

In observing Mrs. Cope performing these activities, it became clear that some of her difficulties were related to a cyclic relationship between her erratic breathing pattern and anxiety. She rushed through activities and became easily frustrated, fatigued, and short of breath. Oxygen desaturation was evident for more strenuous tasks involving lifting, bending, or unsupported arm use, but recovery time was fairly rapid when Mrs. Cope rested. The adapted Borg scale was used to assess her perceived dyspnea and effort, and on most tasks monitored, Mrs. Cope rated her effort and dyspnea in the moderate range.

Managing the Energy Deficiency

Learning New Behaviors

Group Education Sessions. The first stage of treatment with Mrs. Cope involved her participation in group education sessions to facilitate her understanding of the link between respiratory illness, fatigue, and energy limitation. Mrs. Cope's daughter attended as well to better comprehend her mother's situation. For the first time, Mrs. Cope enjoyed having the opportunity to discuss in a group setting the similar difficulties faced by patients with COPD. Hearing the other participants' experiences validated and reinforced her own awareness of her strengths and limitations. She was relieved to know that others shared her environmental sensitivities such as difficulty tolerating less than optimum weather conditions and the smell of perfumes or other strong odors. The principles of energy conservation were explained and presented to the group as one coping strategy to deal with the symptoms of COPD.

Individual Sessions. Mrs. Cope's specific difficulties were the focus of individual treatment sessions. New time management skills helped her in working with the activity void created by both illness and retirement. She created lists and established priorities of which activities she either needed or wanted to do. She learned to categorize her activities as heavy, medium, light, or resting and also created a balance of these activities on daily, weekly, and then monthly schedules. New options for activities oriented toward rest and relaxation were explored.

Breathing principles, learned and practiced with exercise in physiotherapy, were translated in occupational therapy to the functional activities she found particularly difficult in her daily schedule. Mrs. Cope also learned how to break down these activities into manageable steps so that she could better pace and control her energy output. Certain adapted equipment and mobility aids were recommended, and steps were taken to find subsidization for their payment through her private insurance policy. A bath seat, telephone shower, and safety bar enabled Mrs. Cope to decrease the energy consumed involved in bathing. A rollater walker with basket and seat was recommended for outings and errands. Mrs. Cope could use the basket to hold her purse and parcels, and the seat was ideal for rests as needed. Her landlord gave her permission to lock the walker in a cupboard on the main floor of her apartment building to avoid having to negotiate the stairs with it. She planned on looking for another apartment in a building serviced by elevators when her lease was up.

In recognizing her limitations, Mrs. Cope decided to hire cleaning help twice a month to allow herself assistance with the heavier housework. Her daughter agreed to take her grocery shopping once a week. Transportation was a major issue; consequently, adapted transport was arranged for Mrs. Cope through the local transportation commission, which services the handicapped. She was given access to this transport for medical appointments and special outings as needed.

Integrating New Behaviors

Mrs. Cope kept a diary to record difficulties encountered during the re-education phase of her treatment. This diary reflected her growing awareness of her condition and provided her with practice material for problem solving within the occupational therapy practice sessions. Mrs. Cope developed the ability herself to appraise difficult situations realistically and to determine how she could best cope.

Post-testing and Follow-Up

On completion of the education and practical sessions in occupational therapy, Mrs. Cope was re-evaluated with the CRQ and demonstrated a moderate to significant improvement in all four dimensions tested. Although still present, Mr. Copd's fatigue, dyspnea, and anxiety were substantially reduced with increased control and improved illness management.

KEY POINTS

- Have the patient assess his/her own limitations and do a monitored functional assessment to provide both subjective and objective data relevant to the patient's functional status.
- Assist the patient in understanding that fatigue and energy limitations are normal symptoms of a respiratory condition; however, the patient has to learn to cultivate new lifestyle behaviors that enhance his/her capacity to engage in meaningful activity.
- Recommend exercise training regimens as they are known to be beneficial to every patient with COPD; exercise training aims to improve

function for self-care, productive, and recreational activities.
- Assess the patient's resources in terms of human and financial support and transportation availability; assess environmental and architectural barriers to the patient's function.
- Provide opportunities to practice and think through activities using the principles of energy conservation.
- Recommend adapted equipment and community help where appropriate.
- Normalize human "interdependence" and the appropriate times when it is necessary to ask for help.

REFERENCES

1. Chalmers KI. A closer look at how people cope with chronic airflow obstruction. Can Nurse 1984;2: 35–8.

2. Parent LH. Energy: the illusive factor in daily life. In: Cromwell FS, ed. Occupational therapy for the energy deficient patient. New York: Haworth Press, 1986:5–15.

3. Vander AJ, Sherman JH, Luciano DS. Human physiology: the mechanisms of body function. 8th Ed. New York: McGraw Hill, 1998.

4. Killian KJ, Leblanc P, Martin DH, et al. Exercise and ventilatory, circulatory and symptom limitation in patients with chronic airflow obstruction. Am Rev Respir Dis 1992;146:935–40.

5. Barstow RE. Coping with emphysema. Nurs Clin North Am 1974;9:137–45.

6. Atchison B. Cardiopulmonary diseases. In: Trombly CA, ed. Occupational therapy for physical dysfunction. Baltimore: Williams and Wilkins, 1995:875–87.

7. Rashbaum I, Whyte N. Occupational therapy in pulmonary rehabilitation: energy conservation and work simplification techniques. Pulm Rehabil 1996;7:325–40.

8. Small SP, Graydon JE. Perceived uncertainty, physical symptoms, and negative mood in hospitalized patients with chronic obstructive pulmonary disease. Heart Lung 1992;21:568–74.

9. Make BJ. Pulmonary rehabilitation: myth or reality? Clin Chest Med 1986;7:519–40.

10. Trombly CA. Retraining basic and instrumental activities of daily living. In: Trombly CA, ed. Occupational therapy for physical dysfunction. Baltimore: Williams and Wilkins, 1995:289–318.

11. Horne D, Corsello P. Physical and occupational therapy for patients with chronic lung disease. Semin Respir Med 1993;14:466–81.

12. Scanlon M, Kishbaugh L, Horne D. Life management skill in pulmonary rehabilitation. In: Hodgkin JE, Connors GL, Bell WC, eds. Pulmonary rehabilitation: guidelines to success. 2nd Ed. Philadelphia: Lippincott, 1993:246–67.

13. Ream E, Richardson A. Fatigue in patients with cancer and chronic obstructive airways disease: a phemonenological enquiry. Int J Nurs Stud 1997;34:44–53.

14. Falgerhaugh SY. Getting around with emphysema. From grounded theory to practice. Don Mills, ON: Addison Wesley, 1973.

15. Guyatt GH, Berman LB, Townsend M, et al. A measure of quality of life for clinical trials in chronic lung disease. Thorax 1987;42:773–8.

16. Lareau SC, Carrieri-Kohlmon V, Janson-Bjerklie S, Roos PJ. Development of the Pulmonary Functional Status and Dyspnea Questionnaire (PFSDQ). Heart Lung 1994;233:242–50.

17. Nouri FM, Lincoln NB. An extended activity of daily living scale for stroke patients. Clin Rehabil 1987;1:301–5.

18. Bestall JC, Paul EA, Garrod R, et al. The MRC dyspnoea score is a useful measure of disability in patients with severe COPD. Thorax 1999;54:581–6.

19. Wedzicha JA, Bestall JC, Garrod R, et al. Randomized controlled trial of pulmonary rehabilitation in severe chronic obstructive pulmonary disease patients, stratified with the MRC dyspnoea scale. Eur Respir J 1998;12:363–9.

20. Garrod R, Bestall JC, Paul EA, et al. Development and validation of a standardized measure of activity of daily living in patients with severe COPD: the London Chest Activity of Daily Living scale (LCADL). Respir Med 2000;94:589–96.

21. Hogan BM. Pulse oximetry for an adult with a pulmonary disorder. Am J Occup Ther 1995;49: 1062–4.

22. Borg GA. Psychophysical bases of perceived exertion. Med Sci Sports Exerc 1982;14:377–81.

23. Walsh RL. Occupational therapy as part of a pulmonary rehabilitation program. In: Cromwell FS, ed. Occupational therapy for the energy deficient patient. New York: Haworth Press, 1986:65–77.

24. Graydon JE, Ross E, Webster PM, et al. Predictors of functioning of patients with chronic obstructive pulmonary disease. Heart Lung 1995;24:369–75.

25. Berzins GF. An occupational therapy program for the chronic obstructive pulmonary disease patient. Am J Occup Ther 1970;24:181–6.

26. Royal Victoria Hospital Occupational Therapy Department. Tips to help you save energy. Audio visual services and primary services. Montreal, QC: Royal Victoria Hospital, 1998.

27. Stewart C. Retraining housekeeping and child care shills. In: Trombly CA, ed. Occupational therapy for physical dysfunction. Baltimore: Williams and Wilkins, 1995:319–20.

28. Sharp JT, Drutz WS, Moisan T, et al. Postural relief of dyspnea in severe chronic obstructive pulmonary disease. Am Rev Respir Dis 1980;122:201–11.

29. Weiser PC, Mahler DA, Ryan KP, et al. Dyspnea: symptom assessment and management. In: Hodgkin JE, Connors GL, Bell WC, eds. Pulmonary rehabilitation. Philadelphia: Lippincott, 1993:478–511.

30. Haas A, Pineda H, Haas F, Axen K. Pulmonary therapy and rehabilitation: principles and practices. Baltimore: Williams and Wilkins, 1979.

31. McSweeney AJ, Grant I, Heaton RK, et al. Life quality of patients with chronic obstructive pulmonary disease. Arch Intern Med 1982;142:473–8.

SUGGESTED READINGS

Rashbaum I, Whyte N. Occupational therapy in pulmonary rehabilitation: energy conservation and work simplification techniques. Pulm Rehabil 1996; 7:325–40. *This article examines the impact of COPD on quality of life and highlights the importance of a thorough evaluation of basic life management skills and activities of daily living. Steps to facilitate illness management focus on energy conservation and work simplification techniques. Concrete examples are provided.*

Hogan BM. Pulse oximetry for an adult with a pulmonary disorder. Am J Occup Ther 1995;49:1062–4. *This article includes a case study that clearly illustrates the effectiveness of combining monitored functional assessment, energy conservation principles, and activity modification.*

APPENDIX 10–1

Example of a Monitored Functional Assessment Tool

Date:_____

Diagnosis: _____

ACTIVITY	Time	SaO$_2$	Pulse	Perceived Effort 0–10	Perceived Dyspnea 0–10	COMMENTS
Resting supine						
Sitting up on side of bed						
Standing tolerance						
Hygiene and grooming						
Bathing						
Dressing—upper extremity						
Dressing—lower extremity						
Ambulation (30 meters)						
Cooking						
Making bed						
Carrying groceries						
Other:						
Resting 1 min postactivity						
Resting 4 min postactivity						

Observations:

Summary:

Occupational Therapist:

EXERCISE TRAINING IN PATIENTS WITH COPD

François Maltais, Earl S. Hershfield,
David Stubbing, Peter J. Wijkstra,
Ann Hatzoglou, Brenda Loveridge,
Gisele Pereira, and Roger S. Goldstein

OBJECTIVES

The general objective of this chapter is to help allied health care professionals and physicians become more familiar with the use of exercise training in patients with chronic obstructive pulmonary disease (COPD). After reading this chapter, the physician and the allied health care professional will be able to

- recognize the benefits of exercise training in patients with COPD;
- understand the principles of exercise training in patients with COPD;
- recognize the indications of exercise training in COPD;
- select and evaluate patients with COPD for an exercise training program;
- design an effective exercise training program for patients with COPD; and
- refer pulmonary rehabilitation for an exercise training program to patients with COPD.

Based on solid scientific evidence, the practice of regular exercise has been endorsed by numerous official organizations.[1] Performing physical exercise on a regular basis improves fitness,[2] health status,[3] and life expectancy.[4] In elderly individuals, exercise training is also recommended for various reasons[5,6]: it slows or stops the decline in functional status associated with aging,[5] it helps maintain bone[7] and muscle mass,[8] and improves mood status.[9]

Although the idea of using exercise training as a therapeutic modality in patients with COPD was introduced years ago,[10] and despite the fact that earlier studies have suggested that exercise training was indeed beneficial for these patients,[11] the efficacy of this intervention has still been debated until very recently.[12,13] In this context, the research contribution of the last 10 years has been tremendous in the field of pulmonary rehabilitation and exercise training in patients with COPD. The efficacy of exercise training in COPD is now confirmed by well-designed, randomized, and controlled trials.[2,14–18] A better understanding of the physiologic and nonphysiologic effects of exercise training in these individuals has also been obtained.[19–21] As a result, the use of regular exercise as a therapeutic intervention in COPD is gaining widespread acceptance. In fact, exercise training is now recognized as the cornerstone of pulmonary rehabilitation.[2]

In this chapter, we review the evidence supporting the use of exercise training in COPD, examine the different training modalities and settings where this can be performed, and address patient selection and evaluation.

EFFECTS OF EXERCISE IN HEALTHY SUBJECTS

Exercise training can be divided into two broad categories: aerobic/endurance training and strength/resistive training. This distinction is crucial since the specific effects of exercise training depend on the training modality that is being used.

Aerobic training enhances health status and fitness. It is now clear that the level of activity necessary to improve health status is lower than what is required to improve fitness and induce a physiologic response to exercise training.[1] Although low-intensity exercise such as self-paced walking may be sufficient to heighten health status, at least two weekly training sessions of moderately intense exercise are required to induce an adaptive response to training.[1] Therefore, the intensity, duration, and frequency of the training sessions should be selected on the basis of the training objectives.

The physiologic response to training consists of structural changes in the cardiovascular and peripheral muscle systems; this accounts for an improvement in the capacity to transport oxygen and in the respiratory capacity of the trained peripheral muscles.[22,23] As a result, peak VO_2 (oxygen consumption) will be improved with aerobic training. Important structural changes take place within the trained peripheral muscles, which explains why their ability to extract oxygen is enhanced with aerobic training. With aerobic training, there is a conversion from a fast, low oxidative, and fatigable fiber type (type II) to a slow, high oxidative, and fatigue-resistant fiber type (type I).[24–26]

The volume of type I fibers and the mitochondrial numbers are expanded; also, the activities of the mitochondrial enzymes such as citrate synthase and 3-hydroxyacyl-CoA dehydrogenase are enhanced.[5,22,27,28] Improved muscle capillarization and increased myoglobin levels also occur, which, in turn, facilitate oxygen delivery and extraction.[29,30] These structural muscle changes are associated with important modifications in muscle metabolism during exercise; furthermore, they have a lower blood lactate concentration and less CO_2 production for a given level of exercise. Changes in muscle metabolism with exercise training are thought to contribute to the greater tolerance of submaximal exercise,[22] which may be particularly relevant to activities of daily living.

Strength training is also recommended as an integral part of any training program in healthy people.[1] Twice weekly, 8 to 12 repetitions of different exercises involving major muscle groups promote muscle growth and increase strength.[6,8,31] Strength training in healthy adults may also induce a slight improvement in peak exercise performance and in skeletal muscle oxidative capacity.[32] Maintenance of bone mass, reduction in the number of falls, and improvement in depression are other examples of possible benefits derived from strength exercises in elderly individuals.[6,7,9]

One may express concern about the safety of aerobic and strength training, particularly in elderly people. However, in these individuals, aerobic and strength training performed at moderate intensity has been deemed safe, provided that an adequate evaluation is performed at the beginning of the program and that the exercise prescription is individualized.[6]

AEROBIC TRAINING

Aerobic training in COPD results in improvements in endurance,[19] work efficiency,[33] and, to some extent, strength.[34] In patients with COPD, the aim of training is to translate these improvements into a reduction in disability. This should allow improvement in the ability to undertake activities, thereby decreasing the handicap and ultimately improving quality of life. The exercise training regimen should aim to improve function for self-care, productive, and recreational activities.

Benefits of Aerobic Training

Regardless of disease severity, patients with COPD have been shown to benefit from regular upper and lower limb muscle aerobic training programs (Table 11–1).[2,15–21,33–45] Exercise is perhaps the single most important treatment in COPD.

The increased work capacity and decreased breathlessness for a given submaximal effort following exercise training have been well documented.[2,17,35,42,46] Through improved movement efficiency, exercise training also lowers the energy requirements for many activities, resulting in an improvement in exercise tolerance even when no other physiologic changes may be observed.

Recent studies have confirmed that a physiologic adaptation to aerobic training can occur in patients with COPD.[19–21,47] At moderate to high intensity, well-supervised aerobic training regimens in patients

TABLE 11-1 Benefits of Exercise Training

Benefits	Lead Author (Year)
Lessened dyspnea	Goldstein (1994),[17] Ries (1995),[2] O'Donnell (1995),[35] Lacasse (1996)[36]
Increased maximal and submaximal exercise work capacity	Cockroft (1981),[15] Wijkstra (1994),[16] Goldstein (1994),[17] Ries (1995),[2] Casaburi (1991),[19] Lake (1990),[37] Strijbos (1996)[38]
Improved muscle oxidative capacity, strength, and endurance	Casaburi (1991),[19] Maltais (1996),[20] Sala(1999),[21] Bernard (1999),[34] Simpson (1992),[39] Clark (1996),[40] Clark (2000)[41]
Improved neuromuscular coordination	Belman (1993)[33]
Improved functional ability in activities of daily living	Bendstrup (1997)[42]
Enhanced quality of life	Wijkstra (1994),[16] Goldstein (1994),[17] Simpson (1992),[39] Wijkstra (1995),[43] Lacasse (1996),[36]
Lessened anxiety, depression, and assistance to patients in better coping with stress	Toshima (1992)[44]
Decreased health care use	Ries (1995),[2] Griffiths (2000),[18] Guell (2000)[45]

with moderate to severe COPD have been shown to reduce exercise-induced lactic acidosis by improving skeletal muscle aerobic capacity (Figure 11–1) and bioenergetics.[19–21,47] Furthermore, aerobic regimens provide a modest but significant central cardiorespiratory training effect with a decreased heart rate and ventilation (VE) for a given submaximal workload.[48] The degree of benefit that may be derived from an aerobic training program appears to be more related to the patient's ability to participate in more intense and prolonged exercise regimens than to disease severity alone.[19,47–50] This is particularly the case with patients with COPD in their ability to gain substantive physiologic improvement in cardiovascular, respiratory, and musculoskeletal systems.

Since it correlates closely with the reduction in dyspnea and exercise tolerance after training,[35] the reduction in ventilatory requirement during exercise is another important consequence of exercise training in COPD. The fall in ventilatory demand with exercise training is multifactorial. After a few sessions of exercise, patients adopt a more efficient exercise technique, resulting in improved mechanical efficiency and consequently a lessened metabolic cost of exercise.[35,49] The reduction in CO_2 production and in blood lactate for a given level of exercise, which is, in fact, related to the improved muscle bioenergetics, also reduces the ventilatory demand.[19] Some studies have shown a greater breathing pattern efficiency after training with a higher tidal volume and lower frequency and thus a lower VD/VT (dead space to tidal volume ratio) during exercise.[51]

The results show clear evidence of the improvement in quality of life for patients with COPD following an exercise training program.[16,17,39,43]

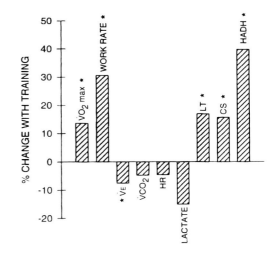

Figure 11–1 The effects of endurance training on VO_2 max; and work rate achieved during exercise, on VE, VCO_2, heart rate (HR), and lactic acid concentration for identical exercise work rate on lactate threshold (LT) and on the activity of citrate synthase (CS) and 3-hydroxyacl CoA dehydrogenase (HADH). Significant changes are indicated by an asterisk. Reported values represent percent changes of the baseline values that occurred after training.[20]

Furthermore, Bendstrup and colleagues have also demonstrated the positive effects that exercise training has on psychosocial well-being.[42]

Several earlier observational studies revealed a decrease in hospital admissions and length of stay following pulmonary rehabilitation.[52,53] Since then, there have been substantial improvements in the management of COPD, as well as a shift to greater outpatient and community-based care. Recent randomized, controlled trials with long-term follow-up of patients documented a trend toward decreased hospital days,[18,54] less exacerbations,[45] and more efficient primary care use.[18]

Lower and Upper Extremity Exercise Training

Studies have conclusively demonstrated that exercise training is specific to the muscle groups trained. A comparison between the effects of upper and lower extremity training has revealed the following: a change occurs in maximum arm workload or endurance only when upper extremity training is used,[37] and an increase happens in lower limb performance only with lower limb training. Thus, both upper and lower extremity training should be included. On the other hand, as the training effect is not task specific or limited to the type of exercise used, lower limb training may include each or all of cycle ergometry, treadmill walking, corridor walking, or weight lifting, whereas upper extremity training is usually performed only by ergometry or weight lifting.

Lower Extremity Exercise Training

For patients with COPD, evidence from several randomized controlled trials is available to support the use of a supervised exercise training regimen (Figure 11–2).[36] These studies of supervised exercise have shown benefits in the intervention group that were unseen in the control group. Improvements in peak exercise and submaximal exercise capacity, as well as in walking distance, have been reported. However, the magnitude of these effects varies from study to study.

Goldstein and colleagues studied 89 patients who were randomized to either 8 weeks of inpatient rehabilitation or to a control group.[17] The exercises used were treadmill and corridor walking. The intervention group showed an increase in 6-minute walking distance and endurance time on a cycle ergometer following rehabilitation that persisted for 6 months. This was not found in the control group. Several

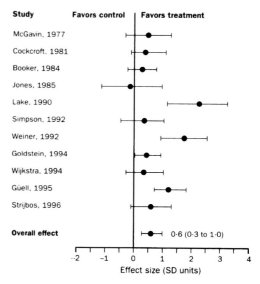

Figure 11–2 Effect of respiratory rehabilitation on functional exercise capacity. (Reproduced with permission from Lacasse, et al. 1996.[36])

other studies have been performed in a supervised outpatient setting or in the home with weekly supervision.[2,16,37,38,55,56] Exercise training included walking,[2,37,38] cycle ergometry,[16,55,56] and treadmill walking.[2,38,55] The intervention groups showed increases in peak exercise capacity,[2,16,38] timed walking distance,[37,38] and submaximal endurance time.[2]

Upper Extremity Exercise Training

As training is specific to the muscle groups used, it is now recommended that upper extremity training be included in pulmonary rehabilitation.[57] Several studies have shown improvements in maximum workload for arm ergometry or in arm endurance following upper extremity training. Lake and colleagues performed a randomized controlled trial in which 28 patients with severe pulmonary impairment were randomized to upper limb training alone, lower limb training alone, or combined upper and lower limb training.[37] Subjects performed three 1-hour supervised exercise sessions each week for the upper limb training involving 20 minutes on a circuit of exercises including ergometry, weight lifting, and throwing. Lower limb training included warm-ups and walking exercises for 15 to 20 minutes followed by cool-downs. All of the intervention groups showed improvement in exercise capacity for the muscle groups trained. With isolated leg training, there was no improvement in arm endurance, but leg endurance increased. Ries and colleagues obtained similar results in a study in which some patients were randomized to upper extremity exercise as part of a rehabilitation program.[54] Arm endurance and maximum workload were increased only in those subjects who undertook arm exercises.

Arm exercises generally include either weight lifting of some form or arm ergometry. Unsupported exercises using weights appear to be more effective than supported exercise using arm ergometry. As part of a rehabilitation program, Martinez and colleagues studied 40 patients randomized to either supported arm exercises using an arm ergocycle or to unsupported arm exercises using a wooden dowel as a weight.[58] Exercise workload and the duration of supported exercise sessions were increased weekly as tolerated up to 15 minutes. The duration of unsupported exercise sessions was increased by half-minute increments to a total time of 3½ minutes, and weights were added as tolerated. Arm endurance increased in both groups, but it was statistically more significant in the group undertaking unsupported arm exercise than the group doing supported exercise. The oxygen consumption during exercise decreased with unsupported arm exercise but not with arm ergometry.

Principles of Aerobic Exercise Training

The general principles used for aerobic training in healthy subjects are applicable to patients with pulmonary impairment. As for healthy subjects, frequency of exercise, duration, and training intensity are all thought to be important. The intensity of training that should be used in COPD has been the subject of many studies. Although it has been thought that breathlessness may limit the workload at which individuals with pulmonary impairment can train, it is now clear that training at moderate to high intensity can be useful.[19,48,50,59] In general, greater improvements in physiologic markers of a physiologic training response, as well as in maximal and submaximal exercise tolerance, have both been reported in subjects training at a high intensity (80% of maximal work rate) compared with low-intensity (below 50% of maximal work rate) exercise.[19,50] However, it is unclear if these additional physiologic benefits of moderate to high training intensity will translate into further improvement in quality of life and clinical outcome.[50] Indeed, a recent randomized

clinical trial has demonstrated that despite marked additional physiologic benefits of a high-intensity treadmill exercise training program, in comparison with a walking exercise program, the quality of life improved similarly in the two groups.[50]

It is generally recommended that aerobic training involve 30 minutes of endurance-specific exercises at least three times per week. Some of the most disabled patients who cannot achieve adequate exercise time seem to tolerate interval training for which 2 to 3 minutes of high-intensity exercise is interspersed with lower-intensity exercise or rest periods. Coppoolse and colleagues compared continuous cycle ergometry, 5 days a week at approximately 60% of maximum for 30 minutes, with interval training; interval training involved 30-minute sessions three times a week.[60] After pedaling for a 3-minute warm-up, the workload on a cycle ergometer was set at 90% of maximum for 1 minute and 45% of maximum for 2 minutes and then repeated nine times. On two other days each week, the subjects in the interval training group performed 30 minutes of continuous cycling at 60% of maximal power output. With interval training, there was an increase in maximum exercise capacity and a reduction in lactic acid production during exercise.

Another strategy to improve tolerance to aerobic training is to use the gas exchange, ventilatory, or dyspnea threshold instead of a fixed proportion of peak exercise capacity to select the training intensity.[61] The idea behind this strategy is to have patients exercising at an intensity lower than that corresponding to ventilatory or dyspnea thresholds, thus avoiding the rapid rise in ventilatory requirement and dyspnea during the exercise sessions. Using this strategy in a small group of patients, Vallet and coworkers reported a greater physiologic improvement after a training program in comparison with patients in whom the level of training was selected using a fixed proportion of their heart rate reserve.[61]

The frequency of exercise sessions and the duration for which each exercise should be performed have not been definitively addressed. A training regimen similar to one that would be appropriate for a healthy individual can be applied to most patients with COPD, with a minimum of two weekly training sessions. The duration for which supervised rehabilitation should occur is also open to debate and varies within programs. The program should probably be long enough for the patient to notice the benefit of the intervention. However, rather than completing rehabilitation after a specified number of sessions or when endurance time has reached a target, it may be more beneficial for the patient in rehabilitation to self-direct a maintenance program prior to discharge.

Prescription and Monitoring Training Intensity

Training intensity can be prescribed and monitored by measuring the work rate on the cycle ergometer or the treadmill and noting how it influences the heart rate and/or dyspnea. In healthy individuals, the intensity of training is most commonly determined and monitored using a fixed proportion of maximal heart rate or of heart rate reserve resting heart rate + 0.5–0.8(peak heart rate − resting heart rate).[1] Because of dyspnea and leg fatigue, this approach is not recommended in patients with COPD, who are exercise limited before they reach their predicted peak heart rate. When the training is performed on a calibrated cycle ergometer or treadmill, the level of intensity can be obtained directly. Another approach is to use the baseline incremental maximal exercise test to determine the heart rate or dyspnea score (using a modified Borg scale) at the chosen exercise level for training. In subsequent training sessions, a target heart rate or dyspnea score can then be used to estimate the training intensity.[62] The possibility for patients with COPD to reproduce a given exercise intensity with reasonable accuracy has been confirmed in previous investigations using a dyspnea score.[62,63] As the training program advances, the intensity of training corresponding to the target heart rate and dyspnea should increase.

Anabolic Hormones and Exercise

Past attempts to improve the effectiveness of an exercise have had two focuses: they have involved either a look at methods that may increase the intensity at which patients are able to exercise (as reviewed previously in the chapter) or have involved the use of potential drugs that might allow exercise to have a greater effect on peripheral muscle. Growth hormone and testosterone are major hormones that affect peripheral muscle. The levels of these hormones may be decreased in COPD, and it has been suggested that these hormones be used in the form of a supplementation as an adjunct to exercise.[51,64–66]

Until now, studies have shown a modest increase in muscle mass with the administration of anabolic corticosteroids[64,65] or growth hormones[51,66] when combined with an exercise training program in patients with COPD. Yet it still remains unclear whether these improvements in muscle mass could translate into further gain in exercise tolerance. However, in most studies, the number of patients has been relatively small, and the dosage of anabolic drugs was probably not optimal. Whether anabolic drugs will prove to be a useful adjunct to exercise training programs is uncertain and requires further study.

STRENGTH TRAINING

Rationale

Muscle wasting is common in COPD, affecting up to 25% of all patients.[64] Using computed tomography (CT), it was found that the reduction in muscle mass averaged approximately 30% in patients with COPD.[67] Not surprisingly, peripheral muscle strength is also reduced in patients with COPD,[67–69] and muscle wasting and weakness may also have important adverse consequences. The perception of leg fatigue, a common symptom limiting patients with COPD during exercise, is inversely proportional to muscle strength; for a given power output, the perception of leg fatigue is greater in weak individuals compared with those who are considered strong.[69] Subjects with stronger muscles have a better exercise capacity, which is also true for healthy individuals and for patients with COPD.[69]

In fact, the strength of the quadriceps has been found to be a significant determinant of exercise capacity independently of impairment in lung function.[68,69] Another potential adverse consequence of muscle wasting is poor survival.[70] In this context, the use of strength training is appealing because it is a better means to improve muscle mass and strength than aerobic training. In addition, because there is less dyspnea during the exercise period,[39] it may be easier to tolerate than aerobic training for patients with severe COPD. Therefore, improving muscle mass and strength appears to be a reasonable therapeutic strategy in patients with COPD.

Different types of strength training can be used depending on the desired objective. High-intensity strength training (90 to 100%) of one repetition maximum (RM) using few repetitions at maximal or nearly maximal tension ameliorates strength, whereas a greater number of repetitions (20 to 30) at lower intensity improves muscle endurance.[71] Moderate-intensity strength training with 10 to 12 repetitions performed at 60 to 80% of one RM seems to be best suited for patients with COPD; it fulfills the objective of improving muscle strength and endurance while avoiding the potential risks of locomotor injuries associated with high-intensity strength training.

Benefits

Few studies on the effects of strength training in COPD have been published. In one study, 34 patients with severe COPD were randomized to 8 weeks of strength training or to a control group.[39] The training program included three weekly sessions of three different exercises (one for the arms, two for the legs). Three series of 10 repetitions were initially performed at an intensity of 50% of the maximal strength, which was progressively increased up to 85%. With this training strategy, muscle strength increased by 16 to 40% depending on the muscle group, whereas the endurance time for submaximal exercise intensity increased by 75%. An improvement in quality of life was also observed in the group submitted to strength training.

In a subsequent study, the efficacy of low-intensity muscle exercises to improve muscle strength, endurance, and exercise capacity was evaluated in 48 patients; the patients involved had moderate COPD[40] and were randomly allocated to exercise training or to a control group. Strengthening exercises were performed daily at home for 12 weeks and consisted of a series of 10 unloaded exercises such as full-arm circling, sitting and standing, and leg straightening. With this training strategy, muscle endurance, as assessed by the number of specific muscle exercises that could be performed before fatigue, increased from baseline; also, a better submaximal exercise capacity was measured by treadmill walking. The same group of investigators also evaluated the effects of peripheral muscle strengthening in patients with mild COPD.[41] Patients were involved in a twice a week program that included three sets of 10 repetitions of eight individual exercises, such as bench pressing for the triceps, body squats, and leg pressing. The load during the exercises represented approximately 70% of the individual maximum values. Improvement in peripheral muscle strength was found as well as an increase in the maximum work that could be sustained for 60 seconds by the quadriceps. Only the patients involved in strength training showed a significant increase in quadricep work capacity. This improvement in peripheral muscle function in the training group was associated with an increase in treadmill walking ability in terms of time and intensity.

Therefore, it is possible to increase peripheral muscle strength and endurance as well as submaximal exercise capacity with strength exercises in COPD. These benefits of strength training can be obtained in a safe and well-accepted manner by the participants.[39–41] However, it should be recognized that an improvement in effort-dependent measures of strength and endurance may not provide definitive evidence of a physiologic muscle adaptation; it may simply reflect an improved motivation and/or a more efficient neuromuscular coupling.[5]

Recently, it has been addressed whether the addition of strength training to aerobic training further improves muscle function and exercise tolerance compared with aerobic training alone.[34] In this study, 36 patients were randomized to aerobic training alone or to a combination of aerobic and strength training. The endurance training consisted of three weekly sessions of leg cycling exercise for 30 minutes at approximately 60% of peak work rate. Using a strategy similar to that of Simpson and colleagues, four muscle strengthening exercises were also performed by the patients included in the combined training modality group.[39] Greater improvements in muscle strength and the mid-thigh muscle cross-sectional area were found in the combined training modality group compared with the endurance training group (Figure 11–3). However, these additional gains in muscle strength and mass in the combined training group did not translate into further improvement in exercise tolerance.

Strength training may also have a number of additional benefits in patients with COPD. Because of advanced age and muscle wasting, patients with COPD may have an increased risk of falling. Strength training for these patients may result, as observed in elderly subjects, in improved gait speed and balance, thus reducing the incidence of falls. Similarly, although no exercise studies with patients with COPD have specifically examined bone loss, there is clear evidence in other elderly populations that weight-bearing exercise is important to minimize the rate of bone loss associated with aging.[6] This effect may be potentially important since osteoporosis is highly prevalent in COPD.[72]

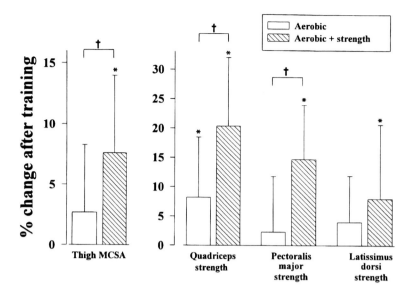

Figure 11–3 Effect of aerobic training and combination of aerobic and strength training, MCSA: muscle cross-national areas.[34]

Can strength training be used safely in patients with COPD? Obviously, there are some potential risks, as with any intervention, but the key elements to remember are the careful preprogram evaluation and the individualization of the training regimen. Strength training should be used cautiously in patients with musculoskeletal disorders and/or osteoporosis to avoid injury such as bone fracture. However, as in other elderly individuals,[6] the experience indicates that when adapted to each patient's condition, strength training can be performed safely in patients with COPD.[34,39–41] Therefore, strength training is feasible and safe in patients with COPD. This training modality improves peripheral muscle function, submaximal exercise capacity, and quality of life and should be included in routine exercise training programs for patients with COPD.

OTHER MODALITIES IN EXERCISE TRAINING

Inspiratory Muscle Training Added to Exercise Training

A few studies have evaluated whether inspiratory muscle training represents a useful addition to exercise training. In representative studies, PI max (maximal inspiratory pressure) and exercise capacity improved compared with exercise training alone.[73–75] In other studies, the addition of inspiratory muscle training did not result in further improvement in exercise per-

formance compared with exercise training alone.[76,77] A systematic review by Lacasse and colleagues was also unable to find conclusive evidence for adding inspiratory muscle training to exercise alone.[78] Still, positive effects have been published with an adequate training load of at least 30%. Therefore, the American College of Chest Physicians/American Association of Cardiovascular and Pulmonary Rehabilitation concluded in their recent guidelines that inspiratory muscle training may be considered in patients with COPD who remain symptomatic despite optimal therapy.[57] Finally, it has been suggested that patients with impaired inspiratory muscle function are especially responsive to inspiratory muscle training. However, this idea has not yet been prospectively determined.[79]

Therefore, the evidence that inspiratory muscle training should be included in rehabilitation programs for patients with COPD remains equivocal. Conceivably, better training protocols with appropriate loads and controlled breathing patterns might yet identify a useful role for this interesting training modality.[57,78,79] The value of inspiratory muscle training must be shown to extend beyond simple improvements in tests of respiratory muscle function. It should include improvements in dyspnea or exercise tolerance or an improved handling of increased loads similar to those sustained during exacerbations.

Supplemental Oxygen during Exercise Training

It has been postulated that by alleviating exercise-induced hypoxemia, the administration of oxygen during exercise training will allow patients to reach a higher training intensity than they would otherwise achieve while breathing ambient air. As with healthy volunteers, the physiologic benefits of training are higher in patients with COPD when they train at a higher power output.

However, the results of two randomized controlled trials have been disappointing. In one study, 24 patients with COPD (mean forced expiratory volume in 1 second [FEV_1] 34% predicted) increased their alveolar-arterial gradient for oxygen during exercise by more than 15 mm Hg[80] and were randomly allocated to breathe either room air or oxygen at 4 L/min during exercise training. After 10 weeks, the intensity of walking, stair climbing, weight lifting, and health status increased in both groups, with no significant between-group differences. In another study, 25 patients (mean FEV_1 30% predicted) were randomized to a similar training protocol with or without supplemental oxygen during the exercise periods.[81] After 6 weeks of training, dyspnea improved in those trained with oxygen, but there was no difference between groups with respect to the shuttle walking distance or in measures of health status. Therefore, although dyspnea during exercise may be reduced with oxygen in some patients, current studies inadequately demonstrate the benefits of prescribing oxygen during training or during transient exercise-induced hypoxemia.

Ventilatory Support during Exercise Training

The severe airflow limitation that characterizes advanced COPD is frequently associated with hyperinflation; it is particularly noticeable during exercise, when the absence of any flow reserve, even at rest, requires the subject to breathe at a higher lung volume to meet the ventilatory requirements of exercise. This, in turn, increases the work of breathing. The increase is initially to overcome the intrinsic end-expiratory pressures (subjects may have to generate a negative pressure of –5 to –15 cm H_2O before any inspiratory flow occurs) and subsequently to sustain ventilation on a flatter part of the pressure volume characteristics of the respiratory system. Hyperinflation also influences the respiratory muscles, placing them in an unfavorable position with regard to their force-length relationship. Thus, the increased ventilatory requirements of exercise may be difficult to sustain. Clinicians are challenged to identify approaches that might improve the neuromechanical

linkages of respiration either by reducing the demand (peripheral muscle training, bronchodilation, oxygen) or by assisting with the mechanical output through the use of ventilatory support.

The application of 4 to 5 cm H_2O of continuous positive airway pressure (CPAP) to patients with COPD (mean FEV_1 1.2 L) decreased their level of dyspnea during steady-state submaximal exercise.[82] Moreover, a similar level of CPAP administered to patients with severe COPD (mean FEV_1 -0.9 L) increased their endurance during constant power cycle exercise by 48%.[83] In contrast, a study comparing inspiratory pressure support (IPS) (mean airway pressure 12 to 15 cm H_2O), CPAP (6 cm H_2O), and oxygen (2 L/min) during exercise noted that only IPS increased walking distance compared with control (62% increase, range +14 m to +533 m, p = .01).[84] Patients experienced less breathlessness at iso-time during IPS than during control exercise. In another study, IPS of 11 cm H_2O applied to patients with a variety of respiratory disorders (mean FEV_1 -0.8 L) improved dyspnea and increased ventilation, presumably by reducing the work of breathing.[85] The influence of proportional assistance ventilation (PAV) has been compared with pressure support ventilation (PSV) and CPAP in 15 stable patients with COPD (FEV_1 32% predicted, mean PaO_2 52 mm Hg, mean $PaCO_2$ 52 mm Hg).[86] The patients underwent randomized submaximal cycle endurance at 80% of their maximal workload, receiving either sham ventilation (1 cm H_2O), CPAP (6 cm H_2O), PSV (inspiratory positive airway pressure [IPAP] 12 to 16 cm H_2O, EPAP 1 cm H_2O), or PAV (8.6 ± 3.6 cm H_2O and 3.0 ± 1.3 cm H_2O of volume and flow assistance, respectively, and EPAP [end-expiration positive airway pressure] 1 cm H_2O). Continuous positive airway pressure, PSV, and PAV were able to increase endurance time over sham ventilation (9.6, 10, and 12 minutes versus 7.2 minutes, respectively). Proportional assistance ventilation also increased endurance more than the other interventions. A second study of very similar design evaluated CPAP plus PAV in normocapnic ($PaCO_2$ 41 mm Hg) patients.[87] Continuous positive airway pressure plus PAV increased submaximal cycle endurance compared with sham ventilation (12.9 minutes versus 6.6 minutes, p < .05). When used separately, neither CPAP nor PAV in-creased exercise time.

Some insight into the mechanism of improved exercise with ventilatory support has come from a recent study in which IPS delayed the rise of serum lactate during exercise in patients with severe COPD.[88] Lactate increased at 2.96 mmol/L during unassisted walking and at 2.42 mmol/L with IPS (p < .01). The duration of exercise was increased with IPS (13.6 minutes versus 5.5 minutes control, p < .01). This observation may be relevant to the application of exercise rehabilitation for patients with severe COPD. In a recent study, the addition of short-term, nasal positive pressure ventilation at home (median 2.1 hours/day, range 0 to 11.4) to an outpatient rehabilitation program had a positve outcome; it improved the shuttle walking distance and quality of life among normocapnic patients (mean $PaCO_2$ 44 mm Hg) to a greater extent than did rehabilitation alone.[89] This randomized study did not include sham ventilation for the control group. In addition, the role of nasal positive pressure ventilation in hypercapnic patients with COPD remains unanswered.

Therefore, ventilatory support during exercise may decrease dyspnea and improve exercise tolerance among patients with COPD; current evidence comes from acute physiologic studies. Therefore, widespread use requires larger clinical trials to identify the most effective approaches to ventilatory support during exercise and to determine whether noninvasive ventilatory support will be a useful adjunct to the exercise training session.

LONG-TERM BENEFITS
OF EXERCISE TRAINING

Many of the benefits of exercise rehabilitation, particularly increased walking distance, decreased dyspnea on activity, and higher scores on quality-of-life measures, all appear to be sustained for several months to at least 1 year following the end of the exercise program.[2,18,38,43,45,46,90–95] Not surprisingly, a common finding of these studies is that the initial improvement is progressively diminished after stopping exercise. As is the case in healthy individuals,[1] a maintenance exercise program is necessary to sustain the initial effects of training. Most studies looking at the long-term effects of training in COPD have offered some form of maintenance to their participants, such as continuation of supervised training at a reduced frequency or the encouragement to continue exercise training at home.[2,18,43,45,91,93,94,96] Since the efficacy of these different strategies has not been compared, it is still uncer-

tain as to which is the best long-term approach.

In healthy individuals, the initial improvement with training was maintained when the duration of training was reduced by as much as two-thirds during the maintenance period and so long as the training intensity was not reduced.[1] Based on this observation, a reasonable maintenance program could consist of one training session every week at least. Further study will be required to determine the optimal maintenance strategy for patients with COPD.

PATIENT SELECTION
AND EVALUATION

Patient Selection

Pulmonary rehabilitation is prescribed for patients with chronic respiratory impairments. The most commonly presented symptoms are dyspnea and a reduced exercise tolerance that influences daily activities. These symptoms persist despite optimal pharmacologic management.[97] Measures of pulmonary function alone will provide some indication as to the severity of the physiologic impairment, but these measurements alone are insufficient as primary indicators of the need for rehabilitation. Patients with severe respiratory impairments might still enjoy an acceptable exercise tolerance. Respiratory impairment as assessed by lung function correlates poorly with dyspnea and exercise tolerance.[98]

Inclusion Criteria

The American Thoracic Society has recently proposed some indications for rehabilitation that include the following: anxiety during activities, breathlessness during activities, limitations in activities of daily living, and loss of independence.[97] Our clinical experience with large inpatient and outpatient programs has led us to take note of the following frequently mentioned reasons as having led to referral for rehabilitation:

1. Dyspnea, especially when it interferes with the patient's lifestyle
2. Reduced exercise tolerance or a reduction in the patient's ability to perform activities or self-care
3. Unexpected increase in symptoms that occurs on a background of long-standing dyspnea
4. Preoperative rehabilitation for lung resection, lung volume reduction surgery, or lung transplantation

5. Initiation, adjustment, and evaluation of home oxygen or elective mechanical ventilation

Although most patients (representative sample of 250 recent patients) do, in fact, complain of dyspnea (85%), decreased exercise tolerance (67%), or difficulties during activities of daily living (53%), patients may also present other characteristics such as mood changes (36%), weight changes (23%), and musculoskeletal soft tissue pain (47%).

In general, with the exception of one study in which it was reported that patients with the best FEV_1 at baseline showed the largest improvement in walking distance,[99] the magnitude of the benefits of exercise training is not related to disease severity.[48,100,101] Since one of the proven outcomes of rehabilitation is an improved quality of life (especially dyspnea), some clinicians try to identify those patients with the worst quality of life and the most severe dyspnea as being the ones who are the most suitable candidates.[57,102] This assumes that rehabilitation remains effective even among very compromised patients (Medical Research Council [MRC] rating of 4 to 5), which may not always be the case, as indicated by Wedzicha et al.[103] Their study reported that patients who were housebound with an MRC dyspnea rating of 5 did not show any improvement in shuttle walking distance or in quality of life compared to a control group. However, their subjects undertook a home-based exercise program involving only walking and did not participate in any group rehabilitation program. Ketelaars and colleagues found that at the start of rehabilitation, patients with the lowest score on the disease-specific health-related quality-of-life questionnaire showed little improvement but then remained stable 9 months postdischarge.[93] This was in contrast to patients with moderate scores on admission, in whom the improvement was more substantial, but their outcomes gradually fell with time. This might suggest that patients with COPD require a differentiated aftercare program (postdischarge rehabilitation) depending on their initial quality-of-life score. These studies underline the importance of starting the rehabilitation process as early as possible in the natural history of the disease. Other issues that may be of equal importance in patient selection are summarized in Table 11–2.[11,48,100,104–111]

Essentially, anyone who is disabled by breathlessness caused by COPD can benefit from pulmonary rehabilitation. Studies that have assessed the impact of exercise and rehabilitation have shown that the benefits occur irrespective of the subject's age,[110] gender,[111] severity of pulmonary impairment,[48,100] severity of disability,[101] or the presence of ventilatory failure as shown by an elevated $PaCO_2$.[112] Altogether, the available data indicate that most patients with COPD can benefit from exercise training even at an advanced stage of their disease. In fact, in North America, most patients enter rehabilitation at this late stage of their disease.[2,17]

Exclusion Criteria

Since exercise is the principal component of pulmonary rehabilitation, the most common exclusion factor is the inability to exercise. Unstable angina, recent myocardial infarction, severe pulmonary hypertension, and disabling arthritis may all make it impossible for a patient to take part in exercise training rehabilitation. On another note, we have been unsuccessful with patients who have an inability to learn, such as dementia. Some patients may not be able to travel the distance required if a program only provides outpatient rehabilitation. In that instance, an inpatient or home-based program should be sought, and the only individuals who must be excluded are those who are unwilling to give consent.

It is always stated that patients should be motivated to take part, yet we are unaware of any studies that have assessed the effect of motivation on outcome or, much less, that have even attempted to scientifically measure motivation. When faced with patients who appear unmotivated, we are challenged to find ways that will change their motivation so that the potential benefits of rehabilitation become available to them. Often when the individual perceives the possible benefits, his/her level of motivation changes.

Patient Evaluation

Patients will enter rehabilitation exercise programs from a variety of referral sources including physician referral, other health professional referrals, or self-referral for some community-based programs. This means that the database that accompanies a patient, and thus makes it available to the health professionals supervising the exercise program, is highly variable. Furthermore, there is a wide variety of health professionals involved in exercise program delivery for patients with COPD. The flowchart and the text for this section consider all types of entry situations and varied health professionals supervising an exercise program.

TABLE 11–2 Important Issues to Consider in the Selection of Patients for an Exercise Training Program

Important Issues	Explanations
Motivation	Those who are motivated are more likely to[104]: Accept assistance Self-improve Commit to the necessary lifestyle changes
Expectations	Realistic expectations as to what they are likely to achieve from the program Unrealistic expectations can be disruptive to the patient, family, and health care team
Comprehension	Language problems can be resolved by interpretation and by printing materials in several languages Simple hearing problems can be addressed with a positive effect Organic brain syndromes preclude a successful rehabilitation program
Situation at home	Reasonable facility for sleeping, cleaning, and washing Social considerations: environmental smoke and pollution Those with supportive families are most likely to succeed than those who are socially isolated[105]
Specific clinical issues[11,106]	
Smoking	Policies vary in that some programs accept only nonsmokers whereas others accept only smokers[107] Adherence to a rehabilitation program is lower in current smokers[105,108] Smoking can be perceived as quite disruptive to other patients However, improvement in quality of life and exercise tolerance is comparable in smokers and nonsmokers[109]
Age and gender	Benefits occur irrespective of the patient's age[110] and gender[111]
Disease severity	Benefits occur irrespective of disease severity[48,100] Rehabilitation is easier in patients who are clinically stable but can be considered during the recovery phase of an exacerbation The severity of a recent exacerbation does not generally influence the outcome of rehabilitation unless there are complications
Medication and oxygen	Pharmacologic treatment and oxygen supplement should be optimized before commencing rehabilitation
Comorbid conditions	Active, associated medical conditions should be treated and stabilized prior to commencing a rehabilitation program Active joint disease or claudication will mitigate against a successful exercise program Malnutrition should be addressed as early as possible

Adherence to exercise is significantly enhanced if the exercise program meets the individual's needs and expectations, if the patient enjoys the exercise activity, and if he/she can continue similar or equally enjoyable activities at home. As well, the appropriate support systems for success from family, peers, and health professionals should be considered.

Physician Assessment and Follow-Up

Communication between the patient's physician and health professionals engaged in exercise program supervision is essential at many stages of the patient's participation. The frequency of interaction is highly dependent on the patient's responses at the various stages of the exercise evaluation and throughout the exercise program delivery process. At a minimum, there should be communication at patient entry to the exercise program and on completion of it. On the flowchart (Figure 11–4), a number of dotted lines indicate where additional communication may be required depending on patient response to exercise evaluations. Whenever a patient exhibits an

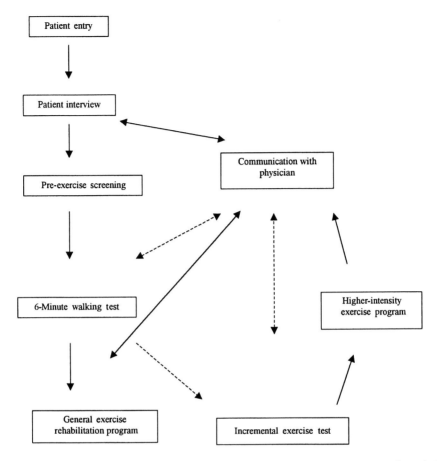

Figure 11–4 Patient evaluation for exercise training. Solid lines (◄——►)indicate patient progression through the exercise evaluation process, and recommended physician communication points. Dashed lines(◄----►)indicate points where additional communication with the patient's physician may be necessary depending on the presence of any abnormal signs and symptoms. These signs could be indicating exercise intolerance and a possible need for further medical investigation prior to proceeding from moderate- to higher-intensity exercises.

abnormal response, which may indicate the need for further medical investigation, it should be communicated to the physician immediately.

If patients enter a program without a referral from a physician and/or if the referral has insufficient information, it is essential that communication occur with the physician prior to any exercise evaluation to confirm the following:
- Respiratory diagnosis and other coexisting medical conditions
- Medications
- Resting 12-lead electrocardiogram (ECG) within past 12 months
- Patient readiness to exercise
- Most recent pulmonary function data

- Oxygen saturation and blood gas data if appropriate

An example of a form that may be provided to a physician for patients entering a community-based program is included in Appendix 11–1.

Initial Interview. Regardless of the referral source, all patients should be interviewed by a qualified health professional prior to commencement of an exercise evaluation. During the interview, the patient's communication and cognition skills should be evaluated, as well as any visual or auditory impairments that may be present.

The interview is aimed at assessing the following information:

1. Confirmation of the patient's respiratory condition and any other medical conditions that may negatively impact exercise training
2. Documentation of exercise history and compilation of activity profile for each patient
3. Identification of psychosocial or other factors that may impact the patient's access or participation in the exercise rehabilitation program

The medical history should document patient knowledge (1) of their respiratory diagnosis, (2) of their respiratory disease management including medication, and (3) of all other medical conditions, with special attention to indicators of coexisting cardiovascular disease and musculoskeletal impairment that may affect exercise performance.

The exercise history (Appendix 11–2 includes examples of questionnaire tools) should document: (1) patient patterns of exercise during early adult life prior to diagnosis of their respiratory disease and current activity patterns; (2) patient access to exercise facilities and equipment at home and in their immediate community; (3) patient exercise likes and dislikes such as exercising in a group or at home or any possible programs that could be built around activities the patient enjoys; (4) patient daily/weekly routine and perceived time and ability to exercise; (5) patient readiness and commitment to regular exercise; and (6) environmental barriers to exercise such as air quality, wind, and temperature at various times of the year, as well as terrain in their home environment.

The psychosocial history should document: (1) any factors that may negatively impact the patient's ability to access the exercise program and facilities and to maintain a home exercise routine at the end of the program and (2) cultural factors that may affect exercise choices.

Pre-exercise Test Screening

Prior to any exercise test, the patient should complete the following test evaluation:
1. Pulmonary function tests. If pulmonary function tests are not available from the referring physician, then, at a minimum, forced vital capacity and FEV_1 should be recorded.
2. Physical examination. A brief musculoskeletal assessment is recommended to identify the normal range of movement at upper limbs, lower limbs, neck, and back; to assess general muscle strength; and to identify any abnormalities/limitations that may impact exercise choices. The

assessment should note any pain on movement and muscle, tendon, or joint stiffness, and assessment of posture and gait should be included as many patients may be using walking aids and/or would benefit from the use of a walking aid.

Advice on appropriate footwear for exercise is essential.

Exercise Evaluation

Six-Minute Walking Test. It is recommended that all patients entering an exercise program for the first time have a 6-minute walking test conducted as a baseline functional exercise assessment.[113–117] Monitoring a patient during the 6-minute test should include recording resting (pre-exercise) heart rate, blood pressure, and respiratory rate. Heart rate should be assessed for 1 minute manually to assess both rate and rythm. If patients have abnormally high blood pressure at rest, blood pressure should be reassessed immediately following the test. At the end of exercise, heart rate should be reassessed manually for 30 seconds to 1 minute, again to ensure that an irregular pulse did not develop during walking. If the patient has an irregular pulse, it is advisable to recheck the ECG record for that patient and discuss ECG monitoring during exercise with the patient's physician. Ratings of perceived exertion for both leg effort and breathing effort should be assessed separately at the end of the test as well.[118,119] A decision regarding the use of pulse oximetry during the 6-minute walking test should be based on interpretation of pre-exercise assessment data. It is advisable to use pulse oximetry during an initial exercise assessment for any patient with severe COPD (as indicated by their pulmonary function test and/or blood gas data) and for those who indicate moderate to severe dyspnea during low-intensity exercise activities. Occasionally, in spite of careful prescreening, a patient will not tolerate a 6-minute walking test and will exhibit signs and symptoms of exercise intolerance, which should warrant further medical investigation. All adverse exercise responses should be communicated to the physician.

A 6-minute walking test is adequate screening for corridor walking–based programs and general arm, leg, and trunk exercises; these exercises can be done without any weights or with the use of very small weights for resistance (eg, 1- to 2-lb weights). However, patients who complete and appear to tolerate a 6-minute walking test are not necessarily safe to exercise at higher intensities. When higher training intensity exercises such as those outlined below are to be a part of the patient's exercise program, it is advisable that further exercise evaluations be conducted. *Submaximal Incremental Exercise.* At a minimum, a submaximal incremental exercise evaluation should precede an exercise prescription of moderate to heavy resistance exercises; for example, these exercises could include aerobic training on bicycles, treadmills, or arm ergometers; stair climbing for which more than one flight of continuous climbing is used as an exercise; stair steppers; rowing machines; and weight-resisted exercise for which weights above approximately 2 to 3 lb will be used. Many patients may develop ECG abnormalities,[120] abnormally elevated blood pressures, and/or oxygen desaturation during resistance exercise. This can happen even at relatively low levels of aerobic exercise, despite the fact that patients may have shown no such responses during the 6-minute walking test.

In the absence of access to a physician-supervised, symptom-limited maximum exercise test, it is possible for other appropriately trained health professionals to administer a submaximal incremental exercise evaluation. The personnel conducting the test should have the appropriate knowledge in training, skills, application, and interpretation of ECG. In addition, emergency procedures should be clearly established, and the guidelines for exercise testing should be adhered to, as outlined by the American College of Sports Medicine.[121] Because patients with COPD are an "at-risk" population, maximum symptom-limited exercise testing should not be performed in settings that are not physician supervised.[121]

The purpose of a submaximal, incremental exercise evaluation in a non–physician-supervised setting is to ensure that a patient may safely exercise within established exercise training parameters. This submaximal exercise evaluation would measure physiologic responses to exercise within the range of intensities used for exercise training, that is, to a maximum dyspnea rating of 5 to 6 on a Borg 10-point scale.[63] Arbitrarily set, submaximal heart rates are not usually very useful with patients with COPD in exercise testing as most patients will stop exercising because of dyspnea and leg fatigue.[116,122] However, even in healthy older individuals, no exercise test in the absence of physician supervision should take patients into heart rate ranges that exceed 85% of predicted maximum.[121]
Maximal Exercise Test. Wherever possible, an incremental, symptom-limited, maximal exercise test

under physician supervision should be undertaken. Details of exercise test protocols and procedures will not be provided here as there are many suitable references for this purpose.[121,123,124] Incremental exercise testing is recommended for all patients in whom moderate to high training intensity is considered part of their exercise training program.[121] This is because of the high incidence of coexisting cardiovascular disease coupled with the older age of most patients with COPD.

SETTING FOR EXERCISE TRAINING

Just as the components of rehabilitation are tailored to the individual, so too should each patient be directed to a type of program that is most appropriate to meet his/her needs. Exercise training can be performed on an inpatient or outpatient basis and in the home. For the majority of patients,[125] a supervised outpatient program seems to offer the best combination of efficacy[50] and cost effectiveness.[91,126] The more disabled patient may find regular travel to an outpatient facility too demanding to make attendance practical. These patients should be directed to an inpatient program, which may also be appropriate for those living far from the facility and when other interventions or specific resources (eg, supplemental feeding or training for home ventilation) are required. For centers that run both inpatient and outpatient programs, the goal should be to offer the same level and frequency of supervision for either program. However, one usually finds that for outpatient programs, attendance is less frequent but often has a greater duration.

Preferably, the rehabilitation program will be in a setting separate from an acute care site, where the environment is especially focused and conducive to wellness over illness. Moreover, the site, staff, and campus are all important. Ideally, the site should include appropriate facilities for clinical and diagnostic assessment, a pulmonary function and exercise testing laboratory, a gym and appropriate equipment for the exercise program, a classroom and educational resources, space for practical testing of activities of daily living, and recreational and relaxation areas for participants. All health professional staff involved in the program should understand the importance on the focus of therapy. A rehabilitation center provides an atmosphere in which the environment, staff, and other patients promote an ethos appropriate to rehabilitation.

Home-based programs are generally used when exercise is of paramount importance, and the other components of rehabilitation remain less significant. These programs may also be very useful in patients who cannot attend a rehabilitation program because of transportation difficulties or when an inpatient program is unavailable. Although home-based programs are effective in improving exercise tolerance and quality of life,[14,16,38,43,127,128] the magnitude of these improvements may be smaller compared to the effects of a closely supervised program.[50] In contrast, Wedzicha and colleagues studied housebound patients who were severely disabled and found no improvement in outcome measures after a home-based program was provided.[103] However, these are the patients who would most benefit from a closely supervised inpatient program. Home-based programs appear to be well suited for highly motivated, self-directed individuals for whom compliance with exercise does not require close supervision.

WHEN TO REFER TO A REHABILITATION PROGRAM

Exercise training is too often considered as a last resort therapeutic modality, and to minimize the consequences of COPD, it would be advisable to consider referring a patient with COPD to pulmonary rehabilitation for an exercise training program as early as possible in the natural evolution of the disease.

Patients should be referred for exercise training rehabilitation if they have impaired peripheral muscle function, decreased exercise tolerance, and reduced quality of life. Medical considerations that will influence the effectiveness of respiratory rehabilitation include confirmation of the diagnosis, maximization of therapy, and the identification and management of associated medical conditions. Other considerations may include patient motivation, smoking status, an adequate home situation and social support, and realistic goals and expectations.[105]

Ideally, a patient should see a physiotherapist as part of a pulmonary rehabilitation program. Referral may be appropriate for patients who have musculoskeletal disorder to design an individualized program based on their specific limitations.

SUMMARY

It is now clear that exercise training is an effective therapeutic strategy in patients with COPD. Despite this, it still remains largely underused.[125,129] Several factors may explain this apparent contrast between the efficacy of rehabilitation and the small number of patients undertaking this therapeutic modality. The poor availability of pulmonary rehabilitation programs is certainly one factor. In Canada, a recent study has shown that there are 36 pulmonary rehabilitation programs that can accept only 4,000 to 5,000 patients with COPD per year, representing less than 1% of all of the COPD population in that country.[125,129] Traveling long distances to find the nearest program is also common. Strategies should be developed to increase the availability of exercise training programs. In selected patients, home-based exercise training is one of these potential strategies that is currently under evaluation to improve accessibility to rehabilitation.

The skepticism of the medical community toward the actual efficacy of exercise training is also a factor preventing this treatment from being used on a larger scale. This skepticism can be attributed to two things: an incomplete understanding of the action mechanisms of exercise training (How can exercise training be effective if it does not improve lung or heart function?[102]) and a common belief that exercise training does not impact the long-term outcome of patients with COPD. These issues have been resolved, at least in part, since the last 10 to 15 years of research in pulmonary rehabilitation have provided strong scientific evidence of the efficacy of this intervention to improve patients' clinical short- and long-term outcome.[2,18,36] Exercise training is also often perceived as a risky procedure in patients with advanced COPD. However, as indicated in recent literature, pulmonary rehabilitation is a safe and effective procedure, even in patients with advanced lung disease.[48]

Another potential explanation for the low popularity of exercise training is the lack of patient motivation. From the patient point of view, it is less appealing to make an effort to adopt newer, more healthful lifestyle habits than to be offered a magic cure with pharmacologic or surgical interventions. Patients are too often passive witnesses of their treatment, and it is important to have them realize how critical it is that they play an active role in the maintenance of their health. In this regard, patient education is an important aspect of rehabilitation that will need to be more extensive if we hope to involve patients directly in their treatment.

In this era in which high technology and expensive drugs are the most valued aspects of medical care, cardiopulmonary rehabilitation should be promoted to

the medical community and the general population; its promotion is crucial because it offers the best chance to prevent respiratory and systemic consequences of COPD, and it optimizes the quality of life for those already affected by these afflicting disorders.

CASE STUDY

Mr. Cope, a 72-year-old patient with COPD, presents to your clinic because of progressive breathlessness with poor exercise tolerance, which has been deteriorating over the past years.

Medical History, Physical Examination, and Test Results

Medical History

- He quit smoking 7 years ago after a 40-pack-year history; he has been stable for many years and was maintained stable with regularly inhaled bronchodilators.
- His dyspnea progressed substantially over a 10-year period, and at the time of presentation to a respiratory specialist, his exercise tolerance was limited to walking slowly on a level surface.
- He still enjoyed a modified game of golf but had required a cart for the last 2 years.
- He started on oxygen at a flow rate of 1 L/min for rest and 2 L/min for exertion and during sleep.
- His medication included: sustained-release verapamil 120 mg/day, ranitidine 150 mg twice daily, salmeterol two puffs twice daily, ipratropium bromide four puffs every 4 hours while awake, and salbutamol two puffs every 4 hours as needed; a theophylline derivative was tried, but the patient could not tolerate the medication because of adverse gastrointestinal effects.
- Comorbid conditions: HBP and GER, no joint disease.

Physical Examination

- He did not have acute respiratory distress.
- His vital signs were as follows: pulse 90 beats/min, respiratory rate 22/min, blood pressure 145/88 mm Hg.
- Accessory muscle used in breathing.
- He had a barrel chest with decreased air entry but no crackle or wheezing.
- His cardiac examination was normal.
- He had no edema or cyanosis on oxygen.

- His musculoskeletal exam was normal.

Test Results

Pulmonary function tests were as follows:
- Forced expiratory volume in 1 second (FEV_1) postbronchodilator 1.0 L (37% predicted) and FEV_1/forced vital capacity (FVC) 38%
- Total lung capacity (TLC) 121% predicted, residual volume (RV) 143% predicted
- Dl_{CO} 33% predicted

Arterial blood gases (room air):
- pH 7.44, PCO_2 36 mm Hg, PO_2 51 mm Hg, SaO_2 87%

Questions and Discussion

This patient with symptomatic COPD, who was already on optimal bronchodilator treatment, could potentially benefit from pulmonary rehabilitation with an exercise program. The patient underwent a pulmonary rehabilitation program after complete pulmonary function tests and an incremental exercise test.

Exercise Program

After warm-up and stretching exercises (Figures 11–5 to 11–11), he initiated aerobic training four times per week on a treadmill, gradually increasing his duration to 12 minutes, and he alternated with cycling on a stationary cycle, which he then gradually increased to 17 minutes per session. Using elastic bands and free weights, he also undertook strengthening exercises for the upper and lower extremities (Figure 11–13 to 11–16). Ten repetitions of each movement were initially performed. The number of repetitions was progressively increased, as tolerated, until 30 repetitions were accomplished.

He participated in all educational activities, and in the psychosocial support groups, he learned breathing control during activities of daily living and panic control and developed relaxation techniques. After the 8-week intensive stage of rehabilitation, he was discharged to continue a home program of leisure walking, interval training, and breathing exercises each morning.

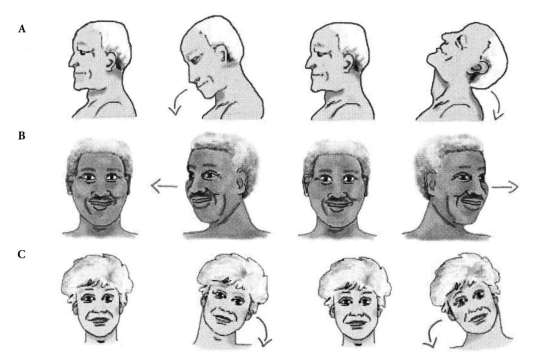

Figure 11–5 Warm-up exercises and stretches of the head and neck *A*, Forward flexion. Flex head forward toward chest and then slightly backward. *B*, Rotation. Rotate head toward the right, and then toward the left. Eyes follow movement. *C*, Lateral flexion. Flex head to the right such that the right ear touches the right shoulder. Repeat, directing left ear to left shoulder. Avoid elevation of shoulders. Incorporate pursed-lip breathing throughout movement. (Adapted from the self-management program "Living Well with COPD©".)

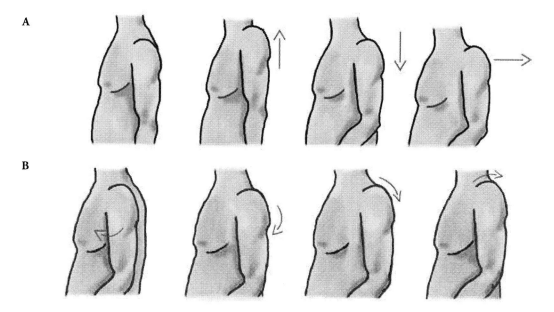

Figure 11–6 Warm-up exercises and stretches of the shoulders. *A*, Elevation and depression. Place shoulders in a neutral position, then elevate upward, downward, and backward. *B*, Rotation. Backward rotation is encouraged over forward rotation to counteract the typical COPD posture of rounded shoulders. Shoulders rotate upward, then backward, and downward and forward (initial position). Pursed-lip breathing is encouraged throughout the movement. (Adapted from the self-management program "Living Well with COPD©".)

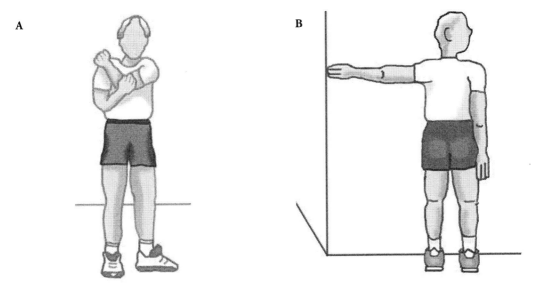

Figure 11–7 Arm and shoulder stretches. *A*, Arm. Hold up right hand with the left elbow pulled in a downward direction, then position left arm toward the right shoulder. Repeat on the other side. It is preferred to hold the position for 4 to 5 breaths using pursed-lip breathing; this discourages the patient from holding their breath during stretches, as this is a common tendency among COPD patients. *B*, Shoulder. This exercise helps to counteract rounding of the shoulders. Rest body with one side of the face up against the wall, position opposite arm outstretched against the wall, then hold position for 4 to 5 breaths using pursed-lip breathing. Repeat on the other side. (Adapted from the self-management program "Living Well with COPD©".)

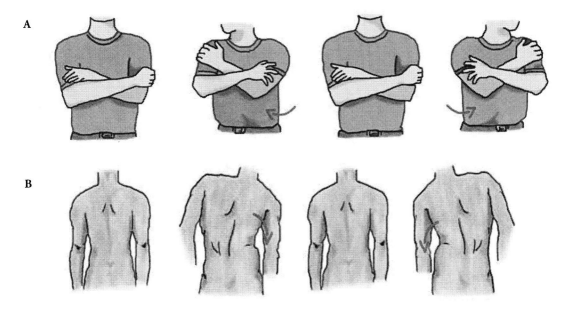

Figure 11–8 Warm-up exercises and stretches of the trunk *A*, Rotation. Cross arms over the chest and rotate trunk toward the right, then return it to the initial position and rotate toward the left. This exercise is recommended in a sitting position in order to isolate trunk mobility. *B*, Lateral flexion. Exercise begins with a straight trunk. Bend trunk to one side (avoid lifting of opposite hip) and return to initial position. Repeat exercise, bending trunk to the opposite side. This exercise is recommended in a sitting position to isolate trunk mobility. Pursed-lip breathing is incorporated throughout the exercise (Adapted from the self-management program "Living Well with COPD©".)

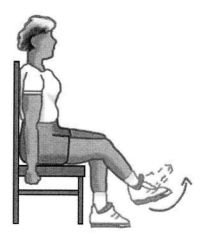

Figure 11–9 Ankle warm-up exercises and stretches. Rotations. Sitting with the back well supported, make circles with one ankle and repeat with the opposite foot. Pursed-lip breathing is incorporated throughout the exercise. (Adapted from the self-management program "Living Well with COPD©".)

A

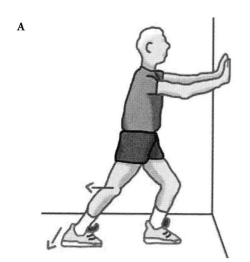

B

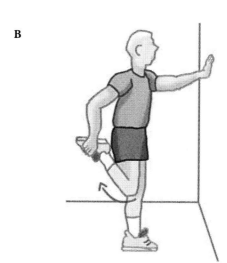

Figure 11–10. Calf and thigh stretches (hip flexors). *A,* Calf. Standing in front of a wall or support, stand with legs in the forward stride position. Keep feet pointing forward; breathe in and during the exhale, move body over the front foot, bending the front knee. The back leg must be straight with the heel on the ground; a stretch behind the knee should be felt. Hold this position for 4 to 5 breaths using pursed-lip breathing, and repeat with the opposite leg. *B,* Thigh. Standing with the left hand on the wall, grasp the right foot with the right hand and pull the right knee backward, while keeping the back straight. Hold for 4 to 5 breaths using pursed-lip breathing. Reverse hands and repeat on the opposite side. (Adapted from the self-management program "Living Well with COPD©".)

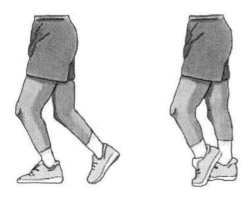

Figure 11–11 Walking on the spot. Walk on the spot for one minute using pursed-lip breathing throughout the exercise. (Adapted from the self-management program "Living Well with COPD©".)

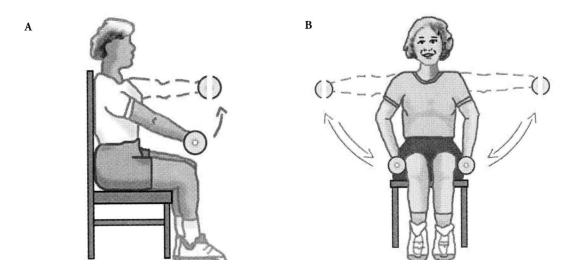

Figure 11–12 Resisted shoulder. *A,* Shoulder flexion. While sitting with the back well supported, raise one arm to shoulder level (keeping the elbow straight) and slowly return to initial position. Repeat using the other arm. *B,* Shoulder abduction. Sitting with the back well supported and arms lowered to the side raise arms to shoulder level then slowly return to initial position. Pursed-lip breathing is incorporated throughout the exercise. (Adapted from the self-management program "Living Well with COPD©".)

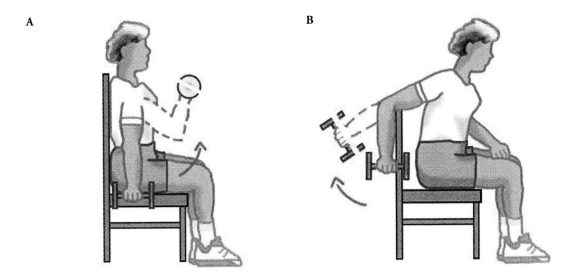

Figure 11–13. Resisted elbow. *A,* Elbow flexion. Sitting with the back well supported, bend the elbow while bringing the hand toward the shoulder and back down. *B,* Elbow extension. Begin by sitting with the arm over the back of the chair and breath in; while blowing out through pursed lips, straighten the elbow. Return hand slowly to the initial position. Pursed-lip breathing is encouraged throughout the movement. (Adapted from the self-management program "Living Well with COPD©".)

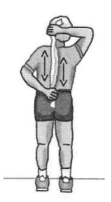

Figure 11–14 Arm exercise using elastic band. Stand while holding plastic band behind the back. The left hand remains stationary at the small of the back while the right hand extends, pulling elastic upward. Reverse hands and repeat. Pursed-lip breathing is incorporated throughout exercise. (Adapted from the self-management program "Living Well with COPD©".)

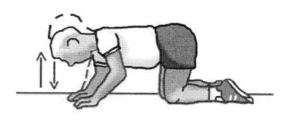

Figure 11–15 Modified push-up. While on all fours, lower body slowly by slightly bending arms at the elbow. Extend arms again, returning to initial position. It is important to avoid holding the breath and to coordinate pursed-lip breathing with movements; in avoiding this "hold," the patient therefore avoids the associated increase in shortness of breath. As an alternative, this exercise may be done in a standing position against the wall. Pursed-lip breathing is incorporated throughout the exercise. (Adapted from the self-management program "Living Well with COPD©".)

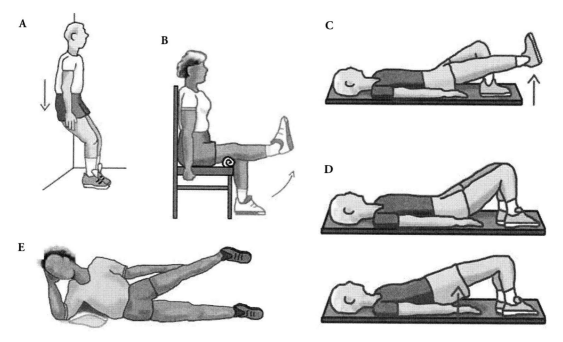

Figure 11–16 Lower body muscle exercises. *A,* Standing. Standing with the back against the wall, bend knees and hold this position for 4 to 5 breaths using pursed-lip breathing. Resume standing position and repeat exercise. *B,* Sitting with knee extension. Sitting with back well supported, raise one foot until knee is straightened. Coordinate pursed-lip breathing with movement. Repeat several times with leg reversal, and add progressive resistance as indicated. *C,* Lying down with straight leg raises. Lying down on the back with arms at the side and one leg bent, raise straight leg off the floor. Hold the position for 5 seconds. Bring the leg down slowly (progressive resistance is added to ankle as indicated). Pursed-lip breathing throughout exercise. *D,* Lying down with bridging. Initial position involves lying down on the back with arms at the side, knees bent, and feet together on the floor. Lift buttocks off the floor, hold position for 5 seconds (pursed-lip breathing), and then slowly return to initial position. *E,* Lying down with hip abduction. Lie down on the side with both legs straight. Raise upper leg making sure heel points toward the ceiling; hold position for 5 seconds (pursed-lip breathing), then slowly lower the leg. Repeat several times and then change sides (progressive resistance is added to raised leg as indicated). (Adapted from the self-management program "Living Well with COPD©".)

He indicated that his confidence had improved and that he was better able to cope with activities of daily living. His 6-minute walking test increased from 398 to 446 meters. His dyspnea scale score (visual analogue scale) decreased from 7 to 5 at the end of the walking test, and he was followed every 3 months by a physical therapist, as well as by his family physician. He was seen every 6 months by a respiratory specialist and had one to two respiratory exacerbations per year but did not require hospitalization.

Follow-Up

Two years later, he complained of a greater decline in exercise tolerance, increased dyspnea, and a decrease in his ability to cope. The patient was still nonsmoking. There was no evidence of active infection or of cardiac disease. He was therefore reconsidered for an abbreviated repeat course of rehabilitation. He still used oxygen at a flow of 1 L/min at rest and 2 L/min during sleep but required 4 L/min to maintain a saturation above 88% during exercise. His medications were essentially unchanged. He had been initiated on an inhaled glucocorticoid with no obvious benefit and had thus discontinued this inhaler.

Repeated lung function tests:
- FEV_1 postbronchodilation 0.9 L (33%) and FEV_1/FVC 35%
- TLC 134% predicted, RV 180% predicted
- DL_{CO} 28% predicted

Arterial blood gases (room air):
- PH 7.46, PCO_2 36 mm Hg, PO_2 48 mm Hg, SaO_2 85%

He completed treadmill, cycle, and upper extremity training but with less success than on the previous occasion. His 6-minute walking test improved from 290 to 320 meters, but his dyspnea scale score at the end of his walking test remained at the prerehabilitation level of 7.

A high-resolution CT scan showed heterogeneous emphysema, with the destruction being predominantly localized to the upper lobes. This was supported by a ventilation/perfusion scan confirming heterogeneity of both ventilation and perfusion, with the greatest reductions being in the upper zones. The patient was accepted for volume reduction surgery and underwent bilateral video-assisted thoracoscopic surgery without any complications. At follow-up, he stated that he observed improvements in both his dyspnea and in his exercise tolerance. At the 3-month follow-up visit, his 6-minute walking test was 448 meters, and his dyspnea scale score was 3 at the end of his walk. His oxygen requirements fell to 1 L/min at rest and 2 L/min for exertion and during sleep. His lung function tests after LVRS were FEV_1 post bronchodilation 1.2 L (41%), TLC 110% predicted, and RV 130% predicted.

This case illustrates the use of rehabilitation to improve dyspnea and exercise tolerance, thereby improving health-related quality of life among patients with chronic respiratory conditions. Regular follow-up is important to monitor and encourage a home exercise program and to identify changes in functional status. The willingness of a patient to re-admit for a repeat (usually abbreviated) course is important for some patients. This case also emphasizes the role of rehabilitation in preparing a patient for surgery such as lung resection, transplantation, or lung volume reduction.

KEY POINTS

- Exercise training is the cornerstone of pulmonary rehabilitation and is one of the most effective therapeutic strategies to improve dyspnea, exercise tolerance, and quality of life in patients with COPD.
- Exercise training is safe and well tolerated in patients with COPD provided that patients are evaluated carefully and that the training program is tailored to the patient's clinical condition.
- A combination of endurance exercise to improve exercise tolerance, dyspnea, and muscle exercises to improve strength appears to be well suited to patients with COPD.
- Despite proven efficacy, pulmonary rehabilitation is largely underused, and the availability of this intervention should be improved. Health care professionals have an important role in promoting this intervention.
- A maintenance exercise program is necessary to sustain the initial effects of training. Long-term adherence to exercise training is therefore an important therapeutic objective.
- Exercise training can be performed in the hospital, on an outpatient basis, in the community, or at home depending on the patient's clinical condition and the availability of the programs.

REFERENCES

1. American College of Sports Medicine Position Stand. The recommended quantity and quality of exercise for developing and maintaining cardiorespiratory and muscular fitness, and flexibility in healthy adults. Med Sci Sports Exerc 1998;30:975–91.

2. Ries AL, Kaplan RM, Limberg TM, Prewitt LM. Effects of pulmonary rehabilitation on physiologic and psychosocial outcomes in patients with chronic obstructive pulmonary disease. Ann Intern Med 1995;122:823–32.

3. Blair SN. McCloy research lecture: physical activity, physical fitness and health. Res Q Exerc Sports 1993;64:365–76.

4. Blair SN, Kohl HW, Barlow CE, et al. Changes in physical fitness and all-cause mortality. A prospective study of healthy and unhealthy men. JAMA 1995;273:1093–8.

5. Rogers MA, Evans WJ. Changes in skeletal muscle with aging: effects of exercise training. Exerc Sport Sci Rev 1993;21:65–102.

6. Evans WJ. Exercise training guidelines for the elderly. Med Sci Sports Exerc 1999;31:12–7.

7. Heinonen AP, Kannus P, Sievanen H, et al. Randomised controlled trial of effect of high-impact exercise on selected risk factors for osteoporotic fractures. Lancet 1996;348:1343–7.

8. Frontera WR, Meredith CN, O'Reilley KP, et al. Strength conditioning in older men: skeletal muscle hypertrophy and improved function. J Appl Physiol 1988;64:1038–44.

9. Singh NA, Clements KM, Fiatarone MA. A randomized controlled trial of progressive resistance training in depressed elders. J Gerontol A Biol Sci Med Sci 1997;52:M27–35.

10. Barach AL, Bicherman H. Advances in the treatment of non-tuberculous pulmonary disease. Bull N Y Acad Med 1952;28:353–84.

11. Petty TL, Nett LM, Finigan MM, et al. A comprehensive care program for chronic airway obstruction. Methods and preliminary evaluation of symptomatic and functional improvement. Ann Intern Med 1969;70:1109–20.

12. Albert RK. Is pulmonary rehabilitation an effective treatment for chronic obstructive pulmonary disease? No. Am J Respir Crit Care Med 1997;155:784–5.

13. Celli BR. Is pulmonary rehabilitation an effective treatment for chronic obstructive pulmonary disease? Yes. Am J Respir Crit Care Med 1997;155:781–3.

14. McGavin CR, Gupta SP, Lloyd EL, McHardy JR. Physical rehabilitation for the chronic bronchitis: results of a controlled trial of exercises in the home. Thorax 1977;32:307–11.

15. Cockroft AE, Saunders MJ, Berry G. Randomised controlled trial of rehabilitation in chronic respiratory disability. Thorax 1981;36:200–3.

16. Wijkstra PJ, Van-Altena R, Kraan J, et al. Quality of life in patients with chronic obstructive pulmonary disease improves after rehabilitation at home. Eur Respir J 1994;7:269–73.

17. Goldstein RS, Gort EH, Stubbing D, et al. Randomised controlled trial of respiratory rehabilitation. Lancet 1994;344:1394–7.

18. Griffiths TL, Burr ML, Campbell IA, et al. Results at 1 year of outpatient multidisciplinary pulmonary rehabilitation: a randomised controlled trial. Lancet 2000;355:362–8.

19. Casaburi R, Patessio A, Iioli F, et al. Reductions in exercise lactic acidosis and ventilation as a result of exercise training in patients with obstructive lung disease. Am Rev Respir Dis 1991;143:9–18.

20. Maltais F, Leblanc P, Simard C, et al. Skeletal muscle adaptation to endurance training in patients with chronic obstructive pulmonary disease. Am J Respir Crit Care Med 1996;154:442–7.

21. Sala E, Roca J, Marrades RM, et al. Effects of endurance training on skeletal muscle bioenergetics in chronic obstructive pulmonary disease. Am J Respir Crit Care Med 1999;159:1726–34.

22. Holloszy JO, Coyle EF. Adaptations of skeletal muscle to endurance exercise and their metabolic consequences. J Appl Physiol 1984;56:831–8.

23. Casaburi R. Physiologic responses to training. Clin Chest Med 1994;15:215–27.

24. Howald H, Hoppeler H, Claasen H, et al. Influences of endurance training on the ultrastructural composition of the different muscle fiber types in human. Pflugers Arch 1985;403:369–76.

25. Simoneau JA, Lortie G, Boulay MR, et al. Human skeletal muscle fibre type alteration with high-intensity intermittent training. Eur J Appl Physiol 1985;54:250–53.

26. Baumann H, Jäggi M, Soland F, et al. Exercise training induces transition of myosin isoform subunits within histochemically typed human muscle fibers. Pflugers Arch 1987;409:349–60.

27. Holloszy JO. Adaptation of skeletal muscle to endurance exercise. Med Sci Sports Exerc 1975;7:155–64.

28. Saltin B, Gollnick PD. Skeletal muscle adaptability: significance for metabolism and performance. In: Peachey LD, ed. The handbook of physiology: the skeletal muscle system. Bethesda, MD: American Physiological Society, 1982;555–631.

29. Pattengale PK, Holloszy JO. Augmentation of skeletal muscle myoglobin by a program of treadmill running. Am J Physiol 1967;213:783–5.

30. Saltin B, Henriksson J, Nygaard E, et al. Fiber types and metabolic potentials of skeletal muscles in sedentary man and endurance runners. Ann N Y Acad Sci 1977;301:3–29.

31. Fiatarone MA, Marks EC, Ryan ND, et al. High-intensity strength training in nonagenarians. Effects on skeletal muscle. JAMA 1990;263:3029–34.

32. Frontera WR, Meredith CN, O'Reilly KP, Evans WJ. Strength training and determinants of VO_2 max in older men. J Appl Physiol 1990;68:329–33.

33. Belman MJ. Exercise in patients with chronic obstructive pulmonary disease. Thorax 1993;48:936–46.

34. Bernard S, Whittom F, Leblanc P, et al. Aerobic and strength training in patients with COPD. Am J Respir Crit Care Med 1999;159:896–901.

35. O'Donnell DE, McGuire M, Samis L, Webb KA. The impact of exercise reconditioning on breathlessness in severe chronic airflow limitation. Am J Respir Crit Care Med 1995;152:2005–13.

36. Lacasse Y, Wong E, Guyatt GH, et al. Meta-analysis of respiratory rehabilitation in chronic obstructive pulmonary disease. Lancet 1996;348:1115–9.

37. Lake FR, Henderson K, Briffa T, et al. Upper-limb and lower-limb exercise training in patients with chronic airflow obstruction. Chest 1990;97:1077–82.

38. Strijbos JH, Postma DS, van Altena R, et al. A comparison between an outpatient hospital-based pulmonary rehabilitation program and a home-care pulmonary rehabilitation program in patients with COPD. A follow-up of 18 months. Chest 1996;109:366–72.

39. Simpson K, Killian K, McCartney N, et al. Randomised controlled trial of weightlifting exercise in patients with chronic airflow limitation. Thorax 1992;47:70–5.

40. Clark CJ, Cochrane L, Mackay E. Low intensity peripheral muscle conditioning improves exercise tolerance and breathlessness in COPD. Eur Respir J 1996;9:2590–6.

41. Clark CJ, Cochrane LM, Mackay E, Paton B. Skeletal muscle strength and endurance in patients with mild COPD and the effects of weight training. Eur Respir J 2000;15:92–7.

42. Bendstrup KE, Ingemann Jensen J, Holm S, Bengtsson B. Out-patient rehabilitation improves activities of daily living, quality of life and exercise tolerance in chronic obstructive pulmonary disease. Eur Respir J 1997;10:2801–6.

43. Wijkstra PJ, Ten-Vergert EM, van-Altena R, et al. Long term benefits of rehabilitation at home on quality of life and exercise tolerance in patients with chronic obstructive pulmonary disease. Thorax 1995;50:824–8.

44. Toshima TM, Blumberg E, Ries AL, et al. Does rehabilitation reduce depression in patients with chronic obstructive pulmonary disease? J Cardiopulm Rehabil 1992;12:261–9.

45. Güell R, Casan P, Belda J, et al. Long-term effects of outpatient rehabilitation of COPD. A randomized trial. Chest 2000;117:976–83.

46. Vale F, Reardon JZ, ZuWallack RL. The long term benefits of outpatient pulmonary rehabilitation on exercise endurance and quality of life. Chest 1993;103:42–5.

47. Casaburi R, Porszasz J, Burns MR, et al. Physiolologic benefits of exercise training in rehabilitation of patients with severe chronic obstructive pulmonary disease. Am J Respir Crit Care Med 1997;155:1541–51.

48. Maltais F, Leblanc P, Jobin J, et al. Intensity of training and physiologic adaptation in patients with chronic obstructive pulmonary disease. Am J Respir Crit Care Med 1997;155:555–61.

49. Belman MJ, Kendregan BA. Exercise training fails to increase skeletal muscle enzymes in patients with chronic obstructive lung disease. Am Rev Respir Dis 1981;123:256–61.

50. Puente-Maestu L, Sanz ML, Sanz P, et al. Comparison of effects of supervised versus self-monitored training programmes in patients with chronic obstructive pulmonary disease. Eur Respir J 2000;15:517–25.

51. Casaburi R, Carithers E, Tosolini J, et al. Randomized placebo controlled trial of growth hormone in severe COPD patients undergoing endurance exercise training. Am J Respir Crit Care Med 1997;155:A498.

52. Hudson LD, Tyler ML, Petty TL. Hospitalization needs during an outpatient rehabilitation program for severe chronic airway obstruction. Chest 1976;70:606–10.

53. Lertzman MM, Cherniak RM. Rehabilitation of patients with chronic obstructive pulmonary disease. Am Rev Respir Dis 1976;114:1145–65.

54. Ries AL, Ellis B, Hawkins RW. Upper extremity exercise training in chronic obstructive pulmonary disease. Chest 1988;93:688–92.

55. Reardon J, Awad E, Normandin E, et al. The effect of comprehensive outpatient pulmonary rehabilitation on dyspnea. Chest 1994;105:1046–52.

56. Weiner P, Azgad Y, Ganam R. Inspiratory muscle training combined with general exercise reconditioning in patients with COPD. Chest 1992;102:1351–6.

57. American College of Chest Physicians/American Association of Cardiovascular and Pulmonary Rehabilitation Pulmonary Rehabilitation Guidelines Panel. Pulmonary rehabilitation. Joint ACCP/AACVPR evidence-based guidelines. Chest 1997;112:1363–96.

58. Martinez FJ, Vogel PD, Dupont DN, et al. Supported arm exercise vs unsupported arm exercise in the rehabilitation of patients with severe chronic airflow obstruction. Chest 1993;103:1397–402.

59. Punzal PA, Ries AL, Kaplan RM, Prewitt LM. Maximum intensity exercise training in patients with chronic obstructive pulmonary disease. Chest 1991;100:618–23.

60. Coppoolse R, Schols AM, Baarends EM, et al. Interval versus continuous training in patients with severe COPD: a randomized clinical trial. Eur Respir J 1999;14:258–63.

61. Vallet G, Ahmaïdi S, Serres I, et al. Comparison of two training programmes in chronic airway limitation patients: standardized versus individualized protocols. Eur Respir J 1997;10:114–22.

62. Mejia R, Ward J, Lentine T, Mahler DA. Target dyspnea ratings predict expected oxygen consumption as well as target heart rate values. Am J Respir Crit Care Med 1999;159:1485–9.

63. Horowitz MB, Littenberg B, Mahler DA. Dyspnea ratings for prescribing exercise intensity in patients with COPD. Chest 1996;109:1169–75.

64. Schols AM, Soeters PB, Mostert R, et al. Physiologic effects of nutritional support and anabolic steroids in patients with chronic obstructive pulmonary disease. A placebo-controlled randomized trial. Am J Respir Crit Care Med 1995;152:1268–74.

65. Ferreira IM, Verreschi IT, Nery LE, et al. The influence of 6 months of oral anabolic steroids on body mass and respiratory muscles in undernourished COPD patients. Chest 1998;114:19–28.

66. Burdet L, de Muralt B, Schutz Y, et al. Administration of growth hormone to underweight patients with chronic obstructive pulmonary disease. A prospective, randomized, controlled study. Am J Respir Crit Care Med 1997;156:1800–6.

67. Bernard S, Leblanc P, Whittom F, et al. Peripheral muscle weakness in patients with chronic obstructive pulmonary disease. Am J Respir Crit Care Med 1998;158:629–34.

68. Gosselink R, Troosters T, Decramer M. Peripheral muscle weakness contributes to exercise limitation in COPD. Am J Respir Crit Care Med 1996;153:976–80.

69. Hamilton AL, Killian K, Summers E, Jones NL. Muscle strength, symptom intensity and exercise capacity in patients with cardiorespiratory disorders. Am J Respir Crit Care Med 1995;152:2021–31.

70. Schols AM, Slangen J, Volovics L, Wouters EF. Weight loss is a reversible factor in the prognosis of chronic obstructive pulmonary disease. Am J Respir Crit Care Med 1998;157:1791–7.

71. American College of Sports Medicine Position Stand. The recommended quantity and quality of exercise for developing and maintaining cardiorespiratory and muscular fitness in healthy adults. Med Sci Sports Exerc 1990;22:265–74.

72. McEvoy CE, Ensrud KE, Bender E, et al. Association between corticosteriod use and vertebral fractures in older men with chronic obstructive pulmonary disease. Am J Respir Crit Care 1998;157:704–9.

73. Dekhuijzen PN, Folgering HT, van Herwaarden CL. Target-flow inspiratory muscle training during pulmonary rehabilitation in patients with COPD. Chest 1991;99:128–33.

74. Weiner P, Azgad Y, Ganam R, Weiner M. Inspiratory muscle training in patients with bronchial asthma. Chest 1992;102:1357–61.

75. Wanke T, Formanek D, Lahrmann H, et al. Effects of combined inspiratory muscle and cycle ergometer training on exercise performance in patients with COPD. Eur Respir J 1994;7:2205–11.

76. Berry MJ, Adair NE, Sevensky KS, et al. Inspiratory muscle training and whole-body re-conditoning in chronic obstructive pulmonary disease. Am J Respir Crit Care Med 1996;153:1812–6.

77. Larson JL, Covey MK, Wirtz SE, et al. Cycle ergometer and inspiratory muscle training in chronic obstructive pulmonary disease. Am J Respir Crit Care Med 1999;160:500–7.

78. Lacasse Y, Guyatt GH, Goldstein RS. The components of a respiratory rehabilitation program. A systematic overview. Chest 1997;111:1077–88.

79. Gosselink R, Decramer M. Inspiratory muscle training: where are we? Eur Respir J 1994;7: 2103–5.

80. Rooyackers JM, Dekhuijzen PN, van Herwaarden CL, Folgering HT. Training with supplemental oxygen in patients with COPD and hypoxaemia at peak exercise. Eur Respir J 1997;10:1278–84.

81. Garrod R, Paul EA, Wedzicha JA. Supplemental oxygen during pulmonary rehabilitation in patients with COPD with exercise hypoxaemia. Thorax 2000;55:539–43.

82. O'Donnell DE, Sanii R, Giesbrecht G, Younes M. Effect of continuous positive airway pressure on respiratory sensation in patients with chronic obstructive pulmonary disease during submaximal exercise. Am Rev Respir Dis 1988;138:1185–91.

83. O'Donnell DE, Sanii R, Younes M. Improvement in exercise endurance in patients with chronic airflow limitation using continuous positive airway pressure. Am Rev Respir Dis 1988;138:1510–4.

84. Keilty SE, Ponte J, Fleming TA, Moxham J. Effect of inspiratory pressure support on exercise tolerance and breathlessness in patients with severe stable chronic obstructive pulmonary disease. Thorax 1994;49:990–4.

85. Maltais F, Reissmann H, Gottfried SB. Pressure support reduces inspiratory effort and dyspnea during exercise in chronic airflow obstruction. Am J Respir Crit Care Med 1995;151:1027–33.

86. Bianchi L, Foglio K, Pagani M, et al. Effects of proportional assist ventilation on exercise tolerance in COPD patients with chronic hypercapnia. Eur Respir J 1998;11:422–7.

87. Dolmage T, Goldstein RS. Proportional assist ventilation and exercise tolerance in subjects with COPD. Chest 1997;111:948–54.

88. Polkey MI, Hawkins P, Kyroussis D, et al. Inspiratory pressure support prolongs exercise induced lactataemia in severe COPD. Thorax 2000;55:547–9.

89. Garrod R, Mikelsons C, Paul EA, Wedzicha JA. Randomized controlled trial of domiciliary noninvasive positive pressure ventilation and physical training in severe chronic obstructive pulmonary disease. Am J Respir Crit Care Med 2000;162:1335–41.

90. Guyatt GH, Berman LB, Townsend M. Long-term outcome after respiratory rehabilitation. Can Med Assoc J 1987;137:1089–95.

91. Troosters T, Gosselink R, Decramer M. Short- and long-term effects of outpatient rehabilitation in patients with chronic obstructive pulmonary disease: a randomized trial. Am J Med 2000;109:207–12.

92. Cockroft AE, Berry G, Brown E, Exall C. Psychological changes during a controlled trial of rehabilitation in chronic respiratory disability. Thorax 1982;37:413–6.

93. Ketelaars CA, Abu-Saad HH, Schlosser MA, et al. Long-term outcome of pulmonary rehabilitation in patients with COPD. Chest 1997;112:363–9.

94. Engström CP, Persson LO, Larsson S, Sullivan M. Long term effects of a pulmonary rehabilitation programme in outpatients with chronic obstructive pulmonary disease: a randomized controlled study. Scand J Rehabil Med 1999;31:207–13.

95. Foglio K, Bianchi L, Bruletti G, et al. Long-term effectiveness of pulmonary rehabilitation in patients with chronic airway obstruction. Eur Respir J 1999;13:125–32.

96. Wijkstra PJ, van der Mark TW, Kraan J, et al. Long-term effects of home rehabilitation on physical performance in chronic obstructive pulmonary disease. Am J Respir Crit Care Med 1996;153:1234–41.

97. American Thoracic Society. Pulmonary rehabilitation. Official statement of the American Thoracic Society Board of Directors. Am J Respir Crit Care Med 1999;159:1666–82.

98. Wijkstra PJ, Ten Vergert EM, Van der Mark TW, et al. Relation of lung function, maximal inspiratory pressure, dyspnoea, and quality of life with exercise capacity in patients with chronic obstructive pulmonary disease. Thorax 1994;49:468–72.

99. Zu-Wallack RL, Patel K, Reardon JZ, et al. Predictors of improvement in the 12-minute walking distance following a six-week outpatient pulmonary rehabilitation program. Chest 1991;99: 805–8.

100. Niederman MS, Clemente PH, Fein AM, et al. Benefits of a multidisciplinary pulmonary rehabilitation program. Improvements are independent of lung function. Chest 1991;99:798–804.

101. Stubbing D, Barr P, Haalboom P, Vaughan R. Is the effect of respiratory rehabilitation in COPD independent of the degree of impairment, disability or handicap. Am J Respir Crit Care Med 1995;15:A151.

102. Celli BR. Pulmonary rehabilitation in patients with COPD. Am J Respir Crit Care Med 1995;152: 861–4.

103. Wedzicha JA, Bestall JC, Garrod R, et al. Randomized controlled trial of pulmonary rehabilitation in severe chronic obstructive pulmonary disease patients, stratified with the MRC dyspnoea scale. Eur Respir J 1998;12:363–9.

104. Haas A, Cardon H. Rehabilitation in chronic obstructive pulmonary disease: a 5 year study of 252 male patients. Med Clin North Am 1969;61:749–58.

105. Young P, Dewse M, Fergusson W, Kolbe J. Respiratory rehabilitation in chronic obstructive pulmonary disease: predictors of nonadherence. Eur Respir J 1999;13:855–9.

106. Agle DP, Baum GL. Psychological aspects of chronic obstructive pulmonary disease. Med Clin North Am 1977;61:749–58.

107. Brooks D, Lacasse Y, Goldstein RS. Pulmonary rehabilitation programs in Canada. A national survey. Am J Respir Crit Care Med 1998;157:A787.

108. Connor MC, O'Driscoll MF, McDonnell TJ. Should patients with chronic obstructive pulmonary disease (COPD) who express a desire to stop smoking be enrolled in pulmonary rehabilitation? Eur Resp J 1999;14:263S.

109. Singh SJ, Vora VA, Morgan MDL. Does pulmonary rehabilitation benefit current and nonsmokers? Am J Respir Crit Care Med 1999;159:A764

110. Roomie J, Johnson MM, Waters K, et al. Respiratory rehabilitation, exercise capacity and quality of life in chronic airways disease in old age. Age Aging 1996; 25:12–6.

111. Stubbing DG, Barr P, Haalboom P, Vaughan R. Gender differences in respiratory rehabilitation. Am J Respir Crit Care Med 1996;153:A153.

112. Foster S, Lopez D, Thomas HM. Pulmonary rehabilitation in COPD patients with elevated PCO_2. Am Rev Respir Dis 1998;138:1519–23.

113. Butland RJA, Pang J, Gross ER, et al. Two-, six-, and twelve-minute walking tests in respiratory disease. BMJ 1982;284:1607–8.

114. Guyatt G, Sullivan MJ, Thompson PJ, et al. The 6 minute walk test: a new measure of exercise capacity in patients with chronic heart failure. Can Med Assoc J 1985;132:919–23.

115. Guyatt GH, Pugsley SO, Sullivan MJ, et al. Effect of encouragement on walking test performance. Thorax 1984;39:818–22.

116. Mahler DA, Franco MJ. Clinical applications of cardiopulmonary exercise testing. J Cardiopulm Rehabil 1996;16:357–65.

117. Redelmeier DA, Bayoumi AM, Goldstein RS, Guyatt GH. Interpreting small differences in functional status: the six-minute walk test in chronic lung disease patients. Am J Respir Crit Care Med 1997;155: 1278–82.

118. Borg G. Psychophysical bases of perceived exertion. Med Sci Sports Exerc 1982;14:377–81.

119. Borg GA. Borg's perceived exertion and pain scales. Windsor, ON: Human Kinetics, One, 1998.

120. Cheong TH, Magder S, Shapiro S, et al. Cardiac arrhythmias during exercise in severe chronic obstructive pulmonary disease. Chest 1990;97:793–7.

121. American College of Sports Medicine. ACSM's guidelines for exercise testing and prescription. Philadelphia: Lippincott, Williams and Wilkins, 2000.

122. Simmons DN, Berry MJ, Hayes SI, Walschlager SA. The relationship between % HR peak and % VO2 peak in patients with chronic obstructive pulmonary disease. Med Sci Sports Exerc 2000;32:881–6.

123. Jones NL. Clinical exercise testing. Lippincott, Williams and Wilkins Philadelphia: WB Saunders, 1988.

124. Wasserman K, Hansen JE, Sue DY, et al. Principles of exercise testing and interpretation. Philadelphia: Lippincott, Williams and Wilkins, 1999.

125. Brooks D, Lacasse Y, Goldstein RS. Pulmonary rehabilitation programs in Canada; national survey. Can Respir J 1999;6:55–63.

126. Goldstein RS, Gort EH, Guyatt GH, Feeny D. Economic analysis of respiratory rehabilitation. Chest 1997;112:370–9.

127. Busch AJ, McClements JD. Effects of a supervised home exercise program on patients with severe chronic obstructive pulmonary disease. Phys Ther 1988; 68:469–74.

128. Debigaré R, Maltais F, Whitton F, et al. Feasibility and efficacy of home exercise training before lung volume reduction. J Cardiopulm Rehabil 1999;19:235–41.

129. Armstrong KL, Wolfe LA, Amey MC. Cardiovascular rehabilitation in Canada. J Cardiopulm Rehabil 1994;14:262–72.

130. Katch VL, Katch FI, McArdle WD. Student study guide and workbook for essentials of exercise physiology. In: Williams, Wilkins, eds. Philadelphia: Lippincott, Williams and Wilkins, 2000:389–90.

131. McArdle WD, Katch F, Katch V. Essentials of exercise physiology. Philadelphia: Lippincott, Williams and Wilkins, 2000:155–9.

SUGGESTED READINGS

American College of Sports Medicine. The recommended quantity and quality of exercise for developing and maintaining cardiorespiratory and muscular fitness, and flexibility in healthy adults. Med Sci Sports Exerc 1998;30:975–91. *A position statement of the American College of Sports Medicine on exercise recommendation for healthy individuals. The rationale of the proposed recommendation is well documented.*

American College of Chest Physicians/American Association of Cardiovascular and Pulmonary Rehabilitation. Pulmonary Rehabilitation Guidelines Panel. Pulmonary rehabilitation joint ACCP/AACVPR evidence-based guidelines. Chest 1997;112:1363–96. *An official statement of the American College of Chest Physician and the American Association of Cardiovascular and Pulmonary Rehabilitation. The evidence supporting the use of several exercise training modalities is reviewed in great detail.*

Troosters T, Gosselink R, Decramer M. Short- and long-term effects of outpatient rehabilitation in patients with chronic obstructive pulmonary disease: a randomized trial. Am J Med 2000;109:207–12. *An excellent recent study published in a general internal medicine journal confirming the short- and long-term efficacy of pulmonary rehabilitation.*

American Thoracic Society. Pulmonary rehabilitation. Am J Respir Crit Care Med 1999;159:1666–82. *The official statement of the American Thoracic Society on pulmonary rehabilitation.*

Guidelines for pulmonary rehabilitation programs. 2nd Ed. American Association of CardioVascular and Pulmonary Rehabilitation 1998. Human Kinetics. *An excellent book reviewing many practical aspects of pulmonary rehabilitation.*

APPENDIX 11–1

Physician Form for Entry to Respiratory Rehabilitation Exercise Program

Patient Name: _____

Patient Date of Birth:_____

Patient Primary Respiratory Diagnosis: _____

Secondary Diagnoses:_____

Medications: _____

12-Lead ECG done in past 12 months. Yes _____ No _____

If yes, please indicate ECG findings: _____

If a 12-lead resting ECG has not been completed in the last 12 months, we request that one be completed and the results forwarded to us prior to our acceptance of your patient into our exercise program.

Number of hospitalizations in past 12 months? _____

Number of emergency room visits in past 12 months? _____

Number of unscheduled physician visits in past 12 months? _____

PFT and blood gas data: _____

I agree that _patient's name___ can participate in the _name of program____.

Signature of Physician:_____

Name of Physician: _____

Address: _____

Phone Number: _____

APPENDIX 11–2

Compiling an Activity Profile

Assessing current, daily exercise abilities of patients provides important baseline information and indicators of the degree of deconditioning and/or respiratory limitation present. This is useful in determining the type and intensity of exercises a patient should commence. At minimum, an activity screening such as that outlined below should be undertaken with all patients.

More detailed assessment tools for determining daily activities and past exercise habits are included and are applicable with many subsets of patients with COPD.

Basic Activity Questionnaire

1. Are you able to make your own meals?
   Yes_____ No_____ Seldom_____

2. Do you do your own grocery shopping?
   Always_____ Sometimes_____ Never_____

3. Do you drive a car?
   Yes_____ No_____ Seldom_____

4. Are you able to do light housework (laundry, dusting, vacuuming)?
   Always_____ Sometimes_____ Seldom_____

5. Are you able to do light yard work (weeding garden, cutting grass)?
   Always_____ Sometimes_____ Seldom_____

6. Is your walking ability limited to: (tick as many as apply)
   _____ Walking any distance is not a problem
   _____ Inside the house or apartment
   _____ 3 to 4 city blocks without stopping
   _____ Short distances outside (weather permitting)
   _____ Leisurely pace in a mall
   _____Other, please describe:_____

7. Do you try to exercise regularly?
   Yes_____ No_____ Seldom_____

8. If yes, what does your exercise program consist of each week?

List Each Activity	Times (weekly)	Minutes (per session)	Perceived Effort During Activity (light, moderate, fairly hard, hard)

8. Are you aware of any other conditions that you have that may limit your ability to exercise?

   Yes_____ No_____

   If yes, please list: _____

9. Please list any other information related to exercising that you feel is important for us to know:

   _____

Patient Signature_____ Date_____

Three-Day Activity Recall

Conduct a three-day activity recall.[130] Construct a chart with activity, time started, and time stopped across the top of the page. Patients then enter every activity they perform over the day from the time they get up each morning until they go to bed at night. From this you can observe, at a glance, the patient's current activity patterns. Knowing the individual's age and body weight in kg allows for estimation of total daily energy expenditure and exercise-related daily energy expenditure.[131]

To estimate lifelong involvement in exercise and changes over time, have the patient complete the following during the interview stage; additional lines under each section should be added. The last column is optional for those who wish to compute estimates of energy expenditure changes over time. Patient body weight and age will be needed for this computation as per the method outlined above.[131]

Patient instructions: Include all exercise activities such as gardening and walking, as well as any recreational and sports activities.

Current Exercise Activities	Times/Week	Minutes/ Session	Perceived Intensity of Effort	Years of Participation	Estimated Energy Expenditure/ Week (kcal)
Activities at age 40 (or some age prior to onset of significant respiratory symptoms)					
Activities at age 18					

PSYCHOSOCIAL CONSIDERATIONS IN COPD

*Diane Nault, Mary Ann Siok,
Elizabeth Borycki, Denise Melanson,
Louis Rousseau, and Yves Lacasse*

OBJECTIVES

The general objective of this chapter is to help physicians and other allied health care professionals assess all of the psychosocial aspects of chronic obstructive pulmonary disease (COPD) and intervene efficiently toward disease adjustment and coping. Both patients' and caregivers' psychosocial needs should be assessed to identify current and potential problems in daily living, social network, family relationships, self-perceptions, coping, and psychological disturbances such as anxiety and depression.

After reading this chapter, the physician and the allied health care professional will be able to

- appreciate the importance of the psychosocial problems of surviving with COPD;
- recognize and understand the psychosocial impact of COPD on the individual, family, and social life;
- recognize the common emotional consequences of COPD, more specifically anxiety and depression;
- assess the psychosocial aspects of COPD such as changes in daily living and self-perceptions, family burden, coping skills, and anxiety and depression;
- choose appropriate interventions to facilitate patient's coping and psychosocial adjustment to the disease; and
- refer to specialized professionals and specific resources when needed.

Having a chronic illness such as COPD means fundamental changes in lifestyle and in quality of life owing to multiple losses and physical disabilities experienced by the individual. The onset of a chronic illness places the individual and his/her family in a state of acute life crisis in which physical, social, and psychological disequilibrium affects ways of coping and brings intense feelings of anxiety, fear, anger, and other emotions.[1] Once the chronic phase takes over, the individual and his/her family try to reestablish and maintain equilibrium by developing a sense of living with a chronic illness, reintegrating the chronically ill person into the family's daily life, and using a variety of adaptive strategies when changes occur during the course of the disease.

Often the individual and the family are under chronic stress and decreased ability to adjust and cope with disease for the following reasons: (1) uncertainty of the future, (2) anger about having a long-term and terminal disease, (3) exacerbation of already existing resentment and ambivalence in relationships, (4) depression related to the numerous losses, and/or (5) substantial changes in life tasks.[2] Chronic obstructive pulmonary disease affects all areas of life, more specifically functional performance.[3–5] Leidy has defined functional performance as "the physical, psychological, social, occupational and spiritual activities that people choose to do in the normal course of their lives to meet basic needs, fulfill usual roles, and maintain their health and well-being."[4] Clinical observations suggest wide differences in the functional performance and perception of dyspnea of patients with COPD despite similarities in the results of pulmonary function tests. Some patients orient themselves toward a life of total dependency on others, inactivity, and social isolation, whereas others continue to carry out some or all of their previous activities and roles.[3] These differences are attributed to various factors such as (1) physiologic (disease severity, exercise tolerance), (2) symptomatic (perception of dyspnea and fatigue), and (3) psychosocial factors (anxiety and depression, internal resources such as self-esteem and self-efficacy, hardiness, well-being, optimism, and mastery).[6–8] The development of well-defined and effective psychosocial interventions is difficult because of the fact that the exact nature of the role of psychosocial factors in functional performance is not well understood. This unclear understanding is probably related to the great diversity in concepts and measures used to explain their influence.[9]

As patients with COPD face multiple challenges of biopsychosocial adjustment in living with the disease, it is very important that health care professionals assess in detail not only physical but also psychosocial stressors occuring at various times in the illness trajectory. They must help patients recognize the factors to which they are adjusting and the strategies promoting effective reactions to those stressors. The choice and the development of psychosocial interventions must aim, on the one hand, at reinforcing the individual's lines of defense and resistance against illness and physical incapacity and, on the other hand, at encouraging the maintenance of many usual activities and roles. In meeting these goals, health care professionals can positively influence the patient's and the family's responses to stressors, functional performance, and coping.

This chapter reviews the general psychosocial impact of COPD in terms of the various problems experienced during the course of the illness, such as gradual losses and changes over time. It then assesses the different psychosocial aspects of the disease, such as changes in activities of daily living, self-perceptions, family interactions, anxiety and depression, and coping. Finally, the appropriate steps in managing psychosocial disorders, including interventions promoting effective coping and adaptation (self-management, rehabilitation/exercise, individualized and group interventions, community resources) and

coping strategies appropriate to use with COPD patients, are discussed.

PSYCHOSOCIAL IMPACT OF COPD

The psychosocial impact of COPD can be defined as the various problems created in all psychosocial aspects of daily life owing to the experience of many personal losses that alter ways of coping. The loss of control over activities of daily living, autonomy, financial status, body image, self-esteem, and interactions with family and friends creates numerous psychosocial life stresses that must be addressed. The trajectory of COPD requires patients and families to consistently modify their activities and lifestyle. Persistent symptoms such as shortness of breath and fatigue in younger adults may precipitate an early retirement or part-time employment, resulting in reduction of financial income. As COPD progresses, the ill person has less and less energy to do his/her usual activities and needs more assistance in managing his/her condition, including transportation, housework, obtaining prescriptions, and buying and cooking food. Roles and responsibilities within the family are changing over time. A decrease in social and family support leads to withdrawal, loneliness, and depression.[10] A comprehensive assessment of all psychosocial aspects of COPD will guide health care professionals in choosing, developing, and implementing psychosocial interventions, allowing patients and families to cope adaptively with the illness.

Life Changes

Daily Living, Lifestyle, and Home Environment

Chronic obstructive pulmonary disease is a devastating illness that gradually, over a period of years, strips or alters the patient's most significant activities and relationships. As the disease and breathlessness progressively become worse, patients' ability to walk, climb stairs, carry parcels, engage in sexual activity, or maintain any kind of physical exertion decreases. They tire easily and require more and more time to recover from any activity. When anxiety and inactivity are added to this situation, then an act as simple as walking down a hall to the bathroom can seem like a day's work.

Graydon and Ross compared oxygen-dependent and non–oxygen-dependent patients with respect to the influence of various symptoms, lung function, mood, and social support on the level of functioning of patients with COPD.[11] In both groups, dyspnea and fatigue had a direct influence on functioning. Both groups also experienced the greatest changes in functioning with respect to recreation, pastimes, and home management. The most frequently expressed mood was tension/anxiety.

The loss of function implies a corresponding loss in the lifestyle of the patients. Socially and professionally active and productive people gradually see these areas of their lives reduced or lost. The implications of these losses are rarely limited to the patient; rather, they affect the whole family. The patients are often unable to replace these activities with others that are perceived to be or, in fact, are equally valuable or pleasant.[12,13]

The progression of the disease often leads to the necessity of modifying the home environment or moving to a more supervised setting. These are difficult decisions for patients and their families and are often financially costly ones. Patients and their families need a great deal of support to explore all of the concrete and emotional issues related to the need for change. We must try to understand patients' values and wishes and how these affect their perception of possible options. Then we can help patients develop a plan for change that responds to their priorities while ensuring their safety and well-being. This means that we must sometimes accept their need to arrive at decisions in their own time and in their own way.

Employment/Work and Financial Burden

The homemaker who had pride in her clean house and her cooking must somehow come to terms with having a less clean house and being displaced in her role by a family member (who is probably less than thrilled with the new role) or by a stranger who is paid to do the work. The truck driver who is no longer able to do the lifting that his job requires may be able for a while to find a more sedentary job, but for how long? These losses have psychological, family, and social impact, as will be discussed.

The financial cost of illness cannot be overestimated. Patients who were earning a salary that supported a certain level of comfort and financial security often find themselves receiving vastly inferior salary insurance, pensions, or social welfare. A dept load that was previously manageable can now be using up financial resources that are necessary for essentials such as rent and food. The decision that someone is no longer fit to work can have enormous consequences, and we should be alert to the possibility that this patient may require financial counseling and, in fact, may have to consider legal processes to manage (eg, bankruptcy). A referral to a social worker is essential for the patient to be informed of the financial resources that could be available. Financial constraints might also be responsible for a lack of stability in the patient's condition. Are they rationing medication or simply not buying it because they cannot afford it? Can they afford a compressor, oxygen, and security bars in the bathroom? We must be alert to these problems to help the patient gain access to needed materials through community organizations or to advocate government and social organizations to work toward filling these unmet needs.

Social Network

Fundamental to the human experience is our need to communicate and belong to a social group. Isolation is one of the worst experiences that a human can endure. One of the effects of advanced COPD is to limit patients' ability to engage in social activities outside the home. In a climate such as Canada's, many patients are essentially prisoners in their homes most of the winter because of their inability to tolerate cold air and wind. In summer, the heat and humidity can be equally limiting. Patients find that they cannot follow their co-workers and friends. They cannot ski, bowl, or play bingo in smoke-filled halls. Relationships become dependent on the telephone or are dropped entirely. This problem is especially critical for patients who live alone, and they are at increased risk of becoming depressed. Treatment plans for patients must take into account the need for social connection of our patients. This issue is discussed in more detail elsewhere.

Chronic obstructive pulmonary disease leads to many losses that increase over the course of the disease. Awareness of these losses can help us be more responsive to the individual and his/her family but can also inform us where we must develop community links to educate and advocate for our client population. It may be necessary to offer special programs within the pulmonary center to meet needs that are specific to that population for which the community does not possess the necessary expertise or client base to incite them to develop one. For example, a pulmonary rehabilitation program is more likely to be developed in a setting in which there are enough patients to justify it and the expertise exists to provide it. Specialized support and stress/management groups might also be most appropriately offered by an expert team in the pulmonary center.

Self-Perceptions

Sense of Control and Personal Integrity

Perception of control and personal integrity can influence functional performance in patients with COPD.[6,14] The Newman systems model defines control as "an intrapersonal component of the hardy personality that interacts with and affects the person's physiologic, socio-cultural, developmental, and spiritual stability."[15] Perception of control strengthens a person's ability to resist or increase resistance to debilitating effects such as symptoms of pulmonary disease, thus promoting adaptation to the illness.[16] Narsavage reported in a group of 124 patients with COPD discharged from hospital following an acute exacerbation that a sense of control could enhance coping with anxiety and shortness of breath by enabling them to anticipate stressors as nonthreatening.[16]

In a recent qualitative study, it was demonstrated that ill individuals face an ongoing challenge of preserving personal integrity, defined as a sense of satisfying wholeness.[6] The two essential features of personal integrity are effectiveness and connectedness. Effectiveness means a sense of being able, expressed through physical being and the perception of competence and involvement through daily activities. Patients with COPD respond to challenges of effectiveness such as maintaining activities through emotional expression, goal setting and trying, and recall of success from past experiences. Connectedness refers to the sense of significant, shared, and meaningful relationships with other people, of which family members are predominant, as well as friends, neighbors, or individuals with whom the person shared similar situations. It seems that patients with COPD experiencing separateness have difficulty in maintaining a sense of connectedness. Familiarity, comfort, shared experiences, understanding of others, and the ability to count on someone else can be sources of encouragement for individuals.

To help patients with COPD develop a sense of control and personal integrity, health care profes-

sionals must work on their motivation as a way of bringing them to identify life stressors and perceive what strategies promote effective reactions and inhibit adverse reactions to these stressors. Assessment can be done through questioning or the use of diaries.[14]

Self-Image

Physical appearance, which is important for everyone regardless of age or sex, can significantly be altered by a chronic illness, such as COPD.[17] The appearance of a barrel chest, swollen ankles, and symptoms of disease such as dyspnea, cough, and sputum production can impair a patient's self-esteem and perceptions of his/her body image.[17] As well, activity intolerance makes the person with COPD unable to spend much time on his/her appearance. Finally, the use of inhalers and oxygen equipment, visual reminders of disease, can lead to feelings of unattractiveness and self-consciousness.[17]

Some patients will attempt to hide their symptoms, visual reminders of disease, or features of their body that have been altered by disease to avoid embarrassment or risk of rejection by others.[18] Frustration with appearance, symptoms, and visual reminders of disease can significantly affect the patient's relationships with others, especially with a spouse. Issues related to sexuality are discussed in Chapter 15. Depression can result in patients who feel physically unattractive.[17]

Health care professionals should assess the patients' self-perception with regard to (1) bodily changes, (2) visual reminders of disease, and (3) symptoms. Helping the patient and his/her family express their thoughts and feelings will encourage them to identify strategies that can be used to enhance their appearance and normalize the changes associated with. If indicated, health care professionals should encourage patients to join a support group.

Self-Efficacy

Self-efficacy is "the belief in one's capabilities to organize and execute action required to manage prospective situations."[19] Simply put, self-efficacy is the individual's perception that he/she is able to perform given actions. Self-efficacy beliefs influence the choices we make, the effort we put into actions, how long we persist in confronting obstacles or failures, and how we feel. They are a reliable predictor of behavior modification. When judging their capabilities, people rely on certain sources of information, such as[20]

1. mastery experience, which depends on the individual's interpretation of previous experiences (successful outcomes such as successful performance in COPD self-management behaviors help to raise self-efficacy, whereas failures lower it);
2. vicarious experience, which refers to the effects of observed action of others or social comparisons with other individuals (peer modeling through self-help groups can be an effective way of enhancing COPD management);
3. verbal persuasion, which involves exposure to verbal judgments made by others (persuasive arguments from health care professionals in regard to management of COPD should aim at small, incremental behavior changes rather than all-or-nothing efforts); and
4. psychological states such as anxiety, stress, arousal, and mood states, which can also have an effect on task performance and subsequently influence efficacy beliefs.

Self-efficacy should be assessed in patients with COPD to predict performance of self-management behaviors and work on patients' motivation and confidence in their capacities.

Self-Esteem

Self-esteem is defined most often as the individual's sense of his/her value or worth or the extent to which a person values, approves of, appreciates, prizes, or likes himself/herself.[21] It means accepting ourselves for who and what we are at any given time in our lives. Low self-esteem leads to self-depreciation and discouragement. One no longer trusts his/her ability to make decisions or effectively cope, consequently leading to a decrease in one's level of self-efficacy and one's performance. Low self-esteem in patients with COPD is related to changes in body image[17] and use of long-term oxygen therapy.[22] In a study of 250 elderly male and female participants, Hunter and colleagues demonstrated that self-esteem did not differ with respect to age, income, education, or living arrangement.[23] However, the low self-esteem group had poorer self-reported health, more pain, more disability, and significantly higher scores on depression, anxiety, and somatization and a more external locus of control. These results resemble what we see clinically in patients with COPD. Health care professionals should question patients about their percep-

tions of self to assist them in redefining the negative idea and, hopefully, improving self-esteem. The questions of interest can be the following[24]:

- Do you have difficulty accepting yourself?
- Do you desperately want to change the way you look?
- Do you think more about your failures than your successes?
- Do you worry a lot that people would not like you if they really knew you?
- Do you feel that everyone is much more competent and confident than you?
- Do you almost always avoid taking on new challenges?
- Are you uncomfortable around successful people?
- Do you avoid making mistakes at all costs?
- Do you worry a lot that you are ineffective and incompetent?

Family Burden

Impact of Disease on Family

Families suffer in many ways when one of their members develops a serious chronic illness.[25] The entire family unit must become the focus of health care professionals. Care-giving responsibilities in the maintenance of the chronically ill person are often identified by the primary caregiver as stressors causing burden. Common problems encountered by families when caring for a chronically ill member have been identified (Table 12–1).[26] To cope with family relationships and changes associated with chronic illness, each member of the family must learn to recognize and use their own personal resources, experiences, knowledge, and skills.[1]

Changes in Roles and Responsibilities

Accepting potential changes in family roles is a major part of adaptation to chronic adaptation.[27] Often domestic roles and responsibilities in families living with COPD need to be reassigned to accommodate the affected family member who has decreased functional capacity.[1] In more severe cases, the healthy spouse must take the role of helping the ill spouse with activities of daily living such as bathing, dressing, or taking medication.[27,28] It seems that one of the most important factors in adjustment to chronic illness such as COPD is the presence of a supportive primary caregiver in the home.[1] For men with COPD, the wife is usually the supportive person

TABLE 12–1 Common Problems Encountered by Families When Caring for a Member with Chronic Illness

Category Characteristic	Specific Problems
Multiple social needs	Lack of transportation
	Inadequate food
	Role changes, etc
	Social isolation (including loneliness and emotional strain)
	Few visitors
	Inability to leave home secondary to need for 7 days/week care needs
	Lack of telephone, etc.
Sexual activity changes	Impotence related to disease, medication
	Feelings of undesirability related to altered body shape, etc
Financial insecurity	Loss of income or health insurance,
	Extraordinary medical bills, etc

Adapted from Stuifbergen.[26]

who, in addition to being a cook and a housekeeper, undertakes the roles of caretaker, decision maker, and finance manager. However, women with COPD seem to experience more stress at home because of their existing central role. Husbands have difficulty assuming the role of caretaker either because of aging, chronic illness, or attribution of the traditional sex role. The number of new roles and associated responsibilities and lack of experience may overwhelm healthy family members and provoke a burden.[1]

Caregiver Burden

According to several authors, caregiver burden can be either physical or psychological.[29,30] Physical burden occurs when the caregiver assumes activities previously performed by the patient. This leaves the healthy caregiver with little time to care for himself/herself or pursue outside activities.[27] Psychological burden or distress occurs within the caregiver when he/she (1) suppresses his/her own needs, thoughts, and feelings, becoming emotionally isolated from the patient; (2) becomes physically and emotionally exhausted, frustrated, and irritable with the patient; and (3) is no longer able to tolerate caring for the patient and becomes neglectful. Miscommunication and tension between the patient and caregiver lead to interactions that provoke attacks of dyspnea in the patient. The unrelieved stress at this point can result in fatigue, loneliness, depression, anxiety, and irritability and can also affect health.[10,27,28,31]

Assessment of Family Interactions and Burden

In cases in which family burden is suspected, the health care professional should assess the roles, responsibilities, and dynamics within the family to understand the underlying causes of burden. Function, communication, and support from one family member to another are key family interactions to be assessed.[32] They should examine and observe the relationships between husband and wife or between child and parent or other caregiver. Patients and families should be asked questions on actual and perceived roles and responsibilities. Expression of satisfaction or disturbances in the family should be encouraged. Assessment of family stressors, family strengths, and family appraisals can also help support family functionning. When burden is identified, the patient and family should be encouraged not to let problems accumulate or overwhelm them. The health care professional should facilitate discussion with patients and their families regarding burden and issues related to disease. He/she may need to speak with family members individually to understand issues and concerns before they are discussed as a group. Throughout these discussions, the health care professional should help family members express their thoughts and feelings in an assertive manner and identify existing solutions to the problems,[31] such as (1) consulting experts, (2) applying for additional home care supports, (3) participating in self-help or advocacy groups, (4) limiting the number of roles undertaken, and (5) planning for outside activities. As COPD is a progressive disease, it is very important that the health care professional continually reassesses burden within the family and helps members identify ways of alleviating or minimizing the level of perceived burden and develop or improve existing strategies and family resources.

EMOTIONAL CONSEQUENCES OF COPD

The emotional consequences of the loss of control over activities of daily living, autonomy, financial status, and self-esteem include irritability, somatic preoccupation, dependency, frustration, and anxiety and depression. As well, reactions to dyspnea, cough, sputum production, and fatigue that accompany COPD can generate anxiety, fear, and depression. These psychological states may, in turn, serve as stimuli, further compromising the patients' physiologic and emotional states. Thus, the close, circular relationship between dyspnea, fatigue, anxiety, and depression makes these phenomena difficult to study.

The following section focuses on the two most devastating emotional consequences of COPD: anxiety and depression.

Anxiety

Prevalence in Patients with COPD

Anxiety and panic are common in patients with COPD. Breathlessness itself provokes anxiety and can make the perception of dyspnea seem more acute, which often results in the patient avoiding even minimal physical activity. The prevalence rates range from 2 to 96%.[33,34] The uncertainty regarding the prevalence of anxiety rate may be attributable to the heterogeneity of the populations or the wide variety of questionnaires used.

Definitions

In the anxiety literature, a distinction has been made between state and trait anxiety.[35] State anxiety refers to an unpleasant emotional arousal in the face of threatening demands or dangers, whereas trait anxiety is conceptualized as the likelihood or predisposition that a person will experience state anxiety in a stressful situation. Spielberger and colleagues also differentiate between anxiety, fear, and panic.[36] Anxiety is an apprehensive anticipation of danger or a stressful situation associated with a feeling of dysphoria or somatic symptoms of tension. Fear is a punctual reaction to a stressful event, whereas panic is an exaggeration of the reaction.

Clinical Presentation

Anxiety is often manifested in various ways, including exaggerated body movements, rapid speech, and physiologic changes such as palpitations, tachycardia, dyspnea, and event sweating. The patient can experience episodes of faintness or difficulty concentrating. In the patient with COPD, anxiety may be triggered by dyspnea; then the anxiety will contribute to further dyspneic episodes. The anxious patient may also develop exaggerated fear such as fear of death and obsessive rumination.

However, there is a distinction to be made between anxiety and fear, which is illustrated by the following story. A man walks down a quiet street and passes a house when, suddenly, a snarling dog charges after him, snapping and growling. The man begins to run as fast as he can, and, finally, after four blocks, the dog abandons the chase and returns home. The man reacted with fear to a situation he perceived as dangerous and called on his flight response to escape the danger. In a similar vein, a patient with COPD has gone to the post office despite being somewhat more short of breath than usual because of a respiratory infection. The wind is stronger than he imagined, and halfway down the block, he becomes more short of breath than he has ever been in his life. He is too short of breath even to speak or call for help. There is no one around to see his distress. He loses control of his bladder and is sure he is going to die. After 20 minutes of leaning against a pole, he regains enough control of his breathing to begin to make his way back home. Our individual was afraid of dying.

Our dog story continues. The same man is walking along the same street and approaching the block where the dog charged him when he remembers the event. He suddenly realizes that the dog may still be loose. He begins to perspire, his heart pounds, his mouth becomes dry, and he begins to shake. When he gets to the corner, rather than advance, he turns right and makes an eight-block detour to avoid the house where the dog was. This is anxiety, a fight/flight response to a thought stimulus. Over time, he may begin to react this way every time he sees a dog. This is an example of a developed phobia. A phobia is an irrational fear response to a real or an imagined stimulus that poses no threat. A few days after the event occurred to our patient with COPD, his respiratory infection has been treated, and he returns to his respiratory baseline and makes a date to meet some friends at a coffee shop. As he begins to dress, he feels more and more short of breath, his heart rate increases, his mouth becomes dry, and he develops a tremor. As soon as he has called his friends to say he is not able to go, he becomes less breathless, and all other symptoms of distress disappear. This too is anxiety, an apprehensive anticipation of danger or stressful situations associated with a feeling of somatic symptoms of tension.

Both of these men have entered the anxiety cycle. Anxious thoughts or images lead to anxious feelings and sensations that, in turn, lead to anxious behaviors. The goal of stress management counseling is to help the patient learn the strategies to help him/her break the anxiety dyspnea cycle.

Furthermore, anxiety in COPD has to be seen in the context of its relationship to dyspnea. Emotionally, patients with COPD describe dyspnea as a fear of suffocating and dying.[37,38] Because physical activity produces dyspnea, anxious patients tend to avoid even realistic tasks. Any dyspnea they experience may be perceived as worse than it actually is because of anxiety. This leads to muscle tension and hyperventilation, which produces inefficient breathing, patterns and impairs gas exchanges. Over a period of weeks, months, or years, this pattern leads to increased anxiety, activity intolerance, physical deconditioning, worsening of cardiovascular and musculoskeletal fitness, and, ultimately, increased dyspnea. In some cases, patients may withdraw altogether, fearful of all activities. This is known as the anxiety dyspnea cycle[39] (Figure 12–1). Controlling anxiety is important when trying to prevent and decrease shortness of breath in patients with COPD.

Assessment

It is essential to the global assessment of the patient with COPD that anxiety and its associated problems be evaluated because of the relationship to morbidity and loss of function. A widely used and validated self-administered questionnaire is the State-Trait Anxiety Inventory (STAI),[36] which has been used extensively in COPD populations and intervention studies.[40,41] Another anxiety questionnaire, the Endler Multidimensional Anxiety Scale (EMAS), has been devel-

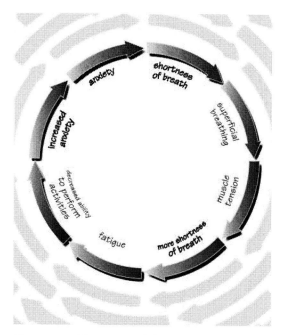

Figure 12–1. The vicious cycle known as the anxiety dyspnea cycle. For many COPD sufferers, emotions, as well as the fear of suffocation can cause shortness of breath. Shortness of breath can lead to anxiety. Anxiety can lead to superficial breathing and muscle tension. This can cause further shortness of breath and anxiety; it can increase fatigue and decrease patient's ability to perform activities. (Adapted from the self-management program "Living Well with COPD©," Module 1: Breathing, Energy Conservation and Relaxation.)

oped to correct the similarity between the STAI and depression measures.[42] The EMAS, however, is a relatively new instrument that has not yet been validated in a COPD population. The health professional's awareness about anxiety represents the initial and most important step in the clinical evaluation.

Although the questionnaires just described to assess anxiety can be used in the clinic, they have been used mostly in research studies. Most of the time, in the clinical setting, the physician or other health professionals of the team will rely essentially on their medical evaluation. Questions should be addressed specifically with respect to the anxiety manifestations just described in the clinical presentation section. It may be of great help to obtain information as well from the spouse or other close family members. If the patient or family reports that his/her functional status is being impaired by anxiety, then treatment possibilities can be discussed, and, if necessary, referral to the appropriate resource can be initiated.

Treatment

Anxiolytics are often used but studies are rare, and it is difficult to favor any one preparation. However, psychosocial support should be favored, and if medication remains an indication for a specific patient, it should be coupled with nonpharmacologic techniques.

The apparent benefits of pulmonary rehabilitation include an exercise program for psychosocial well-being among patients with COPD.[43–45] Based on a recent review on the nature and effects of psychosocial support for patients with COPD (Table 12–2),[46] results from 10 randomized controlled trials were suggestive of the following conclusions:

1. Psychosocial support pertained mostly to relaxation training, with stress management, coping skills training, and cognitive modification as runners-up
2. In virtually all identified studies, significant improvements were observed in outcome variables in the psychosocial domain (eg, self-efficacy, perceived breathlessness, and quality of life)

Although further research is needed on the nature of psychosocial support, we should not underestimate the importance of psychosocial support in managing patients with COPD to contribute to disease control and the patient's well-being.

Depression

Prevalence in Patients with COPD

Irritability and hopelessness are frequent complaints in patients with COPD.[47,48] In a recent systematic review of the literature,[49] depression prevalence rates in patients with moderate to severe COPD ranged from 7 to 42%. The uncertainty regarding the prevalence of depression rate may stem from the heterogeneity of the populations or the measurement properties of the questionnaires used to define depression.[49,50]

The usefulness of most screening questionnaires for depression used in the elderly has been criticized because they include somatic items such as early morning awakening and decreased libido, which may occur as a result of the aging process, with the consequence of overestimating the depression prevalence rate in this population. To overcome the limitations of these questionnaires in the measurement

of depression in the elderly, Yesavage and colleagues developed the Geriatric Depression Scale (GDS) specifically for use with older adults.[51] Using this questionnaire, Lacasse and colleagues found that, in a population of patients with severe, oxygen-dependent COPD, 57% of the patients (95% CI: 47–66) demonstrated significant depressive symptoms; in addition, 18% (95% CI: 12–27) were severely depressed.[52]

Definition

Depression in COPD has been described as being "reactive".[53] In the current classification, depressive symptoms in COPD may range from an "adjustment disorder with depressed mood" when the full criteria for a major depression are not met to "major depression"[54] (Table 12–3). A major depressive episode must be distinguished from a "mood disorder owing to a general medical condition" (such as COPD) as there is no etiologic relationship between depression and COPD. The differential diagnosis between "dysthymic disorder" and "major depression" is difficult because the two disorders share the same symptoms. Both are differentiated on the basis of severity, chronicity, and persistence.[54] In major depression, the depressed mood must be present for most of the days, nearly every day, for a period of at least 2 weeks. Dysthymia must be present for more days than not over a period of at least 2 years. "Major depressive disorder" is diagnosed when at least one major depressive episode has occurred. This classification is important as it may determine the choice of therapy in affected patients.

Clinical Presentation

Signs and Symptoms. Individuals with a depressive episode frequently present with irritability, tearfulness, brooding, obsessive ruminations, anxiety, phobia, and excessive worry over physical health.[54] Depressive disorders in COPD are difficult to recognize in routine clinical practice because symptoms and signs of depression are typically attributed to the disease and often overlooked.[55] The patterns of depression in chronic illnesses may differ from one condition to another. Covino and colleagues found that patients with chronic respiratory diseases are more likely to include low self-esteem, high apathy, and high denial of impulse life as variables in their depression.[56] These features of depression in patients with COPD may bear on the selection of antidepressant drug therapy.

**TABLE 12–2 Core Characteristics of 10 Studies on the Effects of
Psychosocial Support on Psychosocial Outcome Variables for COPD Patients**

First Author (Year)	No. of Patients	Age (yrs)	FEV_1 % Predicted	Psychosocial Intervention	Results
Ashikaga (1980)	E = 25 C = 23	37–82	NR	a. Relaxation, coping b. 6 × 2 h c. Local health care providers d. OP e. Yes	Social disability↓ Perceived chance of improvement↓

Atkins (1984)	E1 = 14
	E2 = 16
	E3 = 16
	C1 = 15
	C2 = 13
		65 ± 8	NR	a. E1 behavior modification
				  E2 cognitive modification
				  E3 combination of E1 and E2
				  C1 attention control
				  C2 no-treatment control
				b. 7 × 2 h
				c. Psychologists
				d. OP
				e. No
					Walking compliance↑
					Exercise tolerance↑
					Quality of well-being↑
					Self-efficacy↑

Blake (1990)	E = 45 C = 49	63	45	a. Stress management, relaxation, cognitive restructuring b. 3 × 2 h c. Nurse d. OP e. Yes	SIP↓
Goldstein (1994)	E = 40 C = 38	66 ± 7	37 ± 10	a. Relaxation b. 20 × 2 h c. Rehabilitation staff d. IP and OP e. No	6MWD↑ Quality of life↑ Dyspnea↓
Lustig (1972)	E = 15 C1 = 15 C2 = 15	NR	NR	a. Relaxation b. 15–20 sessions c. NR d. OP e. No	Vocational activities↑
Prince (1989)	E = 13 C = 18	54–81	(0.3–1.3)*	a. Relaxation, supportive discussions b. 12 × 2 h c. NR d. OP e. No	GHQ↓
Reardon (1994)	E = 10 C = 10	66	67	a. Relaxation, panic control, stress management, symptom control b. 12 × 3 h c. Nurses, physicians d. OP	Dyspnea↓

(continues ...)

Ries (1995)	E = 57 C =62	62 ± 7	44 ± 11	a. Relaxation, coping training b. 12 × 4 h, plus monthly reinforcement	Dyspnea↓ Fatigue↓ Self-efficacy↑
Strijbos (1996)	E1 = 15 E2 = 15	61 ± 6	42 ± 12	a. Relaxation, education b. 24 × 2 h c. Physiotherapist, respiratory nurse d. Hospital setting and OP e. No	Well-being↑
Wijklstra	E1 = 15 E2 = 12 C = 15	62 ±5	44	a. Relaxation b. 12 × 0.5 h c. Multidisciplinary team d. hospital and OP e. No	Quality of life↑

Values given as (range) or mean ± SD unless otherwise stated.

*Value measured as L.

E = experimental group; C = control group; NR = not reported; a = nature of psychosocial intervention; b = duration of intervention; c = providers of psychosocial support; d = setting; e = partners involved?; OP = outpatient; IP = inpatient; SIP = Sickness Impact Profile; 6MWD = 6-minute walking distance; GHQ = General Health Questionnaire; ↑ = significant improvement; ↓ = significant reduction.

TABLE 12–3 DSM-IV Diagnostic Criteria for Major Depressive Episode and Dysthymic Disorder

Major Depressive Episode

A. Five (or more) of the following symptoms have been present during the same 2-week period and represent a change from previous functioning; at least one of the symptoms is either (1) depressed mood or (2) loss of interest or pleasure.

Note: Do not include symptoms that are clearly due to a general medical condition.

1. Depressed mood most of the day, nearly every day, as indicated by either subjective report (eg, feels sad or empty) or observation made by others (eg, appears tearful)

2. Markedly diminished interest or pleasure in all, or almost all, activities most of the day, nearly every day (as indicated by either subjective account or observation made by others)

3. Significant weight loss when not dieting or weight gain (eg, a change of more than 5% of body weight in a month) or a decrease or increase in appetite nearly every day

4. Insomnia or hypersomnia nearly every day

5. Psychomotor agitation or retardation nearly every day (observable by others, not merely subjective feelings of restlessness or being slowed down)

6. Fatigue or loss of energy nearly every day

7. Feelings of worthlessness or excessive or inappropriate guilt (which may be delusional) nearly every day (not merely self-reproach or guilt about being sick)

8. Diminished ability to think or concentrate, or indecisiveness, nearly every day (either by subjective account or as observation by others)

9. Recurrent thoughts of death (not just fear of dying), recurrent suicidal ideation without a specific plan, or a suicide attempt or a specific plan for committing suicide

(continues over...)

TABLE 12–3 DSM-IV Diagnostic Criteria for Major Depressive Episode and Dysthymic Disorder

Dysthymic Disorder

A. Depressed mood for most of the day, for more days than not, as indicated either by subjective account or observation by others, for at least 2 years.

B. Presence, while depressed, of two (or more) of the following:
   1. Poor appetite or overeating
   2. Insomnia or hypersomnia
   3. Low energy or fatigue
   4. Low self-esteem
   5. Poor concentration or difficulty making decisions
   6. Feelings of hopelessness

C. During the 2-year period of the disturbance, the person has never been without the symptoms in criteria A and B for more than 2 months at a time.

D. No major depressive episode has been present during the first 2 years of the disturbance.

Associated Features. Recent evidence demonstrates that depressive symptoms are associated with substantial impairments in psychological, physical, and social functioning.[57] In a recent study of depression in severe COPD, Lacasse and colleagues found profound impairments in all domains of health-related quality of life measured by the 36-Item Short-Form Health Survey (SF-36).[52] The scores were lower in the domains related to physical function. Depression scores correlated with seven of the eight domains of the SF-36. Most correlations were moderate.

Depressive symptoms are also associated with a significant increase in the cost of general medical services.[58] In this 4-year prospective study conducted in Seattle, the increase in cost was seen for every component of health care costs and was not accounted for by an increase in specialty mental health care. The increase in health care costs remained significant after adjusting for differences in age, sex, and chronic medical illness. In an adult population of patients presenting with a primary major depressive disorder, a randomized trial of a depression-specific intervention was followed by a significant improvement in emotional, mental, and social functioning when compared to the usual care.[57] Whether the results of this trial can be generalized to older patients with comorbid conditions such as COPD remains an important and unresolved issue.

Physiologic and Psychological Causes. Although the underlying pathology is initially confined to the lungs, the associated physical deconditioning and the emotional responses to chronic respiratory disease contribute greatly to the resulting morbidity. Increased shortness of breath leads to inactivity and consequent cardiorespiratory and muscular deconditioning, which, in turn, leads to further inactivity, social isolation, fear of dyspnea, and depression.[59] In addition, patients with COPD experience losses in several areas of their life. They often feel useless, have reduced sexual activities, depend on proxies for personal care, and lose interest in future projects. In reaction, many will regress as they focus their energy on a pathologic sick role.

Depression in patients with COPD is more prevalent than depression in an age-matched general population.[52] However, a number of confounding factors may account for this. These include lack of social support characterizing the elderly and chronically ill individuals, past psychiatric and medical history, and low socioeconomic status (72% of our patients had not progressed beyond elementary school). Of note, the findings from community-based studies relating socioeconomic status as a risk factor for depression are mixed.[60] Whether COPD is an independent risk factor for depression largely depends on the selection of the "control group." For instance, depression may not be more prevalent in COPD than in chronic heart failure or rheumatoid arthritis as we hypothesize that depression is more related to the chronicity of a disabling disorder than to COPD itself.

The contribution of chronic hypoxemia and long-term oxygen therapy to depressive symptoms is controversial. On the one hand, several authors have investigated the relationship between hypoxia and neuropsychological function.[61,62] A closer look at this older literature reveals that "neuropsychological function" then defined performances such as abstracting ability, perceptual-motor integration, and coordination. Depression was not addressed in these studies. On the other hand, whether long-term oxygen therapy, in addition to the chronic disease itself, contributes to depression is unknown. It is often suggested that long-term oxygen therapy is a limiting factor in patients' rehabilitation as it is likely to reduce their mobility and their opportunities of social interactions. Both the Nocturnal Oxygen Therapy Trial[63] and the British Medical Research Council[64] trials were conducted before the development of disease-specific quality-of-life questionnaires most likely to capture small but important changes in quality of life and emotional function. Once these trials had demonstrated increased survival from low-flow domiciliary oxygen use in hypoxemic patients with COPD, oxygen therapy became a standard in the management of the disease, with no opportunity to randomize again hypoxemic patients with COPD to receive or not receive long-term oxygen to demonstrate improvement in quality of life. Nevertheless, we did not find any clear relation between depression scores and length of time since the introduction of long-term oxygen therapy.[52]

Impact of Personality Type. Baseline personality will often modulate the way of coping with the disease adopted by the patient with COPD. Those with a dependent personality will often regress and impose a large amount of physical care on their proxies. Those with an anxious personality may become phobic and require their family members to be in continuous attendance. Also, those who have a controlling personality may dictate their will to their family as they lose the ability to perform for themselves daily-life activities. Consequently, the spouse often assumes the social, financial, and family roles, placing the partner under stress and high risk of depression.

Assessment

Use of Case-Finding Instruments for Depression. No laboratory findings that are diagnostic of depression have been identified. The increase in health care providers' awareness about depression represents the initial step in the diagnosis of the disease. Those less familiar with psychiatric disorders often rely on screening questionnaires to identify high-risk patients. Mulrow

and colleagues systematically evaluated the usefulness of case-finding instruments for identifying patients with major depression in primary care settings.[65] Their objective was to familiarize providers with the advantages and disadvantages of nine of these instruments (Table 12–4).

All are written at an easy or average reading level. Almost all can be self-administered within 5 minutes. The overall sensitivity of the questionnaires was 84%, and the specificity was 72%.[65] The authors could not find any significant difference between the instruments. The interpretation of this study, however, was limited in that study samples had to have been composed of primary care patients attending clinic. Those with specific conditions were excluded from the analysis. From the instruments presented in Table 12–4, the Beck Depression Inventory and the Zung Self-Assessment Depression Scale were moderately sensitive and specific in detecting depression in elderly medical inpatients.[66]

To explain the heterogeneity that van Ede et al found in the prevalence rates of depression reported in the 10 studies that met the inclusion criteria of their review, the authors argued that "the most important confounder is an artefact of depression measurement due to an overlap between symptoms of the somatic illness and those indicative of depression."[49] The GDS is a 30-yes/no-item questionnaire that minimizes questions about health concerns. We have successfully used this questionnaire in our clinical research of depression in COPD.[52] It represents a reliable and valid depression screening scale for elderly populations.[67] No special training is required to administer the questionnaire. A score ≥ 11 out of 30 is associated with a sensitivity of 84% and a specificity of 95% for the diagnosis of significant depressive symptoms[67]; a score ≥ 20 out of 30 indicates severe depression. The original 30-item scale has been shortened to the GDS Short Form, which consists of 15 items. This version is even more practical in the clinical or home setting. For clinical purposes, a score of greater than 5 points is suggestive of depression and should warrant a follow-up interview. Scores greater than 10 are almost always depression.

It is important to emphasize that these questionnaires are screening, not diagnostic instruments. The objective of the questionnaires is to enable the clinician to decrease the number of individuals who need more intensive diagnostic interviewing while missing the lowest number of significant depressions

TABLE 12–4 Characteristics of Case-Finding Instruments Used to Detect Depression in Primary Care Settings

Instrument	Scope	Number of Items*	Response Format	Time Frame of Questions
BDI	Depression specific	21	4 statements of symptom severity per item	Today
CES-D	Depression specific	20	4 frequency ratings: less than 1 day to most or all days	Past week
GHQ	Psychiatric illness (several versions)	28	4 frequency ratings: not at all to much more than usual	Past few weeks
HSCL	Multiple versions and multiple components with depression category	25	4 frequency ratings: not at all to much more than usual	Past week
MOS-D	Depression specific	8	Frequency ratings: same format as CES-D	Past week
ID	Depression specific	15	2 items, yes or no; 3 statements of normal, overt, or covert symptomatology	Recently
PRIME-MD	Multiple components with depression category	2	Yes or no	Past month
SDDS-PC	Multiple components with depression category	5	Yes or no	Past month
SDS	Depression specific	20	4 frequency ratings: little of the time to most of the time	Recently
GDS	Depression specific	30	Yes or no	Last week

Instrument	Score Range	Usual Cutpoint†	Literacy Level‡	Administration Time (min)	Monitor Severity or Response
BDI	0–63	10: mild, 20: moderate, 30: severe	Easy	2–5	Yes
CES-D	0–60	16	Easy	2–5	Yes
GHQ	0–28	4	Easy	5–10	Yes
HSCL	25–100	43	Average	2–5	Yes
MOS-D	0–1 (logistic regression)	0.06	Average	< 2	Yes
ID	0–15	10	Easy	2–5	Unknown
PRIME-MD	0–2	1	Average	< 2	Unknown
SDDS-PC	0–4	2	Easy	< 2	Unknown
SDS	25–100 (sum/80 × 100)	50: mild, 60: moderate, 70: severe	Easy	2–5	Yes
GDS	0–30	≥ 11: significant, ≥ 20: severe	Easy	5–10	Yes
Short-Form GDS	0–15	> 5: suggestive, > 10: severe	Easy	2–5	Yes

*Item numbers for the PRIME-MD and SDDS-PC refer to depression questions only; item numbers for the HSCL refer to depression plus anxiety questions.

†Cutpoint is the number at or above which the test is considered positive.

‡Easy = third- to fifth-grade reading level; average = sixth- to ninth- grade reading level.

BDI = Beck Depression Inventory; CES-D = Center for Epidemiologic Studies Depression Screen; GHQ = General Health Questionnaire; HSCL = Hopkins Symptoms Checklist; MOS-D = Medical Outcomes Study Depression Screen; ID = Popoff Index of Depression; PRIME-MD = Primary Care Evaluation of Mental Disorders; SDDS-PC = Symptom Driven Diagnostic System-Primary Care; SDS = Zung Self-Assessment Depression Scale; GDS = Geriatric depression Scale.

Modified from Mulrow, et al.[65]

TABLE 12–5 Effect of the Prevalence of Depression on the Number of Diagnostic Interviews in Two Hypothetical Cohorts of 100 Patients with COPD

	Prevalence of Depression	Number of Interviews Conducted after a Positive Screening Questionnaire*		Missed Cases of Depression
		Questionnaire Was Accurate (true positive)	Questionnaire Was Not Accurate (false positive)	
High-risk patients (eg, patients with severe oxygen-dependent COPD)	20%	17	24	3
Low-risk patients (eg, ambulatory patients with moderate COPD)	5%	4	29	1

*The sensitivity and specificity of the screening questionnaire are assumed to be 85% and 70%, respectively.

possible.[65] Table 12–5 is an illustration of the effect of the prevalence of depression in different cohorts of patients with COPD on the number of interviews to be conducted to diagnose depression, assuming that the sensitivity and specificity of the screening questionnaire are 85% and 70%, respectively. The higher the prevalence of depression, the more efficient are the diagnostic interviews. A strategy to further decrease the number of diagnostic interviewing would be to consider patients having the highest scores on the questionnaire (low sensitivity but high specificity) as being really depressed and to refer for diagnostic interviews those scoring in the mid-range (intermediate sensitivity and specificity). Those scoring below a given threshold (high sensitivity, low specificity) would be considered as not depressed and would not be further investigated.

Predictors of Depression. In the Lacasse and colleagues prevalence study of depression in severe COPD, none of the demographic and clinical characteristics were clearly correlated with depression scores.[52] In addition, mean depression scores were not different in males versus females (15 ± 6 versus 13 ± 6, respectively; p = .05), in those benefiting from a portable oxygen system versus those who did not (14 ± 6 versus 14 ± 6, respectively; p = .89), and in those living with their spouse and those who cannot count on a spouse (12 ± 6 versus 14 ± 6; p = .10).

Treatment

Pharmacologic Therapy. Pharmacologic therapy must be considered when major depression is recognized or when the dysthymic patient does not respond to nonpharmacologic interventions. The ideal antidepressant for use in the typical elderly patient with COPD would have a low side-effect profile, a short half-life, and no active metabolites.[55] It would provoke few drug interactions and could be given once or twice a day.[55,68] Also, the choice of an antidepressant drug also depends on the pattern of depression.

The patterns of depression in chronic respiratory diseases described by Covino and colleagues suggested that the selected antidepressant drug should not include sedation as a potential side effect.[56] The pharmacologic characteristics of selected antidepressant drugs currently used in elderly patients are summarized in Table 12–6. Some of the new highly selective serotonin reuptake inhibitors, a class of antidepressant drugs very active in improving depressive symptoms and anxiety, meet the above-mentioned requirements of an antidepressant drug to be used in elderly patients.

The most important potential side effect to consider in patients with severe COPD is respiratory depression. No report on the effect of the new selective serotonin reuptake inhibitors is currently available. The antidepressant drugs are, however, a class of medication with little effect on ventilatory drive.[69] Other concerns with antidepressant drugs in patients with COPD are related to their potential cardiovascular side effects. The results of two studies in depressive patients and healthy men provided strong evidence that therapeutic doses of paroxetine lack any important hemodynamic and electrophysiologic effects.[43]

Important Considerations for Clinicians. Depression in COPD often remains underdiagnosed and under-

TABLE 12–6 Antidepressant Drug Therapy in COPD:
Summary of the Published Randomized Controlled Trials

Study	Study Design	Intervention	Measurement Instruments	Results
Gordon et al[24]	Randomized double-blind crossover trial (n = 6*)	Desipramine vs placebo (8-wk treatment periods)	Depression: Beck Depression Inventory and Zung Self-Rating Depression Scale	Both treatments (desipramine and placebo) led to a significant improvement in depression scores
Light et al[25]	Randomized double-blind crossover trial (n = 9*)	Doxepine vs placebo (6-wk treatment periods)	Exercise capacity: 12-min walk test Depression: Beck Depression Inventory Anxiety: Spielberger's State-Trait Anxiety Inventory	No significant differences in either exercise capacity or psychological scores was observed
Borson et al[26]	Randomized double-blind parallel groups trial (n = 30*)	Nortriptyline (n = 13) vs placebo (n = 17) (12-wk duration)	Exercise capacity: 12-min walk test; Dyspnea: Pulmonary Function Status and Dyspnea Questionnaire Depression: Hamilton Depression Rating Scale Anxiety: Patient-Rated Anxiety Scale	Nortriptyline treatment was accompanied by improvements in anxiety, certain respiratory symptoms, and day-to-day function; physiologic measures remained unaffected. The clinical significance of these changes is unknown (see text)
Ström et al[27]	Randomized double-blind parallel groups trial (n = 26*)	Protriptyline (n = 14) vs placebo (n = 12) (12-wk duration)	Dyspnea: 6-point scale developed for the purpose of the study Quality of life: Sickness Impact Profile Anxiety and depression: Mood Adjective Checklist; Hospital Anxiety and Depression Scale	No significant difference in the quality-of-life questionnaire scores in either of the two treatment groups; neither protriptyline nor placebo had any impact on the dyspnea score

*Number of patients who completed the trial.

treated. Several factors may explain this situation. First, it is likely that depression remains undetected or overlooked in most patients[55] as it is still often considered an inherent part of the "COPD" syndrome. Perhaps the most important finding of the Lacasse and colleagues study is that depression was undertreated in this group of patients.[52] This situation is not unique to depressed patients with COPD. Redelmeier and colleagues recently provided evidence that in elderly patients with chronic medical diseases, unrelated disorders are indeed undertreated.[70] The authors suggested that, among other factors, time constraints, communication problems, patients' preferences, and the priorities of the specialist involved in the care of the patient may explain the difficulty of addressing more than one problem effectively in any patient.

Second, clinicians may either fear or discount the efficacy of using psychoactive drugs in elderly patients with advanced chronic respiratory failure. Third, and even more importantly, previous trials of antidepressant drug therapy in depressed patients with COPD did not demonstrate significant treatment effect on depression or quality of life (see Table 12–6).[71,72] However, the validity of most health status measure instruments used in these trials was not clearly ascertained beforehand,[50] and those that were used often consisted of generic instruments unlikely to detect small but clinically important changes over time.[73] Examining the efficacy of antidepressant drug therapy in COPD-associated depression represents an area of future research, especially for those patients too handicapped to actively engage in a respiratory rehabilitation program, a treatment modality now known to improve important domains of quality of life in patients with COPD.[43]

Clinicians caring for patients with COPD must have a high level of suspicion regarding the diagnosis of depression. Not only do these patients have COPD, they also live its consequences. Reduced interest for daily-life activities, discouragement, sadness, hopelessness, and loss of appetite and sleep are all symptoms that should prompt an investigation.

Various nonpharmacologic treatment therapies will be discussed in the next section.

COPING WITH COPD

Earlier in this book, COPD was identified as a major contributor to disability, poor quality of life, and death among patients with COPD. Additionally, COPD was described as a respiratory disease characterized by progressive airflow obstruction and symptoms such as cough, dyspnea or breathlessness, and fatigue. Chronic illness such as COPD causes multiple problems of living or stresses for the patient and his/her family. Strauss and his associates provided a framework to help understand the continuous and multiple problems or stressors associated with a chronic illness such as COPD:

1. Prevention of medical crises and their management once they occur
2. Control of symptoms
3. Carrying out of prescribed regimens and the management of problems attendant on carrying out the regimens
4. Prevention of or living with social isolation
5. Adjustment to changes in the course of the disease trajectory
6. Attempts at normalizing both interaction with others and style of life
7. Funding—finding the money necessary to pay for treatments or to survive, despite loss of employment
8. Confronting attendant psychological, marital, and familial problems[74]

In this section of the chapter, we focus on the stressors experienced by patients with COPD, appraisal,

and coping as factors that can affect patient self-management and health outcomes.

Associated Stressors

Numerous stressors are experienced by patients with COPD.[31,75–77] The stressors associated for individuals living with COPD are outlined in Table 12–7. Stress is a natural part of everyday life.[78,79] Stressors can be physiologic, psychological, or social in nature. Psychological stressors have a cognitive aspect as the individual must appraise an event or situation as problematic or threatening. Social stressors arise from changes or disruptions to individual social systems. So although stress and problems are an inevitable part of living, and even more so when living with a chronic illness like COPD, it is the management of these or the coping that makes the difference in adaptational outcome.[78,80] Indeed, the ongoing, effective coping and management of stressors and the processes that enable the individual to function at a perceived maximum capacity and high level of life satisfaction despite the struggles are important aspects of health toward which our activities as health professionals are directed.[81–84]

The patient and his/her family may also be dealing with a number of other life events not related to the COPD, which may potentially or actually be disruptive to them and also exacerbate the patient's COPD. Major life events can be a significant source of additional burden. In the clinical setting, it has been our experience that frequent hospitalizations often correlate with major, positive or negative, life stressors such as a change in living condition (ie, moving) or death in the family. Indeed, there has been extensive life events research on particular health outcomes such as depression, cancer, and cardiovascular disease.[78] In the clinical setting, it is important not only to screen for major life events but also to assess adequacy of social support and resources and the impact on COPD and the caregivers.

Definition of Coping

Coping is a process by which individuals learn to manage the cognitive, emotional, and physical stressors or problems. Coping is reflective of the individual's ability to adapt to an illness and is reflected in his/her self-management strategies.[85] Lazarus and Folkman believe that it is important to distinguish between coping that is directed at managing the specific problem causing the distress and coping that is

TABLE 12–7 Perceived Stressors by Patients with COPD

Author	Perceived Stressors
Graydon and Ross, 1995; McSweeney et al, 1982	Anxiety
Donaldson et al, 1999; Koskela et al, 1989	Cold/humidity
Anderson, 1995; Gift and Austin, 1992; McSweeney et al, 1982	Depression
Tarzain, 2000	Death and dying
Anderson, 1995; Gift and Austin, 1992; Graydon and Ross, 1995; Jonsdottir, 1998; Woo, 2000	Dyspnea
Hahn, 1989	Body image—changes in appearance
Carrier and Janson-Bjerklie, 1986	Environmental pollution
Grayon and Ross, 1995; Kline Leidy and Haase, 1996; Small and Lamb, 1999; Woo, 2000	Fatigue
Thorsdottir et al, 2001	Food consumption—malnutrition
Jonsdottir, 1998; Kline Leidy and Haas, 1996	Maintaining functional ability Household maintenance Ability to exercise and move without limitation
Small and Graydon, 1993	Oxygen equipment
Chalmers, 1984; McSweeney et al, 1982	Powerlessness—in areas such as parenting, work, and management of the household
Chalmers, 1984; Graydon and Ross, 1995; Jonsdottir, 1998; Kline Leidy and Haase, 1996	Reduced ability to participate in recreational activities Family activities Activities with friends who smoke

directed at regulating the emotional response to the problem. The former is referred to as problem-focused coping and the latter as emotion-focused coping. In general, emotion-focused forms of coping are more likely to occur when there has been an appraisal that nothing can be done, whereas problem-focused forms of coping are more probable when such conditions are appraised as amenable to change.[78] Although individual strategies have often been categorized as emotion or problem solving focused, Miller noted that many patients are on problem-focused (approach strategies) and emotion-focused (avoidance strategies) continuums, using combinations of different strategies.[80] Miller suggested five criteria for effective coping:
1. Uncomfortable feelings (anxiety, fear, grief, guilt) contained
2. Hope generated
3. Self-esteem enhanced
4. Relationships with others maintained
5. State of wellness (self-actualized well-being) maintained or improved[80]

Effective mobilization of coping resources is moderated by the processes of appraisal.[78] According to Lazarus and Folkman, there are three types of stressful appraisal:
1. Harm/loss refers to damage the person has already sustained
2. Threat refers to anticipated injury or losses
3. Challenge refers to events that hold the possibility for mastery or gain[78]

The coping strategies used in any particular situation are based on the person's appraisal of the situation or event. This is implicit also in Bandura's work and his theory of self-efficacy.[19] Bandura maintained that efficacy expectancies are principal determinants of behavior: "People fear and tend to avoid threatening situations they believe exceed their coping skills, whereas they get involved in activities and behave assuredly when they judge themselves capable of handling situations that would otherwise be intimidating."[19] Research pertaining to this field is discussed in the next section of this chapter. Lipowski made similar points in his discussion of coping styles and strategies and illness.[86] He contended that coping strategies are directly related to the meaning the individual ascribes to his illness or disability. For example, if illness is viewed as a challenge, then Lipowski theorized that the disease or disability is seen to be mastered, much as previous challenges in that person's life were mastered. The coping strategies or behavior would include seeking medical advice, cooperation, information seeking, finding substitute gratification, and problem solving. If the illness is viewed as an invasion by hostile internal or external forces, Lipowski theorized that the patient would be more anxious, fearful, or angry, feeling helpless, in denial, and displaying regressive dependencies.[86]

Coping Assessment

It is the responsibility of every health professional involved in the care of the patient with COPD to assess the patient and family's perceptions, feelings, and overall effectiveness in dealing with the various aspects of his/her illness. We are also in the privileged position of being able to help patients expand their coping repertoire with respect to COPD. Instruments to evaluate coping in a research context or to validate clinical impressions are limited. The Jalowiec Coping Scale (JCS) has been developed in the general population and used in various research studies involving patients with COPD. In the research setting, the Revised JCS has been found to have construct validity and internal consistency.[87,88] The Revised JSC also offers a framework for the health professional in terms of identifying the overall coping style and the range of coping strategies a patient has implemented specifically with respect to his/her COPD. One important criticism is that it lacks the sensitivity to measure coping changes in patients with COPD. At the present time, the research makes the use of any scale difficult in clinical practice.

Coping Approach and Strategies

There is evidence to suggest that taking an overall problem-focused or solving approach to the stressors associated with chronic illness results in more effective coping than emotion-focused or avoidance strategies. That is, research is attempting to describe the relationship between specific coping strategies to health outcomes. For example, in a recent study by Narsavage and Weaver, a relationship was demonstrated among the use of problem-focused coping strategies, coping, and exercise ability.[89] Patients who employed problem-focused coping strategies were better able to perform exercise. In a more recent study, Buchi and colleagues studied the effect of rehabilitation on forced expiratory volume in 1 second (FEV_1), life satisfaction, and health among participants in a rehabilitation program.[90] What is salient here is that these researchers found that greater improvements in the percentage of FEV_1 predicted correlated with a higher initial quality-of-life score and with lower ratings of wishful thinking as a coping strategy. That is, patients who employed wishful thinking (an avoidance type of coping strategy) were less likely to observe an improvement in FEV_1 and quality-of-life scores.[90] Similar support is found in the literature dealing with other chronic illnesses and coping.

Scharloo and colleagues maintained that specific coping strategies are predictive of mental health, physical and social function, frequency of visits to outpatient clinics, and strength of prescribed medication.[91] Passive coping strategies were associated with worse mental health. Social support seeking strategies were associated with overall poor functioning. Frequent use of distraction was associated with use of milder pulmonary medications and fewer outpatient visits.[91] Weisman and Worden studied 120 patients coping with newly diagnosed cancer.[92] Coping behaviors or strategies included seeking more information (rational inquiry), sharing concerns (mutuality), making light of the situation (affected reversal), doing something else (distraction), taking action regarding the problem (confronting), seeking direction (cooperative compliance), and blaming self. Weisman and Worden concluded that good copers used confrontation, redefinition of the problem (accepting it and looking for positive aspects), and compliance with authority. Poor copers used suppression, passivity, and tension-reducing measures (such as drinking and drugs). Weisman further characterized effective copers as confronting reality, adopting a problem-solving and decision-making process, seeking help, and accepting support.[93]

Traditionally, COPD research on coping has documented the coping strategies of patients. Researchers have described a number of coping strategies that have been employed by patients with COPD and used in the successful management of the disease. This is outlined in Table 12–8. Much of the initial work in this area was qualitative in nature. Many of the coping strategies first described by early researchers such as Barstow are still used by patients

TABLE 12–8 List of Coping Strategies Identified in the Literature

Author	Coping Strategies
Barstow, 1974	Simplification of activities of daily living Pacing activities
Chalmers, 1984	Cognitive strategies Behavioral strategies Expressive strategies or the expression of one's emotions

Carrier and Janson-Bjerklie, 1986	Preventing or controlling dyspnea
	   Immediate strategies (management of acute episodes)
	   Long-term strategies (prevention of future occurrences)

Fagerhaugh, 1986	Planning activities Moving to a location where there is need to use less energy to travel around Asking for assistance Avoiding emotionally charged situations
Parsons, 1990	Emotion-focused coping
Janelli et al, 1991	Blaming others Letting someone else solve the problem
McBride, 1993	Acceptance Determination
Small and Graydon, 1993	Positive thinking Ignoring the future Making positive comparisons Maintaining optimism and hope Accepting illness
Narsavage and Weaver, 1994	Problem solving
Kline Leidy and Haase, 1996	Planning tasks or activities Pacing Using assistive devices to complete tasks (eg, wheelchairs)
Small and Lamb, 1996	Two types of coping strategies were used to manage fatigue Problem focused (ie, energy conservation, use, and restoration) Emotion focused (positive thinking, acceptance of physical limitations, distration and normalizing)
Herbert and Gregor, 1997	Taking medications Trying to maintain a sense of humor Trying to maintain a normal lifestyle Praying Trying to handle things one step at a time
Jonsdottir, 1998	Optimism about one's physical function Isolation to prevent exacerbations of dyspnea Acceptance of one's physical restrictions
Frey, 2000	Optimistic thinking
Scharloo et al, 2000	Avoiding the problem Seeking social support Fostering reassuring thoughts Expressing emotions
Nault et al, 2000	Energy conservation Action plan Pursed-lip breathing Physical exercise

and continue to be taught to patients by health professionals within the context of educational, rehabilitation, and self-management programs.[94–96] Nault and her colleagues carried out a qualitative, 1-year follow-up study of 27 participants in the self-management program "Living Well with COPD©."[97] The participants reported that among the strategies taught in the program, the following were most useful and integrated in their everyday life: (1) energy conservation, (2) action plan, (3) pursed-lip breathing, and (4) physical exercise.

Interventions Promoting
Effective Coping and Adaptation

A number of programs and interventions are effective in improving use of coping strategies and helping patients and their families adapt to COPD. These programs and intervention are presented in the following section.

Fostering a Collaborative Relationship between the Patient and the Health Professional

Self-management and effective strategies are learned and, as such, are contingent on the health professional's structuring learning experiences that are directed toward meeting the needs, goals, and problem-solving styles of patients and their families.[98] Such a relationship encourages patients with COPD to take responsibility in the management of their illness. Thorne proposed that the "rules" that govern relationships between patients and health professionals should be different for acute and chronic illnesses. Adopting sick role dependency is not adaptive in chronic illness, where medical expertise cannot offer a cure. Patients with COPD should be encouraged to "take charge," learn various self-management strategies, and be the "experts" of their illness.

Enhancing self-management through learning is one way of helping the patient with COPD cope not only with the symptoms but also with the multiple physical and psychosocial problems resulting from having this chronic illness. The person with COPD and his/her family must learn new ways to effectively self-manage the consequences of the disease. Self-management of COPD requires the integration in day-to-day life of numerous long-term abilities and skills including smoking cessation, proper use of medications, exercise, energy conservation, anxiety control, healthy life habits, and adequate oxygenotherapy. Preserving or gaining a sense of control and

personal integrity by actively involving themselves o the disease management process and resisting the debilitating effects of COPD can promote patients' efficient coping skills. Increasing the level of self-efficacy can orient the coping of patient and family toward the performance and maintenance of desired self-management behaviors.

Patient Education Directed Toward Self-Management

Patient education directed toward self-management is a central component of pulmonary rehabilitation programs, and the positive impact in patients with COPD has been recognized by the scientific community through these programs.[43,99] However, education seems not to be a sufficient component of pulmonary rehabilitation that can improve the well-being of patients with COPD. Emery and colleagues evaluated the effects of exercise and education on physiologic functioning, psychological well-being, and cognitive functioning among 79 patients with COPD.[100] Subjects were randomly assigned to (1) an exercise training, education, and stress management group; (2) an education and stress management group; and (3) a waiting list group during a 10-week intervention period. The participants in the exercise training group experienced changes not observed in the education or waiting group list, including improved endurance, reduced anxiety, and improved cognitive performance. Only one study examined the effect of education on patients' coping skills, and the results unfortunately showed no benefit.[101] These results suggest that education alone may not be sufficient. However, in a recent randomized clinical trial combined with a qualitative study done in 191 patients with moderate to severe COPD, the net effects of "Living Well with COPD©," including a nonobligatory exercise component, were patients' acquisition and maintenance of new skills and help strategies in activities of daily living,[102] reduction in the use of health care services,[103] and an improvement in health status.[104]

Pulmonary Rehabilitation/Exercise Training

Exercise training in pulmonary rehabilitation is associated with improved use of coping strategies. The effect of exercise training and pulmonary rehabilitation has been discussed in detail in Chapter 11. Exercise training enhances coping with COPD in the following ways:

- It increases the physical stamina and provides the needed reinforcement to cope with physical activity such as activities of daily living and walking by facilitating breathing (ie, reducing dyspnea).
- It decreases anxiety. Dyspnea, dyspnea-related anxiety, and exercise performance have been shown to improve after exercise training in patients with COPD.[105] It is speculated that the procedure of gradually increasing exercise in the presence of specially trained medical personnel leads to a decrease in unrealistic fear of activity and dyspnea. Participants in such a program become "desensitized" to the anxiety associated with activity; therefore, coping with activity is also enhanced.[106]
- There is some evidence of possible cognitive benefits among patients with COPD participating in exercise rehabilitation.[101] In the study referred to earlier, Emery found that the cognitive assessments conducted before and after the exercise intervention period improved significantly on a measure of verbal fluency, involving so-called executive cognitive functions that reflect self-control and self-monitoring. Therefore, this may also have an impact on a patient's overall coping ability.
- It possibly decreases depression. Little is known about the nature and the efficacy of psychological/psychosocial interventions in patients with COPD. Respiratory rehabilitation has gained wide acceptance in the management of COPD as its effectiveness in improving important domains of quality of life was recently recognized in several randomized trials.[43] However, little is known about the nature and efficacy of psychological interventions in patients with COPD. Lacasse and colleagues addressed this issue in a systematic review of the literature conducted to assist physicians and allied health professionals who prescribe rehabilitation and those who allocate resources to promote more widespread availability of this modality for patients with COPD. Depression was never directly addressed in these trials. We can hypothesize that the participation in a pulmonary rehabilitation program would help diminish depression. Through the reduction of dyspnea and improvement in function (activities of daily living) and ambulation, the graduate of such a program would feel less helpless and socially isolated and experience greater self-efficacy with respect to his/her COPD and enhanced physical vitality.

Individualized Interventions

Mind/Body Medicine Techniques: Relaxation, Progressive Muscle Relaxation, and Imagery. Relaxation, imagery, yoga, biofeedback, positive self-talk, meditation, and other techniques belong to this category. The goals of these techniques are (1) gaining mastery over the physiologic effects of the body's stress response and (2) reducing psychological distress such as anxiety. According to Carrieri-Kohlman and colleagues, persons with COPD were able to differentiate their affective response to dyspnea from the intensity of the symptoms.[106] This capacity for insight makes therapeutic interventions such as mind/body techniques likely to be effective.

In a review of the literature of modalities involving mind/body medicine techniques, Barrows and Jacobs concluded that there are enthusiastic case reports and small studies but not large controlled experimental trials.[107] In a systematic review of the literature about the nature and effectiveness of psychological/psychosocial interventions in patients with COPD, Lacasse and colleagues found the following: (1) although relaxation seemed beneficial in acutely relieving dyspnea and anxiety, whether the effect of psychosocial support alone can be maintained at long term remains uncertain; (2) cognitive and behavior modification techniques within the framework of an otherwise, unsupervised program is probably effective in improving both exercise tolerance and important domains of health-related quality of life; and (3) the need for psychological support during exercise training is unclear.[50] A meta-analysis of the effects of psychoeducational care of 65 studies dated from 1954 to 1994[45] also found methodologic weaknesses but relaxation had statistically significant beneficial effects on both dyspnea and psychological well-being. Although there are a number of different relaxation techniques, characteristics common to all of them include rhythmic breathing and decreased muscle tension and also involve an altered state of consciousness. It is beyond the scope of this chapter to discuss all of the various mind/body medicine techniques that could be of benefit to the patient with COPD; however, we will describe three relaxation techniques: deep breathing, progressive muscle relaxation, and imagery.

A deep breathing technique is illustrated in the following exercise (adapted from "Living Well with COPD©," Module 1: Breathing, Energy Conservation and Relaxation, p. 31):

- Put one hand on your abdomen.
- Breathe in deeply.
- Feel your abdomen inflate. Push your abdomen out as much as possible when you are inhaling. This will help your lungs fill with air.
- Exhale through your mouth while keeping your lips pursed.
- Feel your abdomen returning to its normal size.
- Wait after each expiration until you are ready to take another deep breath.
- You will be more relaxed if you close your eyes and think about a quiet place or the word "calm."
- After a few times, you will find your own rhythm: for example; one deep breath for 5 normal breaths.
- If you start feeling dizzy, take a few normal breaths before starting again.

Take your time and don't be too hard on yourself!

Progressive muscle relaxation (PMR) involves systematically tensing and relaxing specific muscle groups with the goals of reproducing skeletal muscle, reducing stimulation of other bodily systems, and increasing perception of the internal locus of control.[108] The goal is to increase the participant's ability to identify tension and to effectively reduce it. Renfoe was able to demonstrate that patients participating in a 4-week PMR training program were able to reduce their perception of dyspnea and anxiety. Progressive muscle relaxation is illustrated in the following exercise (adapted from "Living Well with COPD©," Module 3: Your Symptoms and Plan of Action, p. 25–26):

- Now it's time to relax all of the muscles in your body.
- Start with your feet and go up to your head.
- Relax the muscles in your left foot until you stop feeling any tension. Inhale deeply and exhale using pursed-lip breathing.
- Repeat for the right foot, left leg, right leg, left thigh, and right thigh.
- At this point, make sure that both legs are completely relaxed and inhale deeply. Then exhale using pursed-lip breathing.
- Continue with the buttocks, hips, back, hands, arms, and shoulders.
- Relax the muscles in your neck, face, and scalp.

Go up to the scalp. Keep your eyes closed and inhale and exhale using pursed-lip breathing a few more times before finishing.

The relaxation exercise is developing your ability to concentrate. Be patient with yourself!

Concentrate on only one part of your body at a time. Practice on a regular basis and give yourself time to learn.

Imagery techniques involve the use of fantasy to achieve altered states of awareness, change the participant's perception of the situation, and facilitate control of the autonomic nervous system, thereby helping him/her to increase his/her sense of control.[109] A visualization exercise is provided below (adapted from "Living Well with COPD©," Module 5: Taking Time to Breath in the Good Things in Life, p. 16):

People can picture different images. Our thoughts can generate both positive and negative images. Images can take the form of persons, places, things, or accomplishments. Positive thoughts can make us happy or confident. Negative, stressful thoughts have the opposite effect. They use energy and make you feel tired. As you can see, it is difficult to dispute the power of an image. Now let's create your own positive image using a technique called visualization. Let's see if your positive image will change your thinking:

- Are you ready?
- Picture a positive image.
- Picture an image that makes you feel happy, confident, and relaxed. (You may want to picture a special person, place, thing, or accomplishment.)

Pacing and Energy Conservation Techniques. The impact of dyspnea and fatigue on daily activities was discussed earlier in this chapter. Various energy conservation techniques and the pacing and planning of activities are effective and problem-focused ways of dealing with dyspnea and fatigue. This topic has already been covered in detail in Chapter 10.

Groups

Groups are good for those who employ information seeking as a coping strategy. Attending a group does not necessarily lead to improved coping. Groups enhance the individual's sense of belonging, connectedness, and well-being and encourage socialization. The group process can be useful in helping patients explore the challenges to self-image, isolation, loss of control, and anger, anxiety, and depression, which are the consequences of life with COPD. Group interventions can be a powerful tool in our efforts to help clients regain a sense of mastery over their illness and their lives. Different types of groups exist, and each center must decide which models are appropriate for their

TABLE 12–9 Advantages and Disadvantages of Groups in the Care of COPD

Advantages	Disadvantages
Greater numbers of patients can receive service with more efficient use of staff time	Not all patients are comfortable or interested in participating in groups
Group members have the opportunity to connect socially and emotionally with people who share their experiences and seek the advice of others while finding mutuality	Significant individual issues might be missed that may have a negative impact on that individual's well-being
Groups encourage flexibility in thought and action by demonstrating that there are different ways of seeing difficulties and solving problems	Psychologically fragile patients may be negatively affected by the expressions of distress shared by the other group members
Distorted beliefs can be challenged more easily by fellow patients "who really know what it is like" rather than by health care professionals whose understanding is more theoretical than direct	If group's selection is not thoughtfully managed, some members can be extremely disruptive and the group process can itself exacerbate the distress it is attempting to alleviate
Long-term friendships can be formed that will extend beyond the group and help to restore the patient's sense of connectedness, thus reducing their isolation	
Participation in a group requires effort and discourages passivity	

setting. The advantages and disadvantages of group care of patients with COPD are delineated in Table 12–9.

Self-help groups are voluntary, small mutual aid structures that are designed to accomplish specific goals. These can be open-ended and held regularly over months or years and can be facilitated by a health care professional or a specially trained patient. Caregiver groups can be organized in the same way. Group members choose the topics of discussion, decide on the group's goals and activities, and request expert information on lectures as needed. This type of group contribution to patient well-being might be the social connectedness it helps to restore and the place it allows for patients to take control of the expression of social and educational needs. The loose structure and membership and patient leadership can be problematic, however, when the group's most active members become sick,[110] evaluated the impact of a self-help educational program for individuals with COPD, levels of disability, cognitive distortion, anxiety and depression, somatic symptoms, and hostility were measured pre- and post-treatment. The findings in this study suggest a positive treatment response to the program.

Education Groups. This type of group is time limited and topic based, with a didactic component followed by discussion. The focus is on learning new concepts and skills and encouraging their integration into daily life. Facilitators are chosen for their expertise in the chosen topic but can also include patients who have demonstrated mastery in the area being discussed. Sessions are designed to review the most important issues facing the patient with COPD. The following are examples of possible topics:

1. What is COPD?
2. How is it treated and what are the goals of treatment?
3. What are the benefits of pulmonary rehabilitation?
4. What is energy conservation?
5. Stress management.
6. Caregivers and their questions, needs, and fears.

Stress Management/Coping Groups. These are closed, time-limited groups that can also incorporate some didactic material but focus primarily on sharing personal experiences, discussing life problems, examining group members' current coping strategies, and exploring new ones. These groups are necessarily smaller (between six and eight members). The facilitators of these types of groups should have good knowledge of COPD and be familiar with group dynamics. These groups must be more structured than a support group. Pollen offered a guide to the significant issues facing patients with COPD as their illness progresses. The eight issues are control, self-image, dependency, stigma, abandonment, anger, isolation, and death.

Educational material and exercises related to these issues can be presented by the facilitators to help the participants work through their individual feelings, beliefs, and coping strategies in the face of these challenges. A model of understanding the relationship between dyspnea and anxiety in COPD can be incorporated into the process. Relaxation techniques can be taught and should be practiced at the end of each session. In this way, emotionally charged sessions can be terminated gently and participants taught to regain control of their emotions and breathing. "Observing another individual mastering situations that have been feared can raise one's own expectations of mastering such a situation."[19]

WHEN TO REFER

Psychiatry and Psychosocial Support (Psychologist and Social Worker)

A 1998 survey of pulmonary rehabilitation programs in Canada revealed that social workers and psychologists were respectively involved in only 43% and 9% of the outpatient programs surveyed.[111] Given the enormous psychosocial impact of COPD on the individual and his/her family, it is recommended that these services be more available to this patient population.

Referral for individual or family assessment and psychosocial support to a social worker or psychologist is indicated when

1. on screening, depression is suggested or evident;
2. the individual is experiencing ongoing family dynamic difficulties such as in function/roles, communication, and sexuality;
3. the individual and his/her family are experiencing major life event stressor(s) and are screened to have inadequate social supports and/or are coping poorly;
4. anxiety is having a limiting effect on the patient's physical and social functioning; financial problems;
5. funding for specialized needs such as specialized equipment or services;
6. there is evidence of caregiver fatigue;
7. there is evidence of unresolved grief owing to

multiple losses;
8. there are signs of post-traumatic stress disorder; and
9. vocational training.

Referral to a specialty such as psychiatry, a psychiatrist, or a mental health service is indicated when

1. the diagnosis of depression is unclear;
2. depression is refractory to pharmacologic and/or nonpharmacologic therapy;
3. the choice of antidepressant drug is complicated by the concurrent medication;
4. the patient presents with suicidal ideation;
5. the patient continues to experience high levels of anxiety and other symptoms of psychological distress despite (1) participation in COPD self-management education sessions (either individually or in groups) to manage such symptoms, (2) individual counselling, and (3) medication to control such distress.

Mobilization of Community Resources

The philosophy underpinning the referral process to the community is that patients who receive the community supports they require will be able to maintain a better quality of life and stable health status for longer periods of time and hopefully make less use of emergency and hospital services.

The careful evaluation of the patient with COPD, as described earlier, will have clarified to the patient, family, and staff, patient/family needs and which community resources could complement the nuclear and extended family systems. The extent of potential resources required by the COPD population is impressive. With the family and his/her family in the center of the plan, the hospital resources are mobilized, such as respirology, nursing, physiotherapy, occupational therapy, inhalation therapy, social work, dietary, and pastoral care. At the same time, the community resources can be initiated, such as

- specialized nursing,
- inhalation therapy services,
- psychosocial support such as from a social worker or a psychologist, among others,
- home care support such as Meals on Wheels, housekeeping, shopping, and bathing
- day center,
- caregiver support groups,
- volunteer and adapted transport,
- palliative care.

SUMMARY

Chronic illnesses such as COPD require a comprehensive assessment of the biologic, psychological, and social aspects of the disease. Recognition and identification of the psychosocial components of a person and family's subjective response to COPD allow health care professionals to choose, develop, and implement more effective coping strategies. Coping with COPD requires the patient and family to successfully adapt to variations in the manifestations of symptoms, decline in physical capacity, and changes in all areas of life, including activities of daily living, self-perceptions, family interactions, and

social network. Patients with COPD can have a high level of anxiety and an accompanying depression that interferes with disease management and reduces their quality of life. Health care professionals need to understand how anxiety and depression can be manifested, measured, and treated in this population to promote effective patient and family coping and COPD self-management. Throughout this chapter, we have emphasized the psychosocial considerations of a chronic illness such as COPD, the importance of identifying the stressors that patients with COPD and their families are experiencing, and the concomitant biopsychosocial impact in order to promote effective coping and adaptation to COPD.

CASE STUDY

Mrs. Cope, a 74-year-old woman, has been diagnosed with COPD for 2 years.

Medical History Relative to Psychosocial Aspects of the Disease

She was diagnosed as having COPD, with an FEV_1 of 0.56, when she was hospitalized 2 years ago. She has been experiencing shortness of breath for 5 years, attributing symptoms to her cardiovascular problems and aging. She was followed all that time by a cardiologist and her family doctor. When seen in an outpatient clinic for her posthospitalization appointment follow-up, her PaO_2 was 57% mm Hg and her oxygen saturation at rest was 88%. She was very anxious at that time, and her biggest fear was of becoming oxygen dependent and being placed in a long-term care residence.

Questions and Discussion

Initially, a detailed psychosocial assessment was completed, and information was gathered on
- *Activities of daily living.* The patient had difficulty in performing all activities of daily living such as dressing, taking a bath, banking, laundry, shopping, etc. She lived alone, was retired, and worked as a waitress in the past.
- *Self-perceptions.* The patient had lost control over the symptoms of her disease, especially

shortness of breath, and her limitations to perform daily activities. Consequent to her physical limitations, her sense of effectiveness was altered, and her level of self-efficacy was low.
- *Family interactions.* The patient was divorced from her husband before her illness. She had a grown daughter, who was the most supportive person for her, and was grandmother of two grandchildren whom she loves. She was dependent on her daughter for activities of daily living. She was elder abused by another family member.
- *Anxiety.* The patient had a spectacular history of dyspnea-related anxiety. She felt helpless. She showed no high-risk signs or symptoms of depression according to the GDS.
- *Coping.* The patient had a history of alcohol abuse. She has been a member of Alcoholics Anonymous for 15 years. Until the time of disease diagnosis, she was a smoker of one pack a day for 40 years, which ceased when she was hospitalized for the first time. The patient was not coping very well with her illness because of severe dyspnea, physical limitations, feelings of helplessness, and family difficulties. She was also increasingly homebound.

Once the psychosocial assessment was completed, the health care professional and patient decided which interventions were appropriate to meet her psychosocial needs. The interventions chosen and implemented were as follows:

1. The patient was referred for home care. The referral included nursing, social work, and occupational therapy. These services were quickly initiated.
2. She needed basic education regarding her illness. Medications and a plan of action that included medical prescriptions, breathing techniques, positions of comfort, and pacing activities were addressed efficiently by the appropriate health care professionals and home study. The priority for her was to learn to control dyspnea and increase her muscle strength and endurance to remain autonomous in her own apartment. Reframing of hope was done repeatedly by the members of the COPD team.
3. The patient was referred to a stress management anxiety group.
4. Finally, the patient was assessed for pulmonary rehabilitation and accepted into the program.

The implementation of the psychosocial plan led to successful patient outcomes:

- The patient accepted and was comfortable with home help, especially bath help, shopping, and weekly visits from a community nurse who reviewed her needs, basic control self-management techniques, and the plan of action.
- She participated extremely well in the stress management anxiety group. By the third week, she enlisted her sister to accompany her outside to walk to the corner, something she had not done for more than a year. She developed a close relationship with another group member and maintains a close telephone link with this lady. She also began to assert herself and set limits with the abusive family member.
- Three months after she first attended the COPD clinic and was diagnosed with COPD, she did a pulmonary exercise programme twice a week for a 2 months ½ period. After the rehabilitation program, her oxygen saturation at rest increased at 91%, and she reported a more active and satisfactory social life. The patient still lived in her apartment, remained stable for a year, and successfully used her plan of action twice, thus avoiding hospitalization.

KEY POINTS

- Chronic illness such as COPD affects all areas of life, including activities of daily living, self-perceptions, family interactions, and social network.
- Assessment of life stressors, the patient's and family's perceptions, and usual ways of coping is needed for choosing, developing, and implementing with the patient and family effective illness coping strategies.
- Measure of the patient's anxiety level, identification of the risk of depression, referrals to psychological and social experts, and nonpharmacologic and pharmacologic treatments for anxiety and depression are needed before trying to intervene in coping and self-management in patients with COPD.
- Fostered collaboration between the patient and the family and health care professionals, exercise/rehabilitation, education toward self-management, mind/body techniques, pacing and energy conservation techniques, and self-help groups are strategies that can help patients with COPD and their families cope with illness.

- Referrals to psychological experts and community resources can support patients and families in disease management and promote coping with illness.

REFERENCES

1. Sexton DL, Munro BH. Living with a chronic illness. The experience of women with chronic obstructive pulmonary disease. West J Nurs Res 1988;10(1): 26–44.
2. Small SP, Graydon JE. Perceived uncertainty, physical symptoms, and negative mood in hospitalized patients with chronic obstructive pulmonary disease. Heart Lung 1992;21:568–74.
3. Anderson KL. The effect of chronic obstructive pulmonary disease on quality of life. Res Nurs Health 1995;18:547–56.
4. Leidy NK. Functional status and the forward progress of merry-go-rounds: toward a coherent analytical framework. Nurs Res 1994;43:196–202.
5. Hanson EI. Effects of chronic lung disease on life in general and on sexuality: perception of adult patients. Heart Lung 1982;11:435–41.
6. Leidy NK, Haase JE. Functional status from the patient's perspective: the challenge of preserving personal integrity. Res Nurs Health 1999;22:67–77.

7. Leidy NK. State of science: functional performance in people with chronic obstructive pulmonary disease. Image J Nurs Sch 1995;27(1):23–34.

8. Smith K, Cook D, Guyatt GH, et al. Respiratory muscle training in chronic airflow limitation: a meta-analysis. Am Rev Respir Dis 1992;145:533–9.

9. Leidy NK, Traver GT. Psychophysiologic factors contributing to functinal performance in people with COPD: are there gender differences? Res Nurs Health 1995;18:535–46.

10. Keele-Card G, Foxall MJ, Barron CR. Loneliness, depression, and social support of patients with COPD and their spouses. Public Health Nurs 1993;10:245–51.

11. Graydon JE, Ross E. Influence of symptoms, lung function, mood, and social support on level of functioning of patients with COPD. Res Nurs Health 1995;18:525–33.

12. Carbin, Strauss. Work and care: managing chronic illness at home. 1988.

13. Carbin, Strauss AL. 1984.

14. Narsavage GL. Promoting function in clients with chronic lung disease by increasing their perception of control. Holistic Nurs Pract 1997;12(1):17–26.

15. Newman B. The Newman systems model. In: Newman B, ed. Appleton & Lange; 1995.

16. Narsavage G. Pulmonary functional outcomes after home care nursing in COPD: phase 1. Eur Res J 1996;9(23S):35S.

17. Dudley DL. Coping with chronic COPD: therapeutic option. Geriatrics 1981;36:69–74.

18. Barstow RE. Coping with emphysema. Nurs Clin North Am 1974;9:137–45.

19. Bandura A. Self-efficacy: the exercise control. New York: 1977.

20. Bandura A. Social foundations of thought and action: a social cognitive theory. Englewood Cliffs (NJ): Pentice Hall, 1986.

21. Blascovich J, Tomaka J. Measures of self-esteem. In: JP Robinson PRS, Wrightsman LS, ed. Measure of personality and social psychology attitudes. San Diego (CA): Academic Press,

22. Borak J, Sliwinski P, Piasecki Z, Zielinski J. Physiological status of COPD patients on long term oxygen therapy. Eur Respir J 1991;4:59–62.

23. Hunter KI, Linn MW, Harris R. Characteristics of high and low self-esteem in the elderly. Int J Aging Hum Dev 1981–82;14:117–26.

24. Improve your self-esteem. NSW: Gore & Osement, 1995.

25. Dezzani MS. Coping with chronic illness. Home Health Nurs 1995;13:50–4.

26. Stuifbergen AK. The impact of chronic illness on families. Fam Community Health 1987;4:43–51.

27. Sexton DL, Munro BH. Impact of a husband's chronic illness (COPD) on the spouse's life. Res Nurs Health 1985;8:83–90.

28. Cossette S, Levesque L. Caregiving tasks as predictors of mental health of wife caregivers of men with chronic obstructive pulmonary disease. Res Nurs Health 1993;46:251–63.

29. Bruhn JG. Effects of chronic illness on the family. J Fam Pract 1977;4:1057–60.

30. Cossette S, Levesque L, Bull MJ. Factors influencing family caregiver burden and health. West J Nurs Res 1990;12:758–70.

31. Leidy NK, Traver GA. Adjustment and social behavior in older adults with chronic obstructive pulmonary disease. The family's perspective. J Adv Nurs 1996;23:252–9.

32. Narsavage GL. Families and their relationships. In: Craven R, ed. Fundamentals of nursing: human health and function. Philadelphia: Lippincott, 1996:1441–64.

33. Karajgi B, Rifkin A, Doddi S, Kolli R. The prevalence of anxiety disorders in patients with chronic obstructive pulmonary disease. Am J Psychiatry 1990;147:200–1.

34. Light RW, Merrill EJ, Despars JA, et al. Prevalence of depression and anxiety in patients with COPD: relationship to functional capacity. Chest 1985;87:35–8.

35. Spielberger CD. Anxiety as an emotional state. In: Spielberger CD, ed. Anxiety: current trends and research. Vol. 1. New York: Academic Press, 1972:24–49.

36. Spielberger CD, Gorsuch RL, Lushene R, et al. Manual for the State-Trait Anxiety Inventory (Form Y). Palo Alto (CA): 1983.

37. Gift AG, Austin DJ. The effects of a program of systematic movement on COPD patients. Rehabil Nurs 1992;17:6–10.

38. Skilbeck J, Mott L, Smith D, et al. Nursing care for people dying from COPD. Int J Palliat Nurs 1997;3:100–6.

39. Tames. Breathing to live. Toronto: Grosvenar House Press, 1991.

40. Loo B. The effects of positive mental imagery on hope, coping, anxiety, dyspnea and pulmonary function in persons with chronic obstructive pulmonary disease: tests of a nursing inervention and a theoretical model. Diss Abstr Int 1991;52(1):157-B.

41. Bergeron J. State-trait anxiety in French-English bilinguals: cross-cultural considerations. Series in Clinical and Community Psych: Stress and Anxiety 1983;2:157–76.

42. Endler NS, Parker JDA. Coping inventory of stressfull situations manual. Toronto: Multi-Health Systems Inc, 1990.

43. Lacasse Y, Wong E, Guyatt GH, et al. Meta-analysis of respiratory rehabilitation in chronic obstructive pulmonary disease. Lancet 1996;348:1115–9.

44. Lacasse Y, Guyatt GH, Goldstein RS. The components of a respiratory rehabilitation program: a systematic overview. Chest 1997;110:1077–88.

45. Devine E, Pearcy J. Meta-analysis of the effects of psychoeducational care in adults with chronic obstructive pulmonary disease. Patient Educ Couns 1996;29:167–78.

46. Kaptein AA, Decker FW. Pulmonary rehabilitation: psychosocial support. Eur Respir Soc J 2000;58–69.

47. Kinsman RA, Yaroush RA, Fernandez E, et al. Symptoms and experiences in chronic bronchitis and emphysema. Chest 1983;83:755–61.

48. Guyatt GH, Townsend M, Berman LB, Pugsley SO. Quality of life in patients with chronic airflow limitation. Br J Dis Chest 1987;81(1):45–54.

49. van Ede L, Yzermans CJ, Brouwer HJ. Prevalence of depression in patients with chronic obstructive pulmonary disease: a systematic review. Thorax 1999; 54:688–92.

50. Lacasse Y, Wong E, Guyatt GH, Goldstein RS. Health-status measurement instruments in chronic obstructive pulmonary disease. Can Respir J 1997;4: 152–64.

51. Yesavage JA, Wong E, Guyatt GH. Development and validation of a geriatric depression screening scale: a preliminary report. J Psychiatr Res 1983;17:37–49.

52. Lacasse Y, Rousseau L, Maltais F. Prevalence of depressive symptoms and depression in patients with severe oxygen-dependent chronic obstructive pulmonary disease. J Cardiopulm Rehabil 2001;20:80–6.

53. McSweeney AJ, Grant I, Heaton RK, et al. Life quality of patients with chronic obstructive pulmonary disease. Kango Gijutsu 1989;35:572–82.

54. American Psychiatric Association. Diagnostic and statistical manual of mental disorders. 4th ed. Washington (DC): American Psychiatric Association, 1994.

55. Gift AG, McCrone SH. Depression in patients with COPD. Heart Lung 1993;22:289–97.

56. Covino NA, Dirks JF, Kinsman RA, Seidel JV. Patterns of depression in chronic illness. Psychother Psychosom 1982;37:144–53.

57. Coulehan JL, Schulberg HC, Block MR, et al. Treating depressed primary care patients improves their physical, mental, and social functioning. Arch Intern Med 1997;157:1113–20.

58. Unützer J, Patrick DL, Simon G, et al. Depressive symptoms and the cost of health services in HMO patients aged 65 years and older: a 4-year prospective study. JAMA 1997;277:1618–23.

59. Cooper CB. Determining the role of exercise in patients with chronic pulmonary disease. Med Sci Sports Exerc 1995;27:147–57.

60. Blazer DG II. Mood disorders: epidemiology. In: Sadock BJ, Sadock VA, eds. Philadelphia: Lippincott, Williams and Wilkins, 2000:1298–308.

61. Grant I, Heaton RK, McSweeney AJ, et al. Neuropsychologic findings in hypoxemic chronic obstructive pulmonary disease. Arch Intern Med 1982;142: 1470–6.

62. Adams KM, Sawyer JD, Kvale PD. Cerebral oxygenation and neuropsychological adaptation. J Clin Neurosphychol 1980;2:189–208.

63. Nocturnal Oxygen Therapy Trial (NOTT) group. Continuous or noctural oxygen therapy in hypoxemic chronic obstructive lung disease: a clinical trial. Ann Intern Med 1980;93:391–8.

64. Medical Research Council Working Party. Long term domiciliary oxygen therapy in chronic hypoxic cor pulmonale complicating chronic bronchitis and emphysema. Report of the Medical Research Council Working Party. Lancet 1981;ii:681–6.

65. Mulrow CD, Williams JW, Gerety MB, et al. Case-finding instruments for depression in primary care settings. Ann Intern Med 1995;122:913–21.

66. Rapp SR, Parisi SA, Walsh DA, Wallace CE. Detecting depression in elderly medical inpatients. J Consult Clin Psychol 1988;56:509–13.

67. Brink TL, Yesavage JA, Lum O, et al. Screening tests for geriatric depression. Clin Gerontol 1982;1:37–43.

68. Yesavage JA. Depression in the elderly. Postgrad Med 1992;91:255–61.

69. Steen SN. The effects of psychotropic drugs on respiration. Pharmacol Ther 1976;2:717–41.

70. Redelmeier DA, Tan SH, Booth GL. The treatment of unrelated disorders in patients with chronic medical diseases. N Engl J Med 1998;338:1516–20.

71. Gordon GH, Michiels TM, Mahutte CK, Light RW. Effect of desipramine on control of ventilation and depression scores in patients with severe chronic obstructive pulmonary disease. Psychiatry Res 1985;15:25–32.

72. Ström K, Boman G, Pehrsson K, et al. Effect of protriptyline, 10 mg daily, on chronic hypoxaemia in chronic obstructive pulmonary disease. Eur Respir J 1995;8:425–9.

73. Guyatt GH, Feeny DH, Patrick DL. Measuring health-related quality of life. Ann Intern Med 1993;118: 622–9.

74. Strauss AL, Corbin J, Fagerhaugh S, et al. Chronic illness and the qualify of life. St. Louis: CV Mosby, 1984.

75. Borycki EM. A study of the concerns of people with chronic obstructive pulmonary disease [thesis]. Winnepeg: University of Manitoba, 1996.

76. Johnsdottir H. Life patterns with chronic obstructive pulmonary disease: isolation and being closed in. Nurs Sci 1998;11:160–6.

77. Woo K. A pilot study to examine the relationship of dyspnea, physical activity and fatique in patients with chronic obstructive pulmonary disease. J Clin Nurs 2000;9:526–33.

78. Lazarus RS, Folkman S. Stress, appraisal, and coping. New York: Springer, 1984.

79. Flach F. Pesilience: discovering a new Strength at time of stress. In: Publisher FC, ed. New York: 1988.

80. Miller JF. Coping with chronic illness: overcoming powerlessness. In: Company FAD, ed. Philadelphia: 2000.

81. Audy JR. Measurement and diagnosis of health. In: PSDM, ed. Environmental essays on the planet earth as a home. Boston: Houghton Mifflin, 1971.

82. Bruhn JG, Cordova DA. A developmental approach to learning wellness behavior; part 1. Infancy to early adolescence. Health Values 1977;1:246–54.

83. Gottlieb L, Rowat K. The McGill model of nursing: a practice-derived model. ANS Adv Nurs Sci 1987;9:51–61.

84. Allen M. The health dimension in nursing practice: notes on nursing in primary health care. J Adv Nurs 1981;6:153–4.

85. Wiebe JS, Christensen AJ. Patient adherence in chronic illness: personality and coping in context. J Pers 1996;64:815–35.

86. Lipowski ZJ. Physical illness, the individual and coping process. Int J Psychiatry Med 1970–1971;91–102.

87. Jalowiec A, Murphy SP, Powers MJ. Psychometric assessment of the Jalowiec Coping Scale. Nurs Res 1984;33:157–61.

88. Jalowiec A. Confirmatory factor analysis of the Jalowiec Coping scale. In: Waltz CSO, ed. Measurement of nursing outcomes, measurement of client outcomes. New York: Springer, 1988:287–308.

89. Narsavage GL, Weaver TE. Physiologic status, coping and hardiness as predictors of outcomes in chronic pulmonary disease. Nurs Res 1994;43:90–4.

90. Buchi ST, Villiger B, Sensky T, et al. Psychosocial predictors of long-term success of in-patient pulmonary rehabilitation of patients with COPD. Eur Respir J 1997;10:1272–7.

91. Scharloo M, Kaptien AA, Weinman JA, et al. Physical and psychological correlates of functioning in patients with chronic obstructive pulmonary disease. J Asthma 2000;37:17–30.

92. Weisman AD, Worden JW. The existential plight in cancer: significance of the first 100 days. Int J Psychiatry Med 1976–1977;7:1–15.

93. Weisman A. Coping with cancer. In: New York: McGraw-Hill, 1979.

94. Eiser N, West C, Evans S, et al. Effects of pyschotherapy in moderately severe COPD: a pilot study. Eur Respir J 1997;10:1581–4.

95. Petty TL. Supportive therapy in COPD. Chest 1998;113:256S–62S.

96. Worth H. Self-management in COPD: one step beyond? Patient Educ Couns 1997;32:S105–9.

97. Nault D, Pépin J, Dagenais J, et al. Qualitative evaluation of a self-management program "Living Well with COPD©" offered to patients and their caregivers. Am J Respir Crit Care Med 2000;161:A56.

98. Gottlieb L, Rowat K. The McGill model of nursing: a practice-derived mode. In: Ezer G, ed. A perspective on health, family, learning and collaborative nursing: a collection of writings on the McGill model of nursing. Montreal: McGill School of Nursing, 1997.

99. American Thoracic Society. Dyspnea mechanisms, assessment, and management: a consensus statement. Am J Respir Crit Care Med 1999;159:321–40.

100. Emery CF, Schein RL, Hauck ER, MacIntyre NR. Psychological and cognitive outcomes of a randomized trial of exercise among patients with chronic obstructive pulmonary disease. Health Psychol 1998;17:232–40.

101. Janelli LM, Scherer YK, Schmieder LE. Can a pulmonary health teaching program alter patients' ability to cope with COPD? Rehabil Nurs 1991;16:199–202.

102. Nault D, Dagenais J, Perreault V, et al. Qualitative evaluation of a disease specific self-management program "Living Well with COPD©." Eur Respir J 2000;16:317S.

103. Bourbeau J, Collet JP, Schwartzman K, et al. Integrating rehabilitative elements into a COPD self-management program reduces exacerbations and health services utilization: a randomized clinical trial. Am J Respir Crit Care Med 2000;161:A254.

104. Bourbeau J, Julien M, Rouleau M, et al. Impact of an integrated rehabilitative management program on health status of COPD patients. A multicentre randomized clinical trial. Eur Respir J 2000;16:159S.

105. Carrieri-Kohlman V, Gormley JM, Eiser S, et al. Dyspnea and the affective response during exercise training in obstructive pulmonary disease. Nurs Res 2001;50:136–46.

106. Carrieri-Kohlman V, Gormley JM, Douglas MK, et al. Exercise training decreases dyspnea and the distress and anxiety associated with it. Monitoring alone may be as effective as coaching. Chest 1996;110:1526–35.

107. Barrows KA, Jacobs BP. Mind-body medicine: an introduction and review of the literature. Med Clin North Am 2002;86(1):11–31.

108. Bernstein SA, Berkovec TD, ed. Progressive muscle relaxation: a manual for the helping professions. Champaign (IL): Research Press, 1973.

109. Stephens R. Imagery as a means of coping. In: Miller FJ, ed. Coping with chronic illness. Philadelphia: FA Davis, 2000.

110. Lisansky DP, Hendel Clough D. A cognitive-behavioural self-help education program for patients with COPD. Psychother Psychosom 1996;65:97–101.

111. Brooks D, Lacasse Y, Goldstein RS. Pulmonary rehabilitation programs in Canada: national survey. Can Respir J 1999;6:55–63.

CHAPTER 13

NUTRITION

Marlène Lemieux,
Katherine Gray-Donald, and Jean Bourbeau

OBJECTIVES

The general objective of this chapter is to help physicians and allied health care professionals become familiar with nutritional abnormalities and to develop an approach to screen patients at risk.
After reading this chapter, the physician and the allied health care professional will be able to

- recognize the high prevalence and the consequences of body depletion in patients with stable chronic obstructive pulmonary disease (COPD) and acute exacerbation;
- understand the causes of weight loss and muscle wasting;
- screen the patient for risk of nutritional abnormalities;
- recognize the limitations of the measurements available in the clinic to adequately assess lean body mass; and
- manage patients at risk for nutritional abnormalities (ie, make appropriate and timely referrals to dietitians, social workers, or other allied health professional if needed).

In patients with COPD, underweight, weight loss, particularly loss of lean body mass, can adversely affect physical performance[1,2] and health-related quality of life.[3] Furthermore, weight loss and low body weight are risk factors for poor survival, independent of lung function.[4]

It is generally considered that despite a normal dietary intake,[5] there is an imbalance between energy intake and expenditure in patients with COPD. Increased resting energy expenditure[6] and total daily energy expenditure[6] have been observed in patients with COPD as compared to healthy subjects. It may also be that increased catabolism and muscle proteolysis are involved in the wasting process. In an acute exacerbation, there is more pronounced systemic inflammation, and corticosteroid treatment may also contribute to weight loss and depletion of fat-free mass in addition to an elevated energy expenditure and inadequate dietary intake.[7,8] Despite the limitation for protein-energy supplementation to reverse weight loss,[9,10] in many patients, nutritional status is a problem, especially in elderly or isolated individuals.

The nutritional needs of patients with COPD are often neglected or ignored by health professionals. Many health professionals do not recognize that healthy eating habits among sufferers of COPD work not only to maintain a healthy body weight but also to prevent infections, improve quality of life, and prevent the need for mechanical ventilation should respiratory failure occur.[11]

This chapter reviews the prevalence, consequences, and causes of nutritional abnormalities in patients with COPD, and methods of screening, assessment, and management strategies.

NUTRITIONAL ABNORMALITIES

The term undernutrition or malnutrition is often used whether the condition results from poor food intake or from disease. Nutritional abnormalities in patients with COPD relate to a disturbed energy balance and to altered regulation of substrate metabolism. For many patients, it is more appropriate not to call them undernourished but rather bodily depleted.

Prevalence

The prevalence of the depletion of fat-free mass in patients with clinically stable COPD has been reported to be 20% in outpatients,[12] 35% in patients entering rehabilitation programs,[13] and 62 to 71% in hospitalized patients.[14] The greater the severity of airflow obstruction and hypoxemia, the greater the incidence of weight loss.

Consequences

Consequences of body depletion include respiratory muscle impairment as well as lung structure that leads to disturbances in lung defense mechanisms.[15,16] In turn, disturbances in the defense mechanisms of the lungs lead to increased incidence of infection and subsequent respiratory failure.[4] When weight loss and lung infection occur concomitantly, body depletion, in terms of protein calorie loss, also occurs; protein and lean body mass loss (bone and peripheral muscle) lead to skeletal and diaphragmatic muscle weakness. Moreover, the amount of lean body mass is a significant determinant of peripheral muscle strength,[17] exercise capacity, and exercise response in patients with COPD.[6,18] Decreased exercise tolerance may also have major consequences on health-related quality of life.[3]

It has long been recognized that mortality is increased in patients with COPD whose body weight is reduced. Hospital-based studies[1,4,19] have established that low body weight for height or low body mass index (BMI) is associated with increased mortality independent of forced expiratory volume in 1 second (FEV$_1$) (Figure 13–1). A decrease mortality rate was observed in overweight patients compared with underweight patients and subjects of normal weight.[1,3]

In a recent population-based study of subjects with COPD[20] followed up for an average of 17 years, underweight (BMI less than 20 kg/m^2) was an independent risk factor for COPD-related mortality and all-cause mortality. Furthermore, in severe COPD (FEV$_1$ percent predicted < 50), mortality continued to decrease with increasing BMI in underweight as compared with obese subjects; a similar but weaker association was found in subjects with mild (FEV$_1$ percent predicted ≥ 70) and moderate (FEV$_1$ percent predicted 50 to 70) COPD (Figure 13–2). There is no known pathogenic mechanism that could explain why obesity should protect against mortality in COPD. Since the majority of deaths in subjects with severe COPD are COPD related, a strong association with all-cause mortality was also found in this group, whereas in subjects with mild to moderate COPD, other causes of death, related negatively to overweight such as cardiovascular disease,

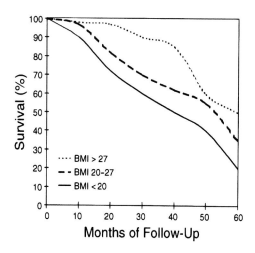

Figure 13–1 Survival curves for patients with COPD by body mass index (kg/m^2). (Adapted from Gray-Donald, et al.[19])

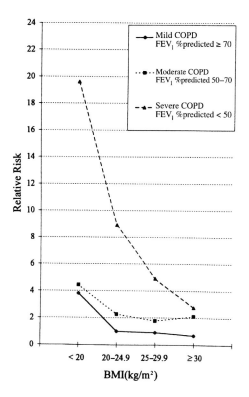

Figure 13–2 Chronic obstructive pulmonary disease–related mortality by body mass index in subjects with mild, moderate, and severe COPD. Normal-weight subjects (BMI 20 to 24.9 kg/m^2) with mild COPD were used for reference. (Adapted from Landbo, et al.[20])

could obscure the association. Therefore, causality should be inferred with extreme caution.

On the other hand, obesity, particularly central obesity, can be conducive to insulin resistance and hyperinsulinemia, hypertriglyceridemia, reduced high-density lipoprotein, and increased number of low-density lipoproteins.[21] In patients with COPD, obesity may lead to sleep-related hypoventilation syndrome,[22] probably owing to the burden placed on the respiratory muscles by the chest wall, with an increased incidence of hypercapnia.[23]

Causes

Increased Energy Needs

Compared to healthy individuals, patients with COPD have increased energy needs,[24,25] as well as an increase in needs during exercise.[26] Increased energy needs may be related to the increased work of breathing, increased dead space ventilation, increased oxygen consumption, and inefficient gas exchange.[27] Patients with COPD expend a great deal of energy on respiration.[24,25] For example, a patient with COPD can expend 30 to 50% more energy on breathing, as compared to individuals who do not have the disease.[15]

Another factor contributing to hypermetabolism is the increased systemic inflammation in patients with COPD. Chronic obstructive pulmonary disease is now considered a systemic disease and not only a lung disease. Studies[28,29] have shown elevated levels of the polypeptide cytokine tumor necrosis factor (TNF), known to trigger the release of different cytokines that mediate an increased energy expenditure and muscle protein catabolism. The elevations of TNF-α levels were demonstrated in patients with COPD, especially those suffering from weight loss.[30]

Hypermetabolism related to acute exacerbation of COPD may also be a factor in body depletion. Factors contributing to weight loss and fat-free mass depletion during exacerbation include an increase in dyspnea,[7] more pronounced systemic inflammation,[31] and the use of systemic corticosteroids.[8]

Suboptimal Dietary Intake

Hypermetabolism can explain body depletion in patients with COPD, but it is not the only cause. Energy balance is often negative during an acute exacerbation because of a dramatic decrease in dietary intake.[7] Energy intake in weight-losing patients is usually lower than in weight-stable patients.[32] The catabolic state may be prolonged unless adequate intake is not rapidly achieved and maintained.

Many factors can affect nutritional intake in patients with COPD.[11,15,25,33] In addition, dietary intake is often reduced during acute exacerbation of COPD when patients experience breathlessness most intensely. Hypoxemia may also impair intestinal absorption of nutrients. The potential factors and rationale to explain suboptimal dietary intake are presented in Table 13–1.

TABLE 13–1 Factors That May Contribute to Suboptimal Dietary Intake

Factor	Rationale
Dyspnea/aerophagia	Gastric distention-induced decrease in functional residual capacity and/or early satiety related to stomach compression by the diaphragm
Chronic mouth breathing	Alters the taste of food and decrease its attractiveness
Thick, foul-smelling sputum	Alters the sensation of taste
Medications	For example, gastrointestinal disturbances related to antibiotics, theophylline, and prednisone
Oral and dental ulcers	May cause mouth pain
Fatigue	May feel tired or lacking in energy to eat; causes some patients to shorten the length of time they will spend eating
Decreased mobility	Unable to walk to the store or do not have the manual dexterity to eat a meal
Social isolation	Difficult to become motivated to shop for food, prepare meals, and eat
Anxiety/depression	Causes appetite suppression Diminishes the ability of an individual to care for himself/herself
Lack of financial resources	May prevent adequate food purchase choices

NUTRITIONAL SCREENING

Nutritional screening is crucial. No parameter is specific to nutritional status, so one must not rely on only one to adequately screen a patient for nutritional depletion. Weight changes and usual intake are of great assistance to the health professional in screening which patients need intervention. Although a parameter such as body weight can underestimate changes in lean body mass, it is still of considerable usefulness. Furthermore, it is simple and clinically applicable.

Body weight at which clinically important depletion occurs is not well known or understood. However, loss of lean body mass in the absence of weight loss and obesity is common in this population and often remains unrecognized. Such patients will suffer from physical impairment to a greater degree than patients with a relative preservation of lean body mass. Body weight can be misleading in the presence of edema caused by severe protein depletion, heart failure, or systemic corticosteroid use.

The health professional can compare the patient's current weight to a healthy weight that is based on current guidelines for height and weight body mass index (BMI). When screening a patient, the health professional should weigh the patient and estimate his/her BMI (Table 13–2). A weight history should also be part of the screening since the patient may have lost a good deal of weight and be at risk nutritionally despite an acceptable actual weight or obesity. The significance of weight loss in relation to the risk of malnutrition can be estimated (Table 13–3).

TABLE 13–2. Body Mass Index and Waist Circumference Ratio*

Body Mass Index (BMI)	Normal
Weight (kg)	• Male (65 yr): 20–25
Height (m^2)	• Female (65 yr): 20–27
	• 65–80 years: 24–29
Waist circumference ratio† (in obese individuals)	
Waist circumference/Hip circumference	• Male 1.0 and less
	• Female 0.8 and less

* Adapted from CPDQ. Manuel de nutrition clinique. Montréal, QC: Guy Connolly, 1991.

† The waist circumference ratio is an indicator of android obesity associated with an increased risk of complications (diabetes, hypertension, dyslipidemia).

TABLE 13–3. Risk Calculation for Malnutrition

Risk of Malnutrition	Mild (%)	Moderate (%)	Serious (%)
% of usual weight _____ %	85–9	75–84	< 75
% of weight loss as a function of time _____ %			
$\dfrac{\text{Usual weight} - \text{present weight} \times 100}{\text{usual weight}}$			
1 wk		1–2	> 2
1 mo		5	> 5
3 mo		7.5	> 7.5
6 mo		10	> 10
% of healthy weight = $\dfrac{\text{present weight} \times 100}{\text{healthy weight}}$			

Well nourished, normal or weight loss (< 10%) followed by weight gain over recent weeks even in the presence of mild subcutaneous tissue loss.

Moderately malnourished, weight loss ≥ 5% over the past few weeks without weight stabilization or weight gain, significant decrease in food consumption, mild subcutaneous tissue loss.

Malnourished, obvious signs of malnutrition (muscle mass loss, serious loss of subcutaneous fatty tissue, edema) in the presence of steady weight loss (often ≥ 10% of usual weight).

As part of the screening, the health professional should also ask the patient about his/her usual daily food intake, number of meals, and snacks. Current diet (Table 13–4), as well as factors that affect dietary intake (see Table 13–1), should be addressed as part of the screening (ie, check if any problem keeps the patient from eating properly such as poor dentition, dysphagia, dyspnea, dyspepsia, allergies to foods, smoking, drug or alcohol consumption, depression, anxiety, physical limitations, and social problems that make food purchasing or preparation a problem).

LABORATORY METHODS AS A MEASURE OF NUTRITIONAL STATUS

Measurement of Body Composition

There is no single parameter that adequately defines body cell mass in all clinical situations. The most accepted and clinically useful parameter is body weight or BMI. However, these measures have been critized because they do not take into account differences in body composition between individuals. As previously mentioned, body weight may be further masked by fluid retention.

Other measurements are presented in the following section. However, it is important to recognize that some of these measurements may not be easily accessible in clinical practice. Furthermore, data are lacking with respect to the clinical impact of using these measurements and their cost benefit.

Skinfold Anthropometry

Studies have shown that body fat is depleted in many patients with COPD. Body fat can be assessed from the triceps skin fold thickness, a noninvasive measurement using a skinfold caliper. The main limitations of this measurement include high interobserver variability[34] and unreliability in edematous patients.[32] Furthermore, it has been shown to overestimate fat-free mass in elderly patients.[35]

Bioelectrical Impedance

The principle of bioelectrical impedance (BI) is based on the conductance through body fluids of an electrical current. Conductivity is higher in fat-free mass, which contains higher body fluids and electrolytes, than in fat. Bioelectrical impedance measurements are believed to provide a means of estimating body composition that takes into account differences in fat distribution. Good correlations of BI measurements with total body water have been demonstrated in patients with stable COPD.[35] However, methods used to compare fat-free mass predictions from BI are open to criticism. Bioelectrical impedance may be a useful measure for the assessment of fat-free mass in patients with severe COPD, and it is preferable to skinfold anthropometry in elderly patients.

Computed Tomography and Magnetic Resonance Imaging

Computed tomography (CT) and magnetic resonance imaging (MRI) have been demonstrated as promising reference methods for quantifying whole body and regional skeletal muscle mass.[36] Computed tomography and MRI are able to detect small differences or changes in soft tissue composition. A single-slice CT measured midthigh appears to be quite useful in the context of muscle strength determinations.[37]

Dual-Energy X-Ray Absorptiometry

Dual-energy x-ray absorptiometry (DEXA) is becoming increasingly popular for measurement of soft tissue composition. Unlike many other methods, DEXA is noninvasive and includes both regional and total-body measurements and peripheral muscle mass. Dual-energy x-ray absorptiometry measures of thigh fat mass correlate extremely well with adipose tissue mass measured by using a multislice CT technique as well as in the abdomen. Nevertheless, there are systematic differences between the two techniques that seem to relate to nonskeletal muscle tissues that are measured as fat-free mass by DEXA. If tissue mass is needed as a denominator for metabolic measurements, DEXA is preferred over a single-slice CT.

Other Laboratory Tests

Nitrogen Balance and Creatinine Height Index

Nitrogen balance is the most common method to assess protein turnover. A negative nitrogen balance usually indicates catabolic state. Nitrogen balance is calculated using the following equation: protein intake (g)/6.25 − [(urinary urea nitrogen[g] + 4 g)].[38] Urinary urea nitrogen has to be measured from 24-hour urine collections. Total urea nitrogen is estimated from urinary urea nitrogen using an adjust-

TABLE 13–4 Daily Dietary Intake Assessment*

Present Weight:	Usual Weight:	BMI:
Height:	Frame:	Healthy Weight:
% Weight Loss:	Time:	% Healthy Weight:

Weight History:	
Appetite:	

Mastication:	Dentition:

Deglutition:	

Digestion:	Nausea/Vomiting:
Elimination:	Laxative Use:

Allergies/Intolerances:	

Mobility:	Activities:

State of Mind:	

Dietary Record	Last Diet:
	Present Diet:

Breakfast Place:	Lunch Place:	Dinner Place:
Time:	Time:	Time:
Morning Snack	Afternoon Snack	Evening Snack

Candy:	
Pastry:	Snack Foods:
Carbonated Drinks:	Alcohol:
Water:	Fiber:
Salt:	Seasoning:
Vitamin and Mineral Supplements:	Tobacco:

*Adapted from Boivin D, Daignault-Gélinas M, Lacroix G. Guide pratique d'évaluation de l'état nutritionnel en gériatrie. Bibliothèque nationale du Québec, 1993.

ment factor of 4 g of nitrogen to account for other nitrogen losses in the urine and from the body (estimated gastrointestinal and cutaneous losses in the absence of malabsorption or severe skin diseases). Incomplete urine collections can introduce error by underestimating urinary urea nitrogen. Any loss in urine would result in even more negative nitrogen balance. Under-reporting of protein intake may also be a concern, especially in elderly patients.

Creatinine height index is a noninvasive method that can estimate lean body mass. The creatinine height index is estimated from the creatinine excreted in the urine normalized for body height (ie, the creatinine/height index).[38] The index is expressed according to a percentage of standards. An index of 100% indicates normal muscle mass as long as urinary function is normal. Overestimation of the creatinine height index because of increased urinary creatinine can be seen when there is an infection, an injury, and a diet high in protein.

Serum Protein, Albumin, Transferrin, and Lymphocytes

The serum protein level is known as an index of visceral protein stores and nutritional status. In patients with COPD, however, there is a tendency to preserve visceral protein stores despite important losses in peripheral muscle mass. A reduction in serum protein can also be secondary to increased capillary permeability as seen in any acute inflammatory process. Serum albumin can be used, but because of a long half-life, it is insensitive to acute nutritional deterioration. Serum prealbumin is better in patients with acute respiratory failure since it has a shorter half-life. Finally, serum transferrin can also be used because its plasma half-life is intermediate between that of albumin and prealbumin. When the serum prealbumin or transferrin level rises, it is a good indicator of positive nitrogen balance. However, it is important to remember that transferrin synthesis is increased with iron deficiency.

Blood lymphocyte count has been used traditionally and can provide some information as to nutritional state. A lymphocyte count of $1,500/mL^2$ or less is abnormal. Refeeding and weight gain increase the absolute lymphocyte count. Delayed hypersensitivity skin testing has also been used, but it can be affected by viral and bacterial infection, uremia, or drugs.

NUTRITIONAL INTERVENTION

Benefit of Nutritional Support

Studies have shown that short-term nutritional repletion leads to an increase in body weight, respiratory function,[39,40] and an increase in lymphocyte count, as well as in reactivity to skin test antigens.[41]

A recent meta-analysis of randomized controlled trials has been done to attempt to answer the question of whether nutritional supplementation improves anthropometric and physiologic parameters such as pulmonary function, respiratory muscle strength, and functional exercise capacity in patients with stable disease.[42] No effect could be demonstrated from nine trials (caloric supplementation for at least 2 weeks), six of which were considered of high quality. The meta-analysis could have been enriched with the measurement of a clinical parameter such as health-related quality of life. Unfortunately, too few study reported dyspnea or health related quality of life for these measurements to be included in the analysis. However, the ability of an aggressive nutritional support regimen to provide a sufficient energy supply in patients with severe COPD is challenging given their high requirements and often poor appetite.

Although nutritional intervention alone has been disappointing for patients with severe COPD, a modality combining nutritional support and exercise has been shown to increase body weight and improve lean body mass and respiratory muscle strength.[43] Despite the variable results on the beneficial effects of nutritional supplementation, the adverse effects of weight loss are such that every effort should be made to prevent or reverse weight loss in the management of COPD.

Most of the studies have investigated the effect of nutritional support in patients with stable COPD. The efficacy of nutritional support during or immediately after an acute exacerbation has not been studied in depth.

Practical Approach to Nutritional Intervention

When addressing the nutritional needs of patients with COPD, the health professional must keep two goals in mind:
1. To prevent or reverse nutritional abnormalities without worsening the disease process and
2. To improve respiratory function, thereby decreasing morbidity and delaying disease-related mortality.

In cases in which the patient's weight is in keeping with that of healthy adults, the health professional should encourage healthy eating habits as outlined in Canada's Food Guide or other food guides. Although Canada's Food Guide addresses many of the issues associated with healthy eating, some other dietary principles need to be considered when addressing the dietary needs of a patient with COPD. Lowering fat intake may not be an issue, as well as use of corticosteroids would influence the needs of the patient and need to be taken into account when assessing and adapting the diet to the patient.

Everything should be done to improve dietary intake in patients with COPD. It is particularly important to work with the patient on increasing nutrient density in quantities well divided during the day to avoid the adverse effects resulting from a high caloric load and avoiding fears about certain foods and remembering that habits are hard to change.

It was long believed that because of ventilatory limitation, provision of more fat-based nonprotein calories to patients with underlying lung disease may lower CO_2 production and ventilatory demand. This issue has been most closely examined in patients with respiratory failure on mechanical ventilation.[44] The clinical benefits of a higher-fat diet (over 50%) are uncertain, and scientific evidence is scarce. Protein intake must be adequate (ie, at least 0.8/kg/day). This is usually sufficient to meet the requirements of the well-nourished patient with COPD. Foods such as cheese, eggs, meats, fish, poultry, tofu, and beans high in protein. The patient should also be encouraged to eat fruits and vegetables.

Patients should participate in an exercise program to stimulate an anabolic response and an increase in fat-free mass rather than fat storage. Exercise improves the effectiveness of nutritional therapy and stimulates appetite. Physical activities, even simple strength exercises combined with breathing techniques, should be encouraged in patients with severe and very limited COPD.

Finally, varying problems may be encountered that are not related to the type of food eaten; rather, they are a function of difficulty obtaining, preparing, or eating food. Table 13–5 provides a list of possible problems that may be encountered as well as potential solutions.

Compliance being difficult should be monitored on a regular basis. Home visits may be indicated for certain patients. Advice and empowerment to the patient and family in the home setting and, more importantly, feedback to the other health care professionals, including the pulmonary physician and the family physician, are of primary importance. A team approach in a continuum of care and service is essential.

WHEN TO REFER TO A DIETITIAN

Even though a clinical nurse specialist or another appropriately trained health care professional can play a valuable role in the clinic or at home, patients may need to be referred to a dietitian.

Patients who are determined to be at risk by screening and those who require any modification to normal diets, are obese, or are experiencing dietary problems should be referred to a dietitian for assessment. A dietitian can develop a plan that will help the patient to replete his/her body's nutritional needs and restore energy and protein intake in a manner that will facilitate weight gain or loss (for obese patients), while taking into account the need for protein and the preservation of muscle strength.[26] For example, in the case of an obese patient, a dietitian can help the patient to eat a low-fat diet, whereas in the case of a bodily depleted patient, the dietitian may suggest a high-energy, high-protein diet. The dietitian can identify the risk of vitamin and mineral depletion and recommend a change to the patient's diet or supplementation.

A consultation with a dietitian is also recommended when there are several coexisting health problems (renal failure, heart failure, etc.). Other candidates include patients with COPD who are on long-term cortisone or corticosteroid therapy.

SUMMARY

Protein depletion with or without weight loss is a common feature in COPD. The consequences include reduction of muscle function and exercise performance, a decrease in health-related quality of life, and an increase in mortality, independent of disease severity.

In patients with COPD, nutritional depletion has been attributed to many factors such as increased energy expenditure, reduced dietary intake, corticosteroid therapy, and an acute exacerbation of COPD.

TABLE 13–5 Problems That the Health Professional May Identify and Proposed Solutions

Problems	Proposed Solutions
Dental problems	Encourage the patient to eat soft, high-calorie-dense foods
Dyspnea/fatigue while eating	Encourage the patient to rest, use bronchodilators, and practice coughing techniques before meals During meals, tell the patient to eat slowly and pursed-lip breathe between taking bites of food Suggest using oxygen (if indicated) while eating
Dyspnea/fatigue while preparing meals/ inability to prepare meals	Provide easy preparation food suggestions (use simple recipes, prepare more than one meal at once) Encourage the patient to stock up on prepared food in the event of worsening of dyspnea, fatigue, or exacerbations of disease Refer to the social worker for arrangements for home-delivered meals (local home care agencies, hospitals, and outpatient clinics provide access to community-delivered meal programs)
Difficulty planning meals and understanding serving sizes	Provide the patient with sample menus and plan a meal together Provide easy to visualize examples of serving sizes (eg, the size, height, and thickness of four fingers excluding the thumb)
Bloating/aerophagia	Encourage patients to eat smaller meals more frequently (5–6 small meals/day), eat slowly, and chew food well Avoid foods that may cause gas, although this may be highly variable (foods such as cabbage, onions, broccoli, cauliflower, etc) Avoid drinking while eating to prevent gas swallowing
Early satiety	Suggest that patients drink fewer liquids during meals (can sip on fluids an hour before meals) Eat cold foods, which provide less of a sense of fullness than hot foods
Constipation	Recommend eating foods high in fiber, drinking plenty of fluids, and exercising as tolerated to prevent constipation (high fiber intake only if the patient drinks a sufficient amount of fluids)

Hypermetabolism is believed to be an important reason why some patients with COPD lose weight despite an apparently normal to even high dietary intake. Nevertheless, it has been demonstrated that dietary intake in weight-losing patients is usually lower than in weight-stable patients. The nutritional status of normal and obese patients should also be assessed since depletion can occur even without weight loss.

Despite the variable results of clinical studies of nutritional supplementation in COPD, efforts to prevent weight loss are warranted as well as healthy eating habits and maintenance of a healthy body weight. Combined treatment modalities including nutritional support and an exercise program, and even simple strength maneuvers, should be encouraged as they are given the most positive results in terms of weight gain and functional improvements.

Screening of nutritional status needs to be monitor in every patient with COPD. A dietitian should be consulted to provide insight into the cause and treatment of patients who experience weight loss.

CASE STUDY

Ms. Cope is a 74-year-old retired nurse who has been hospitalized many times in the last year; she lives alone.

Medical History, Physical Examination, and Test Results

Medical History

- She is an ex-smoker; she smoked a pack of cigarettes per day from the age of 20 to 55.
- She has no cough and sputum except when waking up in the morning. She has had increasing shortness of breath over the past 5 years, which has become worse over the last year to the point that she is limited in doing activities of daily living such as walking or climbing a flight of stairs, making her bed, and taking a shower.
- She has had multiple admissions for COPD exacerbations requiring antibiotic and corticosteroid therapy in the last year; four of six exacerbations required an admission.
- She has other medical/surgical conditions that included bowel resection in 1988 for colon carcinoma, fibrocystic breast disease, atrial fibrillation, osteoporosis, and hospitalization for pneumonia in December last year that was complicated by COPD exacerbation and acute respiratory failure that required noninvasive mechanical ventilation.
- Medications included salmeterol by metered-dose inhaler two puffs twice a day; ipratropium bromide four puffs four times daily (with a spacer device used); inhaled corticosteroids (beclomethasone equivalent of 500 µg twice a day); and calcium carbonate, lanoxin, and hormone replacement therapy; the patient has been on oral corticosteroids many times in the last year (an equivalent of 4 months).

Physical Examination

- She is not in acute respiratory distress; respiratory rate 24/minute; pulse 88 beats/minute (regular), blood pressure 145/70 mm Hg.
- She is underweight with visible evidence of muscle wasting.
- Her skin is dry but no evidence of dehydration.
- Accessory muscle used in breathing.
- Chest examination confirmed the presence of decreased air entry; no wheezing or crackles.
- Cardiac examination is normal.
- No cyanosis or edema.

Weight History

- Height: 160 cm; usual weight: 52.3 kg; BMI: 20.4.
- Her weight went down to 50.8 kg in March last year and to 41.5 kg in December (ie, a weight loss of 20.6% when compared to her usual weight).
- Her BMI was also down to 16.2.

Test Results

- Her spirometry is compatible with severe airflow obstruction without significant reversibility; spirometry postbronchodilator:
  - FEV_1 is 0.70 L (25% of predicted normal)
  - FEV_1/forced vital capacity (FVC) ratio is 40%
- Hemoglobin, hematocrit, lymphocyte count, and serum albumin were all below normal values; December last year, her hemoglobin was 106 g/L, hematocrit 0.34, lymphocyte count 1.92×10^9/L, and albumin 36 g/L.

Questions and Discussion

This patient's management included a pulmonary rehabilitation program. Because of a diagnosis of muscle wasting, a history of weight loss, frequent use of corticosteroids in a patient with osteoporosis, and a decreased serum albumin, hemoglobin/hematocrit, and lymphocyte count, the patient was seen by a dietitian as part of the program for further assessment and intervention. She did not complain of any dyspepsia, dysphagia, problems chewing, constipation, or diarrhea. However, she complained of bloating after the meal. She reported no known food intolerance or allergies.

Subjective Nutritional Assessment

The patient was eating three meals a day, usually small meals as she did not have a very good appetite. She tried to supplement her diet by occasionally drinking a commercial supplement and taking a multivitamin and mineral pill, 400 U vitamin E, and 500 mg calcium carbonate each day.

She consumed two to three servings of cereal products, two to three servings of dairy, two servings of meat and substitutes, and three servings of fruit and vegetables, not meeting Canada's Food Guide recommendations for healthy eating.

Food shopping and food preparation were becoming difficult for her because of fatigue and an increase in shortness of breath on exertion. She was relying more and more on frozen dinners with lesser energy and protein value than her home-cooked meals. As well, she admitted that intake at time was further decreased because of bloating and increased shortness of breath after meals. She consumed few, if any, alcoholic beverages.

Objective Nutritional Assessment

With weight at 79.4% of her usual weight and a weight loss of >10% over 10 months and an albumin of 36 g/L, she was considered as being severely energy depleted as well as protein depleted. Low hemoglobin and hematocrit may, in part, be related to protein depletion and/or to the underlying chronic disease. Further investigation is needed to rule out iron, vitamin B_{12}, or folic acid deficiency. Folic acid and vitamin B_{12} deficiencies are more prevalent in the elderly.

Energy needs were estimated using the Harris-Benedict equation as follows:

$$\text{Women: } [655 + 9.6 \text{ (weight kg)} + 1.7 \text{ (height cm)}] - [4.7 \times \text{age}] = \text{REE} \times 1.5$$

Protein needs were estimated to be at 1.5 to 2 g/kg ideal body weight (IBW).

Since the patient is quite underweight and the goal is to improve her nutritional state without taxing her respiratory system, her present weight of 41.5 kg was used to calculate her needs rather than IBW. Thus, she needs at least 1,466 to 1,500 kilocalories (approximately 6,160 kJ) and 62 g of protein daily.

Education Related to Her Nutritional Condition

The importance of nutritional repletion and the means to achieve this were discussed with the patient. We began by building on what she was already doing to meet goals and discussed various problems that may arise as she was trying to increase her intake.

Small, frequent, nutritionally dense meals were planned with her. Tips included adding skim milk powder to liquids, sauces, minced meats, desserts, and cream soups; adding cheese or chopped egg to salads; frying foods or adding fats and or sauces to dishes. She was given recipes for a variety of easy to prepare high-calorie, high-protein drinks (ie, milkshakes, eggnogs, fruit julep, high-protein "café au lait"). Since she was having difficulty preparing meals because of shortness of breath, the patient was given easy to prepare one-dish meals.

Bloating could be avoided by eating slowly and chewing food well. A list of foods that can aggravate bloating was reviewed with her. Proper use of supplements was discussed with the patient since she tended to rely on them too much and with little success.

Follow-Up and Patient Evolution

A recommendation to do further laboratory tests for anemia as well as biochemistry including albumin, magnesium, and phosphorus was discussed with her physician previous to her next visit for follow-up. Referral to social services was made to arrange for Meals on Wheels and help with food shopping. Then she was given a follow-up appointment and was told to contact the dietitian if any further weight loss occurred before her first appointment or if she was having any problems eating.

Her general condition improved with increased strength, slightly less breathlessness, and better functional capacity and coping with her disease. Her progress was slow, and the patient needed constant encouragement. Six months later, after she completed her 3-month pulmonary rehabilitation program and follow-up with the dietitian, her weight was up to 48.2 kg. Her hemoglobin and hematocrit were within the normal range, and her albumin was 39 g/L. She had not reached her usual or IBW, but there was an improvement in her appetite, and when it was time to eat, she was more hungry. Community services were arranged to her satisfaction and permitted her to stay at home longer.

KEY POINTS

- Protein depletion with or without weight loss is a common feature in COPD; never assume that a normal or obese patient with COPD is well nourished, especially one who is corticosteroid dependent or has lost a significant amount of weight.
- The consequences of body depletion include reduction of muscle function and exercise performance, decreased health-related quality of life, and increased mortality, independent of disease severity.
- No parameter is specific to nutritional status; remember that protein depletion begins before evidence appears in laboratory values.
- Weight changes and usual intake are of great assistance to the health professional in screening which patients need intervention.
- The further deteriorated a patient's nutritional status is, the more difficult it is to reverse.
- Despite the variable results of clinical studies of nutritional supplementation in COPD, efforts to prevent weight loss are warranted as well as healthy eating habits and maintenance of a healthy body weight.
- Combined treatment modalities including nutritional support, an exercise program, and even simple strength maneuvers should be encouraged as they provide the most positive results in terms of weight gain and functional improvements.
- There is no advantage to using commercial supplements alone. They give the patient a false sense of security, and needed changes never occur.
- Follow-up is essential and changes in lifelong food habits require time and patience; constant encouragement and reinforcement are needed.
- Adequate nutritional assessment and therapy by a qualified dietitian are important; involvement of community services is often needed and is the key to success.

REFERENCES

1. Wilson DO, Rogers RM, Wright EC, Anthonisen NR. Body weight in chronic obstructive pulmonary disease. The National Institutes of Health Intermittent Positive-Pressure Beathing Trial. Am Rev Respir Dis 1989;139:1435–8.
2. Gray-Donald K, Gibbons L, Shapiros H, et al. Effect of nutritional status on exercise performance in patients with chronic obstructive pulmonary disease. Am Rev Respir Dis 1989;140:1544–8.
3. Shoup R, Dalsky G, Warner S, et al. Body composition and health-related quality of life in patients with obstructive airways disease. Eur Respir J 1997;10:1576–80.
4. Schols AM, Slangen J, Volovics L, Wouters EF. Weight loss is a reversible factor in the prognosis of chronic obstructive pulmonary disease. Am J Respir Crit Care Med 1998;157:1791–7.
5. Creutzberg EC, Schols AM, Bothmer-Quaedvlieg FC, Wouters EF. Prevalence of an elevated resting energy expenditure in patients with chronic obstructive pulmonary disease in relation to body composition and lung function. Eur J Clin Nutr 1998;52:396–401.
6. Baarends EM, Schols AM, Mostert R, Wouters EF. Peak exercise response in relation to tissue depletion in patients with chronic obstructive pulmonary disease. Eur Respir J 1997;10:2807–13.
7. Vermeeren MA, Schols AM, Wouters EF. Effects of an acute exacerbation on nutritional and metabolic profile of patients with COPD. Eur Respir J 1997;10:2264–69.
8. Saudny-Unterberger H, Martin JG, Gray-Donald K. Impact of nutritional support on functional status during an acute exacerbation of chronic obstructive pulmonary disease. Am J Respir Crit Care Med 1997;156:794–9.
9. Efthimiou J, Fleming J, Gomes C, Spiro SG. The effect of supplementary oral nutrition in poorly nourished patients with chronic obstructive pulmonary disease. Am Rev Respir Dis 1988;137:1075–82.
10. Rogers RM, Donahoe M, Costantino J. Physiologic effects of oral supplemental feeding in malnourished patients with chronic obstructive pulmonary disease. A randomized control study. Am Rev Respir Dis 1992;146:1511–7.
11. Keim NL, Luby MH, Braun SR, et al. Diatery evaluation of outpatients with chronic obstructive pulmonary disease. J Am Diet Assoc 1986;86:902–6.
12. Engelen MP, Schols AM, Baken WC, et al. Nutritional depletion in relation to respiratory and peripheral skeletal muscle function in out-patients with COPD. Eur Respir J 1994;7:1793–7.
13. Schols AM, Soeters PB, Dingemans AM, et al. Prevalence and characteristics of nutritional depletion in patients with stable COPD eligible for pulmonary rehabilitation. Am Rev Respir Dis 1993;147:1151–6.
14. Laaban JP, Kouchakji B, Dore MF, et al. Nutritional status of patients with chronic obstructive pulmonary disease and acute respiratory failure. Chest 1993;103:1362–8.
15. Laaban JP. Nutrition and chronic obstructive pulmonary disease. Rev Pneumol Clin 1991;47:235–50.
16. Rochester DF, Esau SA. Malnutrition and the respiratory system. Chest 1984;85:411–5.
17. Engelen M, Schols AM, Does JD, Wouters EF. Skeletal muscle weakness is associated with wasting of extremity fat-free mass wasting but not with airflow obstruction in patients with chronic obstructive pulmonary disease. Am J Clin Nutr 2000;71:33–8.
18. Palange P, Forte S, Onorati P, et al. Effect of reduced body weight on muscle aerobic capacity in patients

with COPD. Chest 1998;114:12–8.

19. Gray-Donald K, Gibbons L, Shapiro SH, et al. Nutritional status and mortality in chronic obstructive pulmonary disease. Am J Respir Crit Care Med 1996;153:961–6.

20. Landbo C, Prescott E, Lange P, et al. Prognostic value of nutritional status in chronic obstructive pulmonary disease. Am J Respir Crit Care Med 1999;160:1856–61.

21. Lamarche B, Lemieux S, Dagenais GR, Despres JP. Visceral obesity and the risk of ischaemic heart disease: insights from the Quebec Cardiovascular Study. Growth Horm IGF Res 1998;8:1–8.

22. Bonsignore G. Cardio-respiratory function during sleep. Ann Ital Med Int 1991;6:137–47.

23. Bégin P, Grassino A. Inspiratory muscle dysfunction and chronic hypercapnia in chronic obstructive pulmonary disease. Am Rev Respir Dis 1991;143:905–12.

24. Goldstein SA, Thomashow BM, Kvetan V, et al. Nitrogen and energy relationships in malnourished patients with emphysema. Am Rev Respir Dis 1988;138:636–44.

25. Wilson DO, Donahoe M, Rogers RM, Pennock BE. Metabolic rate and weight loss in chronic obstructive lung disease. J Parenteral Enteral Nutr 1990;14:7–11.

26. Donahoe M, Rogers RM. Nutritional assessment and support in chronic obstructive pulmonary disease. Clin Chest Med 1990;11:487–504.

27. Braun SR, Dixon RM, Keim NL, et al. Predictive clinical value of nutritional assessment factors in COPD. Chest 1984;85:353–7.

28. De Godoy I, Donahoe M, Calhoun WJ, et al. Elevated TNF-alpha production by peripheral blood monocytes of weight-losing COPD patients. Am J Respir Crit Care Med 1996;153:633–7.

29. Di Francia M, Barbier D, Mege JL, Orehek J. Tumor necrosis factor-alpha levels and weight loss in chronic obstructive pulmonary disease. Am J Respir Crit Care Med 1994;150:1453–5.

30. Schols AM, Buurman WA, Staal van den Brekel AJ, et al. Evidence for a relation between metabolic derangements and increased levels of inflammatory mediators in a subgroup of patients with chronic obstructive pulmonary disease. Thorax 1996;51:819–24.

31. Creutzberg EC, Schols E, Vermeeren A, et al. The influence of an acute disease exacerbation on the metabolic and inflammatory profile in patients with COPD. Eur Respir J 1999;14:414S.

32. Schols AM, Mostert R, Soeters PB, Wouters EF. Body composition and exercise performance in patients with chronic obstructive pulmonary disease. Thorax 1991;46:695–9.

33. Chapman KM, Winter L. COPD: using nutrition to prevent respiratory function decline. Geriatrics 1996;51:37–42.

34. Fuller NJ, Jebb SA, Goldberg GR, et al. Inter-observer variability in the measurement of body composition. Eur J Clin Nutr 1991;45:43–9.

35. Schols AMWJ, Wouters EFM, Soeters PB, Westerterp KR. Body composition by bioelectrical-impedance analysis compared with deuterium dilution and skinfold anthropometry in patients with chronic obstructive pulmonary disease. Am J Clin Nutr 1991;53:421–4.

36. Mitsiopoulos M, Baumgartner RN, Heymsfield SB, et al. Cadaver validation of skeletal muscle measurement by magnetic resonance imaging and computerized tomography. J Appl Physiol 1998;85:115–22.

37. Schantz PE, Randall-Fox W, Hutchison A, et al. Muscle fibre type distribution, muscle cross-sectional area and maximal voluntary strength in humans. Acta Physiol Scand 1983;117:219–26.

38. Gibson RS. Principles of nutritional assessment. New York: Oxford University Press, 1990.

39. Whittaker JS, Ryan CF, Buckley PA, Road JD. The effects of refeeding on peripheral and respiratory muscle function in malnourished chronic obstructive pulmonary disease patients. Am Rev Respir Dis 1990;142:283–8.

40. Wilson DO, Rogers RM, Openbrier D. Nutritional aspects of chronic obstructive pulmonary disease. Clin Chest Med 1986;7:643–56.

41. Fuenzalida CE, Petty TL, Jones ML, et al. The immune response to short-term nutritional intervention in advanced chronic obstructive pulmonary disease. Am Rev Respir Dis 1990;142:49–56.

42. Ferreira IM, Brooks D, Lacasse Y, Goldstein RS. Nutritional support for individuals with COPD: a meta-analysis. Chest 2000;117:672–8.

43. Schols AM, Soeters PB, Mostert R, et al. Physiologic effects of nutritional support and anabolic steroids in patients with chronic obstructive pulmonary disease. A placebo-controlled randomized trial. Am J Respir Crit Care Med 1995;152:1268–74.

44. Donahoe M. Nutritional aspects of lung disease. Respir Care Clin North Am 1998;4:85–112.

SUGGESTED READINGS

Schols AMWJ, Wouters EFM. Nutritional abnormalities and supplementation in chronic obstructive pulmonary disease. Clin Chest Med 2000;21:753–62. *This is a recent and comprehensive review of the nutritional abnormalities and intervention in patients with COPD. This article also presents the future perspective with respect to anabolic and anticatabolic agents.*

Landbo C, Prescott E, Lange P, et al. Prognostic value of nutritional status in chronic obstructive pulmonary disease. Am J Respir Crit Care Med 1999;160:1856–61. *This is the only population-based study with randomly selected subjects to examine the relation between BMI and mortality in subjects with COPD.*

Ferreira IM, Brooks D, Lacasse Y, et al. Nutritional support for individuals with COPD: a meta-analysis . Chest 2000;117:672–8. *This is a recent meta-analysis of nine randomized, controlled trials of caloric supplementation looking at the improvement in anthropometric measures, lung function, or exercise capacity.*

CHAPTER 14

SLEEP AND COPD

R. John Kimoff and Kathy Riches

OBJECTIVES

The general objective of this chapter is to help physicians and allied health care professionals become more familiar with sleep-related issues and to develop an approach to assess inadequate or poor sleep on which to base their interventions in patients with chronic obstructive pulmonary disease (COPD).

After reading this chapter, the physician and the allied health care professional will be able to

- understand the importance of sleep-related issues in the management of COPD;
- develop a comprehensive approach to assess inadequate or poor sleep related to respiratory and other medical conditions;
- appropriately manage patients with inadequate sleep through the application of some practical interventions;
- recognize that patients can have primary sleep disorders; and
- refer to specialized professionals and specific resources when needed.

Adequate sleep is essential for normal health and well-being. Our bodies are programmed to need sleep, which serves a wide variety of restorative and recuperative functions essential to maintaining wellness.[1–4] Normal sleep is much more than a simple tuning out of the surrounding environment. Rather, it is a highly structured, complex neurologic process that involves many different centers within the brain and that affects the functioning of most major organ systems including the respiratory system.[1,2]

Sleep-related issues can be very important in the management of patients with COPD, in that inadequate or poor sleep can have major consequences for both physical and emotional functioning. Poor sleep can contribute to daytime fatigue and lack of energy, impaired cognitive function, anxiety and a reduced coping ability, reduced exercise tolerance, and a deterioration in lung function.[5–11]

Although the list of potential problems can be long, it is often possible, by taking a careful sleep history and applying some practical interventions, to produce substantial improvements in sleep quality and thereby in the patient's well-being.[5,12–15] Adequate attention to the sleep history is therefore an essential aspect of the integrated care of the patient with COPD.

In this chapter, we review the major problem areas leading to poor sleep in patients with COPD, and for each of these areas, we discuss patient assessment and suggest interventions to improve sleep.

STAGES OF SLEEP

Sleep consists of both rapid eye movement (REM) and non-REM sleep, with the latter divided into four stages. Stage 1, non-REM sleep, normally accounts for less than 10% of the night's sleep, representing a transitional phase from wakefulness to established non-REM sleep. Stage 2 non-REM sleep is the predominant sleep stage for older adults, representing from 50 to 75% of normal sleep. Stage 3 and 4 non-REM sleep are together referred to as delta wave sleep and represent deep, restorative sleep, progressively occupying less of the total sleep time as humans age, such that in older adults, only 5 to 10% of the night may be spent in delta wave sleep. Rapid eye movement sleep, which is deep, dreaming sleep, normally occupies from 15 to 25% of normal sleep, with the relative proportion again decreasing with age.[1,2]

There are normal changes in breathing associated with each of the sleep stages; in these stages, ventilation can be mildly reduced but remains very regular during established non-REM sleep compared with wakefulness. Arterial PCO_2 levels normally rise from 1 to 4 mm Hg during non-REM sleep compared with wakefulness. During REM sleep, particularly at the time of the REM bursts, breathing can become very irregular and shallow because of changes in both the central generation of breathing rhythm and the active inhibition of nondiaphragmatic respiratory muscles.[1,2] In normal subjects, this has relatively minor consequences for breathing, but in patients with COPD, there can be significant blood gas abnormalities that develop as a consequence of this.[5,6,16–19]

The sleep cycle is programmed within the brain to begin at a particular phase of the 24-hour day-night cycle. Once the cycle begins, there is a highly characteristic pattern of appearance in the various sleep stages, going from light to deep non-REM sleep, then into REM, then back into stage 2, then again into REM, and so forth, such that there are normally three or four REM cycles per night. In patients with COPD, a whole host of respiratory and other factors can disrupt the normal pattern or architecture of this very complex process and thus lead to poor quality, nonrestorative sleep.[5–8,20–24]

SLEEP DISTURBANCE

Problems with sleep are common among patients with COPD.[5–7,20] Complaints of insomnia are frequent, with patients reporting difficulty falling asleep, frequent nocturnal awakenings, difficulty returning to sleep once awoken, and a generally short, nonrefreshing sleep. Polysomnographic studies have demonstrated a reduction in total sleep time, sleep disruption with increased number of sleep stage changes and awakenings, and reduced proportions of deeper levels (stages 3 and 4) of non-REM and REM sleep in patients with COPD compared with normals of similar age.[5,6]

It should be borne in mind that factors that may contribute to poor sleep quality are numerous; they include sleep disruption caused by cough, dyspnea or chest pain, gastroesophageal reflux, a sedentary lifestyle with relative physical inactivity and lack of exercise, medication effects, aging-related changes, genitourinary dysfunction, chronic pain syndromes or the effects of other medical illnesses, anxiety and depression, and poor sleep hygiene. Patients with COPD may also suffer from specific sleep-related breathing disorders including obstructive sleep apnea and nocturnal (particularly REM-related) hypoventilation because of sleep-related changes in breathing exaggerated by COPD, as well as other medical sleep disorders such as nocturnal myoclonus, all of which directly affect sleep quality.

GENERAL SLEEP HABITS

Assessment of Sleep Habits

Each patient should be evaluated with a few simple questions to determine whether there is a problem with sleep.[1,2,12–15,25] Although sleep problems are common, some patients with even severe COPD may still sleep quite well. Initial questions would include the following:

- Do you sleep well at night? Do you have problems sleeping at night?
- Do you feel tired or sleepy during the day?

If there appears to be a problem with sleep, pertinent further questions should be addressed regarding sleep patterns, sleep habits, and drug-related and other sleep-disruptive issues (Table 14–1).

The patient should be asked whether he/she takes naps during the day, and, if so, how often and for how long each time. Daytime naps may be helpful in maintaining alertness and daytime function if there are problems with sleep. However, in general, for patients with difficulty sleeping at night, sleep during the day will tend to worsen the problem and should be discouraged.

The extent and pattern of the patient's physical activities need to be assessed as part of the sleep history. Regular exercise is important in promoting good sleep, and lack of exercise is often a contribut-

TABLE 14–1 Sleep Questionnaire for Patients with COPD

Screening questions
  Do you sleep well at night?
  Do you feel refreshed in the morning?
  Are you tired or sleepy during the day?

Sleep patterns
  Do you have difficulty falling asleep?
  Do you wake up at night? How often?
  Do you wake up early in the morning?
  What wakes you up or keeps you awake at night (cough, dyspnea, need to void, pain, etc)?
  What do you do at night if you cannot fall back asleep?
  What helps you to get back to sleep?
  How long have you had sleep problems?

Sleep habits
  Do you go to bed at a regular time? Get up at a regular time?
  Do you stay in bed during the day?
  Do you get dressed each day or do you sometimes remain in pyjamas?
  Do you nap during the day? For how long?
  Do you leave the house each day?
  Do you exercise regularly? How often?
  What time of day do you exercise?
  Do you have indigestion at night?
  Do you eat before going to bed? During the night?
  Is your bed comfortable?
  Is your head elevated at night?
  Is your bedroom well ventilated? A comfortable temperature?
  Is your bedroom quiet?

Drug-related issues
  How much coffee do you drink? Tea? Caffeinated soft drinks?
  Do you smoke in the evening? During the night?
  What medications do you take (eg, evening diuretics, theophyllines, nicotine replacement)?
  Do you take sleeping pills? Which ones, how often, and do they help?

Other sleep-disruptive effects
  Are you feeling stressed or anxious?
  Are you feeling down or depressed?
  Do you have pain at night?
  Are you short of breath or do you cough a lot at night?
  Are your inhalers and/or aerosols always at your bedside?
  Do they relieve your breathing problems?
  Do you use oxygen at night?
  Does the noise of the concentrator bother you?
  Do you need to void frequently at night?

ing factor to poor sleep in patients with COPD. This may be especially marked during winter months when patients are most restricted in their activities.

Feelings of isolation, stress, anxiety, depression, and other psychosocial issues often impact sleep quality in patients with COPD. The assessment of this aspect of the patient's experience is dealt with in further detail in Chapter 12. However, the interaction of these issues with sleep problems should not be overlooked. Indeed, some patients' sleep complaints, such as difficulty falling asleep, early morning awakening, and daytime fatigue, may be impor-

TABLE 14–2 Diary for Sleep Habits

Sleep Habit	Day/Date
Did you nap today?	
When?	
How long?	
Time into bed last night?	
When did you turn out the light?	
What time did you fall asleep?	
Number of awakenings through the night?	
Approximate time awake during the night?	
Time of awakening in the morning?	
What time did you get out of bed?	
Approximate total sleep time?	

tant warning symptoms pointing to the presence of significant depression.

Some patients will have difficulty recalling the details of their sleep habits or may not appreciate certain aspects of their own practices. Asking the patient to keep a sleep diary for a period of one to several weeks can be very useful in this regard (Table 14–2). The patient is simply asked to make a written record of a few daily details concerning bedtime, awakening time, nocturnal sleep quality, and naps. This more objective record of sleep habits can prove very informative and useful in some cases of sleep disorder management. As one questions the patient about sleep habits, the patient's own strategies for inducing a good sleep should be explored; thus, positive habits can be reinforced while the negative ones are modified.

Medication and Dietary Habits

A medication, dietary, and alcohol history is also an important part of the sleep assessment.[1–3,12,15,26] Some medications used in COPD are stimulating and can have sleep-disrupting effects, including theophylline preparations, β_2 agonists, and nicotine replacement preparations.[27,28] Although these medications may be very important for the control of nocturnal respiratory symptoms, they can also disturb sleep. Patients should be questioned as to whether there is any shakiness, agitation, palpitations, or anxiety experienced following medication use as these symptoms would point to the potential for sleep disruption. Oral corticosteroids prescribed in high doses for exacerbations can also produce insomnia with or without associated mood-altering (elevation or depression) effects. Caffeine-containing beverages (many soft drinks as well as colas, coffee, and tea) and chocolate (which is metabolized to caffeine-related products) are stimulating. Although alcohol may initially help with falling asleep, often a rebound insomnia follows. Alcohol also suppresses some stages of deeper, restorative sleep and can worsen nocturnal respiratory problems such as hypoxemia or sleep apnea. An alcohol history should be obtained, remembering that patients quite consistently under-report alcohol use (one rule of thumb is to count on the patient's intake being double that reported). The pattern of food intake through the day should be assessed as large meals late in the evening may contribute to nocturnal dyspnea.

Practical Sleep Hygiene Measures and Treatment

Education on Good Sleep Habits

Patients often need additional education on good sleep habits.[1,2,12–15,25] Their sleep schedule should be regulated as much as possible with a set bedtime and waketime. Late evening should be occupied with calming, relaxing activities, whereas stressful stimuli such as violent or frightening movies, difficult interpersonal interactions, and working on a difficult financial situation should be avoided. Some patients with high anxiety levels may be so bothered by late evening news reports that, ideally, they should be avoided. The bedroom should be used as a place for sleep and intimacy only; paperwork should not be brought into bed, and stressful discussions should not be initiated in the bedroom late at night. The practice of getting into bed early and spending the evening watching television should be discouraged as insomnia may result.

If there is prolonged difficulty falling asleep or returning to sleep when awakened, various relaxation techniques can be used. However, if wakefulness is prolonged, the patient should get out of bed and engage in a quiet activity such as reading, which is often very helpful. Watching television may also be helpful but, in some cases, can prolong the period of wakefulness either because of the bright light effect, stimulating program content, or captivation of the patient's interest with a consequently longer period of wakefulness than would otherwise have occurred. Even if sleep is rated as poor quality, patients should still be encouraged to get up in the morning by a certain time and prepare for the day. This helps entrain the diurnal rhythmn and may also promote increased physical and social activity. Remaining "tied to the bed" throughout the day will tend to produce a more disrupted nocturnal sleep pattern and may also reduce daytime activity, perpetuate depression, and increase social isolation.

If naps are taken during the day, they should be limited to prove beneficial without interfering with nighttime sleep. For instance, if the patient really feels that a nap is essential, setting the alarm for 15 or 30 minutes will ensure that he or she does not oversleep. For patients with marked difficulty sleeping at night, naps should be altogether discouraged in an attempt to better consolidate sleep. If ventilatory assists are prescribed during nighttime sleep (O_2, continuous positive airway pressure [CPAP], etc), they should also be worn during naps. A regular exercise program, obviously tailored to the patient's capacity, can be very beneficial to promote sleep. Since exercise has a stimulating effect and may prevent sleep onset, it should preferably be done during the day and no later than early evening.

Relief of stress and anxiety may help promote sleep quality, and, in turn, improved sleep often helps reduce anxiety. Although not discussed in detail here, these issues are often of paramount importance in the promotion of sleep in patients with COPD. Patients should be encouraged to verbalize these concerns. There may be specific anxieties about going to sleep; for example, the fear of never waking up, concerns about nocturnal respiratory distress, or nervousness about being alone at night or in the dark.

Education on Medication and Good Dietary Habits

Teaching the proper use of bronchodilator and other medications so as to minimize side effects will help reduce treatment-related sleep disruption. Caffeine and chocolate should be avoided from afternoon onward, and in some patients they may need to be eliminated entirely. Patients should be discouraged from using alcohol to promote sleep. If there is evidence of alcohol dependence, a multidisciplinary

approach to this problem should be instituted. Advice should be given on spacing food intake to minimize postprandial respiratory discomfort, especially late in the evening.

Pharmacologic Therapy

Similar to the management of stress and anxiety, behavioral approaches to the management of poor sleep may not produce sufficient improvement, thus making the option of pharmacotherapy a necessity. The use of sleeping pills may be appropriate in some cases.[8,29] The concerns with administering such agents to patients with chronic hypercapnia are very real in terms of producing further hypoventilation and respiratory failure. However, such agents are likely underused in nonhypercapnic patients with COPD because of unjustified concerns in such patients. Ideally, however, sleep should be promoted with the least, most limited use of pharmacotherapy possible.

RESPIRATORY AND OTHER MEDICAL CONDITIONS

There are other factors related to the respiratory disease or other comorbid conditions that may contribute to poor sleep quality. They include sleep disruption caused by cough, dyspnea, chest pain or pain from other origins, gastroesophageal reflux, or urinary dysfunction. It is important to properly assess symptoms that occur at night or symptoms that disrupt the patient's sleep, to provide appropriate advice, and to intervene accordingly.

Nocturnal Respiratory Symptoms

Assessment of Respiratory Symptoms

It is important to assess the frequency and severity of nocturnal cough and/or awakening caused by shortness of breath as these will inevitably disrupt sleep.[5,6,8] A number of simple questions can be addressed:

- How often is the patient awakened by respiratory problems at night?
- Is this caused by cough, secretions, shortness of breath, or a choking sensation?
- What is the patient's sleeping position? How many pillows are used?
- Is the room kept dry or humid, cold or hot, especially in winter?
- Is there any history of allergy, and, if so, does the

patient use feather pillows? Are there carpets in the bedroom? These questions are less of a concern for COPD as they are for asthmatic patients.

- Does a bed partner smoke in the bedroom?
- Is there respiratory equipment in the room (oxygen concentrator, CPAP, etc)?
- What medications are taken prior to retiring?
- Are there symptoms of other medical problems or medical sleep disorders (sleep apnea, restless legs, esophageal reflux, etc)?

Hypoxemia at night may also contribute to sleep disruption and tends to occur in patients with severe lung function impairment and daytime hypoxemia.

Management of Respiratory Symptoms

In general, patients with COPD are relatively asymptomatic when they are asleep. Symptoms such as dyspnea are primarily related to physical activities in patients with COPD. However, increasing nocturnal cough or dyspnea may be the first indication of an impending exacerbation or associated comorbid conditions such as gastroesophageal reflux or congestive heart failure (CHF).

Respiratory symptoms at night can be minimized using bronchodilator therapy. If nocturnal dyspnea and cough is prominent, long-acting agents may be used prior to bedtime such as a long-acting β_2 agonist or evening administration of a sustained-release theophylline. Use of coughing techniques can clear secretions prior to retiring. The patient can also use short-acting bronchodilators to reduce symptoms on awakening at night. As further discussed below, nocturnal oxygen or nasal ventilation is indicated for sleep-related hypoxemia and may improve sleep quality.[10,24,27,28,30-32]

Sleeping in a semisitting position with the use of pillows will help diaphragm movement and consequently reduce dyspnea. Large meals prior to bedtime should be avoided as this also impedes diaphragm movement. Medications including inhalers, and spacers, as well as a box of tissues, should all be kept available at the bedside. The bedroom should be adequately humidified and as free of dust as possible. The ideal room temperature will vary for different patients, but excessive cold and heat may both contribute to a deterioration of respiratory symptoms. Heavy blankets may increase the sense of breathing oppression. Light bedding should be used, with the addition of an electric blanket if the patient is still cold.

Nonrespiratory Medical Conditions

Assessment of Nonrespiratory Medical Conditions

Other medical problems (Table 14–3) may contribute to sleep disruption, and the patient should be questioned regarding these.[1,2,12-14,26] Nonrespiratory medical conditions most commonly seen in patients with COPD are discussed in this section.

Gastroesophageal Reflux. Gastroesophageal reflux disease (GERD) may be associated with indigestion, heartburn, epigastric pain, and reflux of gastric contents into the upper airway with resultant cough, choking, and shortness of breath. Gastroesophageal reflux disease may therefore contribute to sleep disruption and can also contribute to the worsening of lung function and cough during wakefulness.[33]

Congestive Heart Failure. Congestive heart failure can mimic the symptoms of a patient with severe COPD. Patients can present with symptoms of orthopnea, paroxysmal nocturnal dyspnea, and leg swelling in either cases. Furthermore, CHF increases dyspnea by provoking bronchospasm in patients with COPD.

TABLE 14–3 Nonrespiratory Medical Conditions Affecting Sleep

Neurologic
  Dementia
  Parkinson's disease
  Degenerative brain disorders

Psychiatric
  Anxiety
  Depression
  Mania
  Psychosis

Cardiovascular
  Congestive heart failure with nocturnal dyspnea
  Nocturnal cardiac ischemia

Gastrointestinal
  Gastroesophageal reflux
  Peptic ulcer disease

Genitourinary
  Bladder disorders leading to nocturia
  Prostatism

Musculoskeletal
  Fibromyalgia
  Chronic pain syndromes

Bladder or Prostate Problems. Bladder or prostate problems can lead to frequent nocturnal urination or even incontinence. In patients with poor sleep quality, there is often considerable difficulty returning to sleep after getting up to void, thus making nocturia very disruptive to sleep. Underlying factors such as drugs, neurologic conditions, or other symptoms of prostatism such as difficulty initiating urination and a reduced stream should be sought. Nocturia of short duration could be related to urinary tract infection, and symptoms of burning on urination or foul-smelling or cloudy urine should also be looked for.

Chronic Pain. Chronic pain from any source is also a frequent contributor to nocturnal sleep disruption. The location of the pain, its character, and factors that worsen and that relieve it may give helpful clues to management.[1,2,12–14,26]

Management of Nonrespiratory Medical Conditions

Management of GERD includes elevating the head of the bed, avoiding large meals, particularly late at night, and avoiding foods that the patient knows exacerbate symptoms. Although this is beyond the scope of this chapter, pharmacologic treatment of GERD and CHF may be necessary. If there is urinary dysfunction, the patient should avoid liquids late in the evening, diuretics should be taken only in the morning, and a urinal or commode should be kept at the bedside, even at home to make the need to void less disruptive to sleep. The management of chronic pain may vary considerably depending on the cause, but appropriate body positioning at night, use of local therapy (heat, ice), splints, and/or physiotherapy may all be required.

PRIMARY SLEEP DISORDERS

Patients with poor sleep quality and/or daytime sleepiness should be questioned for the presence of other respiratory and nonrespiratory disorders during sleep (Table 14–4).[1–3,26] Primary sleep disorders are discussed in more detail in this section.

Obstructive Sleep Apnea

The most important of these disorders is obstructive sleep apnea (OSA), which is characterized by repeated episodes of upper airway obstruction dur-

TABLE 14–4 Primary Sleep Disorders

Respiratory
  Obstructive sleep apnea
  Central sleep apnea
    Cheyne-Stokes respiration
    Associated with central nervous system
      or neuromuscular disease
    Idiopathic

Nocturnal hypoventilation
  Chronic obstructive pulmonary disease
  Obesity
  Chest wall/neuromuscular disorders

Nonrespiratory
  Restless legs syndrome
  Narcolepsy
  Parasomnias
    REM sleep behavior disorder
    Sleep walking
  Circadian rhythm disorders
    Delayed sleep phase
    Advanced sleep phase

REM = rapid eye movement.

ing sleep, leading to hypoxemia and sleep fragmentation.[34] The typical history for OSA is one of heavy habitual snoring and daytime sleepiness; if these are present together, the patient needs to be assessed for OSA. Other symptoms at night include apneas or breathing irregularity witnessed by the bed partner, restless sleep, nocturnal choking, nocturia, morning headache, and awakening unrefreshed. Obstructive sleep apnea may also contribute to complaints of insomnia, although this is less common. The patient himself/herself is typically unaware of snoring and apneas at night. Daytime symptoms include excessive sleepiness, mood disturbances, problems with concentration and memory, various cardiovascular complications, and altered respiratory control (hypoxemia, hypercapnia during wakefulness). Obstructive sleep apnea is not uncommon in patients with COPD, and the coexistence of the two conditions has been termed the overlap syndrome.[35–37]

Obstructive sleep apnea can be improved with a variety of conservative measures such as weight loss, avoidance of alcohol prior to bedtime, and body positioning in patients for whom snoring and apnea are worse when supine.[34] Definitive treatment for significant OSA usually involves nightly use of nasal

CPAP, and there are a whole series of interventions that may be required to help the patient adapt to this sometimes difficult treatment. Careful attention should be given to issues of mask fit and comfort and placement by the patient. Problems with nasal dryness or congestion, runniness, and sneezing are very common. These can be minimized by use of a humidifier to prevent drying of the nasal mucosa and reflex increases in nasal secretions. Although cold pass-over humidifiers are usually supplied, a heated humidifier may be required to increase humidity. Symptoms of mouth leak, such as morning oral dryness, should be sought as mouth leak increases the machine flow rate and can therefore increase nasal symptoms. Mouth leak is usually controlled with the addition of a chin strap but may require use of a full face mask. Noise from the CPAP machine, although not particularly loud, can be disruptive for some patients or spouses. The machine should be placed on the floor, on a padded surface away from the patient's head. If this is insufficient, various noise barriers can be constructed, or extension tubing can allow the machine to be placed in a cupboard or in the hall outside the room.

Hypoventilation Sleep Apnea

Patients with COPD may also have nocturnal hypoxemia, independent of OSA, caused by hypoventilation during sleep, which is typically worse during REM sleep. This tends to happen in patients with severe lung function and daytime hypoxemia but may also occur in more moderate COPD.[38,39] Nocturnal hypoxemia may be associated with disrupted sleep, nocturnal dyspnea, morning headache, and unrefreshing sleep.[5–8,20–24]

Nocturnal hypoventilation may require administration of oxygen or use of nasal ventilation (eg, with bilevel positive airway pressure [BiPAP]).[10,24,30–32] The approach to optimizing O_2 therapy is discussed in detail in Chapter 7, and issues with nasal ventilation are similar to those with CPAP. One important point to remember is that the disturbance of placing any medical equipment in the bedroom may seem threatening or invasive to the privacy of the bedroom. The patients should be encouraged to verbalize and deal with such concerns. Hands-on teaching by a health care professional concerning the nature and proper use and care of the equipment, with the bed partner present as well, can be very reassuring to the patient and help relieve the very real anxiety that may be engendered by the presence of devices.

Restless Legs Syndrome

The restless legs syndrome can also occur; this typically produces difficulty falling asleep at night with symptoms of restlessness, jumpiness, or pain or numbness of the legs that begins in the late evening or on entering bed.[40] The patient feels a need to move the legs, rub them, get up and walk, or stretch the legs. Symptoms typically resolve after several hours, although they may recur through the night. There are a variety of predisposing factors including medications (caffeine, theophyllines, etc), deficiencies of iron or vitamin B_{12}, electrolyte disturbances (low calcium, magnesium), renal failure, and various neurologic deficits; however, a large proportion of cases have no identifiable cause.

Restless legs syndrome can in some cases be alleviated by avoidance of stimulants or other contributing medication or by the replacement of vitamin and/or electrolyte deficiencies. Stretching and regular exercise may also help reduce symptoms. In some cases, treatment with medication is required (eg, benzodiazepines, dopamine agonists).[40]

Narcolepsy

Narcolepsy is a disorder that typically presents in young adulthood but in some cases goes unrecognized for many years and is diagnosed in older patients.[41,42] Narcolepsy is characterized by the following tetrad: persistent or episodic daytime sleepiness, cataplexy or a sudden loss of muscular tone on strong emotional stimulation; sleep paralysis or being unable to move briefly on awakening, and hypnogogic and hypnopompic hallucinations or dreams with a strong visual component that occur as the patient is falling asleep or near awakening. These symptoms may be present alone or in combination and may vary over time. Some narcoleptics present with complaints of marked daytime sleepiness but nocturnal insomnia.

Narcolepsy is managed by a combination of behavioral and drug treatments. Sleep hygiene with adequate nocturnal sleep is of the utmost importance. Daytime sleepiness is treated with stimulant medications such as methylphenidate hydrochloride (Ritalin) or modafinil (Alertec, Provigil). Some patients may require scheduled daytime naps in addition to stimulants. Cataplexy and sleep paralysis symptoms are treated with antidepressant medications.[41,42]

Parasomnia

A variety of nocturnal behavioral disturbances or para-somnias may present in older patients.[43,44] The most notable is REM sleep behavior disorder, in which patients may vocalize or demonstrate motor activity (thrash about, get out of bed) during sleep. Patients may awaken after such episodes and recall some rela-tion of the activity to dream content. In some instances, patients may injure themselves or the bed partner because of motor activity.[43] Sleep walking is also characterized by nocturnal motor activity, but, typically, the patient is not easily awoken and has no recollection of the episode in the morning. Sleepwalk-ing episodes in adults are more likely to recur at times of emotional stress.[44]

Parasomnias are also managed by a combination of behavioral and drug treatments. Removing injurious objects, locking doors and concealing a key, or patient restraint if safety can otherwise be ensured have all been used for nocturnal behavioral disorders. Drug treatment with clonazepam is often helpful.[43,44]

Other Nocturnal Disorders

The effects of sleep habits and mood disturbances on sleep quality were mentioned above. Some sleep disorders are associated with disturbance of bio-logic rhythmns.[45] For example, some patients with insomnia have difficulty falling asleep before a very late hour; however, if there is no reason for them to get up in the morning, they can easily sleep for 7 or 8 hours once asleep. This represents a delayed sleep phase syndrome, which is caused by a reset-ting of the internal biologic clock. As well, some patients are more prone to depression at various times of the year (fall/winter) (seasonal affective disorder), which may be even more marked in patients with COPD who are even more restricted in their activities at those times of the year. This may, in turn, lead to complaints of poor sleep. Evaluation of the patient should take such factors into consideration.

The approach to delayed sleep phase may be var-ied. There can be attempts to manipulate the sleep phase by programmed advancement of the sleep time and/or use of bright light therapy. The sched-ule for such interventions should be determined with the sleep specialist. Use of medications including melatonin and/or other sleeping medications may also be indicated.[45]

WHEN TO REFER

When to Refer to a Physician

Patients with COPD should be regularly assessed by a physician to ensure that the medical management of respiratory symptoms is optimized. If symptoms are increasing, the strategy for exacerbations should be followed, which may, in turn, necessitate assess-ment for possible adjustment or addition of med-ication. If medication effects are contributing to sleep disruption, a change in prescription may be required. Insomnia with corticosteroids is usually short lived and occurs mainly at high doses, but adjustment of dosing regimens may be required.

If GERD is suspected and conservative manage-ment is unsuccessful, the patient should be referred for possible confirmation of the diagnosis via esophageal pH monitoring or endoscopy and pre-scription of acid-reducing medication. Congestive heart failure needs to be approached with appropri-ate pharmacologic and nonpharmacologic interven-tion; it may also require investigation, especially if it is a new diagnosis. Nocturia requires a thorough medical and urologic investigation, which may lead to drug or surgical treatment, and patients with this symptom should be evaluated at some point. Chronic pain that is not satisfactorily managed by conservative measures should be evaluated by a physician to ensure that the cause has been ade-quately investigated, to select appropriate analgesic treatment, and to obtain surgical consultation.

Uncertain diagnosis or uncontrolled symptoms should be an absolute indication to refer to a physi-cian. When needed, for respiratory problems, the patient should be referred to a respirologist or, for nonrespiratory problems, to the appropriate specialist.

When to Refer to a Specialist in Sleep Disorders

If a medical sleep disorder is suspected, the patient should be referred for evaluation by a physician with training in sleep disorders. In many centers, respirol-ogists perform this function whereas in other cen-ters, neurologists or psychiatrists are responsible. A complete laboratory polysomnogram is the preferred diagnostic procedure for suspected medical sleep dis-orders.[46,47] However, when this is not available, in some cases a partial sleep study or overnight record-ing of respiratory variables may be adequate if inter-preted by an experienced observer. Therapeutic choices for OSA (CPAP, surgery, oral appliances) and nocturnal hypoventilation (ventilatory stimulants, O_2, BiPAP, etc) need to be made by the physician in conjunction with the patient. Restless legs syndrome can be treated with a variety of agents including benzodiazepines, opioids, and dopamine agonists. Symptomatic narcolepsy usually requires stimulant and/or anticataplectic medication in addition to sleep hygiene measures as described above. Thus, medical management of the underlying condition needs to be established by the physician.

SUMMARY

Normal, restorative sleep is important to promote and maintain health in patients with COPD. Sleep problems are common among patients with COPD and can have a substantial impact on well-being and symptoms. A few simple screening questions during patient evaluation can indicate to the caregiver whether a sleep problem should be suspected.

The specific approach will vary between patients, but careful attention to sleep hygiene, optimal management of nocturnal respiratory symptoms, minimizing the adverse effects of medication or dietary habits, optimizing the treatment of other medical conditions that may affect sleep, and recognizing and treating specific primary sleep disorders may all be important in producing improvements in sleep quality. Better sleep may, in turn, have a significant positive impact on the patient's sense of well-being and energy, and it improves activity levels during the day. Treatment of respiratory disorders during sleep may also have a beneficial effect on lung function and the progression of cardiopulmonary disease.

CASE STUDY

Case 1

Mr. Cope, a 72-year-old male patient with COPD, complains of sleeping poorly at night and of always feeling tired during the day.

Medical History, Physical Examination, and Test Results

- He has had a morning cough and sputum present for many years.
- He has breathlessness with poor exercise tolerance (approximately 50 ft on the level); he lives with his wife and rarely leaves the house except for appointments at the hospital.
- He is an ex-smoker (45 pack-years).
- Medications include inhaled corticosteroid, ipratropium bromide and salbutamol inhalers (two puffs each four times daily), furosemide, and omeprazole for reflux symptoms.
- He is on home oxygen at 2 Lpm, 24 hours per day.
- He has a baseline FEV_1 of 0.6 L without significant reversibility after bronchodilator and an FEV_1/FVC of 35%.

Questions and Discussion

When questioned about his sleep habits, the patient responds that he does not have a fixed bedtime. He may turn out the lights anytime between 11 pm and 2 am, usually after watching television in bed. He has difficulty falling asleep, awakens often during the night, and then has trouble falling back to sleep. Nocturnal cough is a frequent problem. This is usually relieved by a short-acting β_2-inhaler, but he often forgets to bring this to bed, so he has to get up and retrieve his puffer from the kitchen. He finds it even harder to get back to sleep after getting up. He is occasionally awakened with heartburn symptoms for which he takes antacids; this appears to be more common if he eats late in the evening, which he likes to do as it seems to help him fall asleep. He voids one to three times per night, which he notes occurs more often if at the end of the day he takes an extra dose of diuretic because his legs are swollen. He is also bothered at night by the noise of his O_2 concentrator, which is in the bedroom. When he has difficulty falling back to sleep, Mr. Cope will often turn on the bedroom television and watch until he feels tired again. If he does not watch television, he often lies awake worrying about family problems and money matters.

The patient typically awakens at 6:30 am and rarely falls asleep again after this. However, he tends to stay in bed for some time after waking up. Because he rarely goes out, he will often remain in pyjamas for the whole day. By the end of the morning he feels tired, and almost every afternoon after lunch he becomes so tired that he gets back into bed and naps for 1 to 1½ hours.

After reviewing this history, the health care team makes some specific recommendations to Mr. Cope and his wife concerning his sleep habits, which they work to implement over the following weeks and months. He tries to maintain a regular sleep schedule, getting into bed no later than midnight and getting out of bed by 7 am at the latest. He finds that keeping a sleep diary over several days helps him to get into this schedule. He gets dressed each day, and for a half hour each morning he does a series of exercises that he was taught in a rehabilitation program. At least 2 days per week, he leaves the house for a short walk or excursion to the local shopping center. He tries to avoid napping in the daytime, but if he is really tired, he will nap with a 30-minute timed limit using an alarm.

He is prescribed a long-acting β_2 agonist, which helps with the nocturnal cough. He also leaves a spare short-acting inhaler at the bedside so he does not have to get up for one if symptoms do occur during the night. He no longer takes extra diuretics in the evening but rather increases his morning dose if his swelling is worse or his weight increases. He avoids eating late at night and notes that he wakes up less often with indigestion. The O_2 concentrator is moved to an adjacent room so that its noise is barely audible in the bedroom, and extension tubing is obtained. The television is moved out of the bedroom. If he does waken at night, he tries to focus on either relaxing or on pleasant thoughts to avoid thinking about problems. If he does not fall back asleep, he will turn on the light and read until he feels tired. He also learns a relaxation technique that he uses if he begins to feel tense or anxious and/or when he is trying to return to sleep.

After several months, Mr. Cope feels that his sleep has substantially improved. He wakens much less often at night and feels more refreshed when he gets out of bed in the morning. He is more energetic during the day and is able to participate more in household duties, which he reports feeling good about.

Main Issues

- Sleep hygiene: regular sleep schedule, avoidance of daytime naps
- Beneficial effects of exercise, change of environment
- Optimize treatment of nocturnal respiratory symptoms
- Coping strategies for stress/anxiety
- Reduce other medical and environmental disruptions to sleep

Case 2

Mr. Cope is a 67-year-old patient followed for moderate to severe COPD.

Medical History, Physical Examination, and Test Results

- He has had a morning cough and sputum present for many years but no previous exacerbations.
- He has had breathlessness on moderate exercise such as walking fast or climbing two flights of stairs, also when exposed to cold air, humid weather, or if there is an irritant in the environment.
- He is a smoker of 25 cigarettes per day for the last 40 years.
- He is overweight and consumes a moderate amount of alcohol.
- Pratrodium bromide, two puffs four times/day
- His medication includes inhaled corticosteroid and salbutamol inhalers, two puffs as needed (usually two times daily).
- He is also treated for hypertension and mild diabetes.
- He has a baseline FEV_1 of 1.6 L (50% of predicted normal) with some reversibility (200 μ) after bronchodilator and an FEV_1/FVC of 65%.

Questions and Discussion

When he is questioned about sleep problems at a routine clinic visit, he denies any difficulty with sleep, stating that he falls asleep as soon as his head hits the pillow and sleeps through the night, getting up only twice to void. However, his wife strongly disagrees. She says that Mr. Cope snores very loudly on most nights and that he sometimes seems to be struggling to breathe or even stops breathing during sleep; at times she shakes him to start him breathing again. She also states that despite sleeping 8 hours a night, her husband is very sleepy during the day. If company visits, he will often nod off during conversations, and whenever he turns on the television or reads the newspaper he falls asleep.

Mr. Cope is referred to a sleep laboratory and is found to have severe OSA, with an apnea-hypopnea index of 68 events per hour of sleep. A second study to titrate nasal CPAP is performed and home CPAP is prescribed at 10 cm H_2O. Mr. Cope adapts to the treatment over a period of several weeks, overcoming some nasal congestion with the addition of a heated humidifier to the CPAP unit. He no longer snores, and his wife notes that his breathing is regular and his sleep is much calmer with the mask in place. The patient says that he feels much better when he wakes up in the morning; his wife notes that he sleeps significantly less during the day and that his activity level is much improved. He uses his short-acting β_2 agonist less often, and his blood pressure medication is able to be lowered after several months on CPAP.

Main Issues

- This is a typical history of OSA with heavy habitual snoring, witnessed apneas, and excessive daytime sleepiness in an overweight patient who ingests alcohol.
- Investigation with sleep studies is preformed and treatment of a primary sleep disorder is prescribed.
- Improvement in daytime sleepiness and activity is seen with treatment.
- Treatment of OSA may improve control of bronchospasm and blood pressure.

KEY POINTS

- Sleep disturbances can have an important impact on the well-being of patients with COPD.
- Significant sleep problems can be suspected from a few simple screening questions.
- Practical sleep hygiene measures can have a major impact on sleep quality.
- Optimizing treatment of nocturnal respiratory symptoms can improve sleep quality.
- Effects of medication and other medical conditions on sleep quality should be assessed and treated appropriately; when needed, the patient should be referred to the physician or to a specialist.
- Primary respiratory or nonrespiratory sleep disorder can be present in patients with COPD; referral to a specialized resource should be done accordingly.

REFERENCES

1. Kryger MH, Roth T, Dement WC. Principles and practice of sleep medicine. Philadelphia: WB Saunders, 2000.
2. Chokroverty S. Sleep disorders medicine: basic science, technical considerations and clinical aspects. 1st Ed. Boston: Butterworth-Heinmann, 1995.
3. Vgontzas AN, Kales A. Sleep and its disorders. Annu Rev Med 1999;50:387–400.
4. Leger D. Public health and insomnia. Economic impact. Sleep 2000;2 Suppl 3:S69–76.
5. Douglas NJ. Sleep in patients with chronic obstructive pulmonary disease. Clin Chest Med 1998;19:115–25.
6. McNicholas WT. Impact of sleep in COPD. Chest 2000;117 Suppl 2:S48–53.
7. Magnusson S, Gislason T. Chronic bronchitis in Icelandic males: prevalence, sleep disturbances and quality of life. Scand J Prim Health Care 1999; 17:100–4.
8. George CF. Perspectives on the management of insomnia in patients with chronic respiratory disorders. Sleep 2000;1 Suppl 23:S31–5.
9. Phillips BA, Cooper KR, Burke TV. The effect of sleep loss on breathing in chronic obstructive pulmonary disease. Chest 1987;91:29–32.
10. Mansfield D, Naughton MT. Effects of continuous positive airway pressure on lung function in patients with chronic obstructive pulmonary disease and sleep disordered breathing. Respirologie 1999;4:365–70.
11. Roehrs T, Merrion M, Pedrosi B, et al. Neuropsychological function in obstructive sleep apnea syndrome (OSAS) compared to chronic obstructive pulmonary disease (COPD). Sleep 1995;18:382–8.
12. Chesson A, Hartse K, Anderson WM, et al. Practice parameters for the evaluation of chronic insomnia. An American Academy of Sleep Medicine report. Standards of Practice Committee of the American Academy of Sleep Medicine review. Sleep 2000;23: 237–41.
13. Sateia MJ, Doghramji K, Hauri PJ, Morin CM. Evaluation of chronic insomnia. An American Academy of Sleep Medicine review. Sleep 2000;23:243–308.
14. Costa E, Silva JA, Chase M, et al. An overview of insomnias and related disorers—recognition, epidemiology, and rational management. Sleep 1996;19:412–6.
15. Kupfer DJ, Reynolds CFI. Managment of insomnia. N Engl J Med 1997;336:341–6.
16. Ballard RD, Clover CW, Suh BY. Influence of sleep on respiratory function in emphysema. Am J Crit Care Med 1995;151:945–51.
17. McKeon JL, Murree-Allen K, Saunders NA. Prediction of oxygenation during sleep in patients with chronic obstructive lung disease. Thorax 1988;43:312–7.
18. White JE, Drinnan MJ, Smithson AJ, et al. Respiratory muscle activity during rapid eye movement (REM) sleep in patients with chronic obstructive pulmonary disease. Thorax 1995;50:376–82.
19. Catterall JR, Claverley PM, MacNee W, et al. Mechanism of transient nocturnal hypoxemia in hypoxic

chronic bronchitis and emphysema. J Appl Physiol 1985;59:1698–703.

20. Klink M, Quan SF. Prevalence of reported sleep disturbances in a general adult population and their relationship to obstructive airways disease. Chest 1987;91:540–6.

21. Cormick W, Olson LG, Hensley MJ, Saunders NA. Nocturnal hypoxemia and quality of sleep in patients with chronic obstructive lung disease. Thorax 1986;41:846–54.

22. McKeon JL, Murree-Allen K, Saunders NA. Supplemental oxygen and quality of sleep in patients with chronic obstructive lung disease. Thorax 1989;44:184–8.

23. Conway WA, Kryger M, Timms RM, Williams GW. Clinical significance of sleep desaturation in hypoxemic chronic obstructive pulmonary disease: studies in 130 patients. Henry Ford Hosp Med J 1988; 36:16–23.

24. Orr WC, Shamma-Othman Z, Levin D, et al. Persistent hypoxemia and excessive daytime sleepiness in chronic obstructive pulmonary disease (COPD). Chest 1990;97:583–5.

25. Morin CM, Colecchi C, Stone J, et al. Behavioral and pharmacologic therpies for late-life insomnia. A randomized controlled trial. JAMA 1999;281:991–9.

26. Diagnostic Classification Steering Committee. International classification of sleep disorders: diagnostic and coding manual. Rochester, MN: American Sleep Disorder Association, 1990.

27. Berry RB, Desa MM, Branum JP, Light RW. Effect of theophylline on sleep and sleep-disordered breathing in patients with chronic obstructive pulmonary disease. Am Rev Respir Dis 1991;143:245–50.

28. Martin RJ, Pak J. Overnight theophylline concentrations and effects on sleep and lung function in chronic obstructive pulmonary disease. Am Rev Respir Dis 1992;145:540–4.

29. Steens RD, Pouliot Z, Millar TW, et al. Effects of zolpidem and triazolam on sleep and respiration in mild to moderate chronic obstructive pulmonary disease. Sleep 1993;16:318–26.

30. Fletcher EC, Luckett RA, Goodnight-White S, et al. A double-blind trial of nocturnal supplemental oxygen for sleep desaturation in patients with chronic obstructive pulmonary disease and a daytime PaO2 above 60 mmHg. Am Rev Respir Dis 1992;145:1070–6.

31. Elliott WM, Simonds AK, Carroll MP, et al. Domiciliary nocturnal nasal intermittent positive pressure ventilation in hypercapnic respiratory failure due to chronic obstructive lung disease: effects on sleep and quality of life. Thorax 1992;47:342–8.

32. Gay PC, Hubmayr RD, Stroetz RW. Efficacy of nocturnal nasal ventilation in stable, severe chronic obstructive pulmonary disease during a 3-month controlled trial. Mayo Clin Proc 1996;71:533–42.

33. Orr WC, Shamma-Othman Z, Allen M, Robinson MG. Esophageal function and gastroesophageal reflux during sleep and waking in patients with chronic obstructive pulmonary disorder. Chest 1992;101:1512–25.

34. Weigand L, Zwillich CW. Obstructive sleep apnea.
Dis Mon 1994;40:197–252.

35. Sampol G, Sagalés MT, Roca A, et al. Nasal continuous positive airway pressure with supplemental oxygen in coexistent sleep apnoea-hypopnoea syndrome and severe chronic obsturctive pulmonary disease. Eur Respir J 1996;9:111–6.

36. Radwan L, Maszczyk Z, Koziorowski A, et al. Control of breathing in obstructive sleep apnea and in patients with the overlap syndrome. Eur Respir J 1995;8:542–5.

37. Chaouat A, Weitzenblum E, Krieger J, et al. Association of chronic obstructive pulmonary disease and sleep apnea syndrome. Am J Respir Crit Care Med 1995;151:82–6.

38. Mohsenin V, Guffanti EE, Hilbert J, Ferranti R. Daytime oxygen saturation does not predict nocturnal oxygen desaturation in patients with chronic obstructive pulmonary disease. Arch Phys Med Rehabil 1994;75:285–9.

39. Chaouat A, Weitzenblum E, Kessler R, et al. Sleep-related O2 desaturation and daytime pulmonary haemodynamics in COPD patients with mild hypoxaemia. Eur Respir J 1997;10:1730–5.

40. Montplaisir J, Boucher S, Poirier G, et al. Clinical, polysomnographic and genetic characteristics of restless legs syndrome: a study of 133 patients diagnosed with new standard criteria. Mov Disord 1997;12:61–5.

41. Mitler MM, Hajdukovic R, Erman M, Koziol JA. Narcolepsy. J Clin Neurophysiol 1990;7:93–118.

42. Krahn LE, Black JL, Silber MH. Narcolepsy: new understanding of irresistible sleep. Mayo Clin Proc 2001;76:185–94.

43. Schenck CH, Mahowald MW. REM sleep parasomnias. Neurol Clin 1996;14:697–720.

44. Kavey NB, Whyte J, Resor SRJ, Gido-Frank S. Somnambulism in adults. Neurology 1990;40:749–52.

45. Richardson GS, Malin HV. Circadian rhythm sleep disorders: pathophysiology and treatment. J Clin Neurophysiol 1996;13:17–31.

46. Connaughton JJ, Catterall JR, Elton RA, et al. Do sleep studies contribute to the management of patients with severe chronic obstructive pulmonary disease? Am Rev Respir Dis 1988;138:341–4.

47. American Thoracic Society. Standards for diagnosis and care of patients with chronic obstructive pulmonary disease. Am J Respir Crit Care Med 1995;152 (5 Pt 2):S77–121.

SUGGESTED READINGS

Douglas NJ. Sleep in patients with chronic obstructive pulmonary disease. Clin Chest Med 1998;19:115–25. *This article is a very readable, comprehensive overview of sleep-related issues in COPD.*

Vgontzas AN, Kales A. Sleep and its disorders. Annu Rev Med 1999;50:387–400. *This reference provides a good general synopsis of sleep disorders.*

CHAPTER 15

SEXUALITY

Ginette Poulin and Diane Nault

OBJECTIVES

The general objective of this chapter is to raise awareness among physicians and allied health care professionals regarding the sexual problems of people with chronic obstructive pulmonary disease (COPD) to encourage professionals to explore their needs and identify interventions that will likely improve their sexual health.

After reading this chapter, the physician and the allied health care professional will be able to

- understand the dimensions of sexual behavior in patients with COPD;
- distinguish the phases of the sexual act, normality of the physiologic manifestations, and subsequent changes owing to age;
- recognize the organic, psychological, and relational factors likely to influence sexuality;
- recognize misconceptions likely to affect people with COPD and propose possible solutions;
- make appropriate use of therapeutic intervention strategies likely to improve the expression of sexuality;
- present a guide for couples wishing to continue having sexual relations; and
- refer to specific professional resources when needed.

Sexuality is as much a basic need for people with COPD as it is for healthy people. At least 50% of people with COPD report that the disease has an effect on their sex life.[1] Hanson also noted that many patients are afraid to express their sexual needs to their partner for fear of triggering a dyspnea attack or a bout of coughing; the root cause of this is based on the dyspnea they experience during daily activities.[1] In addition, they may feel guilty about not responding to their partner's sexual needs because of their illness.[2–4]

Literature concerning the sexuality of people with COPD notes that several taboos, misconceptions, or myths are still widely held by the general population and by health care professionals.[3] These difficulties may be linked to modesty and underlying beliefs about sexuality within the fabric of our culture. However, when a health care professional is caught off guard or does not address the problems expressed by a patient or spouse, the couple may ultimately believe there is no solution for them. A lack of information, or a lack of awareness of the problem, increases anxiety and frustration.[5] On the other hand, an honest and open discussion between the professional, patient, and spouse can help build a relationship of trust and lay the foundation for an improved quality of life for the couple.[3,4]

In this chapter, we define the concept of sexuality, the phases of the sexual act, the problems related to sexual dysfunction, and the myths surrounding sexuality and COPD. Evaluation strategies and interventions that can be used by the health care professional is addressed, and when to refer the client or the couple to a specialist.

DEFINITION OF THE CONCEPT OF SEXUALITY

Sexual health was defined by the World Health Organization in 1975 as being "the integration of the somatic, emotional, intellectual and social aspects of sexual well-being in ways that are positively enriching and that enhance personality, communication and love."[6]

Sexuality is an individual, unique experience leading to a satisfying feeling of well-being. Sexuality comprises two levels of expression. The first is the physical and genital, that is, the sexual act itself associated with pleasure. This is a biologic and instinctive language that takes erotic thoughts and desires into account.[7,8] The second level involves sensuality, psychological needs, emotions, and the ability to communicate with one's partner. This is a more creative and imaginative language, one that invokes sensitivity and the art of giving and receiving pleasure. Sexual maturity is linked to the ability to come to terms with tenderness and genitality. Generally, men and women evolve differently; for men, sexuality is first genital, whereas for women, sensuality comes before sexuality.[9]

Sexual health is a component of general health; it is a holistic experience that encompasses both body and mind. It is also a human reality that includes several dimensions of life in constant interaction. Although there has been little research in this field, the literature points to the importance of this aspect and contains some relevant advice for people with COPD. The literature describes the influence of disabling symptoms of dyspnea, cough, and fatigue not only on the sexual response cycle but also on the psychosocial and relational aspects of the couple.[1,3,10–12]

Corporal or Somatic Dimension

For some people with COPD, physical effort is very demanding; often, they feel they must cease sexual activity out of fear of provoking shortnes of breath. For many people with COPD, sex is one activity among many to be avoided. Their disappointing experiences only serve to reinforce this avoidance behavior. But, just what type of physical effort is involved in sexual relations?

The literature on this subject offers divergent opinions, which, moreover, are not so recent. For Mishara and Riedel, oxygen consumption at the time of coitus with a regular partner is less than that required for fast walking or climbing stairs.[13] This is an often-cited fact in literature on the subject.

There is also an American study that compares sexual activity with exercise obtained through daily activities. According to this study, it appears that the oxygen consumption required during sexual activity is equivalent to exercise of 3 to 5 METs, or 10.5 to 17.5 mL O_2/kg/min (METs represent the energy used by a person at rest), that is, climbing a flight of 20 stairs in 10 seconds without difficulty.[14,15] According to these authors, sexual activity (comprising coitus and orgasm) is therefore demanding as the maximum effort is performed in very little time. It should be noted that this research was mostly done in the laboratory with young, active people, but who, on the other hand, were also likely influenced by a higher stress rate.

Butler and Lewis stated that during sexual activity, the heart rate is approximately 120 beats per minute during orgasm and can vary between 90 and 160 beats per minute during the most strenuous 10 minutes of sexual activity.[7] The systolic blood pressure rises to an average of 160 mm Hg, and respiration can go up to 18 to 60 breaths per minute. People with cardiac or respiratory problems need to be able to recognize signs of excessive shortness of breath.

Other authors suggested four warning signs for cardiac patients indicating the need to avoid initiating sexual activity[15–17]:

1. When the dyspnea or heart rate does not return to normal within 5 minutes following the activity
2. When the person feels extreme fatigue the day after sexual relations
3. When the person experiences insomnia after sexual relations
4. When chest pain is present and unrelieved by rest or the use of relaxation/breathing techniques

According to Kravetz, many people may find it helpful to try masturbation first, the equivalent of 3 to 4 METs, before having complete sexual relations with a partner.[18]

Certain authors also suggest less tiring positions for people with COPD, for example, positions that minimize pressure on the chest or diaphragm.[3,12,19]

Psychoemotional and Relational Dimension

Sexual health also demands an adequate psychoemotional response. It involves communicating one's feelings, needs, desires, and level of satisfaction to one's partner.[8] The most important psychological components in people with COPD are anxiety and depression.[20]

Anxiety stems from the fear of suffocating; this fear increases oxygen consumption, respiration rate, muscular tension, and heart rate.[20] Furthermore, it is heightened when there have been repeated failures because failure is such a strong determining factor in stopping all sexual activity. A lack of understanding of the disease or a lack of information also fuels this anxiety.[3–5]

People with COPD suffer from depression more often than chronic anxiety or any other disorder.[21,22] This situational depression is related to several losses caused by the chronicity of the disease. The appearance of dependence brought on by the disease can lead to frustration, anger, aggression, and resentment when roles are changed.[1] Also, the negative perception of self-image, in turn, negatively affects sexuality.[3]

The transformation of the social situation caused by COPD and its symptoms differs with each individual. For some couples, the problem of the disease can be a pretext to stop intimate relationships that were otherwise unsatisfactory.[12] For others, the disease brings them emotionally closer together.[1]

PHASES OF THE SEXUAL ACT

To understand the possible effects of sexual relations on people with COPD, it is necessary to know the physiologic reactions of the sexual act. The sexual act comprises four phases: excitation, plateau, orgasm, and resolution or relaxation (Table 15–1). Each phase comprises different biologic responses, which are not always absolute. They can be fairly intricate and will vary from one person to another according to the occasion and age.[8,23,24]

Erotic desire is often defined as a drive or potential energy that spurs people into action. This drive varies in intensity depending on sensory stimulation, the individual, and age. It could be considered the engine of the sexual relationship.[23] Desire may be accompanied by romantic foreplay enriched by erotic fantasies.

Table 15–1 shows the physiologic changes that occur during the sexual act. Two phenomena predominate: vasocongestion and an increase in neuromuscular tone.[8] Vasocongestion increases the size of the genital organs and the breasts. In males, there is a relaxation of the smooth muscles of the penile arteries and corpus cavernosum, thus enabling entry of a higher volume of blood.[25] An increase in neuromuscular tone (or myotonia) causes an energy increase in the nerves and muscles, not only in the genital area but throughout the body. This myotonia reaches its peak during orgasm.

SEXUAL DYSFUNCTION

The causes of sexual dysfunction may be organic or physiopathologic, or even psychological and relational. In quantitative terms, one-third of sexual dysfunction cases are thought to be mainly physiopathologic in origin, one-third mainly psychological or relational in origin, and the remaining third of mixed origin.[8,24,25]

Sexual dysfunction may be specific to a phase in the sexual response cycle or to a lack of interest in sexual activity called inhibition or lack of desire; it may be affected by many factors in physical and psychosocial health.[8,24]

The main sexual dysfunction in men is erectile dysfunction, which is now a preferred term to impotence.

The most frequently encountered sexual problems in women are lack of desire, lubrication, coital pain (pain on penetration), vaginitis, and anorgasmia.[8]

Organic or Physiopathologic Factors

There is increasing recognition of the organic factors underlying sexual dysfunction. With a better understanding of sexual function and the aging of the population, a greater emphasis is being placed on identifying these organic factors. After age 50, approximately 50% of men are affected by some form of physical sexual dysfunction.[26] The Viagra (sildenafil citrate) era has shown that sexual problems are more commonplace than first thought.[27]

In men, the most frequent organic causes of erectile dysfunction are blood vessel anomalies and anomalies of the nerves and the central nervous system.[25,28] Additionally, there are hormone and endocrine anomalies.[8,29]

In women, the most frequent organic causes are diabetes and alcoholism, neurologic disorders, hormone deficiencies, and pelvic disorders resulting from an infection or trauma.[30] Other factors, such as aging and its biologic consequences and the side effects of certain medications, can affect both men and women.[8,29]

Blood Vessel Anomalies

Deterioration of the male genitalia is mainly owing to blood vessel anomalies. Any involvement, even benign, of the cavernous arteries is sufficient to produce erectile insufficiency. Arteriosclerosis, hypertension, hypercholesterolemia, and diabetes are the main pathologies involved.[25] Smoking can lead to

TABLE 15–1 Phases of the Sexual Act, Normality, and Changes Owing to Age

Phases of the Sexual Act	Normal Physiologic Signs	Changes Owing to Age
Excitation	*Men*: Erection in two phases: tumescence and rigidity *Women*: Vaginal lubrication, distention of the vaginal wall, engorgement, and sensitivity of the labia minora, clitoris, and breasts	*Men*: A longer time to obtain a firm erection, and a need for direct stimulation, decrease in the engorgement of the scrotum and elevation of the testicles *Women*: Reduced vaginal lubrication, thinning of the vaginal walls in menopausal women who are not on hormone replacement therapy, decreased engorgement of the labia minora and breasts, slower reaction to stimulation of the clitoris
Plateau	Redness all over the body (sexual flush) Increased heart rate, blood pressure, and respiration. Increase in muscle tension *Men*: Increase in the size of the glans, which takes on a more vivid color; the testicles move closer to the body and increase 50% in size *Women*: Retraction of the clitoris, the uterus and the cervix move upward, appearance of sexual flush (color of the labia minora), formation of an orgasmic platform (swelling of the labia minora and elevation of the last third of the vagina), engorgement of the areola, and increase in breast size	*Men*: Complete erection of the penis just before ejaculation, longer time to reach ejaculation, extended plateau phase, change in color of the glans is less likely *Women*: Less expansion of the vaginal wall, decreased sexual flush and engorgement of the areola and breasts, orgasmic platform reduced by half
Orgasm	*Men*: Emission of seminal fluid through the urinary canal and ejaculation, contraction at the base of the penis *Women*: Involuntary contraction of the muscles of the pelvic floor	*Men*: Ejaculation less powerful and less abundant, muscle spasm of the orgasm less intense *Women*: Decreased intensity of muscle spasm during orgasm
Resolution or relaxation	Heart rate, blood pressure, and respiration return to normal. Sweating *Men*: Penis returns to a flaccid state; testicles descend; refractory or recovery period before another orgasm, variable from one man to another *Women*: Possibility of successive orgasms	*Men*: Penis returns to a flaccid state more rapidly, lengthening of the refractory period (longer time between two erections) *Women*: Faster detumescence of the genital organs

Adapted from Masters WH, Johnson VE,[8] Trudel G,[24] Alarie P, Villeneuve R,[25] Kolodny, et al.[29]

constriction of the blood vessels and can decrease blood flow to the penis. This is the main cause of vascular-origin erectile dysfunction.[8,29,31]

Anomalies of the Nerves and Nerve Center

The nervous system plays a major role in sexual behavior and sexual function.[8] Several anomalies may be responsible for the transmission of nerve impulses between the genital organs and the brain. Diabetic neuropathy is the main cause as it leads to nerve degeneration, which, in turn, prevents dilation of the penile arteries. Chronic alcoholism can also affect the nerve pathways to the penis and cause testicular atrophy, as well as an excessive secretion of female hormones in men.[29] Clinical observations show that at least 50% of alcoholics have a problem with desire and sexual function.[29,32,33] In women, alcoholism leads to atrophy of the breasts, uterus, and vaginal wall, and 40% of women say that they have had problems with orgasm or desire.[34]

Other diseases, such as multiple sclerosis, renal failure, or medullary injuries, may cause varying degrees of erectile dysfunction. Some surgeries, such as those on the organs of the pelvis (intestinal, rectal, and prostate surgery), can also be detrimental.

Hormone and Endocrine Anomalies

Blood hormone functioning (follicle-stimulating hormone, luteinizing hormone, prolactin, progesterone, testosterone, estrogen, and the steroid hormones) likely influences sexual desire.[8,29] The research tends to show that hormones play a significant role in desire and sexual activity, both in men and women.[35] But desire remains a difficult concept to quantify, and the causes are often multifactorial.[24]

With a decrease in testosterone, sexual desire and erectile disorders are the symptoms most often identified by men. Lower testosterone leads to a loss of urgent desire, the "drive" to have sexual relations.[36,37]

The most significant endocrine disorder is diabetes. According to the authors consulted, 50 to 70% of diabetics aged 50 and over who have been diabetic for more than 7 years have erectile dysfunction accompanied by various health problems, such as neuropathies and vascular disorders.[29] However, a recent study concluded that improved blood sugar control decreases the risk of microvascular involvement and neuropathy by 33%.[36] It may be possible to extrapolate an eventual decrease in sexual dysfunction among diabetics.

Approximately 40% of women and 70 to 80% of men with pituitary, thyroid, or adrenal disorders complain of loss of desire and dysfunction.[8,29] These problems are nevertheless reversible with treatment.

Aging and Its Biologic Consequences

People in their forties and fifties note the appearance of certain changes. Andropause and menopause start at around age 50, accompanied by an array of clinical symptoms: fatigue, decreased physical strength and muscle mass, sleep disorders, and even symptoms of moderate depression, anxiety, and decreased production at work.[37,38] The genitalia are not immune to these age-induced changes.[39] Table 15–1 shows the main changes owing to age in relation to the phases of the sexual act. Furthermore, according to Butler and Lewis, 70% of people over age 45 have one or more chronic physical illnesses.[7] Clearly, these illnesses will have repercussions on sexuality, and during an acute phase of the illness, all of the couple's energy will be devoted to relieving the symptoms.

In a major study on the sexual behavior of people aged 50 and over, Brecher concluded that sexual function declines gradually from age 50.[26] Nevertheless, it can be seen from his research that behavior and attitudes regarding sexuality are not generalized. In fact, depending on the age group and gender of the respondents, 65 to 98% of people aged 50 to 80 are sexually active. In a couple, the physiologic changes in one necessarily affect the reactions of the other partner. These changes can cause panic in some couples, but for others, they are perceived as offering the possibility of improving their sex life.

Potential Sexual Problems with Medication

Although the literature may be contradictory, medications are responsible for approximately 30% of erectile dysfunction.[25,29] There is little information available on the sexual function of women, but it is thought that women are affected in the same way as men.

The impact of medication on sexuality is very subtle. It is often very difficult to determine whether the medication is actually influencing the sexual function or if there are psychogenic causes.[39]

Given the great complexity and the constant discovery of new medications, we must recall the principles laid out by Badeau and Bergeron concerning medications that can affect sexuality:

- any medication that tends to mimic the action of the parasympathetic or sympathetic nervous system and
- any medication having an effect on neurotransmitters (acetylcholine, adrenaline and noradrenaline, serotonin, dopamine) or acting on the hypothalamopituitary-ovarian/testicular pathway and producing a stimulating or inhibiting effect on the expression of sexuality and the sexual response.[39]

There are, nonetheless, several well-documented effects attributed to certain classes of medications:

hypotensives can decrease the arterial pressure in the corpus cavernosum, thereby inhibiting the rigidity of the erection; psychotropics can decrease libido or sexual desire; and cortisone in a daily dose of more than 20 mg can inhibit the hypothalamus, the pituitary gland, and adrenaline production.[5,29] Patients with COPD frequently have a comorbid condition that links them or makes them susceptible in some way to erectile dysfunction.

Psychological and Relational Factors

Whatever the organic factor at the origin of sexual dysfunction, anxiety overload, stress, and negative ruminations are always present.[9,24] For people with COPD, several factors can accumulate and/or interact with each another. The most frequent psychological causes are a lack of self-confidence, fear of intimacy or failure, preoccupation with sexual performance, previous trauma of a break-up or rejection, and fear of the partner's sexual desire.[8,9,24] Anxiety is, in fact, a cause common to all sexual dysfunction.[23] Accordingly, the sexologist must locate the symptom within the sexual response structure (problem with desire, excitation, or orgasm) to define the treatment. Since sexual desire is very vulnerable to stressful situations, the intensity of the anxiety can lead to avoidance behavior and inhibition of desire.[23]

Other feelings such as guilt, self-depreciation, and shame of not being able to perform can amplify the person's impotence.[24] A decreased self-image is constantly found at the root of these disturbances, and depression is often present after a failure, especially for people with COPD.[40]

Interpersonal conflicts within the couple are frequently associated with sexual dysfunction. The sexual relationship charged with emotion, hostile exchanges, a power struggle, and unresolved conflicts can often negatively affect communication between the couple.[24,40] In addition, daily fatigue, monotony, and the routine of conjugal life can smother desire and the anticipation of pleasure.[23]

Evaluation of Sexual Dysfunction According to the PLISSIT Model

Many professionals do not discuss sexual problems unless the client specifically asks about them. The efforts of health care professionals focus mainly on the physical and psychological aspects of the chronic disease. Allowing patients to talk about their sexual-

ity is, however, a very important aspect because many would like to be able to discuss this with health care professionals.[7,39,41] When patients are referred and guided in re-establishing their sexual function, they often appreciate this openness.[3,42]

Many variables have to be taken into consideration when giving appropriate advice to people with COPD and their spouses. The seriousness of the pulmonary disease affects people differently depending on their age, personality, and social circumstances. In addition, other chronic illnesses frequently complicate the problem.

In their study, Golden and Golden suggested initiating a discussion on sexuality with the client and spouse at different stages of the chronic illness, that is, when first diagnosed, when treatment is started, and systematically during subsequent therapy.[42] A relationship of trust gradually develops, and interventions can be adjusted accordingly.

To help define the problem, a sexologist developed the PLISSIT model.[43] We will use this model to show the activities that a generalist, such as a physician or nurse, can use for people with COPD and their spouses to intervene according to their capabilities. Then, depending on the diagnosis, the client and spouse can be referred to the most appropriate specialist.

PLISSIT Model

The PLISSIT model (permission, limited information, specific suggestions, intensive therapy) is a good guide for a health care professional who wishes to help a client and spouse.[43] The model is described as follows:

Permission. Ask permission to discuss sexuality and evaluate how it is affected by the disease and its symptoms.

Limited Information. Inform the client and spouse about the effects of the disease and its symptoms on their sexuality.

Specific Suggestions. Provide a concrete means of reducing the symptoms and promoting sexual satisfaction.

Intensive Therapy. Following the preceding steps, when complex relational conflicts are present, refer the couple to an appropriate specialist, such as a sexologist.

To facilitate this interview, an appropriate climate of trust for the expression of the couple's concerns must be developed. The health care professional's verbal and nonverbal behavior can contribute to making the client and spouse more comfortable.[23] Alternatively, some types of behavior, such as not making eye contact or insisting on taking notes, can indicate embarrassment and adversely affect the communication of information.

Below is an example of how the model can be used with a person with COPD and his/her spouse:

Permission. Sexuality can be brought up in several ways during the interview. For example, you could say, "Do your respiratory problems affect your sexual life?" This could be followed by, " If so, in what way?"

To provide good information, the health care professional must first evaluate the impact of the disease on the person's activities of daily living and determine the couple's expectations regarding their sexual needs.[20] For example, the spouse of a person with COPD may show a lack of interest in sex to avoid causing the patient an attack of dyspnea. Conversely, the person with the illness may feel less attractive because of the symptoms and thus become withdrawn. By learning how the behavior affects his/her partner, the individual can be more responsive to changing his/her attitude.

When a couple gets along well together, sexual problems are more easily overcome. In contrast, when the couple is dysfunctional, a restructuring of the actual relationship is often necessary before any attempt is made to address the sexual problem. Each member of the couple is responsible for the problem but also for the solution.[9]

Limited Information. At this stage, the health care professional must provide relevant information concerning the possible effects stemming from symptoms of pulmonary disease and the specific treatments likely to affect sexuality.

According to the cognitive behavioral approach, the leading cause of problems related to sexuality is lack of knowledge.[3,8] Among a group of persons with COPD, often over age 50, there is frequently poor knowledge of sexual physiology and the effect of the disease symptoms on sexuality. Moreover, it is necessary to not only consider the impact of other illnesses and the medication used by the client but also the health condition of the spouse.

Armed with the relevant information, the couple will be able to understand the illness, symptoms, and treatment, thereby absolving themselves of guilt by understanding how the illness affects the desire or erectile function of the person with COPD.

Health care professionals must also correct misconceptions and fears by providing the couple with the necessary information.[4,43] At this stage, professionals can normalize the couple's reactions and feelings regarding their fears related to misconceptions. The act of normalizing the couple's intense emotional experience will help them establish a relationship between the illness and their fears and verbalize their respective emotions with the realization that the experienced emotions are not uncommon.[3]

Specific Suggestions. Specific suggestions are aimed at improving sexual behavior by using concrete means to reduce symptoms and improve comfort, while enabling the patient to accept his/her physical limitations.

As the advice given will vary depending on the case, the health care professional must first identify the person's ability to perform activities of daily living; for example, the advice might vary on the significance of the dyspnea after effort, such as climbing stairs. When the person cannot go up three steps without experiencing shortness of breath and then requires resting for several minutes, this could call for advice that suggests limiting sexual activity to affectionate touching and talking about happy memories.[15]

In other circumstances, it is important to teach breathing techniques and less strenuous sexual positions. Discussion must always include suggestions about medications, the temperature of the room, and the time of day when the person is more at rest so as to make the sexual act more satisfactory.[4,44]

Intensive Therapy. Intensive therapy or a referral to a specialist is often necessary.

In situations in which the couple's relationship is disrupted and aggravated by a chronic illness, the intervention of a specialist such as a psychologist or sexologist may facilitate their communication. A more in-depth approach by a sexologist is useful in cases where intrapsychic difficulties dominate, such as inhibitions or perversions, or problems with gender or sexual orientation.[8] A humanistic or behavioral approach that restructures behavior generally produces faster results but is not always ideal when the conflict is superficial.

MISCONCEPTIONS CONCERNING PEOPLE WITH COPD AND SEXUALITY

Several misconceptions prevent the recognition and satisfaction of the patient's needs in regard to sexuality. These misconceptions are held both by professionals and patients.[4] One of the curious elements regarding sexual misconceptions is that they are easily adopted despite the absence of any proof; moreover, they can become a sort of self-fulfilling prophecy.[8] For the people concerned, these misconceptions may often serve as an excuse for abandoning any attempt at improving their sexual life and for the professionals, a pretext for not intervening.[4,8]

Jokes or vague comments concerning sexuality are often precursory indications that the patient or the spouse is experiencing difficulties. The health care professional must be alert to the way a patient talks about his/her problems. First, the professional must identify the patient's fears, attitudes, and possible difficulties and then discredit any misconceptions with adequate teaching. Conversely, the professional may have to get the patient to accept the limitations of the disease and help him/her find a way to satisfy the couple's socioemotional needs.

Misconceptions surrounding COPD are presented in Table 15–2, along with possible solutions for dispelling or correcting them.

TABLE 15–2 Misconceptions Concerning Patients With COPD and Sexuality

Misconception	Scenario	Intervention
1. People who have difficulty breathing are not sexual 2. People with difficulty breathing need to be protected 3. Sexuality is a spontaneous activity in which partners play an active role	Professional: "We have discussed several issues, now we'll talk about sexuality. Is this important to you?" 1. Client: "I had an attack last week, can I resume sexual activities?" 2. Client: "Since I was hospitalized, my husband is afraid of worsening my condition by having sexual relations. What do you think?" "How can I reassure him?" 3. Couple: "For some time, we have had to change our habits and plan in advance for sexual relations, which takes away all the spontaneity."	• Encourage the sharing of emotions to promote dialogue within the couple • Provide information on the effect of any physical activity versus sexual activity. The ability to perform activities of daily living is an indication that sexual relations can be resumed • Explain the vicious cycle to the couple: decreased energy leads to increased fatigue and increased breathlessness • Teach or validate the ability to use coping mechanisms (coughing technique, breathing, medications, relaxation, etc) that improve performance • Emphasize the importance of foreplay, sexual talk, demonstrations of tenderness, caresses, which are all part of sexual relations and satisfy many couples • Explore what each person likes and does not like and encourage creativity • Validate with the couple how they feel about their changing role and its influence on self-esteem
4. Sexual problems experienced by people with COPD are a result of the pulmonary disease	4. Client: "I can't have sexual relations because of my lung disease."	• Validate with the client his/her understanding of the disease and its symptoms

TABLE 15–2 Misconceptions Concerning Patients With COPD and Sexuality (continued)

Misconception	Scenario	Intervention
4.1 Complete abstinence is preferable to the possibility of suffocating or triggering an attack	4.1 Client: "I'm afraid of suffocating or being too tired; so, it's better to abstain from sex in case this happens."	• Ask the couple how they manage the symptoms during sexual activities
4.2 Unpleasant symptoms such as coughing, expectorations, wheezing are unattractive to my partner	4.2 The client tells you about his/her symptoms: "I cough and spit often when I am lying down, so how could I even consider having sex?"	• Explain how individual adjustments to the disease influence behavior, and how to react and think in performing ADL, including sexuality
4.3 Change in self-image. My partner is not attracted by my physical appearance	4.3 Client: "How could a skinny person like me with an oxygen tube in my nose look attractive to my wife?"	• Inform the client that pulmonary disease does not necessarily influence physical ability or capacity to experience pleasure during sex
4.4 Psychological concerns negatively affect sexual relations: • Fear of failure • Fatigue • Personal concerns (family) • Abuse of alcohol or food	4.4. Client: "I could never have complete sexual relations because I am so tired, and my penis isn't as hard as it was before."	• Discuss ways of controlling symptoms and decreasing fatigue, such as trying different positions • Tell them that their fears and anxiety are often the cause of an attack rather than the effort expended • Explain ways of improving self-image: hygiene, dress, etc • Assure them that reactions such as rapid breathing during sexual relations are normal • Validate the significance of the perception of failure and tell them that it is not necessary for the sexual act to always be completed in orgasm • Suggest a referral to a professional, such as a sexologist, when there is a communication problem in the couple, or to a physician when a health problem, other than respiratory, is present
5. Elderly people are not sexual	Professional: "We have discussed several issues, now we'll talk about sexuality. Is this important to you?" Couple A: "We are too old to have sex, we haven't done it for a long time, it no longer interests us. Is this normal?" Couple B: "We're often told that at 60 to 70, we should no longer be thinking about having sex, but for us it's still important, even if it's not the same as before. Are we normal?"	• Ask the couple why they stopped sexual activities • Explain the physiologic changes of aging in men and women • Verify if there are any existing pathologies that could influence sexual desire or one of the phases of sexual response • Explore with the couple the possibility of adopting various ways of expressing tenderness and affection
6. Sexual problems are related to the medications taken for respiratory problems	Client: "I've heard that my medications may be the cause of my impotence problem, and that they decrease desire."	• Explain that the specific medications for respiratory problems do not generally cause sexual problems • Explain the relationship with other medications (antidepressants, hypotensives, etc) and concomitant diseases

ADL = activities of daily living.

THERAPEUTIC
INTERVENTION STRATEGIES

Interventions are aimed at enabling the client and the spouse to express their needs in regard to sexuality and to find solutions to their present problems.

As seen in the PLISSIT model, the lack of knowledge related to the influence of COPD or other pathologies, as well as the effects of aging and medication on sexuality, can influence a couple's behavior concerning sexuality. When the couple understands how these factors affect their sexuality and knows ways to remedy them, they can then have a more satisfying sex life.[3,5]

The following guide, "Guide for the Couple to Breathe Better…During Sexual Activity," summarizes useful suggestions for the couple.[3–5,12,15]

"Showing affection and engaging in sexual activity is an important part of a person's life at any age. People with COPD often express their inability to resume sexual activity. Their fears include shortness of breath, coughing, and fatigue. The partner, in contrast, may fear triggering a coughing bout or shortness of breath in the spouse. The energy required for the sexual act is equivalent to climbing a flight of 20 stairs or fast walking over flat ground for 4 to 6 minutes, while still being able to speak with ease afterward.[15]

The following are helpful suggestions to encourage a couple in their affections and to renew their pleasure during sexual activity:

- Talk to your partner about your concerns, worries, and fears and the ways in which you may be able to prevent the appearance of your symptoms during sexual activity (sexual pleasure depends in large part on satisfying psychoemotional needs).
- Plan your sexual activities for the time of day when your symptoms affect you the least—mid or late afternoon is generally the best time.
- Ensure a relaxed atmosphere; the room should be sufficiently warm (20 to 22°C), with humidity around 40%.
- Avoid having sexual activities if you are tired or have a respiratory infection. Regular bronchial hygiene will help you avoid respiratory infections.
- To build up your tolerance to effort, increase your energy and physical capacity by walking or exercising.
- Wait at least 2 hours after a big meal before any sexual activity.
- Be careful with alcohol, which can act either as a stimulant or a depressant.
- Wait 30 to 60 minutes after using your puffer or bronchodilator to ensure maximum bronchodilation during coitus.
- Avoid perfumed lotions or aerosols likely to trigger a dyspnea attack.
- Keep your aerosol medication close at hand (albuterol), as well as a glass of water and tissues.
- Do your coughing exercises 20 to 30 minutes before sexual activity, thereby freeing up the airways and avoiding a possible coughing attack.
- Use relaxation methods such as breathing techniques with the lips pursed and diaphragmatic breathing to control shortness of breath during sexual activity.
- When oxygen is prescribed, use it as necessary and talk to your physician about the possibility of increasing it by 1 L per minute during sexual relations.
- Use relaxation techniques to reduce anxiety before (eg, take a bath, have your partner give you a massage) or during sexual relations (eg, soft music, rest periods).
- Never rush things, and try to give pleasure to the other person. Demonstrations of tenderness, affectionate touching, caresses, and long massages can provide as much satisfaction for many couples without there being complete sexual relations.
- Allow your partner to play a more active role; tell him/her what you like and do not like in your sexual relations. For example, you could say to your partner,
  - I am sexually excited when…
  - I am most embarrassed and uncomfortable when…
  - the time I like best for sex is…
  - the position I find the most comfortable is…
- Try different positions, the ideal position being the one in which you are most comfortable and which least compresses the chest of the person with the respiratory problem. The partner's health condition must also be considered when choosing a position.
- Give yourself time after an extended period of interrupted sexual relations to readjust. Avoid being discouraged from the outset and explore different techniques and solutions. Self-stimulation (masturbation) or masturbating your partner can also be an agreeable means of experiencing plea-

sure in place of complete sexual relations with a partner.

- Talk to your physician if you are unable to have sexual relations. You may need to have your medication adjusted or your health condition checked. For women, age and some medications can affect vaginal lubrication and sexual desire. In men, some medications, as well as smoking and alcohol or other diseases, can prevent or decrease the ability to have an erection and sexual desire.

It is important to remember that sexual well-being is defined on the basis of what the partners want. Accordingly, a couple can decide to take a break from genitality or the sexual act. They can continue expressing their attachment and sexuality though gestures of tenderness, affection and recall happy memories."

To encourage and improve the expression of sexuality, the couple must adopt a position that they both find comfortable. The most favorable positions are those that cause the least pressure on the chest of the person with COPD and that are less physically demanding on the arms.[3] Consideration must also be given to the partner's health before suggesting certain positions. The couple's cultural and religious beliefs may also limit the positions they could adopt.[15] Figures 15–1 and 15–2 illustrate different positions depicting alternatives for both females and males with respiratory problems.

Among the intervention strategies, we must not neglect the impact of individual or group rehabilitation programs. When a module concerning sexuality is scheduled, the persons concerned about the problem will appreciate having information. In his study, Hahn said that motivation for physical training increased when the program included a module on sexuality.[3] People come to realize that a daily walk can have a significant impact on their sexual performance. In a group, they realized that they shared similar problems. Therefore, it appears that improvement in people's general condition, self-esteem, confidence in their abilities, and better control of the symptoms are likely to lead to a more fulfilling sexual life.

Sexuality is a complex phenomenon. On the physician's part, concern for the quality of the couple's relationship is as important as the pulmonary disease itself. Moreover, it is often beneficial for a couple to consult a physician, sexologist, psychologist, or other therapist to improve the quality of their sexual and emotional relations.

WHEN TO REFER

Anxiety and fear of causing disease symptoms, or failing to perform, can be perceived as a severe blow to self-esteem and thus contribute to potential depression. Depending on the nature of the problem, the patient should therefore be referred to a psy-

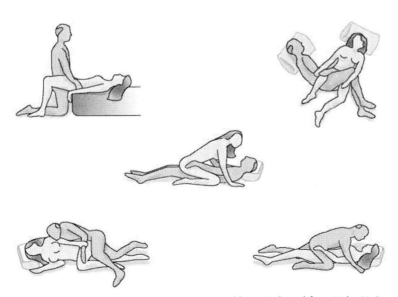

Figure 15–1 Possible positions when the female has respiratory problems. (Adapted from Hahn K. Sexuality and COPD. Rehabil Nurs 1989;14:191–5.)

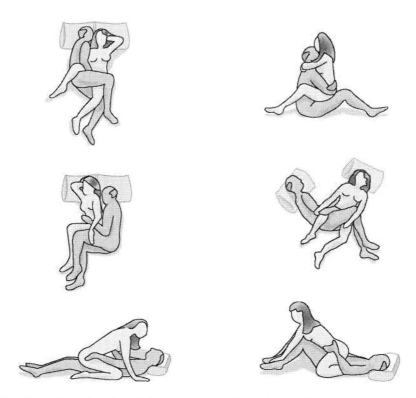

Figure 15–2 Possible positions when the male has respiratory problems. (Adapted from Hahn K. Sexuality and COPD. Rehabil Nurs 1989;14:191–5.)

chiatrist, psychologist, sexologist, or urologist. Sex therapy is not a regulated profession, and the choice of a therapist is sometimes difficult. Information should be obtained from a physician, a university center, or a recognized association.

Concerning the relational aspects, COPD can trigger conflicts in the couple. Consultation with a psychologist or sexologist can help partners learn how to communicate with each other. Based on their shared values, they will be encouraged to express their preferences, needs, and level of satisfaction in their personal and sexual relationships. In this way, the sexologist and the couple can explore ways to express sensuality. Taboos and false modesty can give way to the development of a more stimulating erotic plane. However, according to Masters and Johnson, people referred for sex therapy should feel a genuine need, and the selected goals must be attainable.[8] The level of internal suffering encountered with sexual problems is the most important motivating factor in a desire to change.

For example, intervention by a urologist could be useful in evaluating and treating certain mechanical problems causing erectile dysfunction.

SUMMARY

For people with COPD, the disease can alter both the manner and the opportunity in which sexual needs are expressed. To be effective, health care professionals must be aware of their own sexuality and the prejudices and misconceptions they may hold regarding sexuality in general, as well as the sexuality of people with COPD. They must also be aware of the impact of sexual problems on people with COPD and their partners. The role of health care professionals is to recognize, prevent, and intervene in terms of symptoms likely to influence sexual activity. Health care professionals must also be aware of how anxiety can aggravate symptoms and be able to provide strategies for reducing this anxiety.

The involved partner automatically has a very special place in evaluating and addressing the needs of the person with COPD because he/she is intimately involved in the evaluation of the problem and the proposed solution. The influence of COPD on the sexual behavior of the affected person and his/her partner is a field that has been mostly ignored. Furthermore, no specific research has been done on differentiating how patients with COPD adjust their sexuality.

In the past, sexuality was all but ignored. The development of knowledge appears to have coincided with the proliferation of sexual diseases. With the advent of Viagra, some researchers predict a veritable sexual revolution,[27] while others think this little blue pill is the trigger for generalizing an erotic culture. Will people with COPD be excluded from these possibilities? Will the media create unrealistic expectations and hope, thus fueling the feeling of impotence and anger in people with this disease?

CASE STUDIES

Case Study 1

Ms. Cope, a 68-year-old married woman, is known to have COPD.

Medical History, Physical Examination, and Test Results

- She has had breathlessness on exertion for years, now to the point that she experiences breathlessness just dressing and undressing. Her spouse does all of the daily domestic chores requiring physical effort, such that she feels overprotected. She was previously independent and now feels she is a burden on her husband.
- She has stopped smoking but smoked approximately 20 cigarettes a day for about 30 years.
- She was hospitalized last year, intubated, and on long-term home oxygen, 2 L at rest and 3 L on exertion, since she left the hospital.
- She is known to have cardiomegaly with right predominance and secondary polycythemia.

Physical Examination

- Physical examination revealed this woman to have a barrel-shaped chest with mild accessory muscle use; during the auscultation, she demonstrated reduced breath sounds throughout the chest.

Test Results

- The spirometry is compatible with mild airflow obstruction without significant reversibility. The spirometry pre- and postbronchodilators is as follows:
  - Forced expiratory volume in 1 second (FEV_1) is 1.11 L (45% of predicted normal) prebronchodilator and 2.20 L postbronchodilator
  - Forced vital captacity is 2.95 L (101% of predicted normal) prebronchodilator and 3.00 L postbronchodilator

Questions and Discussion

She visited her physician accompanied by her spouse at the respirology clinic 6 weeks after discharge from hospital. She was intubated during her hospitalization, and her family feared for her life. At home, she requires 2 L of oxygen at rest and 3 L on effort.

Permission. During the second visit, the nurse raises the subject of sexuality with the couple, considering that a trusting relationship is already established.

Nurse: "Physical activity also includes sexual activity. Does this worry you or your husband?"

Ms. Cope answers quickly: "Before my hospitalization, we had sex once or twice a week, but now my husband is afraid to make love to me. When do you think we will be able to start again?"

Nurse to the husband: "Clearly, this is something that bothers you. How do you feel about it?"

At this stage, it is important that the health professional establish a trusting relationship and obtain the couple's permission to talk about sexuality. They should be allowed to express their feelings on this matter and explain why they think it could be a problem. A trusting relationship is more easily established when the professional shows an equal interest in both partners.

Limited Information. The information is influenced by the couple's level of involvement and the time available to the professional.

Nurse: "Ms. Cope, what is it about sex that worries or frightens your husband?"

Ms. Cope: "He's afraid I'll be too short of breath and will start to cough. And I wonder whether I'm still attractive to him with an oxygen tube in my nose. But there's another problem...for my husband, sex is important as he says he will get a prostate problem and become impotent if he doesn't make love at least once a week. Is this possible?"

Nurse: "I understand your concerns and that

you have a lot of questions. Ms. Cope, what do you think is the most serious problem?"

Ms. Cope: "I would like to know how to control my coughing and my shortness of breath so that I don't have any trouble when we make love."

Nurse: "As a reference point, we generally say that if you are able to control your dyspnea after climbing up 20 stairs, it's possible to have full sexual relations."

As Ms. Cope is able to do this, although with a little difficulty, the nurse says to her, "Would you like to know ways of controlling your dyspnea during this specific effort?" The nurse then teaches the importance of exercise as a means of controlling pulmonary disease and making sexual relations possible.

Specific Suggestions. Relevant suggestions concerning sexuality are adapted to the couple's problems.

Nurse: "You may find this leaflet helpful ["Guide for the Couple to Breathe Better...During Sexual Activity"]. We can go through it together."

Ms. Cope: "I see that there are various positions. Which one is the least tiring?"

Nurse: "The main thing to remember is that someone with pulmonary disease must avoid positions that compress the chest."

Then the nurse continues by emphasizing the importance of telling each other what is pleasurable and what requires the least physical effort during sex.

Nurse: "The need to be touched and caressed is essential and often more satisfying than the act itself. Is there something sexual or nonsexual that your husband does that gives you pleasure?"

Ms. Cope: "In the morning, when you touch my stomach and whisper to me, I like that a lot."

Husband: "In the afternoon, I like to lie close to you."

Generally, people who share this type of intimate detail are likely to give each other the pleasure they desire.

Nurse to the husband: "Can you tell me about the fear you have concerning prostate problems and becoming impotent if you do not make love each week."

It is important to show an interest in the couple's beliefs. Some of these may have an unfavorable effect on sexuality and must be discussed early; misconceptions can be cleared up, false beliefs resolved, and positive beliefs reinforced. In addition, depending on expressed interest and need,

the couple can be told about the effects of aging, medication, and certain illnesses on sexuality.

Intensive Therapy. For the couple presenting with more significant adjustment difficulties, or if the health professional notes that the questions are beyond his/her competence, a timely referral to an appropriate specialist must be suggested.

In addition, one partner's problem often causes a problem to arise with the other.[9,24] In the example of Ms. Cope, the urologist could evaluate her spouse and propose treatment, if applicable. Constraining beliefs held by either partner concerning sexuality require that they be correctly informed.

Case Study 2

Mr. Cope age, 65, has emphysema and chronic bronchitis. Today, his spouse, has accompanied him.

Medical History, Physical Examination, and Test Results

- He is dyspneic on virtually any effort (grade 4/5).
- He takes the maximum doses of bronchodilators daily and needs oxygen constantly.
- He takes lorazepam for his anxiety because he is anxious when his wife goes to work and is afraid of dying.
- He also suffers from rheumatoid arthritis, for which he takes 10 mg of cortisone per day.

Questions and Discussion

Permission. The physician notes the patient's distress and asks him, "What can I do for you?" The patient unexpectedly says, "I feel useless; I'm no longer a man. I would like to make love but I'm not able." His wife then adds, "Sex has been very important for my husband. For more than a year, his condition has gotten worse, and he is unable to accept that, even if I tell him that his health is more important for me."

Physician: "I understand your sadness. Can you tell me more about how both of you deal with this?"

Hearing the sadness and anger related to the patient's inability to have sex and his difficulties with activities of daily living creates a favorable climate for continuing the interview. A warm, empathetic therapist facilitates the expression of these intimate details.

Limited Information. The physician asks the couple about their expectations regarding sexuality and the way in which they show their affection.

The physician is also concerned about what they know of the disease and the treatments. It is important to know the couple's perception before making statements that could increase anxiety or prevent any new initiative regarding sexuality.

Physician: "In your current condition, what is more important for you and your spouse: controlling the symptoms or making love?"

Mr. Cope: "If I could control my breathing, I would be less tired and less afraid of being short of breath while making love."

Physician: "With medication, it's possible to have some control over the dyspnea in activities of daily living."

Specific Suggestions. The couple's needs tend toward intervention. They may be cognitive, emotional, or behavioral. The physician believes that at this stage of the patient's disease, the main intervention is to enable the couple to express their sadness and powerlessness. Then he/she can guide them toward a second level of sexuality, that is, tenderness and mutual consideration. The physician notes the couple's closeness and the affection between them.

Physician: "I can see there's a great deal of tenderness between you. That's good. I would encourage you to keep this up and create romantic moments to improve your quality of life. To help, I suggest the following routine: once a day, for example during a nap, lie close to one another and caress each other for 10 minutes, without any genitality. This exercise promotes relaxation."

Then the suggestions in the guide "Guide for the Couple to Breathe Better…During Sexual Activity" are discussed with them.

Intensive Therapy. For this couple, a referral to a social worker was deemed the most appropriate action. The patient was then able to talk about his difficulties living with the losses and fears caused by the disease. His wife was encouraged to continue her work outside the home for her own psychological well-being.

At each new stage in the application of the selected model, it is important to remember that these steps have to be repeated for each new element raised in the discussion, that is, obtain permission to talk about the subject, give limited information, or specific suggestions, and talk about the most appropriate treatment for the client (intensive therapy).

KEY POINTS

- Sexuality is as much a basic need for people with COPD as it is for healthy people.
- Sexuality comprises two levels of expression: (1) the sexual act itself associated with pleasure, and (2) sensuality, psychological needs, emotions, and ability to communicate with one's partner.
- The oxygen consumption required during sexual activity is equivalent to climbing a flight of 20 stairs in 10 seconds without difficulty, which is considered as a big physical effort for patients with COPD.
- Fear of suffocating, repeated failures, and a negative perception of self-image are strong determining factors for stopping all sexual activity.
- Sexual desire is very vulnerable to stressful situations. The intensity of the anxiety can lead to avoidance behavior and inhibition of desire.
- The seriousness of the pulmonary disease affects people differently in their sexuality depending on their age, personality, and social circumstances.

- To be effective in their interventions, health care professionals must be aware of their own sexuality and the prejudices and misconceptions they may hold regarding sexuality in general, as well as the sexuality of people with COPD.
- The spouse has a very special place in evaluating and addressing the sexual needs of the person with COPD. She/he must be involved in evaluating the problems and finding solutions.
- Health care professionals must allow the client and spouse to talk about their sexuality; they must first ask permission to discuss sexuality and evaluate how it is affected by the disease and its symptoms.
- The client and spouse must be informed about the effects of the disease and its symptoms on their sexuality.
- Concrete means of reducing the symptoms and promoting sexual satisfaction must be provided to the client and spouse.
- When complex relational conflicts are present, the couple must be referred to an appropriate specialist.

REFERENCES

1. Hanson EI. Effects of chronic lung disease on life in general and on sexuality: perception of adult patients. Heart Lung 1982;11:435–42.

2. Gilmartin ME. Pulmonary rehabilitation. Patient and family education. Clin Chest Med 1986;7:619–27.

3. Hahn K. Sexuality and COPD. Rehabil Nurs 1989;14: 191–5.

4. Kersten LD. Chapter 18. In: Comprehensive respiratory nursing. Pulmonary rehabilitation and basic self care. Philadelphia: WB Saunders, 1989.

5. Stockdale-Woolley R. Sexual dysfunction and COPD: problems and management. Nurs Pract 1983;8,2: 16–20.

6. World Health Organization. Education and treatment in human sexuality: the training of health professionals. Report of a WHO meeting. Technical Report Series. No. 572. Geneva: WHO, 1975.

7. Butler RN, Lewis MI. L'amour et la sexualité après 40 ans. Montreal: Editions Transmonde, 1987.

8. Masters WH, Johnson VE. Amour et sexualité. Paris: InterEditions, 1987.

9. Poudat FX. Nous n'arrivons pas à nous entendre: mieux vivre sa sexualité. Paris: Editions Odile Jacob, 2000.

10. Dudley DL, Wermuth C, Hague W. Psychosocial aspects of care in the chronic obstructive pulmonary disease patient. Heart Lung 1973;2:389–93.

11. Fletcher EC, Martin RJ. Sexual dysfunction and erectile impotence in chronic obstructive pulmonary disease. Chest 1982;81:413–21.

12. Selecky PA. Sexuality and COPD. In: Hodgkin JF, Petty TL, eds. Chronic obstructive pulmonary disease: current concepts. Philadelphia: WB Saunders, 1987: 215–26.

13. Mishara B, Riedel RG. Le vieillissement. Paris: Presses Universitaires de France, 1984.

14. American College of Sports Medicine. Guidelines for graded exercise testing and exercise prescription. 2nd Ed. Philadelphia: Lea and Febiger, 1980.

15. Thelan LA, Davie JK, Urden LD. Sexuality alterations. In: Textbook of critical care nursing: diagnosis and management. St. Louis: Mosby, 1990:855–69

16. McCauley K, Choromanski JD, Wallinger C, Liu K. Learning to live with controlled ventricular tachycardia: utilizing the Johnson model. Heart Lung 1984;3:633–8.

17. Nemec ED, Mansfield L, Kennedy JW. Heart rate and blood pressure responses during sexual activity in normal males. Am Heart J 1976;92:274–7.

18. Kravetz H. Sexual counseling for the patient with chronic lung disease. Sex Med Today 1981;17:377.

19. Kersten LD. Self-care education. In: Comprehensive respiratory nursing. Philadelphia: WB Saunders, 1989:472–96.

20. Campbell ML. Sexual dysfunction in the COPD. Dimen Crit Care Nurs 1987;6:70–4.

21. Dudley DL, Sitzman J, Rugg M. Psychiatric aspects of patients with chronic obstructive pulmonary disease. Adv Psychosom Med 1985;14:64–7.

22. Monday J. L'nsuffisant respiratoire chronique. Rev Malad Respir 1989;6:311–7.

23. Tordjman G, Cohen J, Kahn-Nathan J, Verdoux C. Le livre de bord de la vie sexuelle. Paris: Marabout, 1998.

24. Trudel G. Les dysfonctions sexuelles: évaluation et traitment par des méthodes psychologique, interpersonnelle et biologique, 2nd Ed. Ste-Foy: Presses de l'Université du Québec, 2000.

25. Alarie P, Villeneuve R. L'impuissance. Montreal: Editions de l'homme, 1992.

26. Brecher EM. Rapport sur l'amour et la sexualité. Montreal: Editions du jour, 1984.

27. Virag R. La pilule de l'érection et votre sexualité: mythes et réalités. Paris: Edition Albin Michel, 1998.

28. Feldman HA, Goldstein I, Hatzichristou DG, et al. Impotence and its medical and psychological corrolates: result of the Massachusetts male aging study. J Urol 1994;151:54–61.

29. Kolodny RC, Masters WH, Johnson VE, Biggs MA. Textbook of human sexuality for nurses. Boston: Little, Brown and Company, 1979.

30. Livingston G, McIntyre M, Forgel C. Sexual dysfunction: etiology and treatment. In: Woods NF, ed. Human sexuality in health and illness. 3rd Ed. St. Louis: CV Mosby, 1984.

31. Hirshkowitz M, Karacan L, Howell JW, et al. Nocturnal penile tumescence in cigarette smokers with erectile dysfunction. Urology 1992;39:101–7.

32. Ackerman MD, Carey MP. Psychology's role in the assessment of erectile dysfunction: historical precedents, current knowledge and methods. J Consult Clin Psychol 1995;60:862–76.

33. Lemere F, Smith JW. Alcohol-induced sexual impotence. Am J Psychol 1983;130:212–3.

34. Browne-Mayers AN, Seelye EE, Sillman L. Psychosocial study of hospitalized middle class alcoholic women. Ann N Y Acad Sci 1976;273:593–604.

35. Brouillette D, Goulet M. Evaluation des difficultés: aspects biologiques. Actual Med 1989;3:29–33.

36. Kaplan HS. The sexual desire disorders. New York: Brunner and Mazel, 1995.

37. Lepine J. La sexualité de l'homme à l'andropause. Le clinicien 1999;3:167–78.

38. Dallaire Y. Pour que le sexe ne meure pas la sexualité après 40 ans. Québec: Option Santé, 1999.

39. Badeau D, Bergeron A. Bien vieillier...en santé sexuelle. Montreal: Editions du Mérédien, 1997.

40. Lefort PE. La sexualité dynamique: à la conquête de sa propre sexualité. Montreal: Editions de l'homme, 1981.

41. Wilson ME, Williams HA. Oncology nurse's attitudes and behaviors related to sexuality of patients with cancer. Oncol Nurs Forum 1988;15:49–55.

42. Golden JS, Golden M. Cancer and sex. Front Radiat Ther Oncol 1980;14:59–65.

43. Annon JS. The PLISSIT model: a proposed conceptual scheme for the behavioral treatment of sexual problems. J Sex Educ Ther 1976;2:211–5.

44. Sexton DL. Nursing care of the respiratory patient. Connecticut: Appleton Lange, 1989.

LEISURE, RECREATIONAL ACTIVITIES AND TRAVEL

Paul Hernandez and Sunita Mathur

OBJECTIVES

The general objective of this chapter is to help physicians and other allied health care professionals counsel patients with chronic obstructive pulmonary disease (COPD) on incorporating leisure, recreational activities, and travel into their daily lives.

After reading this chapter, the physician and the allied health care professional will be able to

- describe the physical and psychological benefits of leisure and recreational activities;
- assist patients with COPD in incorporating leisure and recreational activities into their daily lives;
- provide advice to patients with COPD on minimizing the health risks of travel;
- understand the physiologic consequences of air travel;
- assess and manage potential hypoxemia during air travel; and
- refer to specific professionals from the health care team when needed.

Leisure is usually defined from one of three points of view: as free or residual time, as an activity, or as a state of mind.[1–3] When defined as residual time, leisure refers to the time that remains after having completed necessary daily tasks, namely, work and self-maintenance. From the perspective of activity, leisure refers to those activities in which we participate that we are not compelled to do, or for which we do not receive monetary gain. These are enjoyable pursuits and commonly include hobbies, physical activity, spiritual activity, volunteer work, and travel. Defining leisure as a state of mind refers to the experience of leisure as one's perception as "freedom from obligation."[1] Together, these three concepts define our experience of leisure.

Recreation is the participatory aspect of leisure. It is the actual participation in leisure activities that are enjoyable to the person. It can include both hobbies and more physically active or sporting interests.

Whether for leisure or work, travel has become a common activity of everyday modern life. Patients with COPD face special challenges and risks during travel that can be minimized by careful pretrip plan-

ning. This is especially true for technology-dependent patients, such as those using long-term supplemental oxygen therapy. Having knowledge of the health risks associated with travel, the proper identification of patients at risk, and the management options will allow the health professional to appropriately counsel patients.

In this chapter, we review the benefits of leisure and recreational activities, strategies to incorporate leisure and recreation into daily life, and the health risks and preventive measures associated with travel for the patient with COPD.

LEISURE AND RECREATIONAL ACTIVITIES

The meaning of leisure and the benefits of participating in leisure activities have been studied very little, specifically in the COPD population. Much of the literature from studies done in the elderly may relate to this group and is included in the review of this section.

Benefits of Leisure

The health benefits of leisure in the elderly population have been associated with recreational pursuits involving physical activity such as walking, jogging, or sports. Patients with COPD may be limited in their ability to participate in certain physical activities; however, with appropriate intervention to improve functional capacity, they can engage in physical activities that they previously enjoyed or begin new ones that are consistent with their physical capacity.

The major health benefit of participating in physical activity is the reduction in cardiovascular risk and mortality from cardiovascular disease. Although the American College of Sports Medicine recommends moderate-intensity activity (equivalent to 3 to 6 METs) on most days of the week to gain health benefits, even lower-intensity activity has been found to be beneficial in elderly people.[4] This is an important finding since many patients with COPD may only be able to participate in low-intensity activity. Mensink and colleagues found that older adults (aged 50 to 69 years) participating in light activities such as walking, shopping, and gardening (equivalent to 3 to 4 METs) on most days had lower blood pressure, body mass index, and resting heart rate than sedentary individuals.[5]

Those who participated in moderate to vigorous levels of activity had a further improvement in their cardiovascular risk profile. Hakim and colleagues found that men aged 71 to 93 years who walked more than 1.5 miles per day were at lower risk for developing heart disease than those who walked less than a quarter of a mile per day.[6] Parkkari and colleagues also found similar results in cardiovascular risk reduction (specifically cholesterol and body fat) with men who walked regularly on a golf course.[7] A unique study on the risk for stroke found that leisure-time physical activity was related to a reduced occurrence of ischemic stroke in elderly people. High intensity and long duration of activity were found to relate to a lower incidence of stroke.[8] These studies suggest the importance of encouraging physical activity, such as walking among older adults. Fries provided a good review of the benefits of physical activity in reducing overall morbidity and health care costs.[9]

In addition to the cardiovascular benefit of leisure-time physical activity in the elderly population, physical activity is also associated with a reduced risk of falls. Both sporting activities and tai chi chuan training have been associated with improved postural responses and a reduced risk of falling in the healthy elderly.[10–12] This added benefit is particularly important in the elderly population as balance tends to decrease with age and accidental falls are a common cause of morbidity and mortality.

For the elderly, leisure also has other benefits beyond those affecting health. As people retire from their careers, their self-worth and identity, which were previously associated with their work, may begin to be defined by the leisure activities they pursue.[13] Leisure activities can also provide an intellectual stimulation and social benefit, as well as spiritual satisfaction, all of which are commonly lost after retirement.[13] Satisfaction with leisure activity has been found to be an important determinant of life satisfaction and a meaningful concept in the aging population.[13,14] Satisfaction with leisure activity tends to be higher with participation in self-chosen activities.[3] It is therefore important to incorporate leisure into the lives of patients with COPD for whom quality of life may decline related to changes in health status.

Incorporating Leisure and Recreation into Daily Life

The concept of leisure and each individual's view of it changes with age. Following retirement, a greater portion of the individual's time loses its structure and routine. There is a shift in time spent at work to activities of daily living and recreational pursuits. Leisure takes on a new and more important role following retirement since it may provide the individual with a source of socialization, mental stimulation, sense of usefulness, and belonging to the community.[13,14] Roelofs examined how older adults defined leisure and found that most viewed leisure positively.[3] They enjoyed the freedom in the choice of activity, the time they spent doing it, and the relaxation associated with the leisure activity.

Although the benefits of leisure are well known among health professionals, barriers exist in preventing older adults from participating in leisure activities. Lian and colleagues identified lack of time and poor health as barriers to participating in leisure activity in older adults.[15] Family support and participation in activities, as well as awareness of the benefits to participating in leisure activities, tended to be associated with higher levels of activity. Similarly, Lefrancois and colleagues found health and education to be the most important predictors of participating in leisure activities.[16]

An important relationship exists between leisure and life satisfaction. A person's perception of their leisure activities, rather than the amount of time spent engaged in that activity, appears to be related to life satisfaction.[14] Those individuals who view their leisure experience as positive in terms of self fulfillment and personal growth are also more likely to rate their life satisfaction highly.[14,17,18]

For patients with COPD, disengagement from a previously enjoyed activity may be a problem. Different people derive different needs from their leisure activity including intellectual stimulation, a sense of contribution to the community, health benefits, spiritual satisfaction, and simply passing time; all of these are meaningful aspects of our lives. It is important to allow people to choose their own leisure experiences to gain maximum benefits from the activity. Roelofs found that people who choose their own leisure activities tended to rate those activities in a positive way.[3] This identifies an important message for health care workers seeking to help patients with COPD incorporate leisure into their daily lives. By allowing patients to actively create their leisure experiences based on their own goals, quality of life may be improved.

These findings may provide strategies to increase participation in recreational activities for patients with COPD. To allow these patients to continue an activity that they previously enjoyed, barriers must be identified. Improving functional capacity through an exercise rehabilitation program, education on energy conservation, and adaptations to equipment or a workspace environment may provide strategies by which a health professional can assist a patient in restarting a previously enjoyed activity.

Resources for Health Care Professionals and Patients

Assessment tools have been developed to measure leisure-time physical activity in adults. The Physical Activity Scale For the Elderly is specific to people over 65 years. The Minnesota Leisure Time Physical Activity Questionnaire, which was developed for adults, may be useful in determining the type of activities and the frequency and duration of engagement in these activities. Both forms can be found in their entirety elsewhere.[19]

Measurement tools have also been developed to measure the degree of satisfaction gained from participating in leisure activities. Two such instruments are the Leisure Satisfaction Scale and the Paragraphs About Leisure Form E.[20,21] Both have been applied to older adults and may assist in assessing the older adult with COPD.

The *Physical Activity Guide to Healthy Active Living For Older Adults* is a resource developed by Health Canada and the Canadian Society of Exercise Physiology that provides information about the benefits of physical activity and many options for enjoyable activities for older adults. It is posted on a Web site and can be ordered from <www.paguide.ca> to be supplied to patients at no charge.

TRAVEL

Careful pretrip planning is essential for all travelers. For patients with COPD this should include seeking advice from a knowledgeable health professional well in advance (at least 4 weeks) of the planned departure date. Planning a trip should be seen as an occasion to help the patient and family remember and apply everything they have learned so far in disease self-management. The following questions could be addressed and reviewed with the patient:

- Do you have any concerns?
- Can you assess your strengths, limitations, and abilities to go on a trip?
- Identify if there are things that may make your symptoms worse. How will you face them?
- What precautions would you take before leaving?
- If you feel you can go on a trip, would you start planning now?

Health professionals should inquire about the timing of the trip (eg, departure date, duration of trip), mode of travel (eg, automobile, train, ship, airplane), destination (eg, specific health risks and immunization requirements), and access to medical support systems during the time away from home. At a minimum, patients with COPD leaving on a trip should have the items listed in Table 16–1. These should be carried with the traveler at all times; for example, these items should be packed in a carry-on bag rather than in checked luggage during air travel. When leaving their home country, it is particularly important for travelers to obtain supplementary private health insurance above the coverage provided by their provincial health insurance plan. Many policies will require that travelers provide information from their physician about the presence and stability of any preexisting illness such as COPD.

TABLE 16–1 Essential Items for Patients with COPD Taking a Trip

A list of current medical diagnoses, allergies, and medications (including doses and frequencies)

Enough medication for the duration of the trip

A plan of action, including a supply of prednisone and antibiotics, in case of an acute exacerbation

Updated vaccination status for influenza virus and pneumococcus

Addresses and telephone numbers of medical clinics, hospitals, and pharmacies along the route

Contact numbers of family physician and respirologist

Adequate health insurance

Ground Travel

There are no specific health risks to the patient with COPD associated with ground travel, whether traveling by car, bus, or train. All patients should adhere to general guidelines for trip planning and readiness (see Table 16–1). Patients taking long trips by motor vehicle should plan regular rest stops to stretch and walk to try to prevent venous stasis and blood clot formation. In general, however, ground travel should be well tolerated by the majority of individuals with COPD.

Patients who require supplemental oxygen at ground level will need to plan for an adequate supply during their trip.[22] One option is a portable concentrator that can be plugged into the car battery. Small, pressurized oxygen cylinders can provide a supply for 2 to 8 hours depending on the flow rate. Liquid oxygen tanks can also be used. These devices should be secured tightly in the vehicle. One strategy is to use a concentrator at the destination and tanks, with or without an oxygen-conserving device to prolong the supply period, while en route. Most oxygen supply vendors will provide expert advice and support to clients planning to travel with oxygen.

Cruise Travel

Cruises have been advocated for COPD graduates of pulmonary rehabilitation programs as an enjoyable recreational travel option.[23] However, patients should take the time to consider their own health needs, find out about the medical care on board

the cruise ship, and make any special medical requests prior to departure. Potential passengers might benefit from reading information found on one of the many Internet Web sites dedicated to providing information about health and travel (eg, Liebenstein PJ, Wider J. MedicinePlanet, Inc., <http://www.travelhealth.com/>).

No single authority regulates medical care on board cruise ships; however, many cruise lines have a licensed physician on board. Medical equipment and medications will also vary. Care of complex medical situations is usually provided by affiliated hospitals on shore.

The most common health complaints encountered on cruises relate to sunburn, motion sickness, and gastrointestinal disturbances. Many passengers are elderly, have preexisting medical conditions such as COPD, and eat and drink much more than they usually do at home. In recent years, concern has been raised about the risk in outbreaks of serious communicable diseases. Increased inspection of ship sanitation and water quality by Canadian and American authorities will likely reduce the occurrence of travelers' diarrhea. However, outbreaks of airborne diseases may be more difficult to prevent. Reports of major influenza outbreaks on board North American cruise ships in 1997 and 1998 have led health authorities to recommend that cruise lines vaccinate all crew members, provide antiviral agents to high-risk passengers during outbreaks, and make available rapid diagnostic kits for influenza in the ship's clinics. There have also been reports of legionnaires' disease, in some cases originating from the water supply of the ship's whirlpool. Passengers with COPD should ensure that they seek medical attention on board the ship at the first signs of a respiratory infection. The essential items noted in Table 16–1 are particularly important to enjoy a healthy and less worrisome voyage on the high seas.

Air Travel

The next segment of this chapter deals with the physiologic consequences of air travel, assessment and management of potential hypoxemia during air travel, and other health risks including barotrauma, infection, and economy class syndrome. A number of review articles have recently been published on air travel by persons with lung disease. The Canadian Thoracic Society Standards Committee published an excellent resource of information for health care professionals in 1998.[24] There are also a growing number of Internet Web sites that provide information to patients and health care professionals (eg, <http://www.va.gov/health/pulmonary/clin_prac/module_a/> or <http://www.aircanada.ca/services/medical/>).

Ten to 14 million passengers travel by air in Canada each year.[25] Worldwide, it is estimated that 1 in 10, approximately 40,000 passengers each year, will have a medical incident in flight.[26] One in 150,000 passengers will require the use of in-flight medical equipment or medications.[26] Fortunately, fatalities are a rare event, with an estimated incidence of 0.3 per million passengers.[27] The most common reported causes of death are cardiac (56%), exacerbation of a prior medical condition (19%), respiratory (8%), unknown (15%), and other (2%). Thus, only a minority of in-flight deaths occur in individuals previously certified as being ill.

Most major airlines are members of the International Airline Transport Association (IATA). However, there are no international standards for medical equipment, medications, or crew level of first aid training on board commercial flights. Presently, flight attendants are usually trained in basic first aid; however, the medical kit on board is intended for use only by a physician. Therefore, for serious in-flight medical emergencies, airlines rely on the "good Samaritan" act of physicians from among the passengers on board.

Prior to traveling, it is best for passengers with chronic medical conditions such as COPD to see their own physician, who in some cases will relay information to a member of the airline medical service, for medical clearance. This is always recommended for technology-dependent passengers, such as those who require in-flight oxygen.

Physiologic Consequences

Modern aircrafts cruise at altitudes of up to 12,500 meters (41,000 feet). Ideally for passengers, aircraft cabins should be pressurized to a sea level equivalent, but this would result in difficulties with structural integrity of the aircraft and/or weight problems related to the materials used in aircraft construction that would, in turn, impact the cost effectiveness of air travel. Aircraft cabins are partially pressurized to a variable degree; this depends on the make and age of the aircraft varying in a range of equivalent altitudes between 1,600 and 2,500 meters (5,000 to 8,000 ft).[22] The exception among aircrafts is the Concorde, which is pressurized to the equivalent of 310 meters (1,000 ft). The pressure level will also vary during a given flight with sudden altitude changes related to events such as turbulence. Helicopters and small aircrafts, including commuter planes, often do not have pressurized cabins.

The resulting problems of reduced cabin pressure relate to the expansion of gas trapped in the body cavities of travelers (dysbarisms) and a reduction of the partial pressure of inspired oxygen (PO_2).[28] Dysbarisms occur in accordance with Boyle's gas law, which states that when the pressure exerted on a gas is decreased, the volume of the gas expands proportionally. For example, a passenger taking off at sea level may have gas trapped in certain body cavities, such as the sinus cavities or emphysematous lung bullae, that would be expected to expand by approximately 130% while cruising at a cabin altitude equivalent to 2,500 meters.

Proportionally, the oxygen level in the cabin air of aircraft remains unchanged (FIO_2 approximately 0.21); however, as ambient cabin pressure (PB) falls, so does the PO_2, approximately 4 mm Hg for every 310 meters of cabin altitude equivalent.[28] Therefore, an aircraft taking off at sea level with a PO_2 of 149 mm Hg will have a PO_2 of 117 mm Hg at a cabin equivalent altitude of 2,500 meters. Ultimately, the oxygen level in arterial blood (PaO_2) of passengers will fall in response to a drop in alveolar oxygen (PAO_2). This occurs in keeping with the relationship of PAO_2 and the ambient air oxygen level (eg, the alveolar gas equation: $PAO_2 = FIO_2 (PB-PH_2O) - PaCO_2$/respiratory quotient [RQ]). Although the resultant fall in PaO_2 does not usually pose a problem for healthy passengers, it may present a health risk to individuals with a chronic lung disease such as a patient with COPD with a low resting PaO_2.

Reflex cardiovascular effects of acute hypobaric hypoxia have been studied in young, healthy individuals.[29] Usually, there is an acute increase in heart rate, blood pressure, and cardiac output that is thought to be mediated by the adrenergic system. However, this vasopressor response is attenuated in elderly individuals with COPD. This is potentially beneficial to patients with COPD with coexisting cardiovascular disease. Unfortunately, this means that a simple assessment of heart rate and blood pressure is not likely to be a reliable indicator of hypoxia in elderly patients with COPD during air travel.

The clinical significance of the hypoxic condition of air travel has not been well documented. Medical emergencies are rare events, even in travelers with preexisting cardiac or pulmonary disease. This may be attributable to the relatively short duration of hypoxic exposure or perhaps to the nonspecific nature of the symptoms of acute hypoxemia leading to the infrequent recognition of the association with hypoxemia. In one study, 18 subjects with COPD with forced expiratory volume in 1 second (FEV_1) less than 50% predicted spent 1 hour in a hypobaric chamber simulating air travel at a cabin altitude equivalent to 2,438 meters.[30] This resulted in a PB of 565 mm Hg and a PO_2 of 108 mm Hg. No subjects experienced severe symptoms or arrhythmias that necessitated early termination of the study. However, this was a short flight simulation devoid of other physical and psychological stresses involved in real-life travel.

Additional breathing problems may result from the air quality of aircraft cabins.[25] The relative humidity is usually very low, typically less than 20%, and often as low as 5 to 10%. This may result in dehydration, drying of the skin and mucous membranes of the eyes and respiratory tract. Passengers should avoid beverages containing alcohol or caffeine that may exacerbate dehydration.

Rates of exchange of cabin air vary from 5 to 20 times per hour, and newer aircrafts have ventilation systems that are equipped with high-efficiency particulate air filtration systems. However, no filtration system is 100% effective at removing fumes and particulate matter from air that is recirculated through a common reservoir for the entire aircraft. For example, although smoking is prohibited on many carriers from different countries, this is not necessarily the situation on all international carriers. Also, small pets are allowed to travel with passengers within the cabin. Therefore, airway irritants, aeroallergens, and infectious agents such as second-hand smoke, perfume, animal dander, and airborne viruses may reach passengers sitting anywhere in the cabin. It is not surprising that there have been numerous reports on the transmission of airborne pathogens on commercial aircrafts, such as the highly publicized transmission of multidrug-resistant *Mycobaterium tuberculosis* to passengers and crew on a long flight from Honolulu to Chicago.[31]

Lastly, the nature of modern air travel exposes passengers to cramped and uncomfortable seats. Venous pooling in leg veins and dependent edema place all travelers during prolonged flight segments at increased risk for the development of orthostatic hypotension, syncope, and deep vein thrombophlebitis.[26] This problem is commonly referred to as "economy class syndrome." Patients with COPD with cor pulmonale may be particularly at risk, as are other individuals with risk factors for developing deep vein thrombosis. Passengers should be encouraged to stretch and ambulate regularly during flights. Because of the risk of orthostatic hypotension, they should also be instructed to take care when rising from their seats.

Assessment and Management of Potential Hypoxemia

Not every traveler can be assessed for potential hypoxemia prior to air travel. The Canadian Thoracic Society recommends that health care professionals evaluate patients with certain risk factors (Table 16–2), including individuals with chronic lung diseases such as COPD.[24] A request for in-flight oxygen is the most common reason for preflight medical screening and accounts for 80% of referrals reported by one airline.[32] Furthermore, in that report, 44.3% of the in-flight oxygen requests came from individuals with COPD. The majority (73.3%) were already using long-term oxygen therapy prior to the flight, and one-quarter had previously traveled on a commercial flight with supplemental oxygen.

Various equations and nomograms have been developed to predict a patient's in-flight PaO_2. However, such equations have not been validated for hypercapnic patients or for those using supplemental oxygen at ground level. By combining the FEV_1 percent predicted with the ground level PaO_2 (PaO_2G), Dillard and his colleagues reportedly were able to reliably predict the PaO_2 at a cabin equivalent altitude of 2,438 meters (PaO_2Alt) using the equation below.[30]

TABLE 16–2 Which COPD Patients to Evaluate for Potential Hypoxemia during Air Travel

Known COPD or restrictive lung disease
Known or suspected hypoxemia or hypercapnia
Already using supplemental oxygen
Recent exacerbation of COPD
Prior difficulty with air travel
Those with other health conditions that may be exacerbated by hypoxemia
Patients with severe fear or anxiety of air travel

COPD = chronic obstructive pulmonary disease.
Adapted from Lien, et al.[24]

This equivalent altitude represents the usual worst-case scenario for commercial air travel. The fact that PaO_2Alt is related to FEV_1 highlights the need to optimize treatment of airflow obstruction prior to flying:

$$PaO_2Alt = 0.453(PaO_2G) + 0.386(FEV_1 \% \text{ predicted}) + 2.440 \ (r = .847, p < .0001)$$

Identification of passengers who will develop significant arterial hypoxemia can also be done by exposing the patient to low FIO_2 or by using a hypobaric chamber. Access to a hypobaric chamber is usually impractical; this has led a number of authors to suggest that the hypoxic high-altitude stimulation test proposed by Gong and colleagues is a better alternative.[33] In this test, the arterial oxygen saturation or arterial blood gas is monitored while the potential passenger breathes a hypoxic gas mixture of $FIO_2 = 0.15$, for example, resulting in the lowest expected cabin oxygen level (PO_2) in normal commercial air travel. This test is particularly useful for the hypercapnic patient with COPD but it is not performed in many clinical laboratories and is not recommended for routine use. In contrast to the regression equation approach, it allows for an assessment of the individual's susceptibility to the development of symptoms or electrocardiographic changes during hypoxemia. During the test, it is also possible to administer supplemental oxygen by nasal prongs to determine the necessary oxygen flow rate for air travel. Another practical solution for travelers is to carry a portable pulse oximeter to titrate their own supplemental oxygen during the flight, for example, aiming for an oximetry reading of between 88 and 92%.

Practical Considerations

Some practical advice to help patients prepare for air travel with oxygen is summarized in Table 16–3. Most airlines require prearrangement for in-flight oxygen from 2 to 28 days before departure.[34] Patients should inquire about the charge for in-flight oxygen, which can typically vary from $150 to $400 for each flight. The traveler's physician must complete a medical release form, which specifies the medical diagnosis, treatment, stability of clinical conditions, and oxygen flow needs. However, there is no uniform airline request form; the airline must be contacted by the patient to determine what is required. Airlines are not responsible for oxygen needs on ground while in air-

TABLE 16–3 Practical Considerations for Patients with COPD Planning Air Travel with Oxygen

Travel when COPD condition is stable

Prearrange in-flight oxygen 2–28 days before departure

Passengers are not permitted to carry their own oxygen supply on board aircraft

Bring own nasal prongs

Inquire about the additional charge for in-flight oxygen

Have own physician complete medical release form

Take medications just prior to flight to optimize lung function

Arrive early for the flight to allow for preboarding

Whenever possible, fly direct

For stopovers, arrange oxygen in advance with first aid station at the airport

Ask for an aisle seat

When necessary, prearrange oxygen at final destination

ports. It is best for patients who are oxygen dependent at ground level to fly direct flights. However, when this is impossible (eg, necessary stopover), the patient should check in advance with the first aid station at the airport to arrange for a supplemental oxygen supply. The patient's local oxygen vendor can often assist with these arrangements. Passengers are not permitted to carry their own oxygen equipment on board aircraft. Oxygen cylinders provided by the airline usually have fixed flow options of 2 or 4 L/min, and some airlines use larger cylinders with variable flow meters that allow a wider range of flow rates (1 to 15 L/min).

It is currently recommended that the PaO_2 during air travel should be maintained above 50 mm Hg.[33] As a general rule of thumb, for most travelers who do not need supplemental oxygen at ground level, a flow rate of 2 L/min is sufficient.[35] Patients with COPD on long-term oxygen treatment will require supplementation during flight. For travelers who use supplemental oxygen at ground level, an increase in flow rate by 1 to 3 L/min above their usual setting is generally sufficient.[35] Most airlines will provide either a face mask or nasal prongs. However, it is advisable for patients to bring their own nasal prongs with them.

The American Lung Association provides patient education material for individuals who travel with oxygen (*Airline Travel with Oxygen*). It includes requirements for each commercial carrier, as well as the costs of oxygen during flight, and data that are helpful to both physicians and patients.

High-Altitude Destinations

Health professionals should be aware of the eventual destination of their patient's travels. Individuals who normally live at sea level and travel to high-altitude destinations, such as Denver, are of particular concern. A patient with COPD who has borderline hypoxemia at sea level will likely experience significant hypoxemia at higher altitudes, perhaps necessitating the use of supplemental oxygen. Similarly, an individual who uses supplemental oxygen at sea level may require adjustment in the oxygen flow rate at a higher altitude. Prior to departure, it is advisable to arrange a medical assessment of patients with COPD on their arrival at a high-altitude destination.

WHEN TO REFER

Patients with COPD who are experiencing barriers to participation in their chosen leisure activities will benefit from referral to a knowledgeable health care professional. An ideal setting to begin addressing the physical and psychological constraints to their involvement in leisure activities is a comprehensive pulmonary rehabilitation program. Most programs will have access to specialist physicians, nurses, and physical and occupational therapists as necessary.

All technology-dependent patients with COPD planning to travel should see their physician and equipment vendor well in advance of the trip. Patients with conditions as listed in Table 16–2 should also be seen by their respirologist prior to traveling.

SUMMARY

Leisure and recreation provide benefits to patients with COPD in terms of improving overall health status, self-worth, intellectual stimulation, spiritual satisfaction, and a sense of belonging to a community. Family support and participation in activities, as well as awareness of the benefits of participating in leisure activities, tended to be associated with higher levels of activity. The knowledgeable health care professional can help the patient with COPD overcome barriers to participation in leisure activities.

Travel is an important part of modern life. It is essential for patients, especially those with severe COPD, to obtain advice about travel. The physician and the health professional should inquire about the detail of the proposed trip and then assess the potential problems as well as whether the patient's needs can be met. The physician should ensure that the patient has sufficient medication and may consider providing an emergency supply of antibiotic and prednisone in case of an acute exacerbation. With careful pretrip planning and assistance from a knowledgeable health care professional, even technology-dependent patients with COPD can overcome the specific challenges and health risks that traveling poses.

CASE STUDY

Mr. Cope, a 67-year-old married man, comes to his routine follow-up visit.

Medical History, Physical Examination, and Test Results

Since the age of 57, Mr. Cope has been retired from a 35-year military career as a submarine engineer. His son, daughter-in-law, and their two children have recently moved to live in another part of the country. Prior to the onset of health problems, he enjoyed helping his wife with gardening and landscaping their 1-acre lakeside property. He also spent much of his time working on woodworking projects in the workshop in their detached garage. One day, he had hoped to teach his grandson the skills of making wood furniture using simple tools as his grandfather had once shown him.

His wife expresses concern that her husband does not have much interest in doing the hobbies he once enjoyed. She would like the two of them to visit their grandchildren out west for Christmas, but her husband is concerned about the difficulties associated with the trip.

Medical History

• The diagnosis of COPD was made during hospitalization for an acute exacerbation 5 years ago.

- He was a smoker of one pack per day for 45 years until he quit 4 years ago.
- He has dyspnea with most activities of daily living; he has an occasional cough or phlegm except during frequent (two to three episodes per year) chest infections.
- He was hospitalized 2 years ago with community-acquired pneumonia.
- Medications include regularly inhaled fluticasone propionate 250 µg twice daily, salmeterol 50 µg twice daily, ipratropium bromide 40 µg four times daily, and salbutamol as needed.
- He has had long-term oxygen treatment; 2 L/min nasal prong, for the past 2 years.
- He is not known to have any other medical or surgical condition.

Physical Examination

On examination, he has findings consistent with severe airflow obstruction and limb muscle wasting.

Test Results

- Oxyhemoglobin saturation by pulse oximetry while wearing supplemental oxygen set at 2 L/min by nasal prongs is 92%.
- Last spirometry showed an FEV_1 of 0.7 L (30% predicted) and an FEV_1 to forced vital capacity ratio of 60%.
- His most recent arterial blood gas on room air from 2 years ago showed PaO_2 52 mm Hg, $PaCO_2$ 46 mm Hg, and pH 7.40.

Questions and Discussion

How would you assist your patient in air travel to see his family? What barriers exist for your patient to be able to resume the leisure activities that he had once enjoyed? How can those barriers be overcome? What benefits might your patient enjoy as a result of these changes in his life?

Mr. Cope and his wife received their annual influenza vaccination. Mr. Cope is in a stable medical condition and no changes are necessary in his medical treatments. He carried with him at all times a short written summary of his medical condition and treatments. You review an action plan with him and give him a prescription to be filled prior to departure for his usual medications, plus prednisone and an oral antibiotic. The prednisone and antibiotic were to be taken at the first signs of an acute exacerbation, for example, increased dyspnea accompanied by a change in sputum volume or purulence.

A return appointment is planned for the end of November to complete the medical release form for air travel and to arrange oxygen for the trip. In light of the use of long-term oxygen therapy and presence of hypercapnia, it was not possible, or necessary, to apply a prediction equation for the oxygen requirement during air travel. There was no access to a hypobaric chamber. The respirologist recommended an increase in oxygen flow to 4 L/min during air travel. The trip itinerary involved a 2-hour stopover in Toronto, during which time the airport first aid station was to be alerted to Mr. Cope's need for a wheelchair and portable oxygen supply. The patient contacted his home oxygen provider to assist in setting up an oxygen concentrator for his son's home and a portable oxygen system for any outings during their visit.

Follow-Up Visits and Management

Long term, it is apparent that your patient needs assistance to return to some of the hobbies he had previously enjoyed. Activities such as gardening and woodworking require more physical endurance and strength than he currently possesses. On his return, the patient agreed to enrol in a local pulmonary rehabilitation program. The physiotherapist would develop an individualized exercise training program to target an increase in aerobic capacity, as well as strengthening of the shoulder muscles and hips, which are necessary for gardening and woodworking. An occupational therapist would demonstrate to the patient and his wife the use of tools specifically developed for elderly gardening enthusiasts with physical challenges. The patient also planned to hire the neighbor's son during the summer to help with the heavier jobs in the garden and his workshop (under his close supervision and guidance). During the winter months, he would do the preparatory work at his computer and drawing board, sketching changes to the landscaping, designing a trellis to train a grapevine he had planted 3 years earlier, and planning the timing for planting flowering annuals for that year.

Over the course of the next year, the patient's wife has noted a significant improvement in her husband's physical activity level, mood, and outlook toward life.

KEY POINTS

- Involvement in leisure and recreational activities can improve the overall health and intellectual and spiritual well-being of patients with COPD.
- Ask patients about the impact of their health status on achieving personal leisure goals and enlist the support of family members.
- Health care professionals can and should help patients with COPD overcome barriers to participation in leisure and recreational activities.
- Improved physical functioning following pulmonary rehabilitation may result in greater choice and participation in leisure activities; adaptation of leisure activities may allow patients to continue doing those they previously enjoyed.
- Health professionals should help their patients plan their trip: information regarding patient health status should be provided as well as enough medications for the whole trip and a plan of action in case of an acute exacerbation.
- With careful pretrip planning, even technology-dependent patients with COPD can travel safely. Planning is the key to a good trip.

ACKNOWLEDGMENT

The authors would like to thank Ms. Gredi Patrick for reviewing this chapter.

REFERENCES

1. Cordes KA, Ibrahim HM. Applications in leisure and recreation for today and the future. 2nd Ed. Boston: WCB McGraw-Hill, 1999.
2. Godbey G. Leisure in your life: an exploration. 4th Ed. Pennsylvania: Venture, 1994.
3. Roelofs LH. The meaning of leisure. J Gerontol Nurs 1999;25:32–9.
4. American College of Sports Medicine. ACSM's guidelines for exercise testing and prescription. 6th Ed. Philadelphia: Lippincott, Williams and Wilkins, 2000.
5. Mensink GB, Ziese T, Kok FJ. Benefits of leisure-time physical activity on the cardiovascular risk profile at older age. Int J Epidemiol 1999;28:659–66.
6. Hakim AA, Curb JD, Petrovich H, et al. Effects of walking on coronary heart diseae in elderly men: the Honolulu Heart Program. Circulation 1999;100:9–13.
7. Parkkari J, Natri A, Kannus P, et al. A controlled trial of health benefits of regular walking on a golf course. Am J Med 2000;109:102–8.
8. Sacco RL, Gan R, Boden-Albala B, et al. Leisure-time physical activity and ischemic stroke risk: the Northern Manhattan Stroke Study. Stroke 1998;29:380–7.
9. Fries JF. Physical activity, the compression of morbidity, and the health of the elderly. J Roy Soc Med 1996;89:64–8.
10. Kessenich CR. Tai chi as a method of fall prevention in the elderly. Orthop Nurs 1998;17:27–9.
11. Perrin PP, Gauchard GC, Perrot C, Jeandel C. Effects of physical and sporting activities on balance control in elderly people. Br J Sports Med 1999;33:121–6.
12. Ross MC, Presswalla JL. The therapeutic effects of tai chi in the elderly. J Gerontol Nurs 1998;24:45–7.
13. Hersch G. Leisure and aging. Phys Occup Ther Geriatr 1991;9:55–72.
14. Parker MD. The relationship between time spent by older adults in leisure activities and life satisfaction. Phys Occup Ther Geriatr 1996;14:61–71.
15. Lian WM, Gan GL, Pin CH, et al. Correlates of leisure-time physical activity in an elderly population in Singapore. Am J Public Health 1999;89:1578–80.
16. Lefrancois R, Leclerc G, Poulin N. Predictors of activity involvement among older adults. Activ Adapt Aging 1998;22:15–29.
17. Knox SH. Play and leisure. In: Hopkins HL, Smith HD, eds. Willard and Spackman's occupational therapy. 8th Ed. Philadelphia: JB Lippincott, 1993:260–7.
18. Ragheb MG, Griffith CA. The contribution of leisure participation and leisure satisfaction of older persons. J Leisure Res 1982;14:295–306.
19. Med Sci Sports Exerc 1997;29 Suppl 3:S62–72, S122–9
20. Beard JG, Ragheb MG. Measuring leisure satisfaction. J Leisure Res 1980;12:20–33.
21. Tinsley HE, Teaff JD, Colbs SL, Kaufman N. A system of classifying leisure activities in terms of psychological benefits of participation reported by older persons. J Gerontol 1985;40:172–8.
22. Smeets F. Pulmonary rehabilitation in chronic respiratory insufficiency. 6. Travel for technology-dependent patients with respiratory disease. Thorax 1994;49:77–81.
23. Santoro K. A vacation cruise for COPD patients. Respir Ther 1985;15:31–5.
24. Lien D, Turner M. Recommendations for patients with chronic respiratory disease considering air travel: a statement from the Canadian Thoracic Society. Can Respir J 1998;5:95–100.
25. Skjenna OW, Evans JF, Moore MS, et al. Helping patients travel by air. Can Med Assoc J 1991;144:287–93.
26. Jagoda A, Pietrzak M. Medical emergencies in commercial air travel. Emerg Med Clin North Am 1997;15:251–60.
27. Cummins RO, Chapman PJ, Chamberlain DA, et al. In-flight deaths during commercial air travel. How big is the problem? JAMA 1988;259:1983–88.

28. Gong HJ. Air travel and oxygen therapy in cardiopulmonary patients. Chest 1992;101:1104–13.

29. Berg BW, Dillard TA, Derderian SS, Rajagopal KR. Hemodynamic effects of altitude exposure and oxygen administration in chronic obstructive pulmonary disease. Am J Med 1993;94:407–12.

30. Dillard TA, Berg BW, Rajagopal KR, et al. Hypoxemia during air travel in patients with chronic obstructive pulmonary disease. Ann Intern Med 1989;111:362–7.

31. Kenyon TA, Valway SE, Ihle WW, et al. Transmission of multidrug-resistant *Mycobacterium tuberculosis* during a long airplane flight. N Engl J Med 1996;334:933–8.

32. Gong HJ, Mark JA, Cowan MN. Preflight medical screenings of patients. Analysis of health and flight characteristics. Chest 1993;104:788–94.

33. Gong HJ, Tashkin DP, Lee EY, Simmons MS. Hypoxia-altitude stimulation test: evaluation of patients with chronic airway obstruction. Am Rev Respir Dis 1984;130:980–6.

34. Stoller JK, Hoisington E, Auger G. A comparative analysis of arranging in-flight oxygen aboard commercial air carriers. Chest 1999;115:991–5.

35. Berg BW, Dillard TA, Rajagopal KR, Mehm WJ. Oxygen supplementation during air travel in patients with chronic obstructive pulmonary disease. Chest 1992;101:638–41.

SUGGESTED READINGS

Fries JF. Physical activity, the compression of morbidity, and the health of the elderly. J Roy Soc Med 1996;89:64–8. *This article describes the health benefits and reduction in health care costs associated with participation in physical activity by the elderly.*

Hersch G. Leisure and aging. Physical and occupational therapy. Geriatrics 1991;9:55–77. *This article describes the benefits, beyond improvements in health, for the elderly of involvement in leisure activities.*

Lien D, Turner M. Recommendations for patients with chronic respiratory disease considering air travel: a statement from the Canadian Thoracic Society. Can Respir J 1998;5:95–100. *This article reviews air travel with lung disease and was recently published by the Canadian Thoracic Society Standards Committee. It is an excellent resource of information for health care professionals.*

Smeets F. Travel for technology-dependent patients with respiratory disease. Thorax 1994;49:77–81. *This is a review article in a series of articles published in* Thorax *on the theme of pulmonary rehabilitation in chronic respiratory insufficiency. The author describes the physiologic consequences of air travel and practical considerations for patients with COPD who are planning ground, sea, or air travel.*

CHAPTER 17

PATIENT EDUCATION

Diane Nault, Josée Dagenais,
Vitalie Perreault, and Elizabeth Borycki

OBJECTIVES

The general objective of this chapter is to help physicians and other allied health care professionals from the hospital and community settings, to promote patient learning, and to educate the patient and his/her family on how to manage and cope with chronic obstructive pulmonary disease (COPD). Teaching is essential as the patient and his/her family have to play a centrally active role in the management of the disease. Health care professional educators, patients, and family members have to develop adequate competencies and attitudes to keep the process of learning ongoing and to ideally establish the preset learning goals. After reading this chapter, the physician and the allied health care professional will be able to

- recognize the impact of COPD on patient learning and education provided to the patient and family;
- understand the learning process, principles, barriers, and needs;
- appreciate the use of learning theories and models in the design of educative interventions;
- adopt the different steps to accomplish in patient education;
- recognize the need of the health professional educator's competencies and attitudes; and
- apply the patient education process steps to practice.

In the last decade, ambulatory services have increased rapidly, as well as direct access to health information. Despite the availability of data and the improvement of techniques and programs, it is still not uncommon to witness situations in which patients do not comply with treatment or in which they are unable to manage their diseases. Since numerous authors have proven efficient teaching methods in coping with and controlling diseases, we must devise a way to explain this "relative" performance of teaching intervention. Part of the answer lies within the patient's concept of education.

Patient education is a powerful tool for helping patients gain motivation, attitudes, knowledge, and self-management skills to control and make positive psychosocial adaptations to chronic disease. In diabetes, patient education has emerged as an integral component of disease management during the past 50 years.[1] However, most studies done on diabetes self-management education lacked a theoretical framework[2] and an adequate description of the interventions tested.[3] Much has been learned in terms of the effectiveness on improving knowledge[4] but little on quality of life, attitudes, and self-care behavior changes.[5] Newly explored analyses of the relationship between sense of coherence (active management and emotional state) and treatment results revealed a promising correlation.

More recently, in asthma, on the basis of currently evaluated programs for adult asthmatics, patient education has been shown to reduce the frequency of asthma attacks and decrease patient disability.[6,7] One important aspect sometimes lacking in educational asthma programs is patient compliance. Studies of factors affecting attitudes, beliefs, and self-care behaviors are needed to improve the advice and support given to patients.[5,6]

In COPD, educating patients in self-management has recently become a major challenge in clinical practice. The positive impact of education in COPD is recognized by the scientific community through pulmonary rehabilitation programs.[8,9] Recently, the effectiveness of a comprehensive self-management program has been demonstrated in a randomized controlled trial of patients with COPD.[10] Despite the value recognized in how important a self management-program is, patient education remains a challenge. This is even more pronounced if we consider the aging of the COPD population, the level of education, the disease progression, and associated comorbid conditions.

In this chapter, we define patient education and discuss the impact of COPD on patient learning and education provided by health care professionals. We then examine the learning process by reviewing the principles of adult learning, learning needs, and barriers and through the study of important elements within learning theories and models. Finally, we present each step of the patient education process.

DEFINITION

Patient education involves not only teaching but also promoting learning by helping the patient and his/her family improve knowledge, increase self-confidence, and take charge of the disease by actions that allow prevention or control of disease symptoms and adoption of healthy lifestyles.[11-14] In this sense, patients are able to develop disease self-management and compliance with treatment.[9] Clearly, teaching and learning are part of an interactive process that involves the patient and his/her family, the health care professional educator, the disease itself, and the environment. Teaching does not guarantee learning, and learning can result without a good teacher.[15]

For health care professionals to be effective and efficient as educators, they need to understand learning principles, stimulate patients' motivation to learn and adopt self-care behaviors, be cognizant of patients' learning needs, set mutual learning goals with patients and their families, plan and implement teaching learning interventions, evaluate patient/family learning outcomes, and reinforce successful outcomes.[16-18] Patient education must be tailored to meet individual needs to affect behavioral changes

and cope with the disease. Education enables and empowers patients to live better with their disease. In fact, the three goals of patient education are to help patients gain survival skills, develop the ability to recognize problems, and build the confidence to make the appropriate decisions to benefit their health status.[19]

IMPACT OF COPD ON PATIENT LEARNING AND EDUCATION PROVIDED BY HEALTH CARE PROFESSIONALS

Impact on Patient/Family Learning

A diagnosis of COPD, or anything destabilizing the control of the disease, may act as a catalyst for seeking learning opportunities.[15,20] This aside, learning can be compromised in this equation because patients with COPD are aged, largely low educated, and confronted with many losses that greatly affect their physical, psychosocial, and family lives.[18] They must learn to live with chronic disease on a daily basis, when any symptoms, anxiety, and/or emotions related to diagnosis and illness create situations in which the person is unable to learn productively. There are numerous factors that hinder the lifestyle of a patient with COPD; often, early retirement, the presence of daily symptoms such as dyspnea and fatigue, frequent disease exacerbations, disease complications such as chronic hypoxemia leading to long-term oxygen therapy, comorbid conditions like diabetes, osteoporosis, cardiac or renal failure, inactivity, invalidity, social isolation, depression, important changes in family roles, stigma reducing self-esteem and enhancing dependence on others for care, and caregivers' burden all become the reality of the patient with COPD.[18] To maintain a good quality of life, all of these impacts cause the affected person and involved family to make major lifestyle changes.

Through learning knowledge and skills, patients with COPD have to reconstruct a physical, psychological, and social integrity in which the disease takes its place.[11] Support and involvement from the family is essential in the achievement of this reconstructive process; together, both parties must coordinate to enhance the learning process and take charge of the disease. Self-management of COPD requires that the person suffering from the disease develops and maintains attitudes and skills promoting long-term adherence to a number of different regimens, including smoking cessation, medications, exercise, energy conservation, anxiety control, healthy life habits, and oxygen therapy.[9,11,21–23]

Impact on Education Provided by Health Care Professionals

Physician and health care professionals who educate patients with COPD and their families must learn to orientate their interventions toward disease adaptation because coping and self-management are just as necessary, if not more so, than disease healing.[11] It must be accepted that COPD ultimately has no cure and that educational programs focusing on quality of life, prevention, and control of the disease must be developed as a priority.

To better plan, design, and apply efficient educative interventions, health care professional educators must take into account the following:
1. specific characteristics of COPD patients such as old age, low level of education and literacy, low socioeconomic level, anxious personality with possible low self-esteem and self-confidence and
2. various impacts the disease has on the person/family, such as progressive deterioration of the lung functions, health condition, and functional capacity; social isolation; depression; and burden on the family.[18]

As the presence of dyspnea, fatigue, respiratory infections, anxiety, emotions, or depression affects the capacity of patients with COPD to learn, health care professional educators must intervene. They should evaluate the right time to teach patients with COPD. The environment should be adapted to the patient's condition and learning needs; teaching methods that allow a clear transmission of information, practice of new skills, repetition of information, and constructive feedback should be chosen; and positive reinforcement should be offered.[18] Teaching involves more than transmitting knowledge of the disease to the learner; the health care professional educator has to motivate the patient and the family to be responsible for meeting their own learning needs. This implies helping the patient and the family through the learning process by repositioning them in a context of action that improves their analytic, confrontational, and problem-solving capacities, as well as their focus on the future.[11] In their COPD educational programs, health care professional educators must remember to

use strategies aimed not only at solid control of the disease but also at optimal quality of life for the patient.[14]

Relationship between Patient/Family and Health Care Professional Educators

Patients with COPD, families, and health care professional educators should develop an extensive partnership in the teaching-learning process.[11] The health care professional educator must put faith in the patient's ability, promote a trusting relationship, act as a facilitator and resource person instead of a lecturer, and be willing to take risks and possibly make personal changes. Active patient participation, self-direction, and interdependence that respect the patient's own experiences are more likely to encourage the patient in openness, sharing, risk taking, and adoption and maintenance of new behaviors. Patients with COPD, families, and health care professional educators have to share the responsibilities within a therapeutic contract and cope with the disturbances, crisis, and relapses that can happen during the course of the disease. All parties have to act inside a trajectory constructive process for which the patient goes through several decline phases.[13]

Learning Process

Principles of Adult Learning

In the early 1970s, Malcolm Knowles, influenced by the humanistic education movement, dusted off the word "andragogy" and used it to create a unifying theory of adult learning that is based on four assumptions.[24] Table 17–1 presents the principles of adult learning.[24]

Adult learners need to be active participants in the educational process.[24] They want to be involved in assessing their own needs, setting learning goals and objectives, participating in the learning activity, and evaluating their progress toward idealized goals. They need to have a feeling of commitment toward the learning experience. The desire for individuals with COPD to collaborate with health care professionals in the management of their health should be encouraged.

In addition, the individual's previous experiences should be used as building blocks during the learning process.[24] Techniques such as problem solving and interactive discussions are more effective than passive listening. Adults typically identify learning needs that are generated by real-life experiences.

TABLE 17–1 Principles Of Adult Learning*

1. Adults are independent and self-directed learners who need to be active participants in the educational process.
2. Adults value past life experiences as a rich resource for learning.
3. Readiness to learn for adults is often related to developmental tasks and social roles.
4. Adults are also competency-based learners, meaning that they want to learn a skill or acquire knowledge that they can apply to their immediate circumstance.

*Adapted from Knowles MS. The modern practice of adult education: andragogy versus pedagogy. 2nd Ed. Chicago: Follett, 1980.

They come to new learning situations with many experiences that influence their motivation to seek additional information. For instance, previous encounters with the health care system through hospitalizations and contacts with individuals who suffer from the same or similar diseases act as stimuli and sources of learning.

There are specific times and stages when learning is easier for people because of their developmental readiness. Adults have "their phases of growth and resulting developmental tasks, readiness to learn and teachable moments."[24] Adults engage in learning mostly in response to stimuli or pressures they feel at the moment. For example, as mentioned previously, a diagnosis or an exacerbation of COPD may act as a stimulus for seeking learning opportunities.[15,20] In fact, any type of change in a person's life opens up possibilities for change in other areas of life, including health habits. However, because many barriers can block the readiness to learn, health care professional educators must become more educated in infering life changes that favor a positive change in health habits and learning barriers. Readiness to learn comes into play when the patient can identify a learning need, set a learning goal, and display a willingness to achieve the goal.[18] Should there be an obstacle or any inconsistent verbal or nonverbal behavior, the health care professional educator should take more time to elicit suppressed feelings, questions, fears, and misconceptions about anticipated interventions. Effective communication; an interpersonal relationship of trust, caring, and mutual respect; an optimal physical environment; and the presence of a family member are all enabling factors that help establish a climate in which the patient is ready to learn.

Also, adults will only show interest, invest time, and collaborate with health care professional educators to learn new skills and knowledge when they see the relevance of learning to their own lives.[15,24] Because of their problem-centered orientation, they are motivated by the immediate application of learning, which provides direct feedback and reinforcement. For example, if the patient's condition is stable at the time of COPD diagnosis, and the physical aspect is the chief concern to take into account before any teaching should occur, the provision of immediate useful information at this critical point is ideal to enhance learning at a time when the patient's motivation and interest are high. For adults, useful information and knowledge can reduce stress and anxiety while promoting disease management and coping skills and implementing new behaviors.

Learning Barriers

Learning barriers should be identified and taken into account by health care professionals planning patient education. Adults approach learning in a variety of ways determined by individual lifestyle, personality, and past experiences.[25] Also, intellectual, physical, emotional, environmental, and social barriers can block the capacity to learn and the performance of actions in adult learners.[18,24–26] Comprehension capacity, presence of disease, fears and anxiety, ways of coping, motivation, language and culture, changes in social roles, financial problems, and a lack of resources can all negatively influence learning. Factors related to the educator itself (personality, competencies, style), teaching methods used, and environment and external conditions may further impede the patient's ability to learn. The interaction between the person and the environment is crucial in the learning process. If physical comfort, mutual trust, respect and helpfulness, freedom of expression, and acceptance of differences are not well established, learning cannot occur.[24,25]

As mentioned before, in the COPD population, age, level of education, and physical and psychosocial conditions can become barriers to knowledge acquisition and behavior performance. The nature of the disease and its related treatment, as well as disease complications and comorbid conditions, can leave patients with COPD with little energy, interest, and desire to learn new information and/or alter their lifestyle.[18] In addition, learning can be disrupted by physical and psychomotor changes associated with aging. These changes can include a decline in fluid intelligence and decreased short-term memory, concentration, attention, reaction time, dexterity, hearing, and vision impairments. In the patient with COPD, a progressive loss of autonomy creates a vicious cycle of inactivity, anxiety, isolation, depression, and lack of internal and external resources, which, in turn, decreases self-esteem and the motivation to learn. Early retirement provokes changes in social roles and frequently stirs up financial problems that affect patient learning. Table 17–2 presents what health care professionals should consider while teaching patients with COPD with regard to the common COPD learning barriers and what should be done to assist patients.[18,26–28]

Learning Needs

A learning need is the gap between the information an individual knows and what is necessary for self-management.[15] The identification of learning needs is the first step in teaching patients. Learning needs can be classified into three areas of learning or knowing: cognitive (knowledge), psychomotor (skills), and affective (attitudes).[18,24,25] Table 17–3 presents a synthesis of the learning areas. Health care professional educators must address the three forms of learning (cognitive, psychomotor, and affective); in doing so, they will effectively assist in the determination of learning needs essential for planification, implementation, and evaluation of teaching-learning processes and outcomes.

Cognitive Learning

Cognitive learning refers to knowledge attainment and mental/intellectual processes; more specifically, it pertains to rational thought that comprises basic facts and concepts. Cognitive learning moves from simple to complex concepts so that the patient can apply learned facts to different situations.[24,25] Since they almost immediately forget half of what health care professionals teach them, patients with COPD tend to have a persistent need for reteaching and relearning.[18] Identifying cognitive learning deficits involves assessing patients' current level of knowledge and their ability to receive and process new information and perform skills.

Psychomotor Learning

In contrast to cognitive learning, psychomotor learning is dependent on neuromuscular coordination. Consequently, for psychomotor learning to take place, the patient must have the physical ability to perform the skill, remember how to execute it, and then have several opportunities to practice.[24] The role of the health care professional educator is to evaluate and reassess the learner's ability to perform a skill by correcting deficits, providing feedback and reinforcement, and encouraging practice. In patients with COPD, it is critical to continually reassess inhaler technique because, despite lengthy teaching sessions, it often returns to suboptimal levels.[18]

Affective Learning

Affective learning is also a very important form of learning. Affect refers to the feelings and emotions that proceed from, lead to, accompany, underlie, or give color to a person's experiences and behavior. Affective learning refers to changes in the learner's interests, attitudes, values, and beliefs, which lead to a development or appreciation and appropriate adjustment to new skills.[24,26] Although it may be difficult to assess affective learning, encouraging patients to verbalize their feelings and beliefs is one way of determining patient motivation and attitude toward newly learned skills.[18] Helping patients examine various options, gain support from their significant others, and explore the relationships between values, culture, and beliefs all promote affective learning.

Learning Theories and Models

Patient education programs can help improve health, reduce disease risks, manage chronic illnesses, and improve the well-being of individuals and families. Successful programs are based on a clear understanding of targeted health behaviors and their environmental context. Learning theories explaining health behavior can play a major role in the development of such programs by answering the following questions: Why or why not are people following treatment recommendations or caring for themselves in healthy ways? What do you need to know before developing an intervention program? How do you shape program interventions to reach and impact individuals and families? Learning models are used to support program planning processes in the sense that they help design educative interventions.

Basic Learning Theories

The health care professional educators must understand the strengths and weaknesses of learning theories to maximize their use in the development of patient education programs. However, it is still difficult to differentiate between behaviorism, cognitivism, and constructivism, which make up the basic learning theories.[29]

TABLE 17–2 Common Barriers to Learning In Patients with COPD

Learning Barriers	Solutions
Low reading comprehension level[26]	• Use varying forms of teaching. Use printed material written at a low grade level (not more than grade 6), demonstrate new skills, and observe patient demonstrations.
Poor abstract reasoning and concentration[18,27]	• Concentrate on key information. • Present information in a simple manner. • Break down complex tasks into small steps; teach each step until it is mastered. • Help the patient to identify everyday life situations where teaching can be applied and practice them with him/her. • Use the patient's material during demonstrations. • Teach in an environment where there are few distractions.
Hypoxemia and forgetfulness during teaching sessions[18,27]	• Account for the patient's current activities of daily living; choose a time that will allow the patient to rest prior to teaching. • Allow the patient to choose a time of day when they will feel the least amount of fatigue. • Use short informal discussions supported by comprehensive reading material or illustrations.
Dyspnea, fatigue, and pain[17,25]	• Promote use of breathing techniques, appropriate pain medication, and techniques to help reduce stress and anxiety related to dyspnea and pain before teaching-learning sessions. • Try to teach the patient at home; this will allow the patient to rest prior to the teaching session. • Account for the patient's current activities of daily living; allow the patient to choose a time of day when they will feel the least amount of fatigue. • Use short informal discussions, no more than 10 minutes, supported by comprehensive reading material. • Focus only on the most important information.
Poor nutrition[18]	• Obtain a full nutritional assessment including psychosocial variables, income, food habits, cultural influences, and impaired taste, smell, and chewing ability. • Provide appropriate dietary instruction to the patient and family.
Hearing impairment[18,26]	• Speak directly to the patient, clearly enunciating words. • Encourage the patient to indicate when she/he has difficulty hearing. • Obtain periodic audiology evaluations.
Stress and anxiety[26]	• Try to use humor in teaching. • Make the patient and family talk about their feelings and concerns. • Do a debriefing and give support to the patient and family before teaching sessions.
Finance problems and lack of resources[28]	• Determine patient/family ability to afford and obtain treatment. • Encourage family support. • Identify with the patient/family the community resources that can give helpful services and help them with arangements.

TABLE 17–3   Learning Areas[18,24,25]

Learning Areas	Example
Cognitive (knowledge)	Knowing the name, dosage, and effects of respiratory medications
Psychomotor (skills and performance)	Using inhalers correctly: good hand coordination and inhalation technique
Affective (beliefs, interest, attitudes, values)	Believing that taking inhalers helps to prevent or control respiratory symptoms
	Willing to take inhaled medications regularly

Behaviorism. Behaviorism focuses on the study of observable and measurable changes in behavior.[30] Response to stimulus can be observed quantitatively while completely ignoring the thought processes occurring in the mind before, during, and after action. This means that a new behavioral pattern is repeated until it becomes automatic by the process of conditioning and reinforcement through reward or punishment. In the behavioristic approach, the learner is a reactive rather than an active agent in the learning process. As an example of a conditioned behavior in COPD, learners may use the inhaler when shortness of breath occurs; the patient then becomes conditioned to use the inhaler in response to the occurrence of dyspnea and the fear of dying. The behavior is further reinforced by health care professionals and the family, at which point it becomes learned behavior.

Cognitivism. Cognitivism has been the dominant theory of learning since the 1970s. This theory concentrates on the thought process behind the behavior. Observable changes in behavior are used as indicators as to what is happening inside the learner's mind.[30] Effective learning can be promoted by analyzing the component processes of learning such as motivation to act, knowledge coding and representation, information storage and retrieval, and integration of new knowledge with previous information.[31] Gagne's cognitivist theory of instruction is based on three major elements: (1) classification of learning outcomes including categories such as verbal information, intellectual skills, motor skills, attitudes, and cognitive strategies; (2) internal (learner's skills and capabilities already mastered) and external conditions (learning environments) necessary for achieving learning outcomes; and (3) events of instruction that shape program interventions to reach the learners.[32]

Gagne emphasized that the process of learning occurs in phases:

1. The preparation phase, in which the teacher attracts the attention of the learner (attending), presents the objective of the lesson (expectancy), and asks the learner to recall information learned or previously learned (retrieval);

2. The performance phase, where, on one side, the learner processes the content into short-term (selective perception) and long-term memory (encoding) and, on the other side, the teacher evaluates the learner's ability to perform skills (retrieval and responding) and gives feedback on the quality of skills performance (reinforcement); and

3. The transfer of learning phase, in which the teacher evaluates the ability of the learner to perform new skills or apply new knowledge in a variety of situations (cueing retrieval and generalization).

In 1977, Albert Bandura introduced a key construct of the Social Learning Theory, the concept of perceived self-efficacy, which is an essential indicator of behavior modification.[33] The sense of personal efficacy can enhance or impede the motivation to act; it influences the adoption, initiation, and maintenance of health behaviors. If a person believes that he/she can take action to solve a problem, he/she becomes more inclined to do so and ultimately feels more committed to this decision. A strong sense of self-efficacy leads to better health, higher achievement, and more social integration, whereas a low sense of self-efficacy is associated with depression, anxiety, and helplessness. There are many other names of theorists associated with cognitivism, but the work of Gagne and Bandura had an especially strong impact in the field of cognitive behavior modification. It is important when you educate patients with COPD that you orient them toward the adoption and maintenance of behaviors enhancing disease adaptation, prevention, and control. For example, if the health care professional educator is using a cognitive learning approach to teach patients with COPD inhaled bronchodilator use on the occurrence of dyspnea, he/she must assess any prior knowledge the patient has on the subject and the patient's motivation to act this way. In addition, the educator should set goals and objectives to achieve the proper technique in medication administration; there should be instructions for the patient on performing the skills and making sure that each componant of a skill is mastered through proper sequencing. Also, the educator should evaluate learning outcomes in terms of observable changes in behavior, such as memorization of information related to the medication and its use, attitudes toward the use of the medication, problem-solving abilities showing acquisition, and the mastery of inhalation technique.

Constructivism. Constructivism focuses on the learner's perceptions of experiences in the construction of knowledge. According to Jonassen, "What someone knows is grounded in perception of the physical and social experiences which are comprehended by the mind."[34] Merrill cited five assumptions of constructivism: (1) knowledge is constructed from experience; (2) learning is a personal interpretation of the world; (3) learning is an active process in which meaning is developed on the basis of experience; (4) conceptual growth comes from the negotiation of meaning, the sharing of multiple perspectives, and the changing of our internal representations through collaborative learning; and (5) learning should be situated in realistic settings and testing should be integrated with the task, not a separate activity.[35]

Constructivism is a learner-centered approach in which the teaching is designed to foster but not control learning. The content is not prespecified as direction is given by the learner, and assessment depends on the process and self-evaluation of the learner. Methods and results of learning may not be the same for each learner, and learning outcomes, which are not always predictable, are measured on nonquantitative criteria. Using a constructivist approach in educating patients with COPD means that the health care professional evaluates what the patient already knows about the nature and management of his/her disease, based on the patient's past life experiences and beliefs. The health educator teaches the patient according to what the patient wants to know, and what he/she deems meaningful through authentic contexts, real-life situations, and reflective prac-

tice. The health care professional educator acts more as a facilitator than as a purveyor of knowledge.

In summary, when educative interventions are designed from a behaviorist/cognitivist approach, the educator decides what is important for the learner to know and attempts to do a number of things: he/she tries to transfer that knowledge by analyzing the situation, setting learning goals and objectives, training the individual in the proper sequence of performing desired skills, and evaluating the achievement of the learning objectives criteria. On the other hand, educative interventions based on a constructivist approach require that the educator give the control of the learning aspect to the learner while concurrently acting as a coach or mentor. Content is not predetermined, and the training of skills is done through a variety of real-world situations. Also, outcome evaluations depend more on qualitative rather than quantitative criteria. This kind of approach is appropriate with more advanced learners who already know a lot about the subject, content, and skills.

Learning Models

Patient education programs should be based on learning models that guide program planning and development; assessment of patient readiness and motivation to learn; and orientation, implementation, and evaluation of teaching-learning interventions. Traditionally, COPD and other chronic disease education programs have relied on a review of disease-related information to teach patients and families. Unfortunately, in many cases, a review of information may not ensure that a new health behavior is learned or implemented. In response to this concern, theorists have postulated that behavioral influences such as predisposing, enabling, and reinforcing factors[36]; self-efficacy[37]; stages of readiness[38]; family; health; environment; and caring[39] are all key concepts in planning interventions so that the patient adopts and maintains new behaviors through the learning process. The fundamental components of those theories were used to plan and design the COPD collaborative self-management program "Living Well with COPD©,"[40] which was evaluated in a randomized clinical trial by Bourbeau and colleagues.[10,21]

Green and Kreuter's PRECEDE Model and Bandura's Self-Efficacy Theory

The PRECEDE model is a health promotion planning framework used to design educative interventions that address behavioral and environmental factors that predispose, reinforce, and enable the promotion of healthy behaviors.[36] PRECEDE refers to "predisposing, reinforcing and enabling constructs in educational/environmental diagnosis and evaluation."[36] It consists in making a diagnosis and adopting and maintaining healthy behaviors to improve patient quality of life. This model gives the health care professional educator a mental structure that helps analyze the situation, a quick picture of it, and efficient intervention with the patient and family. For patients, adopting a new behavior is a difficult task. Predisposing factors or the patient's knowledge, attitudes, values, and beliefs all play a role in the success of adopting a new behavior. For instance, the confidence a person has in reaction to specific actions and his/her capacities to perform these actions (self-efficacy)[37] both influence the degree to which new behaviors will be adopted. Enabling factors or the patient's skills, type of personality, and/or personal and environmental

resources also play a role. Finally, reinforcing factors such as successes in actions, improved health outcomes, and the support of friends, family, and the community can strengthen or weaken the patient's self-efficacy and thereby increase or decrease the desire to sustain new behaviors. Therefore, the health professional educator must assess predisposing, enabling, and reinforcing factors in the patient's environment to properly plan and design teaching-learning interventions that will enhance patient implementation and the maintenance of new behaviors. In light of this information, the components of Green and Kreuter's PRECEDE model were used to plan and design asthma and COPD education programs.[21,40–42] Figure 17–1 illustrates the role of the model in designing and planning teaching-learning interventions in COPD.

Prochaska's Stages of Readiness to Learn

Prochaska and DiClemente's learning theory refers to the different stages individuals move through in

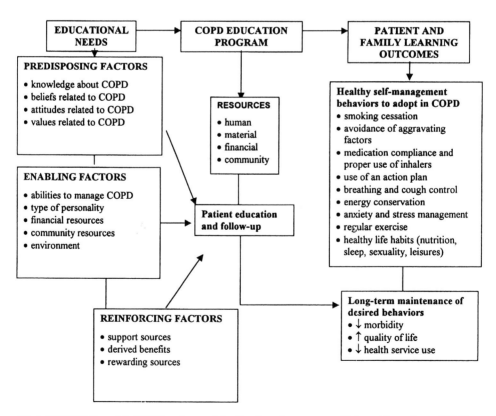

Figure 17–1 PRECEDE model. COPD patient and family education program. (Adapted from Green LW, Kreuter MW. Health promotion planning—an educational and environmental approach. 2nd Ed. Mountainview, CA: Mayfield, 1991.)

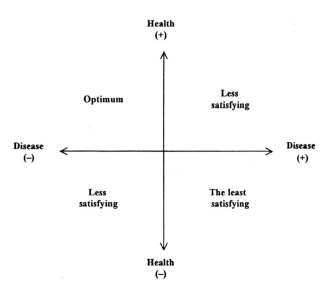

Figure 17–2   McGill Model. Relation between health and disease according to Moyra Allen's model.[45]

making a permanent behavior change: precontemplation, contemplation, action, maintenance, and termination.[38] In the precontemplative stage, the person is unaware of any need to change, and at this stage, education must be oriented to increase patient awareness about his/her condition. In the contemplative stage, the person is considering change but has not taken any action yet. At this point, emphasis should be on reinforcing patient understanding of the need to change and then teaching the skills needed to make these adjustments. In the action stage, the patient starts to change his/her behavior through practice. At this point, education should be aimed at reinforcing new behaviors with modeling and reward tactics to keep the patient engaged in the changes. In the maintenance stage, the person performs the new behaviors regularly. The important point here is to continue reinforcing the new behaviors by providing ongoing education on the importance of maintaining the changes. Finally, in the termination stage, the habits are in place, and the new behaviors are integrated into the person's everyday life. There is no need for further intervention or reinforcement once the change is made.

McGill Model of Moyra Allen

According to the McGill Model, individuals, families, and communities are eager and motivated to increase their health potential.[43] Therefore, the caring given by the health professionals aims to assist those families in their health improvement.[39,44] The first step is an exploration of family perceptions regarding their health and an examination of their environment to identify any potential influences on the learning process.[43] Moreover, the family's readiness must be evaluated prior to the teaching plan to identify their needs.[43] The health care professional must plan the teaching in a stimulating way to motivate and bring effective help to the families throughout their desired health process.

The McGill Model follows four concepts: health, person, environment, and caring. Authors agree that health is the main concept of the McGill Model.[39,43,45] In 1994, Allen stated that health is not an entity but more of a state; it is a process guiding the family to work according to their perceived capacities. Therefore, health and disease are not seen on a continuum because they represent two different concepts.[45] Allen added that health is related to illness on only one matter, and both health and illness state a need to cope with diseases. The McGill Model looks at the person through a family filter; thus, the term "patient" is replaced by "family."[46] The family provides its own solutions to problems, and the health care professional is an assistant in the problem-solving process.[39] Environment refers to the context in which health and health behaviors are learned,[39,43] and caring is based on promoting health to the families by helping them develop better health behaviors.[39,43] Health is a learning process, and the health care professional is a facilitator to the family in that process.[39] Figure 17–2 presents a schema of Allen's conceptual McGill Model.

Globally, the McGill Model uses the strengths and potentials of families to improve their coping and self-management in the health process. Thus, this conceptual nursing model fits perfectly into a self-management program for people with COPD aimed at increasing knowledge and self-efficacy and changing attitudes, beliefs, and behaviors. The McGill Model aims to improve families' capacities to care for their member with COPD at home by receiving support from health care professionals.

PATIENT EDUCATION PROCESS

The patient education process includes important steps that demand strong competencies and appropriate attitudes to be mastered. Table 17–4 summarizes the different steps to accomplish in patient education.

Assessing Learning Needs and Barriers

Various theories consistently identify the proper assessment of learning needs as a critical step in achieving optimal patient learning outcomes. Patients will learn more readily if you teach them what they want to know, in a way suited to their learning style. Health care professional educators should ask themselves the following:

- What is the learner like?
- What are his/her beliefs, attitudes, values, and behaviors?

- What learning needs are unmet? What are the most acute needs of this individual? What does he/she already know?
- What behavior can he/she perform?
- Which are life-threatening problems?

A careful needs assessment facilitates teaching by establishing learning priorities and discovering barriers to learning and doing. Consequently, health care professionals should conduct a learning needs assessment to determine the patient's needs, motivational level, readiness to learn, and ability to perform and maintain new behaviors.[36] However, health care professionals have to remember that learning takes place only when the patient identifies a learning need, and in patients with COPD, learning needs and readiness to learn are often difficult to assess because of coping mechanisms such as denial, repression, and isolation.[15,18,25]

Setting Realistic Learning Goals and Objectives

In addition to assessing learning needs, barriers, and readiness to learn, the health care professional educator needs to use effective communication strategies and foster a trusting, caring, and mutually respectful relationship with the patient and family. Thus, the health care professional educator, COPD patient, and family can develop and set mutually agreeable, realistic, and achievable goals, objectives, and desired outcomes. With teaching interventions being individualized, the three par-

TABLE 17–4 Patient Education Process

Patient Education Steps	Cues For Mastery
Assessing patient's learning needs and barriers	Patient's concerns, attitudes, beliefs, values, knowledge, and learning style
Setting mutual realistic learning goals and objectives	Based on patient's learning needs and barriers Mutual agreement between patient and educator
Planning teaching-learning interventions	Educational plan responding to learning goal and objectives Choice of content and teaching methods according to comprehension level and learning style of the patient
Implementing teaching-learning interventions	Educational plan put into practice Individualized interventions oriented toward patient's integration and maintenance of newly learned behaviors Revision of teaching strategies according to patient's progress
Evaluating patient's learning outcomes	Achievement of learning goal and objectives Test patient comprehension, attitudes, and skills Rewarding and reinforcement are success's key in learning outcomes

TABLE 17–5 Learning Styles

Learner's Style	Teacher's Style	Learning Strategies	Teaching Methods
Diverger Concrete/reflexive learner Likes to discover the "why" of a situation	Motivator	Searching for information Evaluating current information	Information presented in a detailed, systematic, reasoned manner: specific lectures, hands-on exploration
Assimilator Abstract conceptualization/reflective observers Likes to answer "What is there to know?"	Expert or resource person	Predicting outcomes Inferring causes	Information presented in a highly organized format: lectures followed by demonstration, video/audio presentations, laboratories
Converger Abstract conceptualization/active experimenters Likes to understand "how" things work	Coach	Testing theories Designing experiments	Information applied and useful: interactive instruction, case studies, workbooks, computer-assisted learning
Accommodator Concrete experience/active experimenter Likes to ask "What if?" and "Why not?"	Tasks' assigner and supervisor	Trying different solutions Independent learning	Information unstructured: experimentations, active learner's participation

Adapted from Kolb,[47] Litzinger and Osif,[48] Chickering.[49]

ties can successfully overcome learning barriers and effect desired outcomes.

Planning Teaching-Learning Interventions

Planning teaching-learning interventions begins once goal identification and ranking of objectives based on a patient's learning needs are made.[18] An educational plan must contain measurable learning goals and objectives, content to present, and teaching methods.[15] Many factors must be taken into account before choosing a teaching method, including the type of learning objective, the person's learning style (Table 17–5),[47–49] the teacher's knowledge and expertise, amount of available time, teaching resources, and the learner's comprehension level and motivation. People learn through visual, auditory, and verbal stimulation. Audiovisual aids, printed materials, and individual and group discussions are good teaching methods to deliver and reinforce COPD educational content. Demonstration is a teaching method of choice with patients with COPD because of the numerous technical skills required for inhaled medications, oxygen therapy, breathing, cough, and energy conservation techniques. Problem-solving and decision-making techniques

are very efficient in helping the patient with COPD integrate and sustain newly learned behaviors. As an example, notice the teaching in an action plan in which the patient's decisions and commitments are facilitated through his/her participation in scenarios reflecting real-life situations. For example, What do you do when you feel well? What do you do when your symptoms worsen after an exposure to environmental factors, emotions, stressors, or respiratory infections? What do you do when you are in a life-threatening situation?

Implementing Teaching-Learning Interventions

The implementation of teaching-learning interventions means that the proposed educational plan is put into practice.[15,25] While implementing the plan, the health care professional educator must continue to assess and evaluate the progress made by the patient toward the learning goal and achievement of objectives. No progress means that the plan must be changed through a revision of the teaching strategies and content. The health care professional educator should individualize and structure teaching-learning interventions to promote the integration and maintenance of behavior changes.

The following are some important points for individualizing teaching-learning activities with patients with COPD:

1. Printed material (minimum 14 points) must be specific to the patient's disease, comprehension level (grade 6 school level), and interest.
2. Short, informal discussions supported by handwritten comments and diagrams should be used.
3. Family and friends must remain involved throughout the process; demonstrations should be done with the patient's own equipment.
4. Educators should concentrate on one intervention at a time and use simple language.
5. Complex skills must be broken down into small steps, and the mastery of each step is necessary through repetitive skill practice.
6. Patient situation must be taken into account.
7. Consistency and continuity of care should be maintained among health care professionals responsible for teaching the patient and family.[18]

Health care professional educators should also ensure that teaching interventions occur at a time where the patient feels less tired and in an environment that is conducive toward learning; it must be done in a pleasant and comfortable area to allow the patient to concentrate with few distractions.[27]

Evaluating Patient Learning Outcomes

Once teaching is complete, the educator needs to determine if the pre-established goals and expectations were met. Because they assume that the learning needs and objectives are met during the teaching session, health care professional educators are often guilty of not evaluating, or of poorly evaluating, patient learning. This assumption is misleading and dangerous.

It is helpful to consider that there are four levels of learning outcomes that address different increments of learning:

1. patient/family participation during interventions,
2. patient/family performance immediately after learning experience,
3. patient/family performance at home, and
4. patient's overall self-care and health management.

Comprehension and behavior changes take time and practice before occurring, and the presence of barriers slows the process of learning.[26] Some patients are more complex because of multiple learning barriers to overcome, for instance, poor abstract reasoning and any concentration and fatigue related to COPD. These individuals require extra attention in terms of an increased review cycle, repetitive teaching, and different teaching approaches. Constant repetition leads to behavioral changes in creating habits. For these reasons, health care professionals must evaluate learning goals and objectives and teaching strategies used throughout the learning process to supplement information, correct misunderstandings, and reinforce newly learned behaviors. Health care professionals should test patient comprehension, attitudes, and skills through methods such as direct questioning, problem solving, and simulation and observation of behaviors.[18] Such evaluative feedback enables the health care professional to learn about education and the patient to improve their knowledge and skills. If, after evaluating the teaching, the goals and objectives are still not met, the health care professional educator should re-examine and revise his/her teaching-learning strategies and consequently repeat the teaching-learning process.

HEALTH CARE PROFESSIONAL EDUCATOR COMPETENCIES AND ATTITUDES

To be competent in educating patients and families, health care professionals must have the following:

1. *High level of self-confidence.* This means that they have a thorough knowledge of the content to be taught; they can decrease patient/family anxiety, can establish a proper environment for learning, are capable of establishing priorities according to the specific needs of the patient/family, and can help the patient/family acquire the competencies and abilities to perform and maintain new behaviors.
2. *Competence.* Through discussion with the patient and family, they decide what is important to teach and ensure the patient's safety, provide individualized written instructions, and teach home self-management.
3. *Good communication skills.* This involves clear and concise directives; use of simple language, images, and models; and encouragement of patient/family expression and feedback.
4. *A "caring" teaching-learning approach.* This implies empathy, respect, patience and perseverance, recognition of patient/family strengths and concerns, partnership, encouragement, and establishment of time limits.[11]

SUMMARY

The challenge for health care professionals in educating patients with COPD lies in choosing a learning approach (theory) that suits the patient type, situation, and environment and a health promotion framework (model) that will act as a guide in the design of educative interventions.

The patient education process starts with the recognition of what the patient and family already know. It examines barriers and stage of readiness to learn as daily disease self-management strategies and in the identification of a patient's learning needs and style. It proceeds with a set of learning goals and objectives that are mutually agreed on and leads to the planning and implementation of teaching-learning interventions. The process ends with the evaluation of the patient/family learning outcomes, which reflect progress toward pre-established learning goals and achievement of objectives.

Repetition of the information and reinforcement of successful behavior changes are key elements in the achievement of learning goals and objectives for patients with COPD; this is particularly the case considering the severe chronic nature of the disease and owing to specific individual characteristics such as old age, low level of education, anxiety, and associated comorbid conditions. The health care professional must believe in the patient's capacities and persevere in educating patients with COPD. Teaching does not guarantee learning, and learning can result without a good teacher.

CASE STUDY

Mrs. Cope, a 78-year-old woman, has been suffering from COPD for 15 years.

Medical History Relative to Education

The patient already knows a lot about the history and the management of her disease but is skeptical about her actual treatment. In the past year, she went through three exacerbations with no hospitalization. Her level of activity, self-confidence, and autonomy have decreased over the past year. She does not really understand why her condition is deteriorating so rapidly and feels depressed about the whole situation. She lives at home with her son, who is a smoker but is thinking of quitting. She is monitored by a respirologist in an outpatient clinic and has a resource person to contact for questions or respiratory health problems at home.

The last time she visited the clinic was on an unscheduled appointment for an acute exacerbation. She waited 2 days before consulting, hoping that her condition would improve. She came to the clinic with a serious clinical deterioration, reduced lung functions, and oxygen desaturation. She was unable to complete her sentences while speaking. In asking her questions about the exacerbation's onset, duration, and symptoms, she was able to accurately recall the events and identify the factors that contributed to her condition; they were heat, humidity, and arguments with her son. She was also able to describe her symptoms, such as progressive shortness of breath with a decrease in activities and sleep, an increase in secretions but no change in color, and no fever. She was uncertain when asked questions related to medication changes and the use of the action plan at home. She said that she increased her bronchodilator but did not see the need to start her prednisone despite the resistance of the symptoms after 24 to 48 hours. She became very anxious when relaying the arguments she had with her son about smoking cessation. When she met the respirologist, he announced to her that she would need oxygen at home, and he revised the plan of action with her. She became obviously upset about the use of home oxygen. The respirologist asked Mrs. Cope's resource person to see her again for support and teaching.

Questions and Discussion

First, you proceed to an assessment of Mrs. Cope's learning needs including predisposing, enabling, barriers, and reinforcing factors that may or may not promote behaviors preventing exacerbations.

Predisposing Factors

- She does not know why her health condition is deteriorating.
- She is skeptical about her actual treatment and her capacities.

- She does not carefully follow the recommendations in the plan of action.
- She can identify aggravating factors.
- She can describe her symptoms.
- She can initiate her action plan.
- She has low self-confidence.

Enabling Factors

- She has a good follow-up in the outpatient clinic.
- She has a plan of action.
- She has a resource person.
- She is knowledgeable about the disease and its management.
- She does not live alone.

Barriers

- She is depressed and very anxious.
- She has an unstable health condition.
- She must begin long-term oxygen use.
- She has arguments with her son about smoking.
- She has low energy and thus less activity.

Reinforcing Factors

- She has her son's support at home except for smoking cessation.
- She has more exacerbations that are well controlled and without the need for hospitalization.

Second, you assess the stages of readiness:

- Mrs. Cope is in the action stage, for which reinforcement and a reteaching of the action plan are necessary to keep her engaged in the treatment.
- Her son is in the contemplative stage, he is not yet ready to graduate to the smoking cessation stage but is thinking of quitting.

According to the McGill Model, Mrs. Cope's resource person has to involve the son through teaching and follow-up to help them better manage the disease at home.

Learning Needs Emerging from the Resource Person's Assessment

Mrs. Cope wants to

- understand her health condition (decline since a year),
- understand the benefits and the use of long-term home oxygen,
- understand the use of the action plan and its importance in the prevention and control of exacerbations,

- revise her inhalation techniques, and
- understand the role of her son and the way to approach him about smoking cessation.

Second, you determine Mrs. Cope's learning goals and objectives with her. Her learning goals are to

- decrease fear and anxiety related to the deterioration of her health condition and the use of long-term home oxygen,
- learn to properly and safely use home oxygen, and
- regain control over her symptoms and activities.

Her learning objectives are to

- express emotions and feelings about the deterioration of her health condition and the use of long-term home oxygen,
- identify why her health condition is deteriorating,
- identify the benefits of the long-term use of oxygen on her condition,
- properly and safely use oxygen at home,
- properly use the action plan in different real-life situations,
- remember with accuracy the effects of the medications prescribed,
- properly use her inhalers, and
- discuss her relationship with her son and help him in the smoking cessation process.

Third, you plan and complete support and teaching-learning interventions as follows:

- Ensure stabilization of the health condition before any teaching is provided.
- Once the patient's health condition is stabilized, discuss her feelings and emotions related to the deterioration of her health condition and long-term oxygen use.
- Review with Mrs. Cope the events occurring in the previous year using a positive and constructivist approach.
- Explain the decline in lung functions (comparison of the curves from a year ago to now) and discuss ways to maintain a decent activity level (regain confidence in herself and treatment).
- Explain the benefits related to the long-term use of oxygen for her condition (manipulation of equipments) and make arrangements to get oxygen equipment at home.
- Evaluate the patient's previous knowledge and skills used to control symptoms.

- Evaluate the patient's comprehension of the plan of action through her response to questions on situations and prescriptions.
- Reteach the plan of action by putting her in real-life situations and reinforce the importance of preventing and controlling exacerbations.
- Practice the inhalation techniques and evaluate the performance through demonstrations.
- Discuss her dealings with her son (expression of feelings and frustrations).
- Set up the next appointment with the patient and her son to launch a smoking cessation plan.

Finally, you evaluate Mrs. Cope's learning outcomes. Some of the following questions can also serve to evaluate learning needs. The questions ending with an asterisk can also be asked to assess learning needs:

- How do you feel about the past year (focusing on health problems)?*
- Do you believe you can continue to be active even with the deterioration of your lung functions?*
- What are you doing at home to keep active?*
- Do you believe that your treatment can help maintain a stable health condition?*
- Tell me how your treatment can keep your health condition stable.
- Are you still anxious or afraid of using home oxygen?

- Tell me how the use of oxygen can improve your condition.
- Show me your oxygen equipment and how you use it.
- Do you have any problems using oxygen at home?*
- What are the symptoms of an exacerbation?
- Which factors can aggravate your symptoms?*
- What do you do to help control your symptoms?*
- Tell me when you should increase your broncho-dilators.*
- Tell me when you should start your prednisone.*
- Tell me when you should start antibiotics.*
- Tell me when you should increase your inhaled corticosteroids.*
- What can you do other than making changes in your medication to help control your symptoms?
- When should you call your resource person? How do you feel when you have to call her?
- When and in which circumstances should you come to the clinic or the emergency department for an exacerbation?
- Show me how you use your inhaler with a spacer.*
- How is your relationship with your son? Did you have other arguments with him related to smoking cessation? Is he still interested in quitting smoking?*

KEY POINTS

- Recognize the impact of the disease and comorbid conditions on patient learning and education.
- Persevere and believe in the patient's capacities.
- Keep in mind the principles of adult learning.
- Design educative interventions based on (1) a learning theory that fits with the learner's level of knowledge, situation, and environment and (2) a learning model that promotes the adoption, initiation, and maintenance of healthy behaviors.
- Assess the patient/family's learning needs and style, readiness to learn, and learning barriers.
- Set realistic, measurable learning goals and objec-

tives with the patient/family.
- Apply educative interventions that correspond to the specific patient/family needs, learning goals, and fixed objectives; use appropriate teaching methods that suit the learner's style.
- Frequently repeat information to increase comprehension and thus create habits.
- Give lots of positive reinforcement and constructive feedback throughout the learning process.
- Evaluate patient/family learning outcomes in testing their comprehension and capacity to reproduce the newly learned behaviors into daily activities.
- Reward the patient and family.

REFERENCES

1. Dunn SM. Rethinking the models and modes of diabetes education. Patient Educ Couns 1990;16:281–6.

2. Fain JA, Nettles A, Funnell MM, Charron D. Diabetes patient education research: an integrative literature review. Diabetes Educ 1999;25:7–15.

3. Brown SA. Interventions to promote diabetes self-management: state of the science. Diabetes Educ 1999;25:52–61.

4. Graber AL, Christman BG, Alogna MT, Davidson JK. Evaluation of diabetes patient-education programs. Diabetes 1977;26:61–4.

5. Sandon-Ericksson B. Coping with type-2 diabetes: the role of sense of coherence compared with active management. J Adv Nurs 2000;31:1393–7.

6. Worth H. Techniques and impact of education in adult asthmatics. Monaldi Arch Chest Dis 1994; 49:71–5.

7. Kohler CL, Davies SL, Bailey WC. How to implement an asthma education program. Clin Chest Med 1995;16:557–65.

8. Lacasse Y, Wong E, Guyatt GH, et al. Meta-analysis of respiratory rehabilitation in chronic obstructive pulmonary disease. Lancet 1996;348:1115–9.

9. American Thoracic Society. Pulmonary rehabilitation. Official statement of the American Thoracic Society Board of Directors. Am J Respir Crit Care Med 1999;159:1666–82.

10. Bourbeau J, Julien M, Rouleau M, et al. Impact of an integrated rehabilitative management program on health status of COPD patients. A multicentre randomized clinical trial [abstract]. Eur Respir J 2000;16:159.

11. Alvéole-Groupe de Travail Exercice et Réhabilitation de la Société de Pneumologie de Langue Française. La réhabilitation respiratoire. Guide pratique. Paris:, 2000.

12. Make BJ. Pulmonary rehabilitation: myth or reality? Clin Chest Med 1986;7:519–40.

13. Howard JE, Davies JL, Roghmann KJ. Respiratory teaching of patients: how effective is it? J Adv Nurs 1987;12:207–14.

14. Smeets F. Patient education and quality of life. Eur Respir Rev 1997;7:85–7.

15. Gessner BA. Adult education. The cornerstone of patient teaching. Nurs Clin North Am 1989;24: 589–95.

16. Barrass D. The nurse as patient educator. Br J Nurs 1992;1:241–3,245.

17. Bailey K, Hoeppner M, Jeska S, et al. The nurse as an educator. J Nurs Staff Dev 1995;11:205–9.

18. Kersten LD. Self-care education. In: Comprehensive respiratory nursing. Philadelphia: WB Saunders, 1989;472–96.

19. Bennett SJ, Cordes DK, Westmoreland G, et al. Self-care strategies for symptom management in patients with chronic heart failure. Nurs Res 2000;49:139–45.

20. Meillier LK, Lund AB, Kog G. Cues to action in the process of changing lifestyle. Patient Educ Couns 1997;30:472–96.

21. Bourbeau J, Collet JP, Schwartzman K, et al. Integrat-ing rehabilitative elements into a COPD self-management program reduces exacerbations and health services utilization: a randomized clinical trial. Am J Respir Crit Care Med 2000;161:A254.

22. Gallefoss F, Bakke PS, Rsgaard PK. Quality of life assessment after patient education in a randomized controlled study on asthma and chronic obstructive pulmonary disease. Am J Respir Crit Care Med 1999;159:812–7.

23. Gallefoss F, Bakke PS. How does patient education and self-management among asthmatics and patients with chronic obstructive pulmonary disease affect medication? Am J Respir Crit Care Med 1999; 160:2000–5.

24. Knowles MS. The modern practice of adult education: andragogy versus pedagogy. 2nd Ed. Chicago: Follett, 1980.

25. Rankin SH, Duffy Stallings K. Patient education. Issues, principles, practices. 3rd Ed. Philadelphia: JB Lippincott, 1996.

26. Katz JR. Back to basics. Providing effective patient teaching. Am J Nurs 1997;97:33–6.

27. Gilmartin ME. Pulmonary rehabilitation. Patient and family education. Clin Chest Med 1986;7:619–27.

28. Wichowski HC, Kubsch S. Improving your patient's compliance. Nursing 1995;25(Jan):66–8.

29. Ertmer PA, Newby TJ. Behaviorism, cognitivism, constructivism: comparing critical features from an instructional design perspective. Perform Improve Q 1993;6:50–70.

30. Good TJ, Brophy JE. Educational psychology: a realistic approach. 4th Ed. White Plains, NY: Longman, 1990.

31. Saettler P. The evolution of American educational technology. Englewood, CO: Libraries Unlimited, 1990.

32. Gagne RM. The conditions of learning. 4th Ed. New York: Holt, Rinehart & Winston, 1985.

33. Bandura A. Social learning theory. Englewood Cliffs, NJ: Prentice Hall, 1977.

34. Jonassen DH. Objectivism versus constructivism: do we need a new philosophical paradigm? Educ Technol Res Dev 1991;39:5–14.

35. Merrill MD. Constructivism and instructional design. Educ Technol 1991;31(May):45–53.

36. Green LW, Kreuter MW. Health promotion planning—an educational and environmental approach. 2nd Ed. Mountain View, CA: Mayfield, 1991.

37. Bandura A. Self-efficacy mechanism in human agency. Am Psychol 1982;33:344–58.

38. Prochaska JO, DiClemente CC. Stages of change in the modification of problem behaviors. Prog Behav Modif 1992;28:183–218.

39. Allen M. The health dimension in nursing practice: notes on nursing in primary health care. J Adv Nurs 1981;6:153–4.

40. Levasseur C, Beaucage D, Borycki E, et al. Living well with COPD. Toronto: The Piper Group Inc. from Boehringer-Ingelheim Canada, 1998.

41. Ernst P, Fitzgerald JM, Spier S. Conférence Canadienne de Consensus sur l'Asthme. Résumé des recommandations. Can Respir J 1996;3:101–14.

42. Hagan L. Éduquer pour maîtriser l'asthme; principes et méthodes. L'Asthme—otions de base- education-intervention. Québec City: Presses de l'Université Laval, 1997.

43. Gottlieb L, Rowat K. The McGill Model of nursing: a practice-derived model. ANS Adv Nurs Sci 1987;9:51–61.

44. Allen M. Primary-care nursing; research in action. In: Hockey L, ed. Recent advances in nursing; primary care nursing. Edinburgh: Churchill Livingstone, 1983:32–77.

45. Allen M. A developmental health model: nursing as continuous inquiry. Presentation. Nursing Theory Congress 1986. Toronto, 1994.

46. Ford-Gilboe MV. A comparison of two nursing models: Allen's developmental health model and Newman's theory of health as expanding consciousness. Nurs Sci Q 1994;7:113–8.

47. Kolb D. Experimental learning: experience as the source of learning and development. Englewood Cliffs, NJ: Prentice Hall, 1984.

48. Litzinger ME, Osif B. Accommodating diverse learning styles: designing instruction for electronic information source. What is good instruction now? Library instruction for the 90's: papers and session materials presented at the twentieth national LOEX Library Instruction Conference held at Eastern Michigan University 8–9 May 1992 and related resource materials gathered by the LOEX claering house. Ed. Linda Shirato. Ann Arbor, MI: Pierian Press, 1993.

49. Chickering AW. Learning styles and disciplinary differences. The modern American college. San Francisco: Jossey Bass, 1981.

SUGGESTED READINGS

Katz JR. Back to basics. Providing effective patient teaching. Am J Nurs 1997;97:33–6. *This article provides strategies that increase patient compliance and ensure comprehension of educative material. By applying these strategies, health professionals can improve their patient education process to achieve success.*

Gessner BA. Adult education. The cornerstone of patient teaching. Nurs Clin North Am 1989;24: 589–95. *Health professionals can facilitate patient learning by incorporating principles of adult education into their teaching. The patient education process is based on the problem-solving approach, for which the steps include assessment, planification, implementation, and evaluation. This article clearly delineates the steps of the patient education process.*

Kersten LD. Self-care education. In: Jovanovich HB. Comprehensive respiratory nursing. Philadelphia: WB Saunders, 1989:472–96. *This chapter discusses self-care and the teaching-learning needs of respiratory patients. The content focuses on the steps of the patient education process, with emphasis on the needs and problems associated with respiratory clinical applications.*

THE FINAL ILLNESS: PALLIATIVE CARE IN TERMINAL COPD

Peter Warren, Canon Barbara Barnett, Anne Cathcart, and Dawn Chaitram

OBJECTIVES

The general objective of this chapter is to help physicians and other allied health care professionals become more familiar about the palliative care of advanced, terminal chronic obstructive pulmonary disease (COPD) and the management of death from COPD.

After reading this chapter, the physician and the allied health care professional will be able to

- identify the terminal phase of COPD and its prognosis;
- determine goals for relieving suffering during the terminal phase of COPD;
- define what is meant by palliative care;
- demonstrate knowledge and practice of communication with patients and families in the terminal phase of COPD;
- establish advance care planning;
- identify the symptoms and develop a treatment plan for symptoms that are common in end-stage COPD;
- define and provide a "good death" when the time comes; and
- know when to refer to specific professionals from the health care team.

Chronic obstructive pulmonary disease is currently within the five leading causes of death in Canada despite the greatest of efforts, which have been covered in the preceding chapters of this book. For the majority of patients, their COPD is incurable and ultimately, is responsible for their deaths.[1] Once COPD is advanced, patients and their families have to be informed about the process of dying. Death will occur for half of them within 2 years after a hospital admission for respiratory failure. Since exacerbations may come at any time, death can come suddenly and unexpectedly. Meanwhile, the patient will experience the suffering of dyspnea, restricted activity, and feelings of anxiety and depression; this grim message is the reality of the situation. It is not surprising that of over 1,000 patients with COPD, 58% preferred a plan of comfort care over a plan to extend life and that 78% did not want ventilation in intensive care.[2]

Thus, those who manage patients with COPD must become competent and confident in caring for patients in the final phase of their illness. They must assist them and their family to face inevitable death.

In this chapter, we review terminal disease and death from COPD, advance care planning, and managing death. Furthermore, we review relief of symptoms in severe advanced COPD when rehabilitation and all standard therapy no longer seem effective.

TERMINAL COPD

Definition of Advanced, Terminal COPD

It is hard to identify the start of the terminal phase of COPD because it will vary from patient to patient, depending on the state of the lungs, personality, social support, and enjoyment of life. In the terminal phase of COPD, the airflow obstruction is usually severe, with the forced expiratory volume in 1 second (FEV_1) below 0.5 L. As a result, there is often chronic hypoxemia, which can be accompanied by hypercarbia. Some patients with COPD manage to maintain a reasonable oxygenation with a normal or even a low PCO_2 by hyperventilating, thus causing dyspnea, which is often accompanied by anxiety; these have been called "pink puffers." Others tolerate the hypoxemia and often underventilate, thus retaining CO_2. They complain less of dyspnea and, before the days of home oxygen, developed right heart failure; these have been called "blue bloaters." Either way, the patients are very limited in their activities.

They are suffering from symptoms such as dyspnea, inability to perform the activities of daily living, loss of independence, and fear of death. They will usually have had hospital admissions during exacerbations and often will have been in intensive care and ventilated at least once. The patients should already have been enrolled in a rehabilitation program. But despite all efforts, either because of a worsening disease or the inevitable deterioration of aging, there comes a point at which conventional medical care cannot relieve the suffering of the disease or prevent death. Two studies have found that for patients with COPD, compared with patients with lung cancer, the impaired quality of life and emotional well-being are often ignored. The holistic approach is not often taken to their care, and the chosen remedy is to supply aids and appliances that infrequently meet the patient's needs.[2,3]

The transition from the active care of the patient in which we concentrate on the pathophysiology of COPD, as evident by the FEV_1 and the blood gases, to a focus on the quality of life and ensuing death may be difficult for caregivers. This may be particularly hard for those professions in which the more technical aspects of medicine predominate. The professional can feel impotent and a failure, with the conclusion that "nothing more can be done for the patient." In reality, the easier part of the management for COPD has been done: it is relatively straight-forward to administer a bronchodilator, teach oxygen use, increase the 6-minute walk, and correct poor eating habits when the FEV_1 is still above 0.5 L. When the disease deteriorates and these therapies become ineffective, although somewhat paradoxical, there is even more to do. Although all medical care should be holistic, it is particularly paramount now for the patient's physical, psychological, social, and, in particular, spiritual wants to be met. An ideal time to prepare the patient and the family for the last years of COPD is to introduce the subject as part of the rehabilitation program.[4]

The team approach is essential in the achievement of the best quality of life for patients and their families at a time that both affirms life and regards death as a natural process. One major handicap in the management of this COPD phase is that there are few studies of it and so little evidence on which to base one's decisions. For instance, the Global Initiative for Chronic Obstructive Lung Disease ignores the topic or fruitlessly gives as one of its goals an effective program to reduce mortality from COPD[2]; presumably, to die of something else is a success! Once again, the care of the final and difficult phase of this common illness is ignored, although under future research, some of the issues are being addressed.

Prognosis of Advanced COPD

Chronic obstructive pulmonary disease has a poor prognosis once respiratory failure has developed, particularly if this has necessitated admission to intensive care. In a study of 362 cases of intensive care admissions for COPD, for those over 65 years, 41% died within 3 months and 59% within the year.[5] In another study of exacerbations, not necessarily treated in the intensive care unit, the mortality was 43% at 1 year and 49% at 2 years.[6]

Despite these statistics, a major difficulty with end-of-life decisions in COPD is that, even in this advanced stage, the terminal phase is often prolonged, that is, half will live for over 2 years, and the timing of death is almost impossible to forecast. The prognosis is poorly estimated, even within the week of death.[2]

Patients and their families must learn that death can intervene in COPD at any time, most often as a consequence of an infection.[7] Heart failure can compound the problem, and these patients are at an age when heart attacks and strokes are common. Lung cancer is also more common in patients with COPD.

DEATH IN COPD

Facing Death

Patients with advanced COPD, most of whom are elderly, are familiar with death as a natural process of life and thus may not fear it. However, it is common for them to fear the process of dying. They may fear that they will suffocate or choke to death, that they will lose control and/or be abandoned. Watching someone die while gasping for breath is distressing for nurses,[8] and the same can be assumed for the family and other professions. Thus, prevention of this suffocation is crucial for the patient and their caregivers.

A critical decision to be made by patients in the terminal phase of COPD lies in whether they want their caregivers to actively treat the next exacerbation of COPD with the intention of maintaining life or use treatment to ease the passage from life to death:

- If the exacerbation is to be actively treated, how much treatment is appropriate?
- Should intensive care with ventilation be used?
- Should antibiotics be ordered, or should comfort with opiods be the choice?

If the individual has always wanted to die in his/her own home, then a decision as to whether the patient wants admission to the hospital must be considered. If the patient is in a personal care home or chronic care hospital, this is now his/her home; he/she may not wish to be transferred elsewhere to strangers during the last phase of the illness.

These are very difficult and distressing decisions for all concerned. Many factors need to be considered. It takes time to come to a conclusion of which measures to take; thus, it is best done when the patient is not acutely ill. With the support of the family, patients must be asked and assisted in determining what they want when death appears inevitable. Chosen and trusted health professionals should do this when the patient is stable. It is more difficult in a crisis meeting new staff; thus, when possible, these decisions should be made in an outpatient setting such as an office or a rehabilitation program[9] rather than in the emergency department or intensive care unit, however humane and caring their staff may be. If nothing else, the intubated patient will be handicapped from easy final communication with family and caregivers.

A Good Death

Many people wish to die in their own homes surrounded by loved ones. However, most often, death occurs in the hospital, and every assistance must be made for the family to be present. Too often, death with COPD occurs in the intensive care unit, which inevitably adds to the distress of the patient and family and can be a difficult experience for the staff. Studies in the United States have found that such patients are treated aggressively, too often against their previous wishes,[10] and this applies particularly to COPD, in contrast to lung cancer.[2] Turning off a ventilator is an unpleasant experience, although a humane approach has been recommended.[11] Helping patients accept that they are in the palliative phase of COPD and encouraging them to express their wishes in a feasible way can lead to a management plan that avoids death on a ventilator. Often with the support of family, the patient can provide a health care directive that can be translated into an advance care plan that is acceptable to the patient.

Several studies have looked at what patients would like in their last days before death. Singer and colleagues[12] found that at the end of their life, patients identify five issues that they wish to see addressed:

- adequate relief of symptoms such as pain and dyspnea,
- no inappropriate prolongation of life,
- sense of control of their own person,
- relief of the burden to their family, and
- strengthening of family relationships.

Steinhauser and colleagues[13] found six such issues that have a lot in common with those mentioned above:

- pain and symptom management,
- clear decision making,
- preparation for death,
- completion of life,
- contributing to others, and
- affirmation of the whole person.

Recently, Smith, the editor of the *BMJ*, reflected on "a good death" and listed 12 principles of a good death, which are addressed in Table 18–1.[14]

A PLAN FOR THE END OF LIFE

An essential component of caring for patients with chronic lung disease is discussion with them and their families about their preferences for end-of-life care. This includes discussion about prognosis, treat-

TABLE 18–1 Principles of a Good Death*

- To know when death is coming and to understand what can be expected.
- To be able to retain control of what happens.
- To be afforded dignity and privacy.
- To have control over pain relief and other symptom control.
- To have choice and control over where death occurs (at home or elsewhere).
- To have access to information and expertise of whatever kind is necessary.
- To have access to any spiritual or emotional support required.
- To have access to hospice care in any location, not only in hospital.
- To have control over who is present and shares the end.
- To be able to issue advance directives that ensure that wishes are respected.
- To have time to say goodbye and control over aspects of timing.
- To be able to leave when it is time to go and not to have life prolonged pointlessly.

*Adapted from Smith.[14]

ment options, goals of therapy, values, and treatment preferences.[15] The literature suggests that health care professions frequently misunderstand the patient's preferences[16] and that physicians influence the decisions by the patient too much.[17]

Patients with advanced lung disease are faced with difficult decisions, and often confusing dilemmas, as they deal with the essential uncertainty of life with the disease. During acute episodes of respiratory failure, intubation may be chosen, although the patient returns to the chronic state. The alternative is to accept death. Physician-initiated discussion about end-of-life care may be hampered by the lack of reliable predictors that can identify those patients who may be poor candidates for survival or who could regain a reasonable function.[9]

Once a patient has decided what he/she wants, then the production of a health care directive, also called advance directives, living wills, or durable powers of attorney for health care is of value. These have been promoted as documents that allow patients to describe their wishes for end-of-life care in the event that they are mentally incompetent at the time of critical illness and cannot inform their caregivers.[18] Critics of such directives assert that they have not been effective in changing end-of-life decision making in hospitals or in the intensive care unit,[19] but surely the fault lies with these caregivers and not with the process. Professionals must also be aware that family members have been found to inaccurately predict what the patient would choose,[20] even if an advance directive is completed.

Once the patient has decided his/her preferences, then the health care team can begin advance care planning to formulate the management of the patient and his/her death. This planning is an ongoing discussion with the patient, family members, and providers about preferences for end-of-life care. Although no studies have demonstrated this as an effective approach, open, ongoing communication with the patient, family, and the health care team is an essential part of quality care whether the discussion occurs in the intensive care unit, an outpatient clinic, or a pulmonary rehabilitation program.[15] Pulmonary rehabilitation programs have been found to be ideal sites for educating patients about end-of-life decision making; furthermore, they can promote the completion of effective and informed advanced directives.[4] An ongoing dialogue with the physician and other health professionals in the presence of family at a time when decision making can occur outside of a crisis may be the most effective approach.[21] Advanced directives can be an important component of the process. However, they are only as effective as the quality of the preceding discussion between the patient, family as proxy, and health care professionals.

Palliative Care in COPD

The preservation of life is a major beneficence principle in medical care, and active intervention for the good of the patient is paramount in most medical encounters. As more and more medications and technical aids become available, it is tempting to focus on these as the solution to a patient's disorders; how-

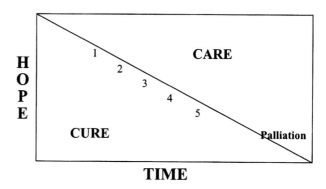

Figure 18–1 Transition from cure to care over time. Vertical axis = hope. Horizontal axis = time. Tangent represents the patient's change from hope of cure to that of care over the duration of COPD. Interventions available are given by the numbers: 1 = smoking cessation focus of treatment, 2 = bronchodilators and rehabilitation, 3 = hospital admissions and possible intensive care, 4 = home oxygen therapy, 5 = lung volume reduction surgery and transplantation. Adapted from the World Health Organization.[23]

ever, there comes a time when COPD is so severe that their effectiveness declines, and new goals and modes of treatment are needed.

Again, through consultation and discussion with the patient, his/her concerns, hopes, and fears should be identified. How best to meet and relieve them follows the advance care plan. At this stage of COPD, a palliative care approach is more appropriate.[22]

The World Health Organization defines palliative care as such:

> The active total care of patients whose disease is not responsive to curative treatment. Control of pain *(for COPD substitute dyspnea)*, of other symptoms, and of psychological, social and spiritual problems, is paramount. The goal of palliative care is achievement of best quality of life for patients and families. Many aspects of palliative care are also applicable earlier in the course of the illness in conjunction with anti-cancer *(COPD)* treatment.[23]

This definition is expanded and clarified by the following: "Palliative care…affirms life and regards dying as a normal process, neither hastens nor postpones death…provides relief from pain and other distressing symptoms…integrates the psychological and spiritual aspects of care, offers a support system to help patients live as actively as possible until death….[and] offers a support system to help the family cope during the patient's illness and in their own bereavement." Too often, palliative care focuses on cancer—hence, the emphasis on pain. But the principles are pertinent to all terminal diseases, and the lessons learnt from the much studied

palliative care of cancer can be applied to them. The transition in the hopes of the patient from curative treatment to comfort care is illustrated in Figure 18–1.[23]

To effectively achieve the palliative care of COPD, two principles are important:

1. The relief of symptoms is the paramount focus of all palliative care. One must improve the quality of life as much as possible from day to day and, for when it happens, to ease the last days of life.
2. Patient-centered care is the method used to plan care. The patient's wishes and instructions, ideally in a health care directive, are what determines the advance care plan.

By determining the purpose and expectations of the therapeutic program with the patient, the methods to achieve the relief of symptoms can be instituted. Patients and their family must be helped to realize the prognosis, what will happen over the next months, and what is possible. A realistic plan of management is essential for success.

End-of-Life Decisions

Ethical Principles

Ethical principles must be the basis for planning end-of-life decisions with a patient, and all health professionals must be familiar with these for they must underlie such decision making. The following definitions are brief but identify the concepts:

1. *Beneficence.* The principle of beneficence is to produce benefit, do good, and act in the best interests of the patient.
2. *Nonmaleficence.* The principle of nonmaleficence is to minimize or do no harm.
3. *Autonomy.* The principle of autonomy acknowl-

edges the rights of self-determination for competent patients to decide what treatment they do or do not want, without influence on the other care given.

4. *Justice*. The health care professional has a duty to act in a manner that is fair and just, ensuring equitable access to the treatment available.

5. *Futility*. The principle of futility is that the health professional cannot be expected to provide investigation or treatment that he/she knows will do harm or will serve no purpose (eg, nonmaleficence). Conversely, futile treatment should not be imposed on the patient.

6. *Double effect*. The principle of double effect is that a treatment is aimed at a specific symptom, but as a result of side effects, it may potentially shorten life.[24] A common example is the use of morphine to relieve pain or dyspnea while knowing that it may depress respiration; this is often the reason that it is not ordered when needed. When the benefits of the patient's suffering outweigh the risks, then such therapy is acceptable and is not considered as euthanasia.

The right of the patient to refuse or discontinue treatment is also founded on sound ethical principles. Respect for a patient's autonomy to refuse life-saving antibiotics or other medications not prescribed for the relief of symptoms enables the health care team to shift the focus to one of comfort care and support to the patient and the family. The disease cannot be reversed or halted. Therefore, although initially soothing and providing false hope, pursuing futile, invasive treatments only heightens patient and family suffering; dying must not be prolonged when death is inevitable.

Cross-Cultural Considerations

Culture will also influence the approach to the final phase of illness of the patient with COPD. One's culture makes up the spectrum of socially transmitted behavior patterns that include art, beliefs, and institutions; it encompasses one's life experiences, values, attitudes, and assumptions. It may not be the same as ethnic origin, but, regardless, it is influenced by it. In advanced COPD, there is little information on how the influence of culture affects the patient and family; however, by borrowing from other palliative care research, it can be considered here.

An individual's interpretation of culture provides a framework for understanding death and dying.

Therefore, health care workers must place the patient's understanding of health and illness within the cultural setting, but they should not automatically assume that because of ethnicity, the individual patient will adhere to all of the values associated with that group. The approach must be tailored to the individual, and communication should be conveyed in a manner that is ethnically, culturally, racially, and linguistically appropriate.

Culture affects the patient's values and beliefs on suffering, relief of symptoms, nutrition, personal care, and alternative therapies. Important factors, such as eye contact, physical touching, and privacy will vary considerably between cultures. Health care workers of a different cultural background must acknowledge that these issues are important in sensitive cross-cultural communication. The patient's own culture must be respected. Most importantly, patterns of decision making vary between cultures, and this can have profound effects on truth telling and management planning.

In Western culture, autonomy and telling the whole truth, thus leading to informed consent are now the generally accepted practice. These discussions are based on the ability of the individual to engage in self-disclosure and to determine his/her own health care preferences.

In some non-Western societies, the concept of self-disclosure may be unfamiliar. Some cultures may rely on the extended family to make end-of-life decisions. In this case, end-of-life directives are thought to be irrelevant since supportive family members will have that responsibility. Also, the patient may not want to hear the reality of the situation or that the burden will be shouldered by the family. A member of the family may be charged with telling the patient the prognosis. If such differences are not recognized or accepted by health care workers, then the management of the patient will be debased.

Issues of mistrust with the health care system may further impede discussions regarding end-of-life decision making. For instance, some cultures are less likely than others to trust health care workers, communicate treatment preferences, or complete advance directives. In some cultures, a lack of knowledge on health care directives, discomfort with death and dying, perceived burden on designated proxies, and lack of potential surrogates may also affect the discussion and completion of advanced health care directives.

A patient who belongs to a culture that is a minority is possibly dispossessed of many of the benefits of Western society through poverty; then there may be concern that the patient will also be deprived of all possible technological aids. In this case, advanced care directives may choose cure over care as the priority for management.[25–27]

The Incompetent Patient

Patients may become incompetent to make end-of-life decisions, that is, to exercise their autonomy because of reversible or irreversible disorders. This problem underlines the lesson that health care directives can never be done too early and that periodic review is valuable, similar to the case of a will. Once a patient appears incompetent, one must make sure that it is not caused by depression, which is very common in severe COPD. Depression could make a patient refuse therapy, even when the disease, or an exacerbation, is still amenable to established therapy. Depression must be assessed if the health professional feels that the decision is inappropriate. Expert psychiatric opinion is needed to assess and treat the depression as well as to determine if the patient is competent to make decisions.

For the permanently incompetent patient for whom there is no end-of-life directive, one must turn for help from the family, ideally the spouse and, if necessary, the children. What one needs to learn is what the patient would have wanted if he/she could communicate: has he/she ever expressed views on resuscitation, the risks of artificially prolonged life, and so on? Unfortunately, in competent patients, it has been learned that the family often incorrectly states a patient's wishes.[20]

Where there is disagreement within the family, they will need guidance to determine who among them will be responsible for the advice. In these situations, the assistance of the social worker and the chaplain may promote consensus. The family may be helped if they are reassured that the life or death decision is not their responsibility but that they are simply guiding the health care professionals in the decision. Each community will have different ethical, legal, and social resources to help the family and health care team make the right decision.

Another issue is that in some jurisdictions, the paramedics will have to ignore health care directives when faced by a dying patient who is now unable to communicate.[28]

Spiritual Care in Managing End of Life

"Breath is not only a physiologic process, it is also a powerful spiritual and religious symbol." In all of the major world religions, "breath" and "spirit" are inextricably linked. The same word is used for both breath and spirit in Arabic, Sanskrit, and Hebrew. In Canadian Aboriginal spiritualities, the gift of wind is one of the four sacred gifts of life; "It is the sacred breath of life, the air we breathe." In the Judeo-Christian religion, breath is not simply the air that enters the lungs; it is the spirit, it is life itself. Meditation practices call for awareness of breathing.

Patients with COPD are conscious of most breaths and are thus constantly reminded of the fragility of their existence and how plainly their life depends on breathing. This awareness may lead them to search for inspiration. They may reflect consciously or subconsciously on their spiritual well-being, their ability to experience life, and their feelings about that experience; they may ask questions about this and search for a meaning in their life and, ultimately, in their impending death.[29]

Suffering may compound the patient's subjective experience of dyspnea and anxiety. Our hospital, à propos pain but equally relevant to dyspnea, defines suffering as "what the patient says it is. It is the human spiritual dimension of physical pain. It is left when physical pain has been alleviated. It is subjective and culturally based." It may include (but is not limited to the following):

- Grief associated with losses (future, life, hope, health/well-being, control, etc, with feelings of anger, sadness, resentment, guilt)
- A person's struggle to resolve issues related to a search for meaning with associated feelings of hopefulness and helplessness
- A questioning of previously held personal or religious values

Spiritual care intervention offers the patient and the family the opportunity to explore and come to terms with some or all of the components of suffering that contribute to the patient's anxiety. Religious teachings, either current or remembered from childhood, may add to the patient's anxiety about death. A patient may need to express feelings about faith that appear to be unacceptable (fear, anger at God). A trusting relationship with a chaplain may also offer the opportunity to express out loud some long-hidden feelings of shame or guilt.

Both patients and family members may have a need to protect each other from the fact that this may be the final illness. Family members may be at different stages in their readiness to face the patient's death and may find this difficult or uncomfortable to contemplate or discuss. Finally, they may all need support as they choose what they want or need to say to each other.

Some patients have special religious or spiritual practices that are important for their well-being. The chaplain can ensure that the interdisciplinary team understands the significance of these. As patients consider what is a good death, they may also wish to plan the details of a funeral or memorial service. This is the completion of their physical life and a final act of control over their destiny.

Facilitate End-of-Life Decision Making

Patients should be educated on the diagnosis, prognosis, and therapeutic choices available for their COPD and should be assisted in stating their final wishes. These can be indicated in a health care directive. This can be the basis of advance care planning by the health care team. There are many approaches to this vital and often forgotten part of the management of patients with terminal COPD. Curtis[15], who works in an acute care hospital setting, has proposed one good model. Depending on the setting and phase of the patient's COPD, his approach may need to be modified, but, nonetheless, the principles expressed are useful. The following is based on his recommendations.

Who Should Do This?

The opinion of all members of the health care team is valuable, and the whole team should be comfortable with the conclusion. The physician is appointed as the one responsible for the decisions since he/she is the person ultimately in charge of writing the orders; in light of this, the involvement of others is still invaluable, particularly as physicians are too often ignorant of this matter. The nurses spend the most time with the patients, but the SUPPORT study revealed that nurses are also often unaware of their patients' preferences.[16] However, patients and their families found that the nurses' communications were the most helpful for helping them decide what they wanted done.[30]

When Should It Be Done?

Hopefully, there is time for the patient to get to know the team and think about these matters. Individual professionals can provide the information from their own area of expertise on patients' problems, therapies, and options to assist in the decision-making process. This does not have to be rushed, although patients and families must be warned that exacerbations can arise at any time. Understandably, patients and their families change their minds over time, progressing from a hope for a cure and a prolonged life to a simple wish for comfort and relief of their suffering. The earlier this process is instituted, the better the chances are of seeing results, thus making the rehabilitation program a good time to start the process.[4]

Where Should It Be Done?

It is preferable to have a large enough room in which all participants can sit comfortably, in privacy (confidentiality), and remain undisturbed. These meetings can be distressing, and a display of intense emotion is not uncommon. Although it is important to have the help of the entire team, it may be inappropriate for everyone to be present since this can dominate the patient. The patient should be asked in private whom they would like to be present at this discussion.[15]

How Should It Be Done?

Traditionally, the physician introduces the subject and is best suited to give a prognosis and describe possible therapies. Health care directives may best be done with someone who will not be responsible for the clinical care of and decisions on the patient; a social worker fills this bill. Most importantly, the essential qualification is that the patient and family have trust in the professional.

The team must know the patient's health care directive, and then advance care planning can be done. Above all, the patient and family must be allowed to express their feelings and ask questions. Good communication is listening as much as telling. The team should prepare for the meeting by clarifying their expectations and coming to a consensus as to what they think can be done; this facilitates clear decision making. First, the patient and the family should be asked what they know and expect about the disease so that autonomy and a sense of control are established. Moreover, the team can now discern in which direction the discussion and decisions may go. Finally, the team leader must summarize the conclusions of the meeting and outline the plan of management.[15]

When reaching decisions for health care directives, four levels of plan are often used (Table 18–2). For COPD, these would include decisions such as the following:

- *Level 4.* All interventions such as full cardiopulmonary resuscitation. Gordon has made the point that resuscitation is effective for a previously "healthy" organ that malfunctions but is of no value for a worn-out organ that is irreversibly damaged by chronic disease such as the lungs in COPD.[31]

For cardiac arrest, the SUPPORT study used the following questions, which can be used as a model by substituting respiratory phrases for cardiac:

As you know, there are a number of things doctors can do to try to revive someone whose heart has stopped beating which usually includes a machine to help breathing. Thinking of your current condition, what would you want your doctor to try to revive you with if your heart ever stopped beating? Would you want your doctor to try and revive you, or would you want your doctors not to try to revive you?

The communication went on: "If you had to make a choice at this time, would you prefer a course of treatment that focuses on extending life as much as possible, even if it means having more pain and discomfort, or would you want a plan of care that focuses on relieving pain and discomfort as much as possible even if it means not living as long?"[16]

- *Level 3.* Intubation and ventilation. Structured decision aids are available to help patients decide what should be done if noninvasive therapy is failing to maintain adequate respiration. Such an aid can provide information on what the processes, risks, and benefits of intubation are and also the probability trade-off to gauge the strength of the patient's preference.[32]

For unremitting dyspnea, lung volume reduction surgery and transplantation are available. To quote Hamlet, "Diseases desperate grown, by desperate appliance are relieved, or not at all." Patients may hope for such measures as a cure. A consultation with the team and a careful evaluation of their suitability will often assuage this uncertainty when it is determined to be of no value. Certainly, for the few for whom these measures are possible, end-of-life

TABLE 18–2 Advanced Care Planning: Examples of Levels of Care, Guided by Patient's Instructions

Level 4	All conditions investigated and treated including cardiopulmonary resuscitation
Level 3	All conditions investigated and treated except cardiopulmonary resuscitation
Level 2	Potentially reversible conditions are investigated and treated
Level 1	Palliative care or comfort care—symptom relief is the focus of all treatment

directives should be prepared for; in some, the operation will hasten death.

- *Level 2.* The patient wants exacerbations treated with antibiotics, corticosteroids, and even noninvasive ventilation. Comfort is important but allows for reversing conditions that have arisen and may respond. The desire to be transferred to an acute care hospital should be clarified.
- *Level 1.* This is palliative or comfort care only, and therapy is given actively and solely for the relief of symptoms. Intravenous therapy, tube feeds, and medications used for conditions that are not adding to the distress are avoided.

MANAGING THE PATIENT'S SYMPTOMS

There is a dearth of studies on the relief of symptoms in the penultimate phase of COPD. It is a modern fad that we must only practice evidence-based medicine; advocates of this school will be thwarted when there are no studies available. Moreover, they should remember the aphorism of Albert Einstein that "Not everything that can be counted counts, not everything that counts can be counted" (Sister Nuala Kenny, personal communication, 2001). The caregivers for these patients must rely on experience. They can borrow from the studies on the symptoms of COPD in earlier stages and from the lessons learned from palliative care research in cancer. Most research on COPD has been done during rehabilitation programs. Very few studies have been done in relieving COPD symptoms once hypoxia and hypercarbia are established.

The major symptoms common in the penultimate phases of COPD are as follows:

- Dyspnea
- Cough and phlegm
- Depression and anxiety
- Insomnia
- Fatigue
- Delirium
- Pain
- Anorexia and weight loss

Since many of these symptoms are covered elsewhere in this textbook, the main focus of the discussion will be on managing patient's symptoms with respect to terminal COPD.

Dyspnea

In the terminal phase of COPD, dyspnea is the dominant symptom; 50% of patients suffer from dyspnea, and this rises to 90% at the end of life.[7]

Dyspnea is only secondary to pain as a feared and distressing symptom that causes suffering. Its underlying mechanism involves a complex series of pathways reflecting the many stimuli to the brain including pulmonary proprioceptors, the chest wall, the respiratory muscles, hypoxemia, hypercarbia and pH, anxiety, and so on[33]. We cannot forget our knowledge of the pathophysiology of COPD for the most effective relief of symptoms is usually based on treatment aimed at relieving the underlying disorder. Chapter 9 of this textbook provides a review of mechanism, assessment, and management.

The circumstances in which dyspnea is worsened need to be identified; these include exercise, anxiety, posture, eating, irritants, or allergies. Dyspnea, like pain, is subjective, and the professional must rely heavily on the patient's account and estimate of its severity as long as they are able to communicate. Dyspnea can be rated on a scale by the patient, and there are several available, although it must be appreciated that these were developed for assessment in earlier stages of the disease and not in the final stage. As for pain, a simple 1 to 10 rating scale can be used.[34]

Relief of this dyspnea must be a priority in the palliative care of COPD. The professional can observe dyspnea in a patient by the distress and use of accessory muscles. Close family members may be the best observers for dyspnea, although they may be more distressed watching it than the patient actually suffering from it. The feeling that the patient's breathing is out of control and that he/she might be suffocating can easily lead to panic and, in turn, a vicious circle of a more rapid struggle to breathe, resulting only in an increased workload. Dyspnea at rest, dyspnea during or after exercise, dyspnea at night, and anxiety all need consideration.[35] It must also be remembered that hypoventilation may be life threatening and easily overlooked since the patient appears comfortable. Dyspnea in a patient who cannot communicate, particularly if intubated, is important and can also be overlooked. Just because the ventilator provides good blood gases and appropriate ventilation it does not mean that the patient does not feel dyspnea.

Pharmacologic Management

Bronchodilators and Standard Therapy. The most effective timing and delivery of bronchodilators should be decided through a critical observation of the patient's symptoms; short-acting dilators as needed, long-acting dilators regularly, and anticholinergics can all be tried separately or together. Theophylline may be of value in some patients in whom side effects are not a problem, and corticosteroids in an oral form may help. Patients often swear by corticosteroids, but it can be hard to show objective improvement, particularly if the focus is on improved lung function. However, in the last months of COPD, when serious side effects will not have time to develop, it means that they can be tried, although depression and confusion must be avoided. Certainly, their euphoric benefit is much used in the palliation of cancer. It is hard to conceive that inhaled corticosteroids have any value.

Opioids. Morphine and its derivatives were much used historically for the symptoms of tuberculosis before it became a curable disease. Opioids are well accepted for the pain and dyspnea of lung cancer. However, fears of respiratory depression and worsening failure have limited their use in COPD. Morphine receptors have been identified in the lungs, and it was hoped that these receptors would produce relief with the use of nebulized morphine without the disadvantages of systemic effects.[36] However, the results are ambivalent.

There have been several studies of morphine in severe COPD, but patients with significant hypoxemia or hypercarbia have usually been excluded. In other words, the studies have looked most at dyspnea in the rehabilitation stage of COPD, not the suffering of its penultimate phase. The initial benefit of morphine is attributable to reduced ventilation and sensation of dyspnea, and this is evident in single-dose studies. The benefits are less evident over several weeks, and side effects are common. Manning identified seven randomized controlled studies on opioids in COPD and concluded that the results were equivocal for clinical practice.[37] The longest study, 6 weeks, with sustained-release morphine, was disappointing.

However, in pain management, the dose is constantly adjusted to control the pain, and the side effects are counteracted as necessary; such an approach might be considered for dyspnea. Constipation causes its own interference with respiration; this is a common side effect, and effective laxative therapy is essential. Nebulized fentanyl has been used for short-duration benefits. Morphine is accepted as the drug of choice for the dying patient.

Anxiolytics. Anxiety often accompanies dyspnea, and dyspnea itself produces anxiety. Anxiolytics are an attractive option for dyspnea in COPD, but, again, the initial promise of these first studies has not been confirmed. The results of several trials with benzodiazepines are mixed; if they are indicated for the anxiety per se, then they are certainly worth trying.

Phenothiazines. There are a few studies of phenothiazines in COPD, suggesting a slight benefit at most.

Antidepressants. There is no evidence that antidepressants improve dyspnea, although it is possible that in an improved mood, the patient may tolerate the dyspnea better.

Nonpharmacologic Management

Oxygen. Certainly, hypoxemia may be responsible for dyspnea and should be relieved by administering oxygen to achieve a saturation of 90%. Higher saturations are not necessary in advanced COPD. Whether oxygen relieves dyspnea in patients in whom there is no severe hypoxemia (eg, a PO_2 of 60 mm Hg or higher) is uncertain. In palliative care for cancer, oxygen is frequently used in this situation, although whether the benefit is attributable to a relief of increased gas flow through the nose, the expectations of the patient, or the pressure on the staff to improve the situation is unclear.

Fresh Air. The simple measure of blowing air on the face by a fan can relieve dyspnea, so fans should be freely available. The relief of a wind across the face and through the nose may explain some of the benefits of oxygen. Open windows may also provide ease.

Noninvasive Ventilation. Noninvasive ventilation (continuous positive airway pressure) seems effective in relieving severe dyspnea in exacerbations. In these cases, nasal cannulae are preferable to the mask, and

low pressures are used. Patients quickly divide into responders or nonresponders, with the latter receiving no feeling of relief or an inability to tolerate the mask. This will not be useful long term for relief of dyspnea but can be used for an hour.[38]

Physiotherapy. Relaxation breathing, in particular, slow deep breaths and pursed-lip expiration, may help; all staff should remind patients of this. Vibration therapy has been tried, but the benefits remain questionable. Relaxation techniques are very important, and exercise may also desensitize patients to dyspnea.

Posture. Patients with COPD may breathe more easily sitting up, or even leaning over a bedtable that they can hold will facilitate the use of accessory muscles.

Blood Transfusion. Significant anemia will produce dyspnea, and transfusion should be given if the anemia is significant (eg, below 60 g/L).

Music Therapy. Considering that, according to Shakespeare, music "soothes the troubled breast," it should be regarded as a potential source of relief in the dyspneic patient. The right tempo may guide breathing patterns, with andante to be favored over allegro.

Alternative Therapy

Acupuncture. There is minimal evidence that acupuncture helps dyspnea in COPD, although one study has shown a benefit in lung cancer.

Herbal Remedies. Not only is there no evidence that these are of benefit, but there is also the possibility that they could do harm. Many of the preparations available in health food stores that are recommended for respiratory disorders contain ephedrine, which is an old-fashioned, weak, sympathomimetic that unfortunately also stimulates the brain and could exacerbate anxiety.

Other Symptoms[39]

Cough and Phlegm

Cough can come in many forms and can lead to distressing side effects that include retching and actual vomiting, a feeling of choking, and syncope. At night, cough can interrupt sleep. Cough may be dry or accompany phlegm production. Factors that exacerbate cough must be sought, as for dyspnea. Phlegm is common in COPD, although except with bronchiectasis, it is not usually of a large volume. It is usually "clear" but can become purulent when it is assumed that there is an infection present. One difficult problem is viscous plugs of phlegm that are hard to clear and lead to dyspnea as they occlude an airway. Phlegm in the throat is responsible for what is known popularly as the "death rattle" and can distress observers of the dying patient.[40]

It is a difficult symptom to cure and may simply need suppression. If simple over-the-counter remedies such as Hall's cough candies do not relieve it, then opioids can be very effective. Corticosteroids may reduce cough if inflammation is contributing to it. If the cough is paroxysmal and unbearable, then an inhaled local anesthetic has been used in the intensive care unit with intubated patients. Whether this would help in regular practice is unknown, and it would also present a serious risk of aspiration.

Secretions can be a problem and are hard to control. Physiotherapy may help clear them and is useful in exacerbations. It is not certain that any medications reduce or help reduce sputum. Hydration must be maintained by drinking enough fluids to reduce viscosity. Humidification will not help the lower respiratory tract unless there is a tracheostomy. If infection is present, then sputum increases and purulent secretions are more viscous and so harder to cough out. Guaifenesin has the reputation of improving sputum control. When close to death, scopolamine is often used as it is thought to reduce secretions and hence diminish the death rattle, to which it is so hard to listen.[40]

Hemoptysis

Blood is not usually coughed up in COPD, even in its advanced stage. Hemoptysis may reveal other diseases, including lung cancer or pulmonary embolism. If distressful, hemoptysis can usually be helped with opioids.

Depression and Anxiety

The SUPPORT study[2] has found that depression is very common in COPD, and, in fact, this is the chronic disease in which it is the most common. Depression that is pathologic is too often overlooked because the patient's situation is naturally depressing; screening for depression using simple questionnaires is important. Depression is associated with mortality, and attempted suicide in the elderly is associated with chronic disease such as COPD.[41]

A feeling of suffocation inevitably induces anxiety, and, in turn, anxiety usually increases ventilation and the perception of breathing. Anxiety is a major problem in COPD, being found in one-quarter of patients. Anxiety often indicates underlying depression and can distract the staff from recognizing that it is the result of the depression.

In a study of potential transplant candidates, Singer and colleagues confirmed these findings and also found that 4% had the antisocial personality tendencies of a psychopathic deviance or hypomanic type.[42]

Depression must be assessed and treated, but one drawback is that antidepressants are slow acting over weeks. In palliative care, the stimulatory methylphenidate (Ritalin) is used; it acts quickly and is short-lived, so that it will not reduce sleep when administered in the morning. Its role has not been studied in COPD. Anxiolytics should be used as indicated and coupled with both nonpharmacologic techniques of reassurance that suffocation is not occurring and relaxation techniques, including deep, measured breaths. A number of medications have been tried for depression or anxiety, but the numbers studied are small, and it is hard to favor any one preparation. Perhaps it is best for the team to become familiar with a few in particular and use just those.

Insomnia

Patients with severe COPD are usually orthopneic and so do not sleep well lying down in a bed; however, other problems, such as obstructive sleep apnea, the stimulant effects of medications such as theophylline, anxiety, and depression all affect sleep. One major cause of fatigue is the sleep disturbance associated with COPD and the loss of a refreshing deep night of sleep.

A hospital bed or "Easy Boy" chair may help as the person can sit up and sleep. The use of oxygen to relieve nocturnal desaturation and long-acting dilators for constriction may help. Sleeping pills may be tried, nocturnal amitriptyline or certain benzodiazepines, and in particular those that are short acting. One must avoid daytime sleepiness and a mixed-up sleep cycle.[43]

Fatigue

Fatigue is more than just being limited by dyspnea. It is a common complaint and again has complex interacting mechanisms responsible for it. These include lack of exercise, loss of body mass, insomnia, and depression. Treatable causes of fatigue, for example, anemia and thyroid abnormalities, should be sought, as well as other, less amenable disorders such as renal failure and chronic heart failure. Psychologically, fatigue saps the will to take part in any therapy, and this compounds the problem.

Corticosteroids, amphetamines, and megestrol have been tried for cancer fatigue, but their value in COPD is unknown. The patient should be informed that the body is often naturally "shutting down." Both physical and mental exercise and activity, by day, will help the patient experience a more profound sleep that is naturally refreshing. Sleep disturbance is a major factor in fatigue; sleep apnea must be ruled out. A proper sleep-wake cycle should be encouraged.

Delirium

Confusion occurs in one-quarter of patients at death. During exacerbations, it is not uncommon for delirium to occur because of hypoxemia or the accompanying acidemia and hypercarbia. Medications or metabolic imbalances (eg, hyponatremia) may compound the problem. Opioid toxicity is a frequent cause and may be controlled by switching to another compound.

Hypoxia and metabolic disorders should be corrected. Haloperidol is a good first-line treatment, and metho-trimeprazine and midazolam can also be helpful. Such therapy may spill over to terminal sedation and should be done only if suffering provides no other choice; moreover, the family and team should be comfortable with such an approach.

Pain

Although pain is not expected as a feature of COPD per se, it was nonetheless reported by one-quarter of patients dying with COPD.[3] It may arise from concomitant bone fractures that are too often one of the complications of corticosteroid-induced osteoporosis. Inevitably, the pain of these impairs respiratory movement and may induce respiratory failure.

Opioids are the mainstay of pain control and must be used when needed, irrespective of fears of respiratory depression. Calcitonin or biphosphonates may relieve the pain of fractures.

Anorexia and Cachexia, Weight Loss

Anorexia may be caused simply in response to the fact that the patient is too breathless to eat, but it is more part of the general change in metabolism, the cachexia, that so often accompanies COPD. The resulting weight loss is a poor prognostic sign. Mouth breathing and the bloating of swallowed air compound the problem. Many people with COPD experience weight loss because of tissue depletion, and this is an indicator of a poor prognosis. The heightened minute ventilation and hence increased basal metabolism need increased caloric intake to maintain the status quo, but this does not explain it all. Reduced respiratory muscle power is one result of the depletion, and this may be compounded by corticosteroids. Malnutrition also affects the immune system and so the ability to combat infections. Potassium, magnesium, and phosphate intake can be inadequate and worsen muscle function. Potassium may also be lowered by the frequent use of sympathomimetic dilator drugs. Depression may add to anorexia.

The nutritionist must review the needs of the patient and devise a diet[44] to meet these with what is fancied. Alcohol can be used judicially to stimulate the appetite. High-calorie supplements such as Ensure may be of value. Corticosteroids may help, although they may actually contribute to muscle wasting. Drugs such as metoclopramide are used in cancer to improve stomach function, and this may help when air swallowing is present. Appetite stimulation with drugs such as megestrol is used in cancer, and anabolic corticosteroids have also been tried. Families should be encouraged to bring in favorite foods; this also enables them to participate in the care of their loved one. The weight loss can be very disturbing to families who see the patient as losing strength and fading away; comfort can be provided by explaining that it is part of the body's natural process of shutting down. However, overloading the metabolism and hence the respiratory system must be avoided.

Constipation

Constipation is the most common side effect of opioids and can become a major problem. A full abdomen and straining at stool will worsen dyspnea. Constipation must be prevented with laxatives, for example, senna (Senokot), bisacodyl, and even lactulose must be given regularly before the problem arises.

Dehydration

Just as eating may be a chore, so drinking adequate fluids may be neglected. This may lead to dryer and more viscous secretions, along with difficulty in clearing sputum. This can be managed with oral or intravenously during exacerbations.

Edema

Edema may develop as the result of heart failure. This can be simply caused by cor pulmonale, right heart failure secondary to the lung disease, or coincidental heart disease. Cor pulmonale is mainly caused by hypoxia producing pulmonary hypertension, and this should be controlled with oxygen therapy. Poor nutrition with low albumin should be excluded, and diuretics should be used to control edema.

MANAGING DEATH

If no resuscitation or potentially active treatment has been the decision of the patient and the family, then the team must be prepared to actively, and appropriately, treat the patient during the time of dying.[10]

Active treatment is established to keep the patient comfortable but fully conscious and in control of the situation for as long as possible. Symptoms should be assessed objectively, and one useful method is the Edmonton Symptom Assessment System,[45] which is used on many palliative units (Figure 18–2).

The treatment is holistic, relying on both pharmacologic and nonpharmacologic means, and some treatment may still seem to be curative. Antibiotics may still be given even when comfort is the primary goal in relieving an exacerbation.

Opioids are the most useful drug for relief of physical and mental suffering in the dying patient. There are several choices, and they can be given orally, subcutaneously, or by patch. A regular dosing timetable with a backup of "as needed" doses is essential. The team must routinely increase the dose of the regularly scheduled drug, depending on the need for breakthrough doses. For anxiety, the benzodiazepines are of value. Haloperidol is often helpful for delir-

SYMPTOM ASSESSMENT

Name: _____

Room No: _____ Time: _____

Please cross the line at the point that best decribes: (For Coding)

No pain	Severe pain
Very active	Not active
Not nauseated	Very nauseated
Not depressed	Very depressed
Not anxious	Very anxious
Not drowsy	Very drowsy
Very good appetite	No appetite
Very good sensation of wellbeing	Poor sensation of wellbeing
No shortness of breath	Very shorth of breath

Assessed by: _____

Figure 18–2 Edmonton Symptom Assessment Score used on many palliative units. Adapted from Brurera, et al.[45]

ium. A delicate balance between relief of symptoms and a sense of control with the patient is the ideal, although the drugs should not add to the confusion that so often occurs at the end. The principle of double effect is exercised. Patients want to communicate and say goodbye to friends and family, so it is advisable to try and maintain consciousness as long as possible. Severe distress does not often happen in COPD since respiratory failure and hypercarbia will produce natural sedation. However, when pneumonia develops, then distress can be severe, and terminal sedation may be needed.

General measures include supportive counseling that involves letting the patient talk, specific relaxation and distraction techniques, simple touch, music, subdued lighting, and quiet. Privacy for the patient must be respected. Families must be able to spend time with the dying in comfortable conditions. Other patients who know the dying should be able to provide support and make themselves useful through their emotional contribution.[13] The presence of the chaplain and, for some, formal religious rituals may be of great comfort wherever the patient is dying.

If the patient has chosen resuscitation and is on an intensive care ventilator, and the decision is made to cease what is now clearly futile therapy, then the steps to accomplish this in an ethical and humane way have been recommended.[10,11]

WHEN TO REFER

As COPD advances, the primary care physician should seek help. The patient should be assessed by a specialist, in particular the rehabilitation team. After the rehabilitation program has ceased to provide meaningful benefits to the patient, then those responsible for the care of the patient must turn their minds to the penultimate phase of the illness and the inevitable death. If the patient is still at home or in a personal care home, then the rehabilitation team in the office or day hospital can fulfill this role. If the patient is an inpatient, the hospital team can do it, and in many cases it will be the intensive care team. Of course, the acute hospital, rehabilitation, and terminal phases overlap, and the same team can do both. The seeds of what will happen must be planted early on in the minds of the patient and the family. In this way, they can identify their hopes and fears to the team and provide directives of what they want to hap-

pen. Whatever may seem obvious to the experts, the patient must still be allowed to take time in accepting the inevitable and in deciding what should be done.

Successful care of the patient in the terminal phase of COPD is dependent on teamwork by professionals, the patient, and the family. Certain members of the team now play a larger role, and all members have to take new approaches to the work; for example, the spiritual care worker now has an important role. The social worker can provide both psychosocial and concrete interventions. The team must communicate by using common records and regular meetings to review a patient's problems and progress. Since it is unlikely that any symptom has just one cause, the solution will involve the expertise of several disciplines. The following professionals should be available.

Physician

Patients still look to the physician for diagnosis, prognosis and treatment, and ultimate responsibility for their care. Ideally, this will be the family physician who has known the patient for years. But our modern world divorces them from institutional work; thus, it may be the respir-ologist in the hospital, rehabilitation program, or chronic care unit who fills this role. The physician need not necessarily be the leader of the team and may be more of a coach than a captain. However, since the physician writes the orders and prescriptions, certain decisions such as "no resuscitation" will be made by the physician. The physician can be a general physician and not necessarily a specialist in respirology.[46] Appropriate use of other specialists such as the psychiatrist and geriatrician may be needed for individual patients and in the development of guidelines and policies.

Nurse

The nurse is the key member of the team, particularly for inpatients. Nurses spend more time than anyone else with the patient, whether it is in the hospital or during home visits. It is the nurse who first hears of and interprets the symptoms of the patients and who is most often present when they draw their last breath. The nurse administers much of the care of the patient.

Social Worker

The social worker is available to provide psychosocial and concrete interventions to patients living with COPD. Social workers may provide individual, family, or group interventions based on the patient's needs. Psychosocial sessions with patients with COPD include providing counseling related to issues of loss, anxiety, and depression. Social workers are also available to assist patients with problem solving around a time of crisis, easing communication between patients, families, and staff, and to assist patients in adjusting to new settings. The social worker may be the person best suited for facilitating the end-of-life directives to the patient in that this profession is not involved in the actual clinical treatment of the patient. Concrete interventions may include admission and discharge planning, providing assistance with financial and legal matters, and accessing community resources and services.

Chaplain

Chaplains support patients and their families in their spiritual struggles, particularly those related to loss, a search for meaning, despair, and dying. Chaplains are trained to work with people from many different religious backgrounds and those with no formal religious beliefs; they can ensure that the religious beliefs, practices, and rituals that provide comfort and meaning to the patient are respected by members of the health care team.

Respiratory Therapist

The respiratory therapist can identify when respiratory function has worsened, administer effective therapy efficiently, and, in particular, ensure that oxygen therapy is adequate and safe. The respiratory therapist can acquaint the patient with procedures when the patient is considering mechanical ventilation, invasive or noninvasive.

Physiotherapist

Physiotherapy is still important, even though at this stage of COPD, exercise may not achieve much in distance walked. Physiotherapy provides the means to attain the limited activities of daily living and has a good effect on relieving depression and achieving a feeling of self-control and independence. Moreover, daily activity can help improve sleep and aids as an effective therapy for mild depression. If cough and phlegm are a problem, then physiotherapy may help clear them; in effect, it is essential in managing exacerbations.

Occupational Therapist

The occupational therapist enables the patient to manage his/her activities of daily living and so maintain independence. Wheelchairs and motorized scooters may enable the breathless patient to enjoy a social life.

Nutrition Therapist

Malnutrition and tissue depletion are major problems in COPD, and the correction of these deficits remains important. Underweight patients have a poor prognosis, and correcting this difficult problem needs experienced expert help. In some patients, obesity simply adds to the symptoms and also requires correction.

Pharmacist

In advanced COPD, many drugs are used both for the COPD itself, for the complications of drug therapy (eg, corticosteroids), and for the accompanying disorders of old age. Careful review of the benefits of each drug, the risk of drug interactions, and the monitoring of doses is necessary. The pharmacist should question whether there is any evidence that the drugs prescribed have any benefit at this stage of the disease; he/she should also remind the physician of their cost to elderly patients on fixed incomes (eg, inhaled corticosteroids).

Music Therapist, Art Therapist

Music and art can help patients cope with their feelings, provide comfort and outlets for their fears and anxieties, and provide relief for their symptoms. Music can influence breathing patterns and hence relieve dyspnea.

Activity Coordinator

Patients with COPD can easily become isolated, thus adding to their depression, inactivity, and insomnia. Activities that appeal to the patient and add to their quality of life are essential.

Health Care Aids

For inpatients or in personal care homes, aids, the individuals who attend the patient's bedside, are usually overlooked as a valuable member of the team. Their experience in handling these patients and their common sense may offer insight into the patient's problems and progress.

Other Patients

No one knows better what COPD means than someone who is experiencing it. Every opportunity should be made for patients and their families to exchange experiences and tips, as well as the mutual support of friendship. This helps the goal of selfless contribution to others at the end of life.

SUMMARY

In the terminal phase of COPD, much needs to be done to reduce suffering and improve the quality of life of the patient. Compassionate care is holistic, and team work to ensure that it is delivered is essential.

Dyspnea is a major problem, and the drugs that may have been effective earlier, such as bronchodilators, are continued, but new ones to reduce symptoms are now being considered, such as opioids. Anxiety, depression, insomnia, fatigue, pain, and cachexia are also common.

Early in severe COPD, for example, in the rehabilitation program, the patient and his/her family must be helped to prepare for death. Like the staff, they must move from a care plan that focuses on the prolongation of life to one that emphasizes the relief of symptoms. Patients must be forewarned of the chronic symptoms of the terminal phase of COPD and that death will probably be caused by it. They should be helped to write a health care directive, and this can be used by the respiratory team for advance care planning. The patient's expectations will change with time as the grim and inexorable final phase of COPD is experienced, and so the team must be available to listen and to support the patient and family. Once the final act of dying has begun, then it is essential that all measures are given to provide relief.

CASE STUDY

Ms. Cope, a 55-year-old widow, first saw her physician for increasing dyspnea on exertion. She was found to have reduced forced expiratory volume in 1 second (FEV_1) and radiology that revealed emphysema. Alpha$_1$-antitrypsin deficiency was detected.

Medical History, Physical Examination, and Test Results

Medical History

- She has cough and breathlessness, which improved initially with bronchodilator therapy.
- Dyspnea was 5/5 on the Medical Research Council scale (ie, patient has breathlessness dressing or undressing).
- Smoking was discontinued 10 years ago (10 pack-years).
- She has no relevant past medical history other than COPD.
- Medications included ipratropium bromide, four puffs four times daily, and albuterol (Ventolin), two puffs five times daily (with a spacer device used).
- Oral corticosteroids made her feel better but did not improve her FEV_1.

Physical Examination

- She was in no respiratory distress.

- She had a barrel-shaped chest with vigorous accessory muscle use.
- Auscultation revealed reduced breath sounds throughout; she appeared in respiratory distress during the minimal activity of walking over to the examination couch.

Test Results

- Her body mass index was 25.6 kg/m^2.
- Pulmonary function tests showed an FEV_1 of 37% predicted of normal; residual volume 210% predicted of normal, and diffusion capacity 40% predicted of normal; at rest, PaO_2 is 64 mm Hg, $PaCO_2$ is 41 mm Hg, and pH is 7.4.

Questions and Discussion

She lived 24 years from diagnosis. Her pulmonary function tests inescapably worsened. She continued to live at home and travel abroad but after 7 years became hypoxemic and was accepted by the Home Care Oxygen program. She was able to drive, with her handicap documented in her license. She attended an ambulatory rehabilitation program and benefited both physically and mentally; however, she lived on the outskirts of the city, and as she slowly and inexorably deteriorated, she found it more and more difficult to manage at home, resulting in her giving up driving.

The constant dyspnea became intolerable and her exacerbations became more frequent, often taking her to the emergency department despite the use of an action plan with customized antibiotic and prednisone prescription. Her oxygen needs rose, and she found her life depressing but did not have frank depression. Anxiety and fear of each exacerbation dominated her existence. She attended an in-hospital rehabilitation program after a recent hospitalization for pneumonia with COPD exacerbation. She benefited physically and mentally but not as much as she did years ago. She hoped for relief and reassurance.

In due course, it was clear that she could no longer manage at home, but she was still reluctant to leave it. She would expect admission and hoped that some drug would relieve her suffering. After 2 years of managing at home with increased community care and services, she accepted the inevitable and wrote an end-of-life directive that asked that her next exacerbation be treated solely for comfort.

She was admitted to a terminal care unit for COPD. Dyspnea, thick sputum, and nonspecific lower chest pain were the dominant symptoms. A discussion was held, and she agreed to receive morphine for curbing of the dyspnea and pain control. She was aware that it could produce respiratory failure, but her main fear was confusion and loss of consciousness. However, every week, the morphine needed to be increased, with some apparent relief of symptoms and without side effects. She was a religious person, and her church provided the sacrament of the sick. Finally, an infection, as judged by purulent sputum, intervened, and she died with increasing morphine to relieve distress. She asked for antibiotics, hoping that they would relieve her symptoms and that this phase would not drag on. Her daughters and son knew of the impending death. She slipped into unconsciousness and died 1 month after her final admission.

KEY POINTS

- Patients with severe COPD usually die of it and certainly with it.
- The terminal phase is often protracted, and the patient is symptomatic, mainly dyspneic, every minute of the day.
- Depression and anxiety are common developments in terminal COPD.
- Death, usually from an exacerbation, can occur at any time.
- Patients favor comfort care over life-prolonging care.
- The sooner that health care directives are produced, the better will be the advance care planning for the terminal phase of COPD for the patient.
- Death should be comfortable. Respiratory depression by opioids is of no consequence in the naturally dying patient.

REFERENCES

1. Pauwels RA, Buist S, Calverley PMA, et al., on behalf of the Gold Scientific Committee. Global strategy for the diagnosis, management and prevention of chronic obstructive pulmonary disease NHLBI/WHO. Global Initiative for Chronic Obstructive Lung Disease (GOLD) Workshop summary. Am J Respir Crit Care Med 2001;163:1256–76.
2. Claessens MT, Lynn J, Zhong Z, et al. Dying with lung cancer or chronic obstructive pulmonary disease. Insights from SUPPORT. Study to Understand Prognoses and Preferences for Outcomes and Risks of Treatments. J Am Geriatr Soc 2000;48:S146–53.
3. Gore JM, Brophy CJ, Greenstone MA. How well do we care for patients with end stage chronic obstructive pulmonary disease (COPD)? A comparison of palliative care and quality of life in COPD and lung cancer. Thorax 2000;55:1000–6.
4. Heffner JE, Fahy B, Hilling L, Barbieri C. Outcomes of advances directive education of pulmonary rehabilitation patients. Am J Respir Crit Care Med 1997;155:1055–9.
5. Seneff MG, Wagner DP, Zimmerman JE, Knaus WA. Hospital and 1-year survival of patients admitted to intensive care units with acute exacerbations of chronic obstructive pulmonary disease. JAMA 1995;274:1852–7.
6. Connors AFJ, Dawson NV, Thomas C, et al. Outcomes following acute exacerbation of severe chronic obstructive lung disease. The SUPPORT investigators (Study to Understand Prognoses and Preferences for Outcomes and Risks of Treatments). Am J Respir Crit Care Med 1996;154:959–67.
7. Lynn J, Ely EW, Zhong Z, et al. Living and dying with chronic obstructive pulmonary disease. J Am Geriatr Soc 2000;48:S91–S100.

8. Tarzain AJ. Caring for dying patients who have air hunger. J Nurs Scholarship 2000;32:137–43.

9. Heffner JE. Role of pulmonary rehabilitation in palliative care. Respir Care 2000;45:1365–71.

10. Brody H, Campbell ML, Faber-Langendoen K, Ogle KS. Withdrawing intensive life-sustaining treatment—recommendations for compassionate clinical management. N Engl J Med 1997;336: 652–7.

11. Eschun GM, Jacobsohn E, Roberts D, Sneiderman B. Ethical and practical considerations of withdrawal of treatment in the intensive care unit. Can J Anesth 1999;46:497–504.

12. Singer PA, Martin DK, Kelner M. Quality end-of-life care. Patients' perspectives. JAMA 1999;281:163–8.

13. Steinhauser KE, Clipp EC, McNeilly M, et al. In search of a good death: observations of patients, families and providers. Ann Intern Med 2000;132:825–32.

14. Smith R. A good death. An important aim for health services and for us all. BMJ 2000;320:129–30.

15. Curtis JR. Communicating with patients and their families about advance care planning and end-of-life care. Respir Care 2000;45:1385–94.

16. Covinsky KE, Fuller JD, Yaffe K, et al. Communication and decision making in seriously ill patients; findings of the SUPPORT project. The Study to Understand Prognoses and Preferences for Outcomes and Risks of Treatments. J Am Geriatr Soc 2000;48:S187–93.

17. Schneiderman LJ, Kaplan RM, Pearlman RA, Teetzel H. Do physicians' own preferences for life-sustaining treatment influence their perceptions of patient's preferences? J Clin Ethics 1993;4:28–33.

18. Singer PA, Siegler M. Advancing the cause of advance directives. Arch Intern Med 1992;152:22–4.

19. Teno JM, Licks S, Lynn J, et al. Do advance directives provide instructions that direct care? SUPPORT Investigators. Study to Understand Prognoses and Preference for Outcomes and Risks of Treatments. J Am Geriatr Soc 1997;45:508–12.

20. Layde PM, Beam CA, Broste SK, et al. Surrogate's predictions of seriously ill patient's resuscitation preferences. Arch Fam Med 1995;4:518–23.

21. Pfeifer MP. End-of-life decision making: special considerations in the COPD patient. Respir Care 1998;2:5.

22. Rubenfeld GD, Curtis JR. Palliative respiratory care. Respir Care 2000;45:1318–9.

23. World Health Organization. Cancer pain relief and palliative care. Technical Report Series 804. Geneva: WHO, 1990.

24. Quill TE, Dresser R, Brock DW. The rule of double effect—a critique of its role in end-of-life decision making. N Engl J Med 1997;337:1768–71.

25. Masi R, Mensah L, McLeod KA. Health and cultures: exploring the relationships. Oakville, ON: Mosaic Press, 1995.

26. Braun KL, Peitsch JH, Blancette PL. Cultural issues in end of life decision making. CA: Sage, 2000.

27. Morrison RS, Zayas LH, Mulvihill M, et al. Barriers to completion of healthcare proxy forms: a qualitative analysis of ethnic differences. J Clin Ethics 1998; 9:118–26.

28. Guru V, Verbeeck PR, Morrisson LJ. Response of paramedics to terminally ill patients with cardiac arrest: an ethical dilemma. Can Med Assoc J 1999;161: 1251–4.

29. Purvis-Smith TA. Breaking the power of Ondine's curse. Pastoral Care 2000;54:55–62.

30. Kennard MJ, Speroff T, Puopolo AL, et al. Participation of nurses in decision making for seriously ill adults. Clin Nurs Res 1996;5:199–219.

31. Gordon M. In long-term care the "R" in CPR is not for resuscitation. Ann RCPSC (Royal College Physicians and Surgeons of Canada) 2001;34:441–3.

32. Dales RE, O'Connor A, Hebert P, et al. Intubation and mechanical ventilation for COPD: development of an instrument to elicit patient preference. Chest 1999;116:792–800.

33. American Thoracic Society. Dyspnea mechanisms, assessment, and management: a consensus statement. Am J Respir Crit Care Med 1999;159:321–40.

34. Sorenson HM. Dyspnea assessment. Respir Care 2000;45:1331–8.

35. Luce JM, Luce JA. Perspectives on care at the close of life. Management of dyspnea in patients with far-advanced lung disease. "Once I lose it, it's kind of hard to catch it." JAMA 2001;285:1331–7.

36. Zebraski SE, Kochenash SM, Raffa RB. Lung opioid receptors: pharmacology and possible target for nebulized morphine in dyspnea. Life Sci 2000; 66:2221–31.

37. Manning HL. Dyspnea treatment. Respir Care 2000;45:1342–50.

38. Janssens JP, de Muralt B, Titelion V. Management of dyspnea in severe chronic obstructive pulmonary disease. J Pain Symptom Manage 2000;19:378–92.

39. Brurera E, Neumann CM. Management of specific symptom complexes in patients receiving palliative care. Can Med Assoc J 1998;158:1717–26.

40. Sorenson HM. Managing secretions in dying patients. Respir Care 2000;45:1355–63.

41. Frierson RL. Suicide attempts by the old and the very old. Arch Intern Med 1991;151:141–4.

42. Singer HK, Ruchinskas RA, Riley KC, et al. The psychological impact of end-stage lung disease. Chest 2001;120:1246–52.

43. Hansen-Flaschen J. Advanced lung disease. Palliation and terminal care. Clin Chest Med 1997;18:645–55.

44. Donahoe M. Nutritional support in advanced lung disease. The pulmonary cachexia syndrome. Clin Chest Med 1997;18:547–61.

45. Brurera E, Kuehn N, Miller M, et al. The Edmonton Symptom Assessment System (ESAS): a simple method for the assessment of palliative care patients. J Palliat Care 1991;7:6–9.

46. Regueiro CR, Hamel MB, Davis RB, et al. A comparison of generalist and pulmonologist care for patients hospitalized with severe chronic pulmonary disease: resource intensity, hospital costs and survival. SUPPORT Investigators. Study to Understand Prognoses and Preferences for Outcomes and Risks of Treatment. Am J Med 1998;105:366–72.

SUGGESTED READINGS

Clin Chest Med 1997;18 September. *Covers a wide range of topics including prognosis, measurement of dyspnea and quality of life, psychology, nutrition, long-term ventilatory support, and palliative care.*

Doyle D, Hanks GWC, MacDonald N. Oxford textbook of palliative medicine. 2nd Ed. Oxford, UK: Oxford University Press, 1998. *An encyclopedic multiauthor textbook on palliative care. Cancer dominates the whole book but provides many lessons of value for the management of the many other fatal diseases that deserve palliation. There is a very useful chapter on the palliation of respiratory symptoms.*

Molloy W. Let me decide. The health and personal care directive that speaks for you when you can't. 3rd Ed. Toronto: Penguin Books, 1996. *A guide to patients and their families on how to prepare a health care directive that will direct health care workers. It is written by an experienced geriatrician and a nurse.*

CHAPTER 19

PROGRAM EVALUATION AND OUTCOME MEASUREMENT

Judith Soicher, Tanya Dutton, and Jean Bourbeau

OBJECTIVES

The general objective of this chapter is to help physicians and other allied health care professionals become more familiar with the theoretical and practical aspects of program evaluation and outcome measurement. After reading this chapter, the physician and the allied health care professional will be able to

- appreciate the importance of program evaluation in the clinical setting;
- take the appropriate steps in planning and implementing a program evaluation;
- understand the theoretical basis of outcome measurement with respect to scaling, classification, and psychometric properties;
- differentiate and select among measuring instruments to assess clinically relevant domains in chronic obstructive pulmonary disease (COPD); and
- refer to experts for assistance in planning and implementing program evaluation and in selecting appropriate measurement tools.

Comprehensive management of COPD represents a global care approach for chronic disease and has been shown to be both clinically[1,2] and cost effective.[3] Programs integrating education, self-management, and rehabilitation components have been and will continue to be implemented in different clinical settings for various COPD patient groups. When planning and introducing a new clinical program, it is important to implement a program evaluation process using standardized measuring instruments. However, time and resources are seldom devoted to the processes of evaluation and measurement. Unfortunately, these processes are often regarded as a burden rather than necessary for and beneficial to the patient, program, institution, and health care system.

Program evaluation involves establishing program goals and objectives and evaluating whether they have been met using outcomes measured before and after program administration. Following completion of a program, changes in individual outcome scores are used to provide objective feedback to the patient, family members, and other health professionals. Qualitative methods can also be used to capture patients' perspective and impressions of the program. Overall results from a program evaluation can be used by health professionals and administrators to justify the program's existence and to allocate appropriate staff and equipment resources within an institution or care setting. At a regional or national level, findings from a large-scale evaluation can influence health policy for a particular patient group or care setting.

Finally, with increasing awareness of the need for cost-effective interventions, economic evaluation is an additional systematic evaluation strategy needed to assist decision makers in making rational choices.

In this chapter, we review the ABC's of program evaluation and the theoretical basis of outcome measurement and discuss measuring instruments that capture clinical domains relevant to patients with COPD. Research methodology and economic evaluation will not be covered as they are beyond the scope of this book.

THE ABC'S OF PROGRAM EVALUATION

Structure-Process-Outcome Model of Program Evaluation (A)

Health program evaluation is simply the process of determining the degree to which the objectives of a program have been met.[4] Feedback from a program evaluation provides valuable information to plan and manage health resources to maximize outcomes. Donabedian's structure-process-outcome model is an appropriate and feasible model for evaluating health care programs[5]; the following sections review the definitions of structure, process, and outcome.

Structure refers to the physical setting in which health care services are delivered and the tools required to deliver that care (eg, space and equipment).[5–7] *Process* pertains to how the care is delivered from the perspectives of both the patient and the health care professionals; furthermore, it includes the clients' entry into the health care program, how the health care service is carried out, and the health care professional's activities in diagnosis, goal setting, and treatment.[6] *Outcomes* represent important end points of health care such as reducing disability or improving quality of life. Other key outcomes for program evaluation include patient satisfaction and improvement in the patient or family's understanding of the disease.[6,7] It is also important to choose some outcomes that are meaningful to the wider health care and research communities, such as health service use and cost. The choice of outcomes may differ according to the program stakeholder (eg, patient, physician, or health care manager) and his/her individual perspective. Each of these stakeholders brings to the program evaluation different expectations; therefore, it is important for team members to agree on the most relevant outcomes for the program as a whole.

Goals and Objectives (B)

You first have to evaluate the structure, process, and outcome of your program to ensure that it has defined goals and objectives for all three aspects.[4] Goals and objectives must cover the range of services to be provided and have consensus from the health care team as to their appropriateness.

Goals are general statements that reflect the intent of the program,[8] and they should be created from the purpose or mission of the program. Goals must be stated clearly and should be realistic; they need not be directly measurable but must be attainable. An example of a goal would be to decrease disability in the group of patients with COPD who visit the emergency department often or require frequent hospitalization.

Objectives are operational statements detailing the ways in which the goal will be attained and the criterion or standard expected.[4,8] In other words, the objective outlines the specific changes necessary to achieve the goal. A goal can consist of several objectives, and each objective should have four components:

- Outcome measure that will be changed
- Direction and magnitude of anticipated change
- Time period involved
- Group of individuals who will experience the change (target group)

For the goal "to decrease disability," an example of an objective would be to improve performance on the 6-minute walking test (6-MWT) by 50 meters over an 8-week treatment period in 80% of the group of COPD patients who visit the emergency department or require hospitalization. Although the target group is an essential component of both goals and objectives, it does not have to be repeated for each goal and objective if the program is designed for a specific population.

Five Basic Steps to Program Evaluation (C)

Step 1: Analyze the Program's Processes

Understanding how your program presently functions, from client admission to discharge and follow-up, is an important first step in program evaluation. A diagrammatic representation of the program's processes should be created to outline a client's progression through the program. This diagram or pathway may help identify redundant or inefficient processes. An example is provided in relation to the case study at the end of the chapter. It is important to map not only the client's progress through the program but also the behind the scenes meetings and the documentation related to the client's care. Timelines are then established either through existing policy (eg, "the initial assessment must be completed in three visits") or by the best guess of the program team (eg, "I think our team meetings usually occur within 3 weeks of the program start").

Once completed, the pathway or map should be tested. Randomly choose one or two clients and describe their actual progress through the program. Then compare this "real" map to the initial "ideal" map; discrepancies may reflect errors in mapping the processes or an atypical client. It is essential to have an intimate understanding of a program before an evaluation can begin. Mapping provides a deeper understanding of the program's structure, process, and outcomes.

Step 2: Refine and/or Create Goals and Objectives

Goals and objectives are the cornerstone of health program evaluation. As the goals stem from the program's mission or purpose, the program *must* have a mission statement before the program evaluation process can begin. If one does not exist, it must be developed. A mission statement should reflect the program's overall mandate in terms of the program's impact on the target group. Next, the consumers of the program's services must be identified. Are the consumers of the program solely the clients (target group), or are they also family members, caregivers, or other community health providers?

Once the mission statement has been reviewed and the consumers identified, a list of the important components of the program is generated. At this stage, the team identifies key words or phrases that reflect their goals. These phrases must be expanded into program goals that reflect what the program is striving to achieve. An example of a program goal would be "to decrease disability" within the population being served.

Once the goals have been established, the next step is to construct for each goal measurable objectives with specific criteria. Criteria for objectives are

established from the research literature or, in its absence, from a clinical "best guess." For the goal "to decrease disability," recall that the objective was "to improve performance on the 6-MWT by 50 meters over an 8-week treatment period in 80% of clients." The measure chosen, the 6-MWT, must reflect the construct of the goal (disability), and the criterion (a change of 50 meters in 80% of clients within 8 weeks) should represent a clinically meaningful and realistic change within the specified time frame.

One of the most challenging aspects of setting objectives is to identify clinically meaningful change for the clientele served by the program. Additionally, the measurement tools used (eg, the 6-MWT) must be reliable and valid in that population. Furthermore, each goal and objective should be classified according to whether it relates to structure, process, or outcome to ensure that all aspects of the program are covered. Program evaluation is an ongoing process; thus, limiting the number of goals and objectives will facilitate quick and effective evaluations in the future.

Even after all of this is complete, the team needs to review the goals and objectives and confirm that they do capture the important components of the program. If not, adjustments need to be made. Involvement of the team throughout the goal and objective development process will minimize the number of revisions made and subsequently increase the compliance of the team when data collection begins. More importantly, ongoing team input will promote acceptance of the results and will motivate change within the program.

Step 3: Collect Data or Review Existing Data

Data can come from existing records or from assessing clients prospectively. A form outlining the data to be collected is essential. These data must be entered into a computer database using a program that is user friendly. Efforts have been made in some settings to implement computerized data collection and patient record systems. The most practical data collection systems are those that are part of the natural process of patient care.

Missing data pose a major problem and therefore should be minimized by proper data form design and data entry procedures. Data may be missing when the health care professional fails to record the information or when the client is absent. It is important to distinguish between these two sources of missing data as they will affect program evaluation results. For example, if only the improving clients return for all evaluations, the program will have an artificially high success rate.

Step 4: Determine Whether Each Goal Has Been Met

A goal has been achieved if its objective has been met. For the goal "to decrease disability" and the objective "to improve performance on the 6-MWT by 50 meters over an 8-week treatment period in 80% of clients," calculate the percentage of clients who have achieved a change of at least 50 meters on the 6-MWT. If the percentage exceeds 80%, then the objective and its corresponding goal have been met.

To determine whether goals and objectives have been met, it is more meaningful to look at percentages rather than averages and ranges of test scores. An average score can be pulled up or down by extreme values and is often inaccurate in telling the real story. In contrast to factory-type settings, where it is acceptable to report the average number of units produced per day, it is more meaningful in a clinical setting to know what percentage of clients attained the pre-established criterion.

Step 5: Review and Reflect

Review the results from an initial program evaluation with team members and then use the results to modify program components as is feasible within your clinical setting. Explore the possible reasons why goals were not met. The team could reflect on the interventions (type, intensity, frequency, duration), the target population, the criterion chosen as representing a clinically important change, the quality of the data, or a combination of these factors. For example, perhaps the duration of the intervention was insufficient to produce a clinically meaningful change in a particular client population.

Qualitative Methods for Program Evaluation

The five steps outlined above describe the procedures for *quantitative* program evaluation using measurable objectives and outcome criteria. It is important to realize, however, that *qualitative* research methods can also be used for program evaluation. In fact, a combination of qualitative and quantitative methods is the optimal method for health research on the management of chronic conditions, such as COPD, which have a major and ongoing impact on patients' everyday life.[9] For example, one COPD self-management program, "Living Well with COPD©," was evaluated quantitatively through a randomized clinical trial[1] and qualitatively by doing semistructured interviews with participants having received the program in the clinical trial.[10]

Qualitative research is primarily concerned with the patient's point of view. Detailed interviews and observation allow researchers to appreciate the patient's perspective of the program being evaluated. The purpose of a qualitative study is to understand participants' experiences within the context of objects, persons, and events encountered in their everyday life.[11] The emphasis of the research is therefore on describing processes and meanings rather than causal relationships between variables.[12] Qualitative research is summarized below with respect to sampling, data collection, and data analysis.

Sampling in qualitative research is not done by random selection, as in quantitative research, but is instead intentional.[13] Rather than using specific inclusion criteria for selecting participants, qualitative researchers seek "good" informants who can describe the experience under study. A good informant is willing to participate, is able to reflect on and articulate his impressions, and has the time to be interviewed.[13] In qualitative research, there is no set "formula" to determine the sample size. To ensure that sufficient data have been collected, the investigator continues to sample until multiple patients provide similar or redundant information.[14] There are two principles to remember in qualitative sampling: (1) there is an inverse relationship between the amount of data collected from each informant and the number of informants, which means that small samples require more data from each informant, and (2) if there is a greater diversity inherent in the research topic, a larger sample size is required for sufficient data collection.[14]

Data collection can be done through different formats or types of qualitative interviews. In an unstructured format, the interviewer presents the topic for discussion and asks open-ended questions but leaves most of the talking to the interviewee. When specific information is desired, a semistructured format can be used combining open-ended and specific questions.[15] The aims of qualitative evaluation interviews are to obtain in-depth participant views on the strengths and weaknesses of a program[15] and to understand patient health behaviors taught in the program.[11] Therefore, it is important that the interviewer refrains from imposing his/her point of view on the interviewees. Finally, qualitative interviews should be tape recorded to facilitate written transcription of the content for data analysis.

Data analysis is not as rigorous as in quantitative research in terms of computational methods. However, comprehensive descriptive data are required to capture the essence of the participants' experience in the program and the meaning of this experience in their lives. Content analysis is the process of determining from the interviews themes and categories, relationships among categories, and indices of behavior that occur throughout the program. Also, any areas of patient tension or conflict will emerge through this process and are important in providing a true reflection of participants' experience. Coding, a method of content analysis, is used to classify the written content of each interview into categories that bring together similar ideas, concepts, or themes.[15] It is recommended that two or more individuals code the data independently and that the final coded categories be reached by consensus among these individuals. Once the data have been coded and entered into a database, a computer program such as NUD*IST (Nonnumerical Unstructured Data Indexing, Searching, and Theorizing) can be used to group the data by category code, thereby greatly reducing the time spent on data analysis.[16] The validity of qualitative research ultimately depends on how closely the final results correspond to the patient descriptions obtained by interview. Therefore, in analyzing the data, the qualitative researcher must remain true to both the content and the feelings expressed by the patients.

THEORETICAL BASIS OF OUTCOME MEASUREMENT

A standardized measure is a published measurement tool, designed for a specified purpose in a given population; it has detailed instructions provided as to administration, scoring, interpretation of scores, and evidence of reliability and validity. Standardized measures include outcome measures, which are tools (instruments, questionnaires, rating forms, etc) used to document change in one or more patient characteristics over time.[17] Therefore, an outcome measure is a scale or test that measures the effect of a treatment, program, or policy on individuals, groups, or populations.

Outcome and standardized measures are used to measure clinical domains. A domain is a physical, psychological, or sociopersonal attribute. Measuring patient attributes or domains is necessary for identifying problem areas, setting treatment goals, and implementing appropriate interventions in the clinical setting. Furthermore, if implemented in an objective and standardized manner, these measures can also be used for program evaluation and clinical research. In this section, several common outcome measures are used as examples to clarify theoretical concepts. These measures, if not already familiar to the reader, are covered in detail later in this chapter.

Scales Used in Outcome Measurement

The first step in choosing and implementing an appropriate outcome is to understand that there are different types of measurement scales. The most fundamental distinction is whether a scale is continuous or categorical.[18] A continuous measure can have any value within a reasonable range, an example is the distance walked during a specified time interval. A categorical measure, however, can take on only certain values.

Both continuous and categorical measures can be further subdivided into interval and ratio scales. An interval scale is one with an arbitrary "zero" point, for example a Celsius or Fahrenheit temperature scale. A ratio scale is one where the zero point is meaningful in that it theoretically represents the absence of an attribute. For example, a score of zero on the mastery subscale of the Chronic Respiratory Questionnaire (CRQ), although unlikely to occur in practice, would theoretically mean that a patient has no feeling of control over his/her disease.

A categorical outcome is one for which the measurement scale has a limited number of values or responses. There may be only two possible responses, as in a dichotomous scale. An example of a dichotomous outcome is a single question with a yes/no response, representing the presence/absence of a symptom such as pain. Categorical outcomes can also have multilevel scales, for which more than two responses are possible. *Ordinal* multilevel outcomes have a limited number of responses, which have an inherent ranking or order. An example of an ordinal multilevel outcome is the Medical Research Council (MRC) dyspnea scale, which is graded from 1 to 5. Grade 1 corresponds to a mild level of exertional dyspnea, whereas grade 5 represents a higher or more severe level of exertional dyspnea. A *nominal* multilevel outcome has responses that are labeled but do not have an inherent order. An example is discharge destination, where the possible choices, for example, are home, rehabilitation facility, nursing home, or other.

Classification of Outcome Measures

Functional, Descriptive, or Methodological Types of Classification

Outcome measures can be organized according to functional, descriptive, or methodological types of classification. Functional classifications focus on the purpose or application of the measures, descriptive classifications focus on their scope, and methodological classifications consider technical aspects, such as methods used to record information.[19]

Within each classification type, different schemes have been put forth. An example of a functional classification scheme is that of Kirshner and Guyatt,[20] which distinguishes between discriminative, evaluative, and predictive purposes of health measures. A *discriminative* instrument is one that, when administered at one point in time, can discriminate between people with different levels of a particular attribute or disease. A *predictive* instrument classifies people according to an external criterion. Predictive measures include diagnostic tests that correspond with a clinical diagnosis and prognostic tests that predict the likelihood of a future event, such as the development of a disease. An *evaluative* instrument, when administered at several time points, measures change over time in the same person.

Most measures have discriminative, predictive, and evaluative properties to varying degrees. The choice of measure and the extent to which it should be discriminative, predictive, or evaluative depend on the purpose(s) for which it will be used. Suppose the coordinator of a comprehensive self-management or rehabilitation program wants to screen patients, according to level of dyspnea, to put them in one of two levels of a dyspnea education class. The measure chosen should be one that is primarily discriminative, such as the MRC dyspnea scale. If the coordinator instead wants to implement a measure that will evaluate the effect of a particular intervention on dyspnea, then an evaluative instrument should be chosen. An example would be the dyspnea subscale of the CRQ.

Descriptive and methodological classifications have a large number of categories or distinctions by which outcome measures can be organized. A descriptive classification can categorize measures by the domain evaluated, such as dyspnea or quality of life, or according to whether a measure is generic or specific. Generic measures can be used in a variety of conditions or age groups and are useful in epidemiologic and health services research. Disease-specific instruments focus on a particular disease (eg, COPD), problem (eg, sleep disturbance), or population (eg, geriatric) and are designed to detect change over time or following an intervention. Examples of methodological distinctions are objective versus subjective, performance versus self-report, and interviewer- versus self-administered questionnaires. Although comprehensive, both descriptive and methodological classifications potentially have a large number of categories.

International Classification of Functioning, Disability and Health

Alternatively, measures can be classified in a smaller number of broad categories or dimensions using the International Classification of Functioning, Disability and Health (ICF).[21] Functioning is an umbrella term for the positive or neutral aspects of dimensions at body, individual, and society levels, whereas disability is an umbrella term for the problems in these dimensions. This classification is the revised version of the International Classification of Impairments, Disabilities and Handicaps (ICIDH) commonly used in rehabilitation and presented in Figure 19–1.[22]

In the original version (ICIDH), impairment refers to the loss or abnormality of psychological, physiologic, or anatomical structure or function (eg, anxiety), whereas disability is defined as the resultant restriction or lack of ability to perform an activity in the manner or within the range considered normal for a human being (eg, decreased functional exercise capacity). Handicap is a disadvantage, caused by impairment or disability, that limits or prevents fulfilment of a normal role (eg, reduced social functioning). In the ICF as presented in Figure 19–2, impairment is further subdivided into body functions and structures, whereas activities and participation replace the terms disabilities and handicaps, respectively. Another modification to the original classification is that the ICF includes environmental and personal factors as integral components that interact with the

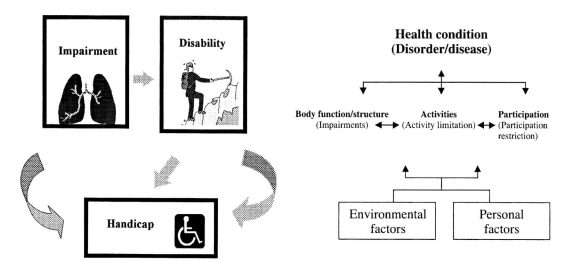

Figure 19–1 International Classification of Impairments, Disabilities and Handicaps.[22]

Figure 19–2 Interactions between the components of the ICF.[21]

dimensions of body functions and structures, individual activities, and participation in society.

The ICF covers a continuum from the basic organ level (body functions and structures) through to tasks (activities) and life situations (participation). The usefulness of this scheme is that domains and their measures can be classified according to body function, body structure, activity, or participation (functioning dimension), whereas the corresponding clinical problem can be classified as an impairment, activity limitation, or participation restriction (disability dimension). Definitions for each of the functioning and disability dimensions are provided in Table 19–1. For each functioning dimension and its corresponding disability, a clinical example is given of a domain, outcome measure, and problem. By analyzing clinical problems within this framework, the clinician can determine the contributing causes and the most appropriate interventions.

In the clinical examples in Table 19–1, the participation restriction of reduced social functioning is complex and difficult to treat directly but may be partly attributable to the presence of decreased exercise capacity (impairment) and physical functioning (activity limitation). Therefore, social functioning can be treated indirectly by implementing a cardiovascular conditioning program to improve exercise capacity and by teaching principles of energy conservation and body mechanics to improve physical functioning. The

effectiveness of these interventions in improving social functioning is evaluated by administering the 6-MWT and the 36-item Medical Outcomes Short-Form Health Survey (SF-36) (which includes social functioning and physical functioning subscales) before and after intervention. Suppose that exercise capacity and physical function improve, whereas social function remains unchanged; the treatment has been successful in addressing two of the clinical problems (reduced exercise capacity and physical function). However, other contributing causes of reduced social functioning, such as contextual factors, need to be explored. Therefore, the ICF provides a framework in which clinical assessment, problem identification, treatment planning, and outcome measurement can be approached in a logical and systematic manner.

Psychometric Properties

Psychometrics is the science of using standardized tests or scales to measure attributes of a person or object. After a new measuring instrument is developed, its reliability and validity must be tested. Reliability or reproducibility is the degree to which a score is repeatable either between evaluators (interrater) or between separate administrations of the test (test–retest). Internal consistency, often considered a form of reliability, is the extent to which items on a scale correlate with each other and with the scale's total score. Validity is the degree

TABLE 19–1 Clinical Examples of ICF Dimensions*

Functioning Dimension (WHO ICF, 2001)	Clinical Example			Disability Dimension (WHO ICF2, 2001)
	Domain	Outcome Measure	Problem	
Body function Physiologic function of body systems (including psychological functions)	Functional exercise capacity	Six-minute walking test	Decreased functional exercise capacity	Impairment Problem in body function or structure, such as a significant deviation or loss
Body structure Anatomical part of the body such as organs, limbs, and their components	Structure of lung tissue	Chest radiograph findings	Scarring of lung parenchyma	
Activity Execution of a task or action by an individual	Physical functioning	Physical function subscale of the 36-item Short Form Health Survey (SF-36)	Reduced physical functioning	Activity limitation Difficulty an individual may have in executing activities
Participation Involvement in a life situation	Social functioning	Social function subscale of the SF-36	Reduced social functioning	Participation restriction Problem an individual may experience in being involved in life situations

*Dimension: level of functioning at body, individual, or society level. Each dimension has two poles, one indicating nonproblematic (neutral or positive) functional states and the other problematic states.

ICF = International Classification of Functioning, Disability and Health; WHO = World Health Organization.

to which the instrument measures the attribute under study. The different types of validity are summarized in Table 19–2.

Once reliability and validity are established, an instrument must show evidence of sensitivity and responsiveness. Sensitivity is the ability of an instrument to measure the change of an attribute or health state, irrespective of whether the change is relevant to the patient or clinician.[23] Responsiveness, however, is the ability of a measure to detect a minimal clinically important difference (MCID) over time. The MCID is a clinical change that is meaningful to the patient, caregiver, and/or health care professional. Interpretability is the ability of a measure to distinguish between trivial and important changes in patient status[24] and to describe what the change in score means. For example, for a given domain of the CRQ, a change of 0.5 represents a minimal clinically important change, 1.0 represents moderate change, and 1.5 or more represents a large change.[25]

The psychometric properties of a measure are established through multiple studies in the patient population of interest. Therefore, if a measure was developed and tested in patients with congestive heart failure, its psychometric properties cannot be assumed for a COPD population. Also, if a measure is modified, translated into another language, or used in a different cultural environment, repeated psychometric testing is necessary before using the measure for either clinical or research purposes.

From Theory to Practice

An outcome may be psychometrically sound and may thoroughly assess the domain of interest. Its ultimate usefulness, however, will be decided largely on the basis of practical considerations. The following questions should be asked before implementing a measure in either clinical or research settings:

• Is the measure feasible with respect to both time and equipment?
• Is it appropriate to the setting and time frame of the therapeutic intervention?

TABLE 19–2 Types of Measurement Validity

Content validity	Degree to which the components of an instrument represent a particular subject area; evaluated by literature review, clinical experience, consensus of experts
Construct validity	Degree to which the instrument measures an abstract concept (construct) or attribute; evaluated by comparison with instruments measuring related constructs
Criterion validity	Degree to which the instrument predicts the score on an established instrument that measures the same construct
Concurrent	New and established instruments are administered on the same day
Predictive	New instrument predicts score on a health state or event in the future (eg, death, institutionalization)

- Are testing instructions or guidelines available?
- Is the questionnaire available in the language(s) of the patient population, and has psychometric testing been carried out on the translated version?
- If self-administered, do patients find the questionnaire difficult to complete?
- If a patient has poor literacy skills, can the questionnaire be easily administered by an interviewer?
- Is the questionnaire easy to score or is a computer program required?
- Can the results be easily communicated to patients and health care professionals?

Careful consideration of these questions, together with a trial implementation, is recommended to identify the practical aspects of a measure that will either facilitate or hinder its use.

CLINICAL DOMAINS AND MEASURING INSTRUMENTS

This section describes key clinical domains in COPD, and the instruments commonly used to measure each domain. The definition and clinical importance of each domain are presented. For each instrument, the practical aspects of administration and scoring are discussed, and the psychometric properties are summarized.

Dyspnea

Dyspnea is the unpleasant sensation of labored or difficult breathing and is synonymous with the terms breathlessness or shortness of breath.[17] It is among the most frequent complaints in COPD and is an

important determinant of physical functioning.[26–28] Although dyspnea is a complex psychophysiologic process, techniques to reduce the sensation of dyspnea are a standard component of treatment (see Chapter 9). It follows that dyspnea should be routinely measured as it is a meaningful and modifiable outcome.[29] Methods to measure dyspnea range from patients' subjective reports and descriptions to reliable and valid scales.[30] These scales are divided into two main types: those that measure dyspnea during daily activity and are in a questionnaire format and those that measure exertional dyspnea and are administered during exercise. Common dyspnea measures are summarized in Table 19–3, and each is discussed in detail in the following sections of this chapter.

Dyspnea with Activity

The complaint that commonly brings patients to the attention of respiratory health professionals is their breathlessness in performing activities of daily living (ADL). Patients report shortness of breath that either prevents or limits them from carrying out a specific activity. Furthermore, the level of dypnea is usually out of proportion to the activity being performed. For example, a patient may report that his level of breathlessness requires him to stop at least once while climbing a normal flight of stairs and that it takes him 3 to 4 minutes to recover once he has reached the top of the staircase. This type of disability is often a major complaint, and a decrease in this disability is an important goal of treatment. Therefore, this domain should be measured to assess patients' level of breathlessness in ADL and any change following treatment. Since these activities are not usually performed in a clinical setting, it is nec-

TABLE 19–3 Measures Commonly Used to Measure Dyspnea

Type of Dyspnea	Measure	Scoring	Administration Time
Dyspnea with activity	Medical Research Council scale American Thoracic Society scale	Grades 1–5	3–5 min
	Baseline Dyspnea Index	Items: 0–4 Total: 0–12	10 min
	Transitional Dyspnea Index	Items: –3 to +3 Total: –9 to +9	10 min
	University of California, San Diego, Shortness of Breath Questionnaire	Items: 0–5 Total: 0–120	10 min
	Oxygen Cost Diagram	0–100	< 2 min
	Dyspnea subscale of Chronic Respiratory Questionnaire	1–7 (converted) or 5–35 (raw)	5–10 min
Exertional dyspnea	Borg rating of perceived dyspnea scale	0–10	< 30 s
	Visual analogue scale	0–100	< 30 s

essary to use questionnaires that rely on the patient's self-report of his/her experience.

Medical Research Council Dyspnea Scale. A commonly used tool is the MRC dyspnea scale, which assesses the type and magnitude of activity that elicits dyspnea. It is a self- or interviewer-administered ordinal scale on which patients rate their dyspnea according to five grades of increasing severity as presented in Table 19–4.

The MRC scale is easy to administer and requires very little time to complete. It has demonstrated construct validity as it is correlated with other mea- sures of dyspnea and with lung function.[31] Because it is primarily a discriminative tool, sensitivity to change is not relevant to the MRC scale as it is not intended to measure change over time.

ATS Dyspnea Scale. The dyspnea section of the ATS Respiratory Questionnaire[32] is similar to the MRC scale in both items and scoring as presented in Table 19–4. The ATS dyspnea scale consists of five yes/no questions that generally correspond to the five grades of the MRC scale.

On the ATS scale, the final question assesses whether the patient is too breathless to leave the

TABLE 19–4 Medical Research Council (MRC) and American Thoracic Society (ATS) Scales

Grade	MRC Scale	ATS Scale
1	I only get breathless with strenuous exercise.	No to question for grade 2.
2	I get short of breath when hurrying on the level or walking up a slight hill.	Yes to Are you troubled by shortness of breath when hurrying on the level or walking up a slight hill?
3	I walk slower than people of the same age on the level because of breathlessness, or I have to stop for breath when walking at my own pace on the level.	Yes to Do you have to walk slower than people of your age on the level because of breathlessness or do you ever have to stop for breath when walking at your own pace on the level?
4	I stop for breath after walking about 100 yards or after a few minutes on the level.	Yes to Do you ever have to stop for breath after walking about 100 yards (or after a few minutes) on the level?
5	I am too breathless to leave the house.	Yes to Are you too breathless to leave the house or breathless on dressing and undressing?

house (corresponding to MRC grade 5) and the additional component of breathlessness on dressing/undressing. This added component may lessen the discriminative ability of this scale. Patients with COPD often complain of breathlessness during upper extremity functional tasks, including grooming activities and dressing. Therefore, a patient may answer "yes" to the question for ATS grade 5 even though he is able to leave the house. Therefore, the dressing/undressing component in grade 5 can misclassify some patients into an artificially high level of disability. If a patient answers yes to this question, the interviewer should clarify whether the patient is indeed unable to leave the house, breathless on dressing/undressing, or both. If only the dressing/undressing component is problematic, the interviewer needs to look at the response to previous questions. If the patient has also answered "yes" to questions for grades 1 to 4, then the patient clearly has a high level of disability and should be classified as grade 5. However, if the patient has answered "no" to previous questions, then his/her true level of disability is unclear.

Baseline Dyspnea Index and Transitional Dyspnea Index. The Baseline Dyspnea Index (BDI)[33] was developed to assess the magnitude of activity that provokes dyspnea, the magnitude of effort required to execute an activity, and functional limitations in work and ADL. The BDI is an interviewer-administered questionnaire that evaluates patients' baseline status in each of three categories: magnitude of task, magnitude of effort, and functional impairment. The index is administered by an interviewer, experienced in history taking for respiratory disease, who asks open-ended questions about the patient's breathlessness. Based on the patient's responses, the interviewer rates each category from grade 0 (very severe impairment) to grade 4 (unimpaired). For example, grade 0 for the category "Functional Impairment" corresponds to the criterion "Very Severe Impairment. Unable to work and has given up most or all usual activities, due to shortness of breath." The category ratings are then summed to give a baseline focal score ranging from 0 to 12, with a lower score indicating a more severe level of dyspnea. The Transitional Dyspnea Index (TDI) is the accompanying evaluative tool to the BDI and evaluates change over time in each of the three categories. The TDI is administered in a manner similar to the BDI through a series of open-ended questions. Change from baseline status is rated according to seven grades, ranging from –3 (major deterioration) to +3 (major improvement), with 0 representing no change. In the category "Change in Functional Impairment," for example, a score of –3 corresponds to the criterion "Major Deterioration. Formerly working and has had to stop working, and has completely abandoned some of usual activities due to shortness of breath." Category ratings are again summed to give a transition focal score ranging from –9 to +9, with a lower score indicating a larger deterioration in dyspnea.

The BDI and TDI can each be administered by an experienced interviewer in under 10 minutes. As the questions are not standardized, it is essential for research purposes that evaluations be done by the same interviewer or interviewers with comparable levels of experience. Otherwise, ratings may depend on the interviewer's skill or interpretation of patient responses. For clinical purposes, however, the BDI/TDI provides a detailed picture of the magnitude of activity and effort that provokes dyspnea (BDI) and the way in which this changes over time or in response to treatment (TDI). Psychometric testing of the BDI and TDI provides evidence of reliability, validity,[31,33] and sensitivity to change.[34]

The University of California, San Diego, Shortness of Breath Questionnaire.[35] The Shortness of Breath Questionnaire (SOB-Q) is a self-report instrument that assesses dyspnea during ADL. The SOB-Q consists of 24 items, 21 of which assess the severity of dyspnea associated with specific ADL on an average day during the past week. The three remaining items assess the extent of limitation in ADL caused by shortness of breath, fear of harm from overexertion, and fear of harm from shortness of breath. Each item is graded on a scale ranging from 0 (not at all) to 5 (maximal or unable to do because of breathlessness). Item scores are summed to generate a total score that can range from 0 to 120. It is recommended that a health care provider or research assistant review the questionnaire instructions and a few items with the patient. Patients can then complete the questionnaire independently, usually in under 10 minutes. Some patients have difficulty estimating their breathlessness for activities they no longer perform. In this case, they should give an estimate of their breathlessness if they were to perform the activity (Prewitt L, UCSD Medical Center, Pulmonary Rehabilitation Program, personal communication, 2001). The SOB-Q appears to be valid [35,36] and sensitive to change.[37]

London Chest Activity of Daily Living Scale. The London Chest Activity of Daily Living (LCADL) scale was developed specifically to evaluate ADL performance in patients with severe COPD.[38] The LCADL is a 15-item self-administered questionnaire that covers the following types of activities (number of items in brackets): self-care (four), domestic (six), physical (two), and leisure (three). Items are rated from 0 to 5, with grade 5 representing the greatest level of disability. Grades 1, 2, and 3 correspond to different levels of breathlessness during activities performed by the patient during the past few days. Grade 4 is reported when a patient is unable to perform an activity because of breathlessness and no one is available to help. Finally, grade 5 corresponds to the situation in which someone else either helps or does the activity for the patient. Scores can range between 0 and 60. In addition to the 15 items, there are two additional questions that are not scored. One question asks whether the patient lives alone and the second asks whether the patient's breathing affects their normal ADL "a lot," "a little," or "not at all." The questionnaire can be completed in under 10 minutes. Although a relatively new instrument, the LCADL shows evidence of construct and concurrent validity, internal consistency[38] test–retest reliability, and sensitivity to change.[39]

Oxygen Cost Diagram. The Oxygen Cost Diagram (OCD) is another instrument used to assess dyspnea with daily activities. The OCD is a 100-mm line on which 13 activities are indicated, with their position proportional to the oxygen cost or requirement (Figure 19–3). The patient is asked to mark the point above which their breathlessness will not allow them to go when at their best. The score is recorded as the distance (in mm) from the bottom of the line.[40] The OCD has shown evidence of validity[33,41] and sensitivity to change.[42] A practical limitation of this scale, however, is that patients may not carry out some of the listed activities, potentially affecting the accuracy of responses. For this reason, the OCD is used less often than the other measures discussed.

Dyspnea Subscale of the CRQ. The dyspnea subscale of the CRQ is another evaluative instrument that can be used to measure dyspnea associated with daily activities. This scale is based on five activities, selected by the patient as being most important in his/her day-to-day life. The scoring, practical considerations, and psychometric properties are discussed in the section on health-related quality of life (HRQL).

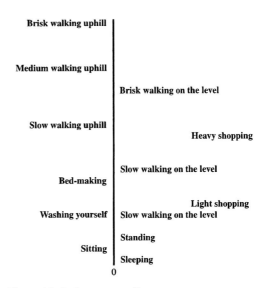

Figure 19–3 Oxygen cost diagram.

Exertional Dyspnea

Borg Scale. The Borg scale is a categorical scale consisting of numbers and a set of verbal qualifiers. It is used to measure exertional dyspnea during cardiopulmonary exercise testing and training and is also referred to as a Rating of Perceived Dyspnea (RPD) scale. Originally, the Borg scale was developed to measure exertion and for this use is referred to as the Rating of Perceived Exertion (RPE) scale. The original RPE scale ranges from 6 to 20.[43] This version is still used, particularly for measuring exertion in cardiac patients, as ratings correlate well with heart rate.[44] A 10-point ratio scale was subsequently developed[45] (Figure 19–4) and is the version most commonly used to quantify dyspnea (RPD) and exertion (RPE) in COPD. The verbal qualifiers may differ from those shown, depending on the setting or the specific parameter being measured (eg, shortness of breath, generalized exertion, or leg fatigue). It is essential, though, that the same set of qualifiers be used within the same program or research project for a given parameter.

The Borg scale should be reproduced in a large and easy-to-read format and explained to the patient prior to the exercise test or training session. The explanation should be standardized, particularly if results are being used for research or program evaluation purposes. If the dyspnea scale is being used during a graded exercise test, the standardized explanation might read as follows:

The purpose of this scale is to measure your shortness of breath during the exercise test. Zero corresponds to "no shortness of breath," whereas 10 represents "maximal shortness of breath." It is important that you respond according to what *you* are feeling. At 1-minute intervals and at the end of the test, I will ask you to point to the number that best represents your shortness of breath.

There is considerable evidence of the reliability,[46–48] validity,[41,49] and sensitivity to change[50] of the Borg 10-point dyspnea scale in patients with COPD. *Visual Analogue Scale.* Exertional dyspnea can also be measured using the Visual Analogue Scale (VAS) for dyspnea. The VAS consists of a vertical or horizontal line, usually 100 mm in length, with verbal anchors at each end indicating extremes for the sensation of dyspnea (Figure 19–5). The anchor at the bottom (or left) of the scale is "no breathlessness," and the anchor at the top (or right) is "greatest breathlessness." Patients are asked to indicate the point on the scale that corresponds to their sensation of breathlessness. The score is obtained by measuring the distance (mm or cm) from the bottom or left side of the scale to the point indicated by the patient. In administering the VAS, the same practical considerations must be taken into account as for the Borg scale. The VAS for dyspnea has shown evidence of reliability,[47,49,51] validity,[52] and studies suggest that it may be more sensitive to change than the Borg scale.[47,51]

Exercise Capacity

Exercise capacity or cardiorespiratory fitness is an individual's ability to perform large-muscle, dynamic, moderate-to-high intensity exercise for prolonged periods.[53] Exercise capacity can be assessed by various testing procedures, some of which are relatively complex and require expensive laboratory equipment and highly skilled technicians. This is the case for assessing incremental maximal exercise capacity and submaximal constant exercise capacity with workload monitoring and continuous measurement of exhaled gases. Incremental exercise testing is usually done in a laboratory setting to formulate the initial exercise training program; it is also used to detect any cardiac or pulmonary abnormalities before starting an exercise program. Since these testing procedures are beyond the textbook's scope, the main focus of the discussion will be on the measurement of functional exercise capacity.

Functional exercise capacity is an individual's ability to undertake physically demanding ADL. It is a subcategory of submaximal exercise capacity and is measured using performance tests.[54] Functional exercise capacity is generally measured by standardized walking tests, with the most common being the 6-MWT.

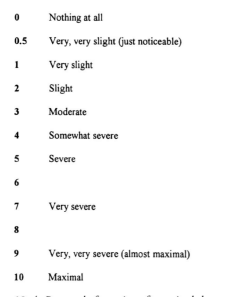

0	Nothing at all
0.5	Very, very slight (just noticeable)
1	Very slight
2	Slight
3	Moderate
4	Somewhat severe
5	Severe
6	
7	Very severe
8	
9	Very, very severe (almost maximal)
10	Maximal

Figure 19–4 Borg scale for rating of perceived dyspnea and exertion.

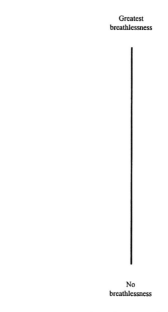

Greatest
breathlessness

No
breathlessness

Figure 19–5 Visual Analogue Scale for dyspnea.

Six-Minute Walking Test

The 6-MWT can be carried out on a track or pre-measured hospital corridor. Inconspicuous markings should be made along the course at 5-meter intervals to aid in measurement of the final distance. If carried out in a corridor, the course should be at least 20 meters in length, marked by a chair or pylon at either end, and located in a relatively quiet area. Patients are instructed to cover as much distance as possible in 6 minutes, and encouragement should be provided at 30-second intervals.[55]

Because of a learning effect,[56] it has been recommended that a total of three tests be performed (two practice and one test), preferably on different days or with sufficient rest periods between tests. It is often not feasible, however, to carry out three tests because of either patient fatigue or lack of staff availability to administer the test. Therefore, often only two tests will be done for practical reasons. There is evidence, however, that most of the learning occurs between the first and second tests.[56]

Recommended procedures and equipment for the 6-MWT are given in Table 19–5. Suggested standardized instructions are as follows:

The purpose of this test is to find out how far you can walk in 6 minutes. You will start from this point (indicate pylon) and follow the corridor to the pylon at the end. You will walk back and forth between the pylons as many times as you can in the 6-minute period. If you need to, you may stop and rest. Just remain where you are until you can go on again. However, the most important thing about the test is that you cover as much ground as you possibly can during the 6 minutes. I will tell you the time every 2 minutes, and I will let you know when the 6 minutes are up. When I say "STOP," please stop and stand right where you are."[57]

The Borg RPD and RPE should be measured immediately following test completion. The standardized instructions for the Borg scale are those given in the section on exertional dyspnea.

The result should be reported in meters as the maximum of the two or three trials. Using prediction equations developed in healthy adult volunteers, the percentage of predicted normal value can also be reported.[58,59] Prediction equations should be used with caution, however, as they are dependent on the methodology of the study through which they were developed. In the studies cited, the characteristics of the participants and the administra-tion of the 6-MWT may be different from the pop-ulation and/or 6-MWT procedures in your clinical or research setting.

The 6-MWT is reliable,[56,60] valid,[61,62] and sensitive to change[63]; it also appears to be responsive to clinical change, as one study showed that a "just noticeable" change in patients' perception of their walking ability was 54 meters.[64] Therefore, the MCID for the 6-MWT is commonly cited as being approximately 50 meters.

Incremental Shuttle Walking Test

The incremental shuttle walking test (ISWT) is a standardized, progressive walking test used to measure functional exercise capacity in patients with cardiorespiratory conditions. The patient walks up and down a 10-meter course, equivalent to one shuttle, and the pace is externally controlled by a series of signals from an audiocassette. The test consists of 12 levels, with each level lasting 1 minute and separated by a triple "bleep" signal. Each level is carried out at a progressively faster speed, controlled by a series of single "bleeps," with each one corresponding to the completion of one 10-meter shuttle. The test is stopped either by the patient, when he or she is too breathless to maintain the required speed, or by the clinician, when the patient falls behind the external pacing by more than 0.5 meters for two consecutive 10-meter shuttles. The test result is recorded in meters, calculated by multiplying the total number of completed shuttles by 10 meters/shuttle. Table 19–6 summarizes the walking speed, time per shuttle, and number of shuttles (per level and cumulative) for each of the 12 levels, all of which are externally controlled by the audiocassette. Recommended procedures and equipment for the ISWT are given in Table 19–7, and the course layout is illustrated in Figure 19–6.

In patients with COPD, the ISWT is reliable after one practice test.[65,66] Evidence of validity is provided by high correlations with VO_{2max} (maximum oxygen uptake) on both maximal treadmill[66] and cycle ergometer tests.[67] Performance on the shuttle walk improved significantly following pulmonary rehabili-tation,[68,69] providing evidence of sensitivity to change. The MCID of the ISWT has not yet been determined.

Endurance Shuttle Walking Test

The endurance shuttle walking test (ESWT) is a mod-ification of the ISWT to measure endurance capacity.

TABLE 19–5 Recommended Procedures and Equipment for the 6-Minute Walking Test

Phase of Test	Procedure	Equipment
Course set-up	Pylons placed at either end of 20 to 50 meter course (if track unavailable)	Pylons
	Markings placed at 5-meter intervals	Measuring tape
		Colored tape or marker
Prior to test	Record	
	Oxygen saturation	Oxygen saturation monitor
	Heart rate	Stop watch
	Respiratory rate	
	Blood pressure	Blood pressure cuff
Instructions	Standardized instructions	Printed instructions for
	Walking test	walking test and Borg scale
	Borg RPD/RPE scales	Printed RPD/RPE scales
Test	Record number of laps walked	Paper and pen
	Encouragement provided at 30-second intervals, using phrases such as "You're doing well," "Keep up the good work"	Stop watch
	Notify patient when 2, 4, and 6 minutes have elapsed	
After test	Record distance walked	Paper and pen
	Record	
	RPD/RPE	Printed RPD/RPE scales
	Oxygen saturation	Oxygen saturation monitor
	Heart rate	Stop watch
	Respiratory rate	
	Blood pressure	Blood pressure cuff

RPD = rating of perceived dyspnea; RPE = rating of perceived exertion.

The ESWT is also carried out over a 10-meter course (see Figure 19–6) and is externally paced using signals from an audiocassette. The walking speed for the ESWT is constant throughout the test and corresponds to 85% of VO_{2max}, established from the ISWT distance using a predictive equation. The ESWT result is recorded in minutes. The ESWT was also found to be reliable after one practice test and was comparable to a treadmill endurance test with respect to post-test heart rate and rating of perceived exertion and breathlessness. The ESWT was also sensitive to change following rehabilitation to a greater degree than was the ISWT.[70] However, the ESWT is a relatively new measure and requires further psychometric testing and use in clinical trials. The cassette and instructions for the ISWT and ESWT can be obtained from the Pulmonary Rehabilitation Department, Department of Respiratory Medicine, University Hospitals of Leicester NHS Trust, Glenfield Hospital, Groby Road, Leicester LE3 9QP, UK, fax: 0116 2367768.

Although the 6-MWT is the more established and commonly used walk test in COPD, the ISWT is being used with increasing frequency for both clinical and research purposes. It has been suggested that the 6-MWT is a steady-state measure of exercise endurance, whereas the ISWT is an incremental measure of exercise capacity. Furthermore, 6-MWT performance is potentially affected by self-pacing, whereas this effect is eliminated in the ISWT.[71] In studies that have compared the two walk tests, the maximal heart rates attained were higher for the ISWT,[66,72] suggesting that it assesses exercise capacity in a more strenuous manner than the 6-MWT. Ongoing studies are needed to further elucidate the differences between the two tests and the contexts in which each is indicated. The MCID for the ISWT also needs to be determined if this test is to continue to gain more widespread use.

TABLE 19–6 Externally Controlled Walking Parameters for the Incremental Shuttle Walking Test*

Level	Speed (m/s)	Time/Shuttle (s)	Number of Shuttles	
			Per Level	Cumulative
1	0.50	20.00	3	3
2	0.67	15.00	4	7
3	0.84	12.00	5	12
4	1.01	10.00	6	18
5	1.18	8.57	7	25
6	1.35	7.50	8	33
7	1.52	6.67	9	42
8	1.69	6.00	10	52
9	1.86	5.46	11	63
10	2.03	5.00	12	75
11	2.20	4.62	13	88
12	2.37	4.29	14	102

*Adapted from Singh, et al.[66]

TABLE 19–7 Recommended Procedures and Equipment for the Incremental Shuttle Walking Test

Phase of Test	Procedure	Equipment
Course set-up	Pylons placed at 0.5 and 9.5 m 10-m course	Pylons Measuring tape
Prior to test	Record Oxygen saturation Heart rate Respiratory rate Blood pressure	 Oxygen saturation monitor Stop watch Blood pressure cuff
Instructions	Standardized instructions Played from audiocassette Borg RPD/RPE scales	 Audiocassette and cassette player Printed instructions for Borg scale Printed RPD/RPE scales
Test	Record number of shuttles completed	Paper and pen
After test	Record RPD/RPE Oxygen saturation Heart rate Respiratory rate Blood pressure Reason for stopping	 Printed RPD/RPE scales Oxygen saturation monitor Stop watch Blood pressure cuff

RPD = rating of perceived dyspnea; RPE = rating of perceived exertion.

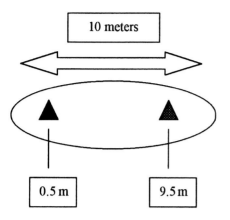

Figure 19–6 Course for incremental and endurance shuttle walking tests. Triangles indicate pylons inset 0.5 meters, to minimize abrupt changes in direction.

Functional Status

Although walking tests are very useful in evaluating exercise capacity, they may not give a true picture of how a patient is performing in daily activities. Functional status is the extent to which individuals perform their usual behaviors and activities. This ability is severely compromised in COPD largely because of dyspnea and fatigue. Currently, there is only one disease-specific instrument that assesses functional status in relation to both dyspnea and fatigue. The Pulmonary Functional Status and Dyspnea Questionnaire—Modified (PFSDQ–M) is a 40-item questionnaire that assesses functional status through three domains: activity, dyspnea, and fatigue.[73] This questionnaire was modified from its original 164-item format, which was considered too long for routine clinical use. The PFSDQ–M is a self-administered evaluative questionnaire and takes less than 10 minutes to complete. The content and scoring of the PFSDQ–M are summarized in Table 19–8. A number of scores can be calculated; however, the individual and total scores are those most often reported clinically. Although patients sometimes have difficulty differentiating between fatigue and shortness of breath because they are similar sensations, the questionnaire is generally well understood by patients.[74]

The PFSDQ–M shows evidence of reliability[73,75] and validity for the activity and dyspnea domains.[73] Total scores for activity, dyspnea, and fatigue improve significantly following pulmonary rehabilitation,[74] suggesting that the PFSDQ–M is sensitive to change. Preliminary work on the scale's responsiveness shows that a change of 1.9 in "Most Days" dyspnea rating represents a minimal clinically important difference.[76] Further studies are needed to verify the PFSDQ–M's sensitivity to change following clinical intervention and the responsiveness of activity and fatigue components.

Self-Efficacy

Self-efficacy is an individual's confidence in his/her ability to execute behaviors to achieve specific outcomes.[77] Bandura's Theory of Self-Efficacy states that self-efficacy is the important link between knowing what to do (knowledge) and actually doing it (self-management).[78] Examples of self-management behaviors discussed in previous chapters include smoking cessation, correct use of inhaler medications, breathing techniques, and exercise training. Self-efficacy is an important domain to measure in COPD; it is associated with dyspnea,[79] it plays a mediating role between disease state and activity restriction,[80] and, finally, it has a positive effect on exercise behavior.[81]

Self-efficacy assessment helps the health care personnel to implement interventions specifically designed to increase the patient's self-efficacy in a given situation. Bandura suggested that scales of perceived self-efficacy should be tailored to the particular situation or activity of interest. In the standard methodology for measuring efficacy beliefs, individuals are presented with items representing different levels of task demands and are asked to rate their belief in their ability to execute the different tasks.

There is one published self-efficacy questionnaire specific to COPD. The COPD Self-Efficacy Scale (CSES) is a 34-item self-administered questionnaire. Items are scored on a 5-point scale, with 1 representing "not at all confident" and 5 representing "very confident" in managing or avoiding breathing difficulty in a specific situation. The items aggregate into five domains or subscales: negative effect (12 items), emotional arousal (8 items), physical exertion (5 items), weather or environment (6 items), and behavioral risk factors (3 items). Total and domain scores are calculated by dividing the summed responses by the number of items. The CSES has shown evidence of reliability,[80] and there is evidence of sensitivity to change following pulmonary rehabilitation.[82] More extensive psychometric testing is required, however, if the CSES is to be used more widely.

TABLE 19–8 Pulmonary Functional Status and Dyspnea Questionnaire—Modified Content and Scoring

Domain	Items	Scale	Scores (Range)
Activity	10 common activities rated according to patient's involvement now as compared to before developing breathing problems	0–10 scale 0: as active as I've ever been 10: have omitted entirely Patient can also choose the response "Has never been an activity"	Total score: sum of individual activity scores (0–100) Mean score: total score divided by number of activities rated (0–10) Individual activity scores (10 scores): change in each of the 10 activities (0–10)
Dyspnea	5 general survey questions evaluating the frequency and severity of dyspnea	0–10 scale 0: no shortness of breath 10: very severe shortness of breath	Frequency score: number of times per month patient experiences severe to very severe dyspnea (0–30) General scores (3 scores): severity of dyspnea on most days, today, and with most day-to-day activities (0–10)
	10 common activities rated according to degree of shortness of breath caused by each activity	0-10 scale 0: no shortness of breath 10: very severe shortness of breath	Total score: sum of dyspnea scores for each activity (0–100) Mean score: total dyspnea score divided by number of activities rated (0–10) Individual activity scores (10 scores): degree of dyspnea reported for each of the 10 activities (0–10)
Fatigue	5 general survey questions evaluating the frequency and severity of fatigue	0–10 scale 0: no tiredness 10: very severe tiredness	Frequency score: number of times per month patient experiences severe to very severe fatigue (0–30) General scores (3 scores): severity of fatigue on most days, today, and with most day-to-day activities (0–10)
	10 common activities rated according to degree of fatigue caused by each activity	0–10 scale 0: no tiredness 10: very severe tiredness	Total score: sum of fatigue scores for each activity (0–100) Mean score: total fatigue score divided by number of activities rated (0–10) Individual activity scores (10 scores): degree of fatigue reported for each of the 10 activities (0–10)

Disease Knowledge

A potential limitation of assessing disease knowledge is the fact that some people can learn and memorize information but are unable to apply it to themselves. Although it is recognized that knowledge change may not translate into behavior change, knowledge is an important parameter to measure as it is the basis on which behavior change is made.[83] It is sometimes useful in COPD to evaluate the patient's knowledge of his/her disease process and management. Suppose that a new teaching technique is being implemented in a group education session. It would be important to compare the change in knowledge between patients attending the session using the new teaching technique to those attending a standard education session.

There is one published instrument to measure knowledge in patients with COPD, the Pulmonary Rehabilitation Knowledge Test.[83] This questionnaire is a self-administered multiple-choice test consisting of 40 questions, and it covers areas of knowledge identified as common to rehabilitation programs. The Pulmonary Rehabilitation Knowledge Test was developed to assess change in knowledge following participation in a pulmonary rehabilitation program.

The questionnaire can be completed in under 15 minutes and assesses knowledge in the following areas (number of questions in brackets): ADL (four), anatomy and physiology (three), COPD definitions (three), diet and nutrition (two), emergency care/panic control (two), exercise (three), keeping airways open (six), medicines (four), mental health (two), pathophysiology (one), sex education (two), sleeping (one), stress and relaxation (five), support groups/organizations (one), and tests (one).

An increase in Pulmonary Rehabilitation Knowledge Test scores between pre- and postrehabilitation provides evidence of information retention over time. The items on the test demonstrate internal consistency and content validity, and there is also preliminary evidence of construct validity.[83] However, the scale's test–retest reliability has not been documented. As with the CSES, more extensive psychometric testing is required for the Pulmonary Rehabilitation Knowledge Test to be used for either clinical or research purposes.

Health-Related Quality of Life

Health-related quality of life is the subjective experience of the impact of health on quality of life[84]; it is usually measured in the domains of somatic sensation (eg, symptoms such as dyspnea or pain), physical function, emotional state, and social interaction. As defined by Guyatt and colleagues,[85] it consists of "all those things that one might want to measure about the health of an individual beyond death and physiologic measures of disease activity." In COPD, there are important decrements in HRQL.[26,86] Because of the chronic and mainly irreversible nature of the disease, the therapeutic goal of many interventions is to improve quality of life. Therefore, HRQL is routinely measured in COPD, particularly in measuring the effects of multidisciplinary interventions such as rehabilitation.

Health-related quality of life instruments can be designed to measure overall HRQL (generic) or only those aspects related to a particular disease (disease-specific). The choice of instrument will depend on the program goals and objectives. Generic instruments cover a wider breadth of HRQL issues than disease-specific instruments. Also, generic instruments are routinely administered in a wide variety of clinical settings and patient groups. Therefore, they are able to pick up problems that may be missed by disease-specific instruments, such as treatment side effects. Furthermore, patients with COPD commonly experience comorbid conditions, the symptoms of which may not be covered by COPD-specific questionnaires. Generic instruments can also be used to compare scores between different populations. However, when evaluating the impact of treatment, generic measures may not be as responsive to small changes in quality of life in COPD. Disease-specific quality of life questionnaires are needed because they have a content specific to COPD and are more sensitive to change following an intervention.

This section will focus on the two most commonly used disease-specific questionnaires, the CRQ and the St. George's Respiratory Questionnaire (SGRQ). The SF-36 will also be discussed as it is the most widely used measure of generic HRQL and is commonly used for patients with COPD.

Chronic Respiratory Questionnaire

The CRQ is a disease-specific evaluative tool developed to measure HRQL in COPD.[86] It is an interviewer-administered questionnaire that assesses the domains of dyspnea, fatigue, emotional function, and mastery. Administration of the dyspnea section differs between initial and follow-up testing. Initially, the patient generates a list of activities that have caused breathlessness during the past 2 weeks. These activities are either reported spontaneously or selected from a list of 26 items often associated with dyspnea. The patient is then asked to choose the five activities most important in his/her day-to-day life. This portion of the questionnaire requires the most attention and patience on the part of the interviewer as patients often take time to decide on and prioritize activities. Once the five activities are selected, the patient rates each one according to its associated shortness of breath from 1 (extremely short of breath) to 7 (not at all short of breath). Although dyspnea items are individualized, they remain the same for a given patient on repeated questionnaire administration. Therefore, the dyspnea section requires less time on repeated administration.

At both initial evaluation and follow-up, the remaining domains (fatigue, emotional function, mastery) are evaluated by standardized questions rated on a 7-point scale. The response choices, however, differ according to the nature of the question. Responses are printed on color-coded cards, with the corresponding color indicated below each item on the questionnaire. Therefore, after a question is read by the interviewer, the patient selects his/her response from the appropriate card. The CRQ takes approximately 15 to 25 minutes to complete, and the time often decreases with repeated administration. Clinically, the CRQ is usually scored by converting domain scores to a 7-point scale, permitting uniform comparison between domains. Converted scores are obtained by dividing the raw score by the number of items in each domain. For research purposes, the 7-point scale or the raw score can be used. Raw scores allow a greater numerical range, an advantage for statistical analyses, and allow consideration of overall HRQL (out of 140). For both converted and raw scores, a higher score represents a better HRQL.

Studies to date have provided strong evidence of the test–retest reliability, internal consistency,[87–89] and construct validity,[26,88,89] of the CRQ. Evidence of the responsiveness of the CRQ has been demonstrated by studies evaluating the effects of pulmonary rehabilitation[90–92] and other interventions.[24] A change in score of 0.5 represents an MCID for a given domain of the CRQ.[25,93] Similarly, a change in score of 1.0 represents moderate change, whereas 1.5 or more represents a large change.[25] In summary, there is strong evidence of the psychometric properties of the CRQ, thereby supporting its use as an outcome measure in COPD.

St. George's Respiratory Questionnaire

The SGRQ is another evaluative measure of HRQL, developed for use in patients with fixed (COPD) and reversible (asthma) airway obstruction.[94] The SGRQ is an interviewer- or self-administered questionnaire consisting of 76 weighted items. The SGRQ takes approximately 15 minutes to complete and assesses three domains: symptoms (frequency and severity), activity (activities that cause or are limited by breathlessness), and impact (social functioning and psychological disturbances resulting from airway disease). Individual questionnaire items are rated either by choosing the most applicable response from four or five choices or by a true/false answer. Responses are then scored using weights, which differ for each item. Domain and total scores are converted to a percentage, with higher scores indicating a lower quality of life. The scoring process is tedious and is therefore a practical limitation to using this questionnaire in a clinical environment. For research purposes, the SGRQ is scored by computer using a statistical or database application.

The SGRQ shows good test–retest reliability and construct validity.[94] Also, the SGRQ was sensitive to change over time in a randomized controlled trial of nasal positive-pressure ventilation in hypercapnic patients with COPD[95] and in studies investigating the effects of medication.[96] The SGRQ also appears to be responsive to clinically important change, as 4 points represent a slight change or MCID, 8 points represent moderate change, and 12 points represent a large change.[94] Therefore, the SGRQ demonstrates strong psychometric properties in a COPD population.

36-Item Medical Outcomes Short-Form Health Survey

The SF-36 is a discriminative and evaluative measure of generic HRQL, developed for a wide range of disease populations. It is self- or interviewer-administered in under 15 minutes and assesses the following eight health domains: physical functioning, social functioning, role limitation—physical, role limitation—emotional, pain, mental health, vitality, and general health perceptions. The scale consists of a total of 36 items, with the number of items per domain varying between two and eight. Item scaling is on a yes/no or 2-, 3-, 5-, or 6-point scale. Domain scores are transformed to a scale ranging from 0 (worst) to 100 (best). Total scores are reported as physical and mental health component scores, standardized to have a mean of 50 and a standard deviation of 10 in a healthy U.S. population. For both domain and total scores, patient values can be compared to age- and sex-matched norms generated from a healthy sample of the general Canadian[97] or U.S. population.[98]

The psychometric properties of the SF-36 have been extensively studied in nonpulmonary populations. Although fewer studies have been done in patients with COPD, the SF-36 appears psychometrically sound in this population. Internal consistency, test–retest reliability, and construct validity were acceptable.[88] In patients reporting a self-perceived health change over time, the responsiveness of the SF-36 was moderate for the domains of physical and social functioning.[88] For a given domain, a 5-point difference between groups or a 5-point change over time is considered to be significant[99]; however, the MCID for patients with COPD has not been determined.

A disease-specific COPD module for the SF-36 has recently been developed. This module is intended for use with the SF-36 to provide a more comprehensive evaluation of HRQL in patients with COPD. The 21-item COPD module assesses the domains of symptoms (4 items), feelings (7 items), and function (10 items). Preliminary psychometric testing indicates good internal consistency, test–retest reliability, and construct validity.[100] Further testing is required, however, before the new module is ready for either clinical or research use.

Which HRQL Questionnaire Should Be Used?

Deciding on which HRQL measure to use is a topic of ongoing debate. It is generally recommended that both a generic and a disease-specific instrument be used to cover all important aspects of quality of life. In choosing a disease-specific instrument, the most important consideration is that it captures the constructs addressed by the intervention and is sensitive enough to detect small changes within a given time frame. For example, if the intervention addresses primarily functional or activity restrictions caused by dyspnea, then either the SGRQ or CRQ would be appropriate. However, if the intervention focuses on emotional issues and coping skills, the CRQ would better capture any changes resulting from the intervention. Items relating to emotional functioning were intentionally excluded in the development of the SGRQ as a number of established instruments already assessed this domain.[94] Within the same pulmonary rehabilitation program, the physiotherapist might use the SGRQ, whereas the occupational therapist could use the CRQ to measure change resulting from their respective interventions. It is important within any program, however, that the most pertinent information be obtained from the least possible number of measures. Patients with an already reduced energy level and functional capacity often feel overwhelmed by the many tests and questionnaires required. Outcome measurement is a mechanism for evaluating and refining treatment, and the time and energy demanded of the patient should reflect this purpose.

WHEN TO REFER

Although the individual clinician is the expert in program content and treatment delivery in his/her specific area of expertise, other health care and research professionals are needed for a comprehensive and well-designed program evaluation. In creating program goals and objectives, all members of the multidisciplinary team should be involved to ensure that the important clinical domains are covered. In establishing specific objectives with outcome measures and criteria, consultation with researchers specializing in measurement theory is recommended. This combination of clinical and research expertise will ensure a balance between practical considerations and scientific rigor in formulating program objectives and choosing outcome measures.

SUMMARY

The planning of all new programs of care should include a program evaluation process. Program evaluation is about setting standards and assessing whether they are met; formal research training provides many of the skills that are useful for program evaluation. The process of program evaluation is complex and should be done in collaboration with experts in research methodology (quantitative and qualitative) and statistical analysis; it is a dynamic process that requires a constant feedback loop to ensure continuing program improvement.

Unfortunately, program evaluation is not often considered, or, when it is, the resources are not available to realistically support it. If health professionals are to improve the effectiveness of their work, they need not only to plan it according to the best available evidence; they also need information about their program's performance. This information is best provided through a well-designed program evaluation and routine administration of objective measurement tools.

The choice of outcome measurement tools will depend on the goals and objectives of the program. However, for both clinical and research purposes, the most important considerations are that a measure captures the specific domain being treated or studied and that its psychometric properties are thoroughly documented in the literature. A further consideration for clinical use is that the measure is of a reasonable length and can be easily understood by the patient. Choosing and implementing measurement tools is an ongoing learning process, and the clinician should not hesitate to contact experts in the field to assist in this process.

CASE STUDY

Choosing and implementing outcome measures should generally be done for a group of patients rather than individuals. The following case study describes the choice of outcome measures in a COPD outpatient rehabilitation group for two different scenarios: program evaluation and evaluation of intervention effectiveness.

Program Evaluation

Because of budgetary constraints, your hospital is considering eliminating the outpatient rehabilitation program for patients with COPD. It is necessary to carry out a program evaluation to support the need for and effectiveness of this service.

The first step is to document the pathway by which the patients flow through the program. This pathway, consisting of a sequence of processes, will give you a clear picture of how the program truly works and if there are any redundant processes to address. An example of the initial pathway for an outpatient rehabilitation program is outlined in Figure 19–7. The second step is to look at the established purpose or mission of this program, for example, "to provide comprehensive outpatient pulmonary assessment and rehabilitation and to prevent or delay hospital admission." The next step is to refine and/or create goals and objectives.

Suppose that the overall program goals and corresponding interventions are those outlined in Table 19–9. If the established goals truly reflect the programs's purpose, then achieving these goals should have an impact on hospital admission. Functional exercise capacity, dyspnea, and mastery are all associated with quality of life.[28,101] As quality of life is, in turn, associated with health resource use,[102] the goals of "improving functional exercise capacity," "reducing shortness of breath," and "improving a patient's sense of control and ability to cope with their disease," it could indeed prevent a hospital admission. It is important to note, however, that these are all outcome goals, therefore, structure and process goals would also be necessary for a complete program evaluation. To operationalize these goals, objectives with specific outcome measures and criteria for change need to be created. From the information available on program goals and interventions, an objective with a

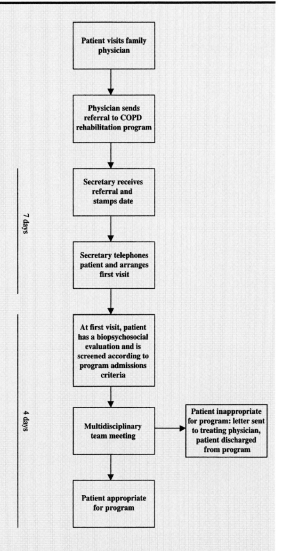

Figure 19–7 Initial pathway for an outpatient rehabilitation program.

specific outcome measure and criterion can be developed for each goal (see Table 19–9).

The choice of outcome measures should reflect the domains being addressed in the goals, namely, functional exercise capacity, dyspnea with activity, and mastery. Data from the 6-MWT should be analyzed for changes in functional exercise capacity, whereas the CRQ data should capture changes in dyspnea and mastery. Once the goals and objectives have been established, the next three steps of program evaluation can take place: collect data or

TABLE 19–9 Program Goals, Interventions, and Objectives for a Pulmonary Rehabilitation Program

Program Goals	Interventions	Objectives
To improve functional exercise capacity	Aerobic conditioning program (cycle ergometer and treadmill) Upper and lower extremity strengthening exercises	To improve the distance walked on the 6-minute walking test by 50 meters, in 80% of clients.
To reduce shortness of breath associated with activities of daily living	Instruction of controlled breathing techniques and principles of self-pacing and energy conservation	To achieve a 0.5-point increase on the CRQ dyspnea 7-point scale in 80% of clients
To improve the patient's sense of control and ability to cope with their disease (mastery)	Support group including group counseling and instruction of specific behavioral and relaxation techniques	To achieve a 0.5-point increase on the CRQ mastery 7-point scale in 80% of clients

CRQ = Chronic Respiratory Questionnaire.

review existing data, determine whether each goal has been met, and, finally, review and reflect.

Evaluation of Intervention Effectiveness

As mentioned previously, it is necessary to put in place a method of evaluation when a new intervention is implemented. A group of patients receiving the new intervention should then be compared with a group receiving the standard treatment. Suppose that within the outpatient rehabilitation program, a new treatment component is being implemented by the psychologist and occupational therapist. The goals of this component are for patients to acquire practical strategies to control dyspnea and to incorporate these strategies into ADL. Specific interventions include group and individual counseling on controlling fear associated with dyspnea and practicing these techniques during functional tasks. The

domains being addressed are therefore dyspnea with activity and fear associated with dyspnea. The SOB-Q is an evaluative instrument that captures changes in these domains as it focuses on dyspnea with ADL and includes items relating to fear.

For both program evaluation and assessing intervention effectiveness, data analysis should be done in consultation with a statistician, to ensure the accuracy and assist in the interpretation of results. If the results are not as expected, then the interventions and measures need to be examined more closely, and the following questions addressed: Are the interventions of sufficient duration, intensity, and frequency to produce the desired results? Do the measures include items relating to the specific type and time frame of the interventions? The choice of outcomes should be reviewed regularly as new research findings emerge and as new measures are developed and validated.

KEY POINTS

- The structure-process-outcome model is a framework for identifying the key components of a health care program to carry out an evaluation.
- The five steps to carrying out a program evaluation are (1) analyze the program's processes, (2) refine and/or create goals and objectives, (3) collect data or review existing data, (4) determine whether each goal has been met, and (5) review and reflect. Program evaluation, using quantitative methods, can be combined with qualitative

research methods to provide a comprehensive program assessment.
- Outcome measures can have continuous or categorical scales and can be classified according to functional, descriptive, or methodological types of classification.
- The ICF can be used to classify clinical problems and the corresponding outcome measures according to body functions and structures, activities, and participation.
- The psychometric properties of an instrument, together with the practical aspects of adminis-

tration and scoring, must be considered before implementing a measure for either clinical or research purposes.

- Dyspnea is a frequent complaint in COPD and a modifiable outcome. Dyspnea scales are of two main types: questionnaires in which patients report on their level of dyspnea with different activities, and simple scales or diagrams that assess exertional dyspnea used during or immediately after exercise.

- Functional exercise capacity is measured using standardized walking tests. The 6-MWT is a self-paced test that measures the distance in meters covered in 6 minutes. The ISWT is a progressive test of exercise capacity in which the pace is externally controlled by an audiocassette and the total walking distance is recorded. The ESWT is a modification of the incremental test and measures the time walked at a pre-established pace.

- The PFSDQ–M, CSES, and Pulmonary Rehabilitation Knowledge Test are questionnaires for measuring functional status, self-efficacy, and disease knowledge, respectively. More psychometric testing is needed, however, for these instruments to gain more widespread use.

- Measures of HRQL can be either generic or disease specific. The most commonly used COPD-specific questionnaires are the CRQ and SGRQ. The SF-36 is a generic instrument commonly used in patients with COPD. A COPD-specific module has recently been developed for the SF-36.

REFERENCES

1. Bourbeau J, Collet JP, Schwartzman K, et al. Integrating rehabilitative elements into a COPD self-management program reduces exacerbations and health services utilization: a randomized clinical trial. Am J Respir Crit Care Med 2000;161:A254.
2. Bourbeau J, Julien M, Rouleau M, et al. Impact of an integrated rehabilitative management program on health status of COPD patients. A multicentre randomized clinical trial. Eur Respir J 2000;16:159S.
3. Bourbeau J, Schwartzman K, Collet J-P, et al. Economic impact if a disease specific self-management program in the management of patients with COPD. Am J Respir Crit Care Med 2001;163:A13.
4. Timmreck TC. Planning program development, and evaluation: a handbook for health promotion, aging and health services. Boston: Jones and Bartlett, 1995.
5. Donabedian A. Evaluating the quality of medical care. Milbank Q 1966;44:166–203.
6. Donabedian A. The quality of care: how can it be assessed? JAMA 1988;260:1743–8.
7. Donabedian A. Quality assesment and assurance: unity of purpose, diversity of means. Inquiry 1988;25:173–92.
8. Rossi PH, Freeman HE. Evaluation, a systematic approach. 5th ed. New York: Sage, 1993.
9. Casebeer AL, Verhoef MJ. Combining qualitative and quantitative research methods: considering the possibilities for enhancing the study of chronic diseases. Chronic Dis Can 1997;18:130–5.
10. Nault D, Pépin J, Dagenais J, et al. Qualitative evaluation of a self-management program "Living Well with COPD©" offered to patients and their caregivers. Am J Respir Crit Care Med 2000;161:A56.
11. Field PA, Morse JM. The application of qualitative approaches. Qualitative approaches: an overview. Rockville, MD: Aspen Publishers, 1985.
12. Denzin NK, Lincoln YS. Strategies of qualitative inquiry. Thousand Oaks, CA: Sage Publications, 1998.
13. Morse JM. Strategies for sampling. Qualitative nursing research. A contemporary dialogue. Rockville, MD. Aspen Publishers. 1989;117–31.
14. Morse JM. What's wrong with random selection? Qual Health Res 1998;8:733–5.
15. Rubin HJ, Rubin IS. Qualitative interviewing. The art of hearing data. Thousand Oaks, CA: Sage Publications, 1995.
16. Richards L, Richards T. Computing in qualitative analysis: a healthy development. Qual Health Res 1991;1:234–62.
17. Cole B, Finch E, Gowland C, Mayo N. Physical rehabilitation outcome measures. Canadian Physiotherapy Association. Toronto: Publishing, Supply & Services Canada, 1994.
18. Streiner DL, Norman GR. Health measurement scales: a practical guide to their development and use. 2nd Ed. New York: Oxford University Press, 1995.
19. McDowell I, Newell C. Measuring health: a guide to rating scales and questionnaires. 2nd Ed. New York: Oxford University Press, 1996.
20. Kirshner B, Guyatt GH. A methodological framework for assessing health indices. J Chron Dis 1985;38(1):27–36.
21. World Health Organization. International Classification of Functioning, Disability and Health. Geneva: World Health Organization, 2001
22. World Health Organization. International Classification of Impairment, Disabilities and Handicaps: a manual classification relating to the consequences of disease. Geneva: World Health Organization, 1980.
23. Liang MH. Longitudinal construct validity: establishment of clinical meaning in patient evaluative instruments. Med Care 2000;38:1184–90.
24. Lacasse Y, Wong E, Guyatt GH. A systematic overview of the measurement properties of the Chronic Respiratory Questionnaire. Can Respir J 1997;4:131–9.
25. Jaeschke R, Singer J, Guyatt GH. Measurement of health status. Ascertaining the minimal clinically

important difference. Control Clin Trials 1989; 10:407–15.

26. Alonso J, Anto JM, Gonzalez M, et al. Measurement of general health status of non-oxygen dependent chronic obstructive pulmonary disease patients. Med Care 1992;30:MS125–35.

27. Mahler DA, Faryniarg K, Tomlinson D, et al. Impact of dyspnea and physiologic function on general health status in patients with chronic obstructive pulmonary disease. Chest 1992;102:395–401.

28. Moody L, McCormick K, Williams AR. Psychophysiologic correlates of quality of life in chronic bronchitis and emphysema. West J Nurs Res 1991;13:336–47.

29. American College of Chest Physicians/American Association of Cardiovascular and Pulmonary Rehabilitation. Pulmonary Rehabilitation Guidelines Panel. Pulmonary rehabilitation: joint ACCP/AACVPR evidence-based guidelines. J Cardiopulm Rehabil 1997;17:371–405.

30. American Thoracic Society. Dyspnea mechanisms, assessment, and management: a consensus statement. Am J Respir Crit Care Med 1999;159:321–40.

31. Mahler DA, Wells CK. Evaluation of clinical methods for rating dyspnea. Chest 1988;93:580–6.

32. American Thoracic Society. Recommended respiratory disease questionnaire for use with adults and children in epidemiological research. Am Rev Respir Dis 1978;118:1–53.

33. Mahler DA, Weinberg DH, Wells CK, Feinstein AR. The measurement of dyspnea: contents, interobserver agreement, and physiologic correlates of two new clinical indexes. Chest 1984;85:751–8.

34. Mahler DA, Matthay RA, Snyder PE, et al. Sustained-release theophylline reduces dyspnea in nonreversible obstructive airway disease. Am Rev Respir Dis 1985;131:22–5.

35. Eakin EG, Resnikoff PM, Prewitt LM, et al. Validation of a new dyspnea measure: the USCD Shortness of Breath Questionnaire. Chest 1998;113:619–24.

36. Mapel DW, Allen RE, Picchi MA, et al. Validation of a new dyspnea questionnaire in patients with chronic obstructive pulmonary disease. Am J Respr Crit Care Med 2000;161:A58.

37. Make B, Tolliver R, Christensen P, et al. Pulmonary rehabilitation improves exercise capacity and dyspnea in the National Emphysema Treatment Trial (NETT). Am J Respr Crit Care Med 2000;161:A254.

38. Garrod R, Bestall JC, Paul EA, et al. Development and validation of a standardized measure of activity of daily living in patients with severe COPD: the London Chest Activity of Daily Living scale (LCADL). Respir Med 2000;94:589–96.

39. Garrod R, Wedzicha JA. Reliability and sensitivity of the London Chest Activity of Daily Living Scale. Am J Respir Crit Care Med 2001;163:A57.

40. McGavin CR, Artvinli M, Naoe H, McHardy CJR. Dyspnea, disability, and distance walked: comparison of estimates of exercise performance in respiratory disease. BMJ 1978;2:241–3.

41. Mahler DA, Rosiello RA, Harver A, et al. Comparison of clinical dyspnea ratings and psychophysical measurements of respiratory sensation in obstructive airway disease. Am Rev Respir Dis 1987;135:1229–33.

42. O'Donnell DE, McGuire M, Samis L, Webb KA. The impact of exercise reconditioning on breathlessness in severe chronic airflow limitation. Am J Respir Crit Care Med 1995;152:2005–13.

43. Borg GAV. Perceived exertion as an indicator of somatic stress. Scand J Rehabil Med 1970;2:92–8.

44. Noble BJ, Borg GA, Jacobs I, et al. A category-ratio perceived exertion scale: relationship to blood and muscle lactates and heart rate. Med Sci Sports Exerc 1983;15:523–8.

45. Borg. GA. Psychophysical bases of perceived exertion. Med Sci Sports Exerc 1982;14:377–81.

46. Silverman M, Barry H, Hellerstein J, et al. Variability of the perceived sense of breathing during exercise in patients with chronic obstructive pulmonary disease. Am Rev Respir Dis 1988;137:206–9.

47. Wilson RC, Jones PW. A comparison of the visual analogue scale and modified Borg scale for the measurement of dyspnoea during exercise. Clin Sci 1989;76:277–82.

48. Wilson RC, Jones PW. Differentiation between the intensity of breathlessness and the distress it evokes in normal subjects during exercises. Clin Sci 1991; 80:65–70.

49. Leblanc P, Bowie DM, Summers E, et al. Breathlessness and exercise in patients with cardiorespiratory disease. Am Rev Respir Dis 1986;133:21–5.

50. O'Donnell DE, Lam M, Webb KA. Measurement of symptoms, lung hyperinflation and endurance during exercise in chronic obstructive pulmonary disease. Am J Respir Crit Care Med 1998;158:1557–65.

51. Muza SR, Silverman MT, Gilmore GC, et al. Comparison of scales used to quantitate the sense of effort to breathe in patients with chronic obstructive pulmonary disease. Am Rev Respir Dis 1990;14 (4 Pt 1):909–13.

52. Gift AG. Validation of a vertical visual analogue scale as a measure of clinical dyspnea. Rehabil Nurs 1989; 14:313–25.

53. American College of Sports Medicine. ACSM's guidelines for exercise testing and prescription. Philadelphia: Lipincott Williams and Wilkins, 2000.

54. Noonan V, Dean E. Submaximal exercise testing: clinical application and interpretation. Phys Ther 2000;80:782–807.

55. Guyatt GH, Pugsley SO, Sullivan MJ, et al. Effect of encouragement on walking test performance. Thorax 1984;39:818–22.

56. Knox AJ, Morrison JFJ, Muers MF. Reproducibility of walking test results in chronic obstructive airways disease. Thorax 1988;43:388–92.

57. Steele B. Timed walking tests of exercise capacity in chronic cardiopulmonary disease. J Cardiopulm Rehabil 1996;16:25–33.

58. Enright PL, Sherrill DL. Reference equations for the six-minute walk in healthy adults. Am J Respir Crit Care Med 1998;158:1384–7.

59. Troosters T, Gosselink R, Decramer M. Six minute walking distance in healthy elderly subjects. Eur Respir J 1999;14:270–4.

60. Guyatt G, Sullivan MJ, Thompson PJ, et al. The 6 minute walk test: a new measure of exercise capacity in patients with chronic heart failure. Can Med Assoc J 1985;132:919–23.

61. Mak VH, Buglar JR, Roberts CM, Spiro SG. Effect of arterial oxygen desaturation on six minute walk distance, perceived effort, and perceived breathlessness in patients with airflow limitation. Thorax 1993;48:33–8.

62. Guyatt GH, Berman LB, Townsend M, Taylor DW. Should study subjects see their previous responses? J Chron Dis 1985;38:1003–7.

63. Lacasse Y, Wong E, Guyatt GH, et al. Meta-analysis of respiratory rehabilitation in chronic obstructive pulmonary disease. Lancet 1996;348:1115–9.

64. Redelmeier DA, Bayoumi AM, Goldstein RS, Guyatt GH. Interpreting small differences in functional status: the six-minute walk test in chronic lung disease patients. Am J Respir Crit Care Med 1997; 155:1278–82.

65. Hernandez E, Fernandez Guerra J, Toral Marin J, et al. Reproducibility of a shuttle walking test in patients with chronic obstructive pulmonary disease. Arch Bronconeumol 1997;33:64–8.

66. Singh SJ, Morgan MDL, Scott S, et al. Development of a shuttle walking test of disability in patients with chronic airways obstruction. Thorax 1992;47: 1019–24.

67. Hernandez E, Ortega Ruiz F, Fernandez Guerra J, et al. Comparison of a shuttle walking test with an exertion test with cycloergometer in patients with COPD. Arch Bronconeumol 1997;33:498–502.

68. Singh SJ, Smith DL, Hyland ME, Morgan MD. A short outpatient pulmonary rehabilitation programme: immediate and longer-term effects on exercise performance and quality of life. Respir Med 1998;92: 1146–54.

69. White RJ, Rudkin ST, Ashley J, et al. Outpatient pulmonary rehabilitation in severe chronic pulmonary disease. J R Coll Phys Lond 1997;31:541–5.

70. Revill SM, Morgan MD, Singh SJ, et al. The endurance shuttle walk: a new field test for the assessment of endurance capacity in chronic obstructive pulmonary disease. Thorax 1999;54:213–22.

71. ZuWallack R. Outcome assessment. In: Hodgkin JE, Celli BR, Connors GL, eds. Pulmonary rehabilitation. Philadelphia: Lippincott Williams & Wilkins, 2000:363–87.

72. Morales FJ, Martinez M, Agarrado A, et al. A shuttle walk test for assessment of functional capacity in chronic heart failure. Am Heart J 1999;138:291–8.

73. Lareau SC, Meek PM, Roos PJ. Development and testing of a modified version of the pulmonary functional status and dyspnea questionnaire. Heart Lung 1998;27:159–68.

74. Lareau SC, Wilhite C, Specht NL, Pettis JL. Effects of pulmonary rehabilitation on activities, dyspnea and fatigue. Am J Respir Crit Care Med 1999;159:A763.

75. Lareau SC, Meek PM. Testing of a modified version of the Pulmonary Functional Status and Dyspnea Questionnaire. Am J Respir Crit Care Med 1996; 153:A421.

76. Meek PM, Lareau SC. Important differences in ratings of dyspnea from the client's perspective: when is it worse and when do you treat. Am J Respir Crit Care Med 1998;157:A867.

77. Bandura A, Adams NE. Analysis of the self-efficacy theory of behavioral changes. Cogn Ther Res 1977; 1:287–308.

78. Bandura A. Self-efficacy mechanism in human agency. Am Psychol 1982;33:344–58.

79. Fishman AP. Pulmonary rehabilitation research. Am J Respir Crit Care Med 1994;149(3 Pt 1):825–33.

80. Wigal JK, Creer TL, Kotses H. The COPD Self-Efficacy Scale. Chest 1991;99:1193–6.

81. Kaplan RM, Atkins V, Reinsch S. Specific efficacy expectations mediate exercise compliance in patients with COPD. Health Psychol 1984;3:223–42.

82. Scherer YK, Shmieder LE. The effect of a pulmonary rehabilitation program on self efficacy, perception of dyspnea, and physical endurance. Heart Lung 1997;26:15–22.

83. Hopp JW, Lee JW, Hills R. Development and validation of a pulmonary rehabilitation knowledge test. J Cardiopulm Rehabil 1989;7:273–8.

84. Curtis JR, Deyo RA, Hudson LD. Pulmonary rehabilitation in chronic respiratory insufficiency. 7. Health-related quality of life among patients with chronic obstructive pulmonary disease. Thorax 1994;49: 162–70.

85. Guyatt G, Feeny D, Patrick D. Issues in quality-of-life measurement in clinical trials. Control Clin Trials 1991;12(Suppl 4):81S–90S.

86. Guyatt GH, Berman LB, Townsend M, et al. A measure of quality of life for clinical trials in chronic lung disease. Thorax 1987;42:773–8.

87. Waterhouse JC, Harper R, Marsh F, et al. Measuring quality of life in chronic obstructive pulmonary disease. Can we assess change? Eur Respir J 1994;7 Suppl:419S.

88. Harper R, Brazier JE, Waterhouse JC, et al. Comparison of outcome measures for patients with chronic obstructive pulmonary disease. Thorax 1997;52: 879–87.

89. Wijkstra PJ, TenVergert EM, Van-Altena R, et al. Reliability and validity of the chronic respiratory questionnaire (CRQ). Thorax 1994;49:465–7.

90. Goldstein RS, Gort EH, Stubbing D, Randomised controlled trial of respiratory rehabilitation. Lancet 1994;344(8934):1394–7.

91. Guell R, Morante F, Sangenis M, Casan P. Effects of respiratory rehabilitation on the effort capacity and on the health-related quality of life of patients with chronic obstructive pulmonary disease. Eur Resp J 1995b;(8 Suppl):356s.

92. Wijkstra PJ, Van-Altena R, Kraan J, et al. Quality of life in patients with chronic obstructive pulmonary disease improves after rehabilitation at home. Eur Resp J 1994;7(2):269–73.

93. Redelmeier DA, Goldstein RS, Min ST, Hyland RH. Spirometry and dyspnea in patients with COPD. When small differences mean little. Chest 1996;109: 1163–8.

94. Jones PW, Quirk FH, Baveystock CM, Littlejohns P. A self-complete measure of health status for chronic airflow limitation. The St. George's Respiratory Questionnaire. Am Rev Respir Dis 1992;145:1321–7.

95. Meecham Jones DJ, Paul EA, Jones PW, Wedzicha JA. Nasal pressure support ventilation plus oxygen compared with oxygen therapy alone in hypercapnic COPD. Am J Respir Crit Care Med 1995;152: 538–44.

96. Jones PW, Lasserson D. Relationship between change in St. George's Respiratory Questionnaire scores and patients' perception of treatment efficacy after one year of therapy with nedocromil sodium. Am J Respir Crit Care Med 1994;149:A211.

97. Hopman WM, Towheed T, Anastassiades T, et al. Canadian Multicentre Osteoporosis Study Research Study Group. Canadian normative data for the SF-36 health survey. Can Med Assoc J 2000;163:265–71.

98. Ware JE, Kosinski M, Keller S. SF-36 Physical and Mental Health Summary Scales: a user's manual. Boston: The Health Institute, New England Medical Center, 1994.

99. Ware JEJ. Health survey manual and interpretation guide. Vol. SF-36. Boston: The Health Institute, New England Medical Center, 1993.

100. Spajiha J, Collet JP, Bourbeau J, et al. A new module for measuring quality of life in COPD patients. Am J Respir Crit Care Med 2000;161:A823.

101. Ketelaars CAJ, Schlosser MAG, Mostert R, et al. Determinants of health-related quality of life in patients with chronic obstructive pulmonary disease. Thorax 1996;51:39–43.

102. Osman IM, Godden DJ, Friend JA, et al. Quality of life and hospital re-admission in patients with chronic obstructive pulmonary disease. Thorax 1997;52: 67–71.

SUGGESTED READINGS

Timmreck TC. Planning, program development, and evaluation: a handbook for health promotion, aging and health services. Boston: Jones and Bartlett, 1995. *This book describes the steps of a health program evaluation and includes a detailed section on the creation of goals and objectives. The rationale for program evaluation and the resulting impact on health service delivery are also discussed.*

Rubin HJ, Rubin IS. Qualitative interviewing. The art of hearing data. Thousand Oaks, CA: Sage Publications, 1995. *Chapters 1 and 2 present the foundation of qualitative interviewing with respect to its rationale, participants, and data collection procedures. The process of qualitative data analysis is described in detail in Chapter 10.*

Zuwallack R. Outcome assessment. In: Hodgkin JE, Celli BR, Connors GL, eds. Pulmonary rehabilitation. Philadelphia: Lippincott Williams & Wilkins, 2000: 363–87. *This chapter provides a comprehensive overview of outcome measures used in pulmonary rehabilitation, with extensive discussion on research findings to support their use. The domains covered include dyspnea, functional exercise capacity, HRQL, functional status, and ADL. Additional sections on incremental and endurance exercise testing, nutritional status, survival, and health care use discuss specific testing methods.*

Lacasse Y, Wong E, Guyatt G, Goldstein R. Health status measurement instruments in chronic obstructive pulmonary disease. Can Respir J 1997;4:152–64. *This review article presents extensive data on the psychometric properties, structure and scoring, and administration of commonly used measurement tools in COPD. Detailed information is presented in tables, allowing easy comparison between instruments. Measures of dyspnea, HRQL, functional status, and self-efficacy are covered.*